IFFS

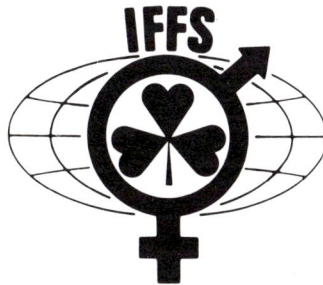

FERTILITY and STERILITY

The Proceedings of the XIth World Congress on Fertility and Sterility, Dublin, June 1983, held under the Auspices of the International Federation of Fertility Societies

Edited by
R. F. Harrison
J. Bonnar W. Thompson

MTP PRESS LIMITED

a member of the KLUWER ACADEMIC PUBLISHERS GROUP
LANCASTER / BOSTON / THE HAGUE / DORDRECHT

Published in the UK and Europe by
MTP Press Limited
Falcon House
Lancaster, England

British Library Cataloguing in Publication Data

Advances in fertility control and the treatment of sterility.
1. Contraception—Congresses
I. Rolland, R.   II. Harrison, R. F.
III. Bonnar, J.   IV. Thompson, William, 1937-
V. World Congresses on Fertility and Sterility (*11th: 1983: Dublin*)
613.9′4   RG136

ISBN 0–85200–768–X

Published in the USA by
MTP Press
A division of Kluwer Boston Inc
190 Old Derby Street
Hingham, MA 02043, USA

Library of Congress Cataloging in Publication Data

Main entry under title:
Advances in fertility control and the treatment of sterility.
Bibliography: P.
Includes index.
1. Oral contraceptives – Congresses. 2. Infertility, Female – Treatment – Congresses. I. Rolland, R. II. World Congress of Fertility and Sterility (11th: 1983: Dublin, Dublin) [DNLM: 1. Fertility – Congresses. 2. Infertility – Therapy – Congresses. 3. Contraceptives, Oral – Congresses. QV 177 A244 1983]
RG137.5.A38 1983   618.1′78   83-22258
ISBN 0–85200–768–X

Copyright © 1984 MTP Press Limited

Phototypesetting by Titus Wilson, Kendal
Printed in Great Britain by
Butler & Tanner Limited, Frome and London

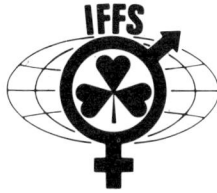

IFFS

FERTILITY
and
STERILITY

To our long-suffering wives and families

Contents

PART III: SPECIAL SYMPOSIA

Section 1: Prolactinomas and Pregnancy

ix

Section 2: Advances in Fertility Control and Treatment of Sterility

Section 4: Reproductive Health in Adolescence

Preface

The International Federation of Fertility Societies XI World Congress on Fertility and Sterility took place in Ireland at the Royal Dublin Society from the 26th June–1st July, 1983. Some 1900 delegates representing 54 countries attended the social and scientific programme in glorious weather that showed off the unsurpassable rare beauty of Dublin and Ireland, so often hidden in mist and rain.

The book begins with the full inaugural address to the Conference by Dr A. Kessler, Head of the WHO Special Programme of Research, Development and Research Training in Human Reproduction. It then records scientific contributions presented in the main themes of the Congress, followed by synopses of deliberations from workshops held during the course of the meeting. Papers from four special symposia are included, which acknowledge the debt IFFS Dublin '83 owes the World Health Organization and our colleagues in the pharmaceutical industry. The large number and excellent standard of the related communications is such that they deserve publication in separate appropriate volumes. These are already in preparation.

If the published proceedings of scientific meetings are to have any merit at all, data must be as up-to-date as possible with emphasis on new advances and research. This can only be achieved by producing the record as complete as possible in the minimum time. Such a task needs the total co-operation of delegates who submit to a standardised format, complete manuscripts by the due date, thus allowing sufficient time for editorial refereeing to be directed to the all-important scientific content. To this end we are indebted to the magnificent co-operation of the large majority of the participants and the publishing expertise, friendly advice and efficiency of MTP Press. It has thus been possible for this record from a large World Congress to appear so soon after the meeting.

We trust you will agree that these efforts have been worthwhile and find this volume of the proceedings of IFFS Dublin '83, as rewarding for you to read as we found it to edit, and a valuable addition to the world literature on Fertility and Sterility.

Robert F. Harrison
John Bonnar
William Thompson

Ireland, October 1983

List of Contributors

A. A. ACOSTA
Department of Obstetrics and
  Gynecology
Eastern Virginia Medical School
Norfolk, VA 23507
USA

P. ADELASCO
III Department of Obstetrics and
  Gynecology
University of Milan
Via M. Melloni, 52
I-20120 Milano
Italy

A. J. M. AUDEBERT
Institut Aquitain d'Etude et de
  Recherche en Reproduction
  Humaine
40, Cours de Verdun
33000 Bordeaux
France

S. AYDINLIK
Schering Aktiengesellschaft
Postfach 65 03 11
D-1000 Berlin 65
West Germany

M. BARTELLONI
Postgraduate School of Andrology
1st Medical Clinic
University of Pisa
Ospedale S. Chiara
I-56100 Pisa
Italy

B. N. BARWIN
Department of Obstetrics and
  Gynecology
University of Ottawa
501 Smyth Road
Ontario K1H 8L6
Canada

A. BELANGER
Departments of Medicine and
  Molecular Endocrinology
Laval University Medical Center
2705 Laurier Boulevard
Quebec G1V 4G2
Canada

M. A. BELSEY
Maternal and Child Health
World Health Organisation
Geneva
Switzerland

T. BERGH
Department of Obstetrics and
  Gynecology
University Hospital
S-751 85 Uppsala
Sweden

G. BETTERNDORF
Universitäts Frauenklinik und
  Poliklinik
Martinistrasse 52
D-2000 Hamburg 20
West Germany

M. BOGHEN
II Department of Medicine
Fatebenefratelli Hospital
Corso di Porta Nuova 23
I-20121 Milano
Italy

J. BONNAR
Department of Obstetrics and
  Gynaecology
Trinity College Unit
Rotunda Hospital
Dublin 2
Ireland

G. BRAMBILLA
III Department of Obstetrics and
  Gynecology
University of Milan
Via M. Melloni, 52
I-20129 Milano
Italy

M. H. BRIGGS
Department of Biological and
  Health Sciences
Deakin University
Victoria 3217
Australia

K. BROGAARD HANSEN
Department of Gynecology and
  Obstetrics
Kommunehospitalet, Århus
DK-8000 Århus C, Denmark

A. D. G. BROWN
Department of Obstetrics and
  Gynaecology
Eastern General Hospital
Seafield Street
Edinburgh EH6 7LN
Scotland

G. J. BRUINING
Scientific Development Group
Organon International BV
PO Box 20
5340 BH Oss
The Netherlands

R. BULLOCK
Institute of Neurological Sciences
Southern General Hospital
Glasgow G51 4TF
Scotland

G. BURGER
Medical Research Centre and
  Department of Endocrinology
Prince Henry's Hospital
St. Kilda Road
Melbourne, Victoria 3004
Australia

D. CANALE
Postgraduate School of Andrology
1st Medical Clinic
University of Pisa
Ospedale S. Chiara
I-56100 Pisa
Italy

W. CATES
Division of Venereal Disease
  Control
Centers for Disease Control
Atlanta, GA 30333
USA

J. COHEN
Société Francaise Pour L'Etude de
  la Fertilité
3 rue de Marignan
F-75008 Paris
France

J. COMHAIRE
Endocrinology Section
Academisch Ziekenhuis
De Pinlelaan 185
B-9000 Gent
Belgium

W. P. COLLINS
Department of Obstetrics and
  Gynaecology
Kings College Hospital Medical
  School
Denmark Hill, London SE5 8RX
England

I. D. COOKE
Department of Obstetrics and
  Gynaecology
Jessop Hospital for Women
Sheffield S3 7RE
England

E. M. COUTINHO
Department of Human
  Reproduction
Federal University of Bahia
Maternidade Climerio de Oliveria
Rua do Limoeiro, No. 1 – Nazaré
Salvador 40,000
Bahia
Brazil

P. CROSIGNANI
III Department of Obstetrics and
  Gynecology
University of Milan
Via M. Melloni, 52
I-20129 Milano
Italy

G. CULLBERG
KK. Östra Sjukhuset
S-416 85 Göteborg
Sweden

O. DE ACOSTA
Institute of Endocrinology and
  Metabolic Diseases
Hospital "CMDTE Fajardo"
Havana 4
Cuba

L. DE CECCO
Department of Obstetrics and
  Gynecology
University of Genoa
Italy

P. N. M. DEMACKER
Department of Internal Medicine
St Radboud University Hospital
Nijmegen
The Netherlands

E. DICZFALUSY
Reproductive Endocrinology
  Research Unit
Department of Obstetrics and
  Gynecology
Karolinska Sjukhuset
Box 60500
S-104 01 Stockholm
Sweden

M. DOCKER
Medical Physics Department
Birmingham Maternity Hospital
Queen Elizabeth Medical Centre
Edgbaston, Birmingham B15 2TG
England

W. H. DOESBURG
Department of Statistical
  Consultation
University of Nijmegen
Nijmegen
The Netherlands

R. DOROW
Department of
  Neuroendocrinology and
  Neuropsychopharmacology
Schering AG
Postfach 65 03 11
D-1000 Berlin 65
West Germany

A. DUPONT
Departments of Medicine and
  Molecular Endocrinology
Laval University Medical Center
2705 Laurier Boulevard
Quebec G1V 4G2
Canada

R. G. EDWARDS
Physiological Laboratory
Cambridge University
Cambridge CB2 3EG
England

M. ELSTEIN
Department of Obstetrics and
  Gynaecology
University Hospital of South
  Manchester
West Didsbury
Manchester M20 8LR
England

W. FEICHTINGER
Institute of Reproductive
  Endocrinology and In Vitro
  Fertilization
Hadikgasse 76
A-1140 Vienna
Austria

C. FERRARI
II Department of Medicine
Fatebenefratelli Hospital
Corso de Porta Nuova, 23
I-20121 Milano
Italy

A. M. FLYNN
Department of Obstetrics and
  Gynaecology
Birmingham Maternity Hospital
Queen Elizabeth Medical Centre
Edgbaston, Birmingham B15 2TG
England

S. FRANKS
Department of Obstetrics and
  Gynaecology
St Mary's Hospital Medical School
London W2 1PG
England

T. K. FUJII
Department of Obstetrics and
  Gynecology
Nihon University School of
  Medicine
30-1 Oyaguchi-Kamimachi
Itabashi-Ku, Tokyo 173
Japan

J. GARCIA
Department of Obstetrics and
  Gynecology
Eastern Virginia Medical School
Norfolk, VA 23507
USA

J. GASPARD
Department of Obstetrics and
  Gynecology
State University of Liège
Boulevard de la Constitution 81
B-4020 Liège
Belgium

D. J. GILLAIN
Department of Obstetrics and
  Gynaecology
State University of Liège
Boulevard de la Constitution 81
B-4020 Liège
Belgium

K. HALL
Department of Neuroradiology
Regional Neurological Centre
Newcastle upon Tyne
Tyne and Wear NE4 6BE
England

R. F. HARRISON
TCD Unit
Rotunda Hospital Dublin
Dublin
Ireland

C. HARVENGT
Laboratoire de Pharmacothérapie
    Clinique
Université Catholique de Louvain
53 Avenue E. Mourid
B-1200 Brussels
Belgium

H. S. HATHAWAY
Maternity, Infant, Children and
    Youth Program
Tri-County District Health
    Department
4857 South Broadway
Englewood, CO 80110
USA

F. R. HELLER
Laboratoire de Pharmacothérapie
Université Catholique de Louvain
53 Avenue E. Mourid
B-1200 Brussels
Belgium

O. K. HOFFMANN
Medical Committee of Pro Familia
Hallervordenweg 7
D-4540 Lengerich
West Germany

R. HOROWSKI
Department of
    Neuroendocrinology and
    Neuropsychopharmacology
Schering AG
Postfach 65 03 11
D-1000 Berlin 65
West Germany

T. HJORT
Institute of Medical Microbiology
University of Århus
DK-8000 Århus C
Denmark

P. L. IZZO
Postgraduate School of Andrology
1st Medical Clinic
University of Pisa
Ospedale S. Chiara
I-56100 Pisa
Italy

H. S. JACOBS
Department of Endocrinology
Middlesex Hospital
Mortimer Street
London W1
England

A. JASPER
Universitäts-Frauenklinik
D-7400 Tübingen
West Germany

P. M. JOHNSON
Department of Immunology
University of Liverpool
Liverpool L69 3BX
England

G. E. S. JONES
Department of Obstetrics and
    Gynecology
Eastern Virginia Medical School
Norfolk, VA 23507
USA

H. W. JONES
Department of Obstetrics and
    Gynecology
Eastern Virginia Medical School
Norfolk, VA 23501
USA

W. R. JONES
Department of Obstetrics and
  Gynaecology
Flinders Medical Centre
Bedford Park, SA 5042
Australia

E. KAWAGUCHI
Department of Obstetrics and
  Gynecology
Nihon University School of
  Medicine
30-1 Oyaguchi-Kamimachi
Itabashi-Ku, Tokyo 173
Japan

C. R. KAY
Manchester Research Unit
Royal College of General
  Practitioners
9 Barlow Moor Road
Manchester M20 0TR
England

E. KELLER
Universitäts Frauenklinik
D-7400 Tübingen
West Germany

P. KEMETER
Institute of Reproductive
  Endocrinology and In Vitro
  Fertilisation
Hadikgasse 76
A-1140 Vienna
Austria

A. KESSLER
Special Programme of Research in
  Human Reproduction
World Health Organisation
CH-1211 Geneva 27
Switzerland

H. J. KLOOSTERBOER
Scientific Development Group
Organon International BV
PO Box 20
5340 BH Oss
The Netherlands

D. M. DE KRETSER
Department of Anatomy
Monash University
Clayton, Victoria 3168
Australia

P. KRUPP
Pharmaceutical Department
Clinical Research
Drug Monitoring Centre
Sandos Ltd
CH-4002 Basle,
Switzerland

F. LABRIE
Departments of Medicine and
  Molecular Endocrinology
Laval University Medical Center
2705 Laurier Boulevard
Quebec G1V 4G2
Canada

U. LACHNIT-FIXSON
Schering Aktiengesellschaft
Postfach 65 03 11
D-1000 Berlin 65
West Germany

L. LEFROY
Adoption Advice Service
Barnardo's
244 Harolds Cross Road
Dublin 6
Ireland

J. LEHNERT
Schering Aktiengesellschaft
Postfach 65 03 11
D-1000 Berlin 65
West Germany

L. LUND
Salakunta Central Hospital
Pori
Finland

B. LUNENFELD
Institute of Endocrinology
Chaim Sheba Medical Centre
Tal Hashomer
Israel

S. LYNCH
Steroid Laboratories
The Birmingham and Midland
  Hospital for Women
Showell Green Lane
Sparkhill, Birmingham B11
England

R. M. MACLEOD
Department of Internal Medicine
University of Virginia School of
  Medicine
Charlottesville, VA 22908
USA

E. M. MARTIN
Diplomatic Liaison
Population Crisis Committee
Room 550, 1120 19th Street
Washington, DC 20036
USA

C. D. MATTHEWS
University of Adelaide
The Queen Elizabeth Hospital
Woodville, SA 5011
Australia

L.-A. MATTSON
K. K. Östra Sjukhuset
S-416 85 Göteborg
Sweden

A. McCORMACK
Population and Development
  Office
St Joseph's College
Lawrence Street
Mill Hill
London NW7 4JX
England

G. MENCHINI FABRIS
Postgraduate School of Andrology
1st Medical Clinic
University of Pisa
Ospedale S. Chiara
I-56100 Pisa
Italy

P. MESCHINI
Postgraduate School of Andrology
1st Medical Clinic
University of Pisa
Ospedale S. Chiara
I-56100 Pisa
Italy

L. METTLER
University of Kiel
Frauenklinik
Hegewischstrasse 4
D-2300 Kiel 1
West Germany

R. MORRIS
Steroid Laboratories
The Birmingham and Midland
  Hospital for Women
Showell Green Lane
Sparkhill, Birmingham B11
England

F. MÜLLER
Carnegie Laboratories of
  Embryology
California Primate Research
  Center
Davis, CA 95616
USA

H. NAKAMURA
Department of Obstetrics and
  Gynecology
Nihon University School of
  Medicine
30-1 Oyaguchi-Kamimachi
Itabashi-Ku, Tokyo 173
Japan

A. NEGRO-VILAR
Section on Reproductive
  Neuroendocrinology, LRDT
NIEHS, PO Box 12233
Research Triangle Park, NC 27709
USA

N. C. NEVIN
Department of Medical Genetics
The Queen's University of Belfast
Institute of Clinical Science
Belfast BT12 6BJ
Northern Ireland

J. R. NEWTON
Department of Obstetrics and
  Gynaecology
Birmingham University Hospital
Edgbaston, Birmingham B15 2TG
England

S. J. NILLIUS
Department of Obstetrics and
  Gynaecology
University Hospital
S-751 85 Uppsala
Sweden

S. NITSCHKE-DABELSTEIN
Department of Obstetrics and
  Gynaecology of the Ludwig
  Maximilian's University
Klinikum Grosshadern
Marchioninstrasse 15
D-8000 München 70
West Germany

S. NUMMI
Satakunta Central Hospital
Pori
Finland

A. M. O'MOORE
TCD Unit
Rotunda Hospital
Dublin 1
Ireland

R. R. O'MOORE
TCD Unit
Rotunda Hospital
Dublin 1
Ireland

R. O'RAHILLY
Departments of Human Anatomy
  and Neurology
University of California
Davis, CA 95616
USA

A. PARACCHI
II Department of Medicine
Fatebenefratelli Hospital
Corso di Porta Nuova, 23
I-20121 Milano
Italy

M. R. N. PRASAD
World Health Organisation
Special Programme of Research in
  Human Reproduction
CH-1211 Geneva
Switzerland

R. N. V. PRASAD
Department of Obstetrics and
  Gynaecology
National University of Singapore
Kandang Kerbau Hospital
Hampshire Road
Singapore 0821

J. P. PRYOR
Department of Urology
St Peter's Hospital
Henrietta Street
London W11
England

P. RAMACHANDRAN
Department of Reproductive
  Physiology
National Institute of Nutrition
Hyderabad
India 500007

P. RAMPINI
II Department of Medicine
Fatebenefratelli Hospital
Corso di Porta Nuova 23
I-20121 Milano
Italy

S. S. RATNAM
University Department of
  Obstetrics and Gynaecology
National University of Singapore
Kandang Kerbau Hospital
Singapore 0821

A. RICHARDS
Institute of Neurological Sciences
Southern General Hospital
Glasgow G51 4TF
Scotland

D. ROBB
TCD Unit
Rotunda Hospital
Dublin 1
Ireland

S. ROBERTSON
Alan Grant Fertility Clinic
St Margaret's Hospital
Bourke Street
Sydney 2010
Australia

R. ROLLAND
Department of Obstetrics and
  Gynecology
St Raboud University
Nijmegen
The Netherlands

A. ROMUS
Department of Obstetrics and
  Gynecology
State University of Liège
Boulevard de la Constitution 81
B-4020 Liège
Belgium

M. J. ROSENBERG
Centers for Disease Control
4676 Columbia Parkway
Cincinnati, Ohio
USA

P. J. ROWE
Special Programme of Research
Development and Research
  Training in Human
  Reproduction
World Health Organisation
CH-1211 Geneva 27
Switzerland

P. ROYSTON
Division of Computing and
  Statistics
MRC Clinical Research Centre
Harrow, Middlesex HA1 3UJ
England

H. N. SALLAM
Department of Obstetrics and
  Gynaecology
Kings College Hospital Medical
  School
Denmark Hill, London SE5 8RX
England

B. SANDOW
Department of Obstetrics and
  Gynecology
Eastern Virginia Medical School
Norfolk, VA 23507
USA

J. SANDOW
Hoechst AG
Pharmacology H 821
D-6230 Frankfurt 80
West Germany

C. P. Th. SCHIJF
Department of Obstetrics and
  Gynecology
St Radboud University Hospital
Nijmegen
The Netherlands

A. E. SCHINDLER
Universitäts-Frauenklinik
D-7400 Tübingen
West Germany

L. E. M. SCHIPHORST
Department of Obstetrics and
  Gynaecology
King's College Medical School
Denmark Hill, London SE5 8RX
England

W. H. F. SCHNEIDER
1 Universitäts Frauenklinik Wien
Wien
Austria

A. SCHOLZ
Department of
  Neuroendocrinology and
  Neuropsychopharmacology
Schering AG
Postfach 65 03 11
D-1000 Berlin 65
West Germany

T. SCHUMACHER
Universitäts-Frauenklinik
D-7400 Tübingen
West Germany

K. SEMM
Universitäts-Frauenklinik und
  Michaelis-
  Hebammenschule Kiel
Hegewichstrasse 4
D-2300 Kiel 1
West Germany

M. SMITH
UK Family Planning Association
27-35 Mortimer Street
London W1N 7RJ
England

J. M. SPIELER
Research Division, Office of
  Population Agency for
  International Development
Washington, DC 20523
USA

T. STANDLEY
World Health Organisation
Avenue Appia
CH-1211 Geneva 27
Switzerland

R. ST ARNAUD
Departments of Medicine and
  Molecular Endocrinology
Laval University Medical Center
2705 Laurier Boulevard
Quebec G1V 4G2
Canada

V. C. STEVENS
Department of Obstetrics and
  Gynecology
Ohio State University
163 Upham Hall
473 W. 12th Avenue
Colombus, OH 43210
USA

S. TAKAGI
Department of Obstetrics and
  Gynecology
Nihon University School of
  Medicine
30-1 Oyaguchi-Kamimachi
Itabashi-Ku, Tokyo 173
Japan

P. TALBOT
Biology Department
University of California
Riverside, CA 92521
USA

H. TAUBERT
Abteilung für Gynäkologische
  Endokrinologie
Johann-Wolfgang-
  Goethe Universität
Theodor-Stern-Kai 7
D-6000 Frankfurt am Main
West Germany

G. TEASDALE
Department of Neurosurgery
Institute of Neurological Sciences
Southern General Hospital
Glasgow G51 4TF
Scotland

S. TEPER
Social Statistics Research Unit
Department of Mathematics
The City University
Northampton Square
London EC1V 0HB
England

C. M. G. THOMAS
Department of Obstetrics and
  Gynecology
St Radboud University Hospital
Nijmegen
The Netherlands

J. THOMPSON
Institute of Neurological Sciences
Southern General Hospital
Glasgow G51 4TF
Scotland

W. THOMPSON
Department of Midwifery and
  Gynaecology
Queen's University Belfast
Belfast BT9 7AE
Northern Ireland

C. THORNER
Department of Internal Medicine
University of Virginia School of
  Medicine
Charlottesville, VA 22908
USA

K. TSUBATA
Department of Obstetrics and
  Gynecology
Nihon University School of
  Medicine
30-1 Oyaguchi-Kamamachi
Itabashi-Ku, Tokyo 173
Japan

Y. TSUKAHARA
Department of Obstetrics and
  Gynecology
Nihon University School of
  Medicine
30-1 Oyaguchi-Kamamachi
Itabashi-Ku, Tokyo 173
Japan

I. TURKALJ
Pharmaceutical Department
Clinical Research
Drug Monitoring Centre
Sandoz Ltd
CH-4002 Basle
Switzerland

H. UNTERBERG
Universitäts-Frauenklinik
D-7400 Tübingen
West Germany

W. H. UTIAN
Department of Obstetrics and
  Gynecology
Mt Sinai Medical Center of
  Cleveland
University Circle
Cleveland, OH 44106
USA

M. L. VANCE
Department of Internal Medicine
University of Virginia School of
  Medicine
Charlottesville, VA 22908
USA

E. V. VAN HALL
Department of Obstetrics and
  Gynaecology
University Hospital
University of Leiden
Rijnsburgerweg 10
2333 AA Leiden
The Netherlands

L. VEECK
Department of Obstetrics and
  Gynecology
East Virginia Medical School
Norfolk, VA 23507
USA

T. G. WEGMANN
Department of Immunology
University of Alberta
Edmonton, Alberta
Canada T662H7

M. J. WEIJERS
Medical Research Development
  Unit
Organon International BV
PO Box 20
5340 BH Oss
The Netherlands

C. ZAVAGLIA
III Department of Obstetrics and
  Gynecology
University of Milan
Via M. Melloni 52
I-20129 Milan
Italy

M. ZWIRNER
Universitäts-Frauenklinik
D-7400 Tübingen
West Germany

Inaugural Address: trends and prospects for research on fertility and sterility in the 1980s

A. KESSLER

I have great pleasure in bringing to the eleventh World Congress on Fertility and Sterility the best wishes of the Director General of the World Health Organization, Dr Mahler. The Organization has close links with the International Federation of Fertility Societies, which is one of the non-governmental organizations in official relations with WHO.

For WHO, the Federation's Fourth Congress in Rio de Janeiro in 1962 represented an important landmark, since this was the forum chosen by the then Director General of WHO, Dr Marcolino Candau, to call for much greater world-wide activity in the area of research on fertility and sterility. He pointed to the many biological, clinical and social issues relating to fertility and sterility in which knowledge was deficient. He concluded that 'the understanding of reproduction, especially human reproduction, demands no less attention than that given to specific diseases and public health problems'.

It may be difficult for many of the younger participants in this Congress to realize how politically courageous were his statements as this was a time when the majority of governments and policy makers still preferred to leave aside this controversial area.

It would be presumptuous to attempt, in this address, to take stock of what has happened in research since then, but it should be possible to pull out some trends, some tensions, and from these to extrapolate

1

to what may occur in the next decade or so to research in fertility and sterility.

Since the early 1960s there has been a profound change, probably one of the most significant social revolutions of the century, both in thinking and in action in this whole area. The majority of governments have established national programmes to allow individuals to control their fertility, including measures to help them overcome unintended infertility. The change of attitude is epitomized in the Alma Ata Declaration of the 1978 International Conference on Primary Health Care organized by WHO and UNICEF in which family planning was identified as an integral part of health care and social development, a declaration endorsed unanimously in 1979 by the 156 Member States of WHO.

Research, starting in the mid-1960s and during the early 1970s, grew apace with this increase of interest in fertility and sterility. Funding to the field is one measure of activity: in the decade 1965–74, expenditures world-wide in relevant reproductive biology, contraceptive development, safety evaluation of birth control methods and in infertility more than doubled in constant dollar terms, i.e. allowing for inflation with 1970 taken as a baseline. This doubling of expenditures must, however, be seen against the 1965 funding level to the field, which was about US $40 million, an extremely low one for biomedical research, for instance in comparison with the cancer field or infectious diseases. The reason for this is that in the two decades that followed World War II the reproductive sciences had been virtually excluded from the rapid expansion of support to biomedical research. In the mid-seventies, the rise in overall funding to research in fertility and sterility, that had begun in the sixties, came to an end. In fact funding decreased by about 20% in constant dollar terms and has remained more or less at that level since then.

The sources of funding too have changed in the past two decades. Industry's interest waned in the seventies. It was receiving high returns on its earlier investment in contraceptive development, and drug testing requirements for fertility control methods had become so demanding as to inhibit research on innovative approaches. Recently, however, there appears to be a slight rekindling of interest on the part of industry. Nevertheless, its share of funding to the field has decreased from about 40% in 1965 to roughly 15% at present. There has been a similar decline in interest on the part of the philanthropic foundations. They played a very significant role in the 1960s and early seventies in stimulating reproductive biology and training scientists in it. Their share of the funding has reduced from about 20% to less than 5%.

As a result of the growing recognition by governments of the importance of this research, the greatest change has been in their financial contributions to the field, which now account for 80% of the funding. Of that 80%, three-quarters comes from the US Government. The other sources of support are mainly European research councils and technical assistance agencies of European governments. The latter, through contributions to WHO, have played a major role in setting up the WHO Special Programme of Research, Development and Research Training in Human Reproduction, which is also financially supported by such developing countries as Cuba, India, Nigeria, the People's Republic of China and Thailand. These, and a few other developing countries have, in the past decade, begun to give substantial support to research on fertility and sterility within their own countries. This, in itself, is a very significant development.

Over the past 20 years, the proportion of funds allocated to basic studies and to applied research has remained fairly constant with about 50% going to each. Within applied research, safety studies on birth control methods are now receiving an increased proportion of the funding. The distribution at present stands roughly at 15% for safety studies, 30% for research and development of new methods, 5% for infertility research and 50% for basic research. A noteworthy change in the past few years is the sharp rise in activity in research relating to male reproduction, an attempt to catch up in an area that had lagged far behind that of research into female reproduction.

Overall, however, the field is still receiving less than 1% of the funds going to biomedical research. This seems a small amount to devote to problems that affect 1500 million people, that is all persons of reproductive age, or one third of the world population.

One can think of several possible reasons for this state of affairs:

(1) Achievement in research has been poor, which has discouraged funding.
(2) Other areas of biomedical research deserve higher priority.
(3) There are political constraints to funding.
(4) The absorptive capacity for funds is lacking.
(5) The problems encountered in fertility and sterility no longer require research.

3

I shall discuss these points below.

ACHIEVEMENT IN RESEARCH HAS BEEN POOR, WHICH HAS DISCOURAGED FUNDING

On the whole, the field can point to solid achievement in the past 20 years, whatever the criteria used, whether they be knowledge acquired, papers published, or technology developed. There is quasi-unanimous agreement that our understanding of reproductive biology has progressed very significantly in these two decades. One can take as examples the advances in knowledge of releasing factors, gonadotrophins, hormone receptors, prostaglandins and sperm maturation. These advances and others have been reflected in an increasingly large volume of publications and new journals devoted to specialized aspects of research on fertility and sterility.

There have also been many positive achievements in technology. *In vitro* fertilization is the one that first comes to mind, and one should also include major progress in assay techniques and in drugs for the treatment of infertility in women. Most of the development work on the contraceptive pill had been done before 1960, but in the subsequent years considerable refinements, including reduction of the steroid dosage, were introduced. The past 20 years have seen the development and introduction of entirely new types of IUDs, injectable contraceptives, new techniques for female sterilization and non-surgical methods of abortion. Hopefully, several other techniques for the regulation of fertility, which are at various stages of clinical testing, should become available within the next 5 years. These include vaginal rings, long-acting implants and non-surgical methods of sterilization.

Despite, however, this apparently impressive list there is some evidence of dissatisfaction with achievement in the area of contraceptive development. Certain funding agencies point to the fact that there is still no drug available for fertility regulation by men, that a birth control vaccine is still a long way from availability and that there is still no reliable and simple way to predict ovulation for couples wishing to practise natural family planning methods. The long time it takes to develop new fertility regulating methods, because of the intrinsic difficulty and the stringent drug testing requirements, is – it must be recognized – leading to a certain disenchantment and to what has been called 'donor fatigue'.

On the whole, however, one can say confidently that the achievements have been such that they cannot have discouraged funding.

OTHER AREAS OF BIOMEDICAL RESEARCH DESERVE HIGHER PRIORITY

Discussing priorities, particularly other people's priorities (which are notoriously difficult to understand), is an area where angels fear to tread. Tentatively, however, one can identify some criteria for priority ranking upon which to base a non-controversial argument; for instance the extent to which the research will affect mortality, morbidity, or the quality of life, and the number of people it will benefit.

Number of people has already been mentioned, and here our field scores high, with 1500 million potential customers for the results of the research. On mortality and morbidity, however, it scores low. With two-thirds of deaths in developed countries due to cancer and cardiovascular disease, and a rapidly rising percentage of deaths in developing countries from these causes, it is clear where the politicians' interest is going to lie, particularly as they themselves tend to belong to the older age groups. Other areas that account for high morbidity or mortality and where research is needed are mental disorders, parasitic and other infectious diseases, and diseases of ageing.

On the other hand, infertility, which is a morbid condition, does affect 5–10% of the world's population and is therefore a problem of public health dimension. Probably half the cases suffer from infertility of unexplained origin or for which adequate treatment is not known, and here clearly there is a case for research. However, infertility is not a life-threatening condition, it does not affect a person's work capacity and it does not cause substantial hospital-bed occupancy, so it tends to be given lower priority on the research agenda.

Much of the research on fertility and family planning will find its application in preventive rather than in curative medicine and unfortunately this automatically gives it a lower ranking. Nevertheless, with the present increasing concern for the quality of life, the temper of opinion is changing and the legitimate demands for better methods of fertility control are likely to get a more sympathetic hearing. The problem of abortion – which, in developing countries particularly, entails a sizeable mortality and morbidity – is significantly related to dissatisfaction with available birth-control methods.

5

A point we should not forget is that some countries, such as China and India, which after all together account for nearly 40% of the world's population, do give highest priority, within all research, to that on fertility. They consider that limiting population growth is an issue the importance of which outweighs all others. However, although they are committing substantial funds and manpower to this research, they need the help of developed countries in research and in building up their research facilities.

Thus it would seem fair to conclude that, although there are many other very important problems requiring investigation, certainly the area of fertility and sterility deserves more than 1% of the biomedical research pie.

THERE ARE POLITICAL CONSTRAINTS ON FUNDING

As already mentioned, this area of research has been considerably defused over the last two decades. Compared, however, with leprosy, arthritis or cancer, fertility research remains harassed by controversy. It may spring from moral, religious or political origins. This is not surprising, given the fact that sex and reproduction are not just biological phenomena but also intimately personal as well as social and cultural issues. Not only do they affect everyone, but everyone feels an 'instant expert' on the matter, entitled to full participation in any debate. The discussions that have surrounded research on *in vitro* fertilization and the heat of the depate on Depo-Provera are ample evidence of the power of vocal minorities in limiting scientific investigation.

An even more far-reaching effect on research has been the US Government's moratorium on the use of federal funds for studies relating to abortion, a situation confused by the absence of agreement on a biological definition of what constitutes an abortion. Given the important role of US scientific institutions in reproduction research, the moratorium is a serious blow world-wide, since it sharply reduces development of methods such as postcoital drugs or drugs for termination of pregnancy which are in great demand from governments such as those of China and India. At the same time, the hot-gospellers of population control have caused a revulsion in part of public opinion which fears infringement of human rights. This has understandably led many politicians to adopt a low profile when budgets for reproduction research are discussed.

THE ABSORPTIVE CAPACITY FOR FUNDS IS LACKING

At first sight, given the number of scientists present at the Congress, this would hardly seem to be the case. Moreover, we are told that the US National Institutes of Health can only find funds for 20% of the projects in this field that they have technically approved. There would therefore seem to be spare absorptive capacity, at least in the developed countries. In most developing countries where there is interest, the lack of trained manpower and facilities is sorely felt. Funds are needed in the first place to strengthen and build up their capabilities for research in fertility and sterility and then to support such research. The decreased funding in developed countries is not only affecting their own research output but also their capacity to train their own scientists and those of developing countries.

There is no doubt that, were the less than 1% of biomedical research funds currently allocated to fertility and sterility to be doubled or trebled, there would be no problem in absorbing these increases.

THE PROBLEMS ENCOUNTERED IN FERTILITY AND STERILITY NO LONGER REQUIRE RESEARCH

Many unresolved problems requiring research have already been mentioned. At the basic level, some of the areas of particular importance to an understanding of fertility and sterility include the immunological aspects of reproduction, factors affecting the maturation of oocytes and sperm, those regulating implantation, the hypothalamic control of gonadotrophin synthesis and release, and the mechanism of action of hormones at the cellular level. Advances in basic research are likely to be of benefit to both infertility and birth-control technology.

To those present at the Congress, the case for sustained research on the short- and long-term safety of birth control methods does not need to be stressed. With these methods being used by millions of persons, most of them healthy individuals, the need for monitoring is self-evident and will continue as long as new methods are introduced. Much more work is required in this area in developing countries as extrapolation of safety data obtained in developed countries is questionable, since the populations in developing countries differ in health status, genetic constitution, diet, reproductive patterns, lactation practices, etc. Some problems are specific to developing

7

countries, for instance the effect of contraceptive drugs in the presence of endemic malaria or schistosomiasis.

Research in new birth-control technology is clearly called for to improve present methods, for instance to further diminish the metabolic effects of the daily pill or the bleeding disturbances associated with IUDs and injectable contraceptives, or to reduce the period of abstinence required of users of natural family planning methods. More appropriate methods are needed for adolescents and for lactating women. I have already referred to such major gaps in technology as drugs for men, postcoital pills and chemical abortifacients. To this list could be added simple reversible methods of sterilization for men and women, birth control vaccines, and weekly or monthly pills. One element in facilitating this research and development would be a more scientific approach to toxicological testing. Research is needed to give a sounder basis to the requirements of the nature of the tests to be used, the species of animals to be employed, the numbers and duration of tests and the dose to be administered.

In the area of infertility, much more needs to be done in basic research in order to reduce the proportion of cases presently diagnosed as of unknown aetiology. Hopefully, terms such as idiopathic testicular failure will disappear from textbooks printed in the 1990s. The field is plagued by questionable diagnostic procedures and therapeutic measures of doubtful value. They need to be subjected to prospective, comparative controlled clinical trials. They also need to be simplified for use in the primary health-care context of developing countries.

This brings us to an area of research that so far has gone unmentioned in this address and that tends to be neglected: the psychosocial aspects of fertility and sterility and the delivery of family planning care, including infertility services. However good the technology, it must be appropriate to the requirements of different age groups or segments of the population, it must be explained in suitable terms and it must be delivered in a manner that is acceptable and convenient. The delivery must also be cost-effective. This area of research suffers from methodological difficulties, as do many of the social sciences. It is one of particular importance to developing countries which are attempting to add another form of care, which must reach large numbers of people, to an already over-extended service infrastructure.

Hopefully, this condensed catalogue shows that if research workers in the areas of fertility and sterility fall out-of-work, it will certainly not be for lack of challenging problems.

INTERNATIONAL COLLABORATION

In summary, the field has a sound record of achievement, it has absorptive capacity for considerable additional funding and it is alive with questions that it wishes to address, at both the fundamental and at the applied level. It can claim a higher level of priority than it has so far received. I am sceptical, however, whether any significant expansion can be expected at present given the economic situation and the political obstacles. We should therefore consider how best to make use of available resources.

One approach is through international collaboration. WHO has pioneered this through the setting up of its Special Programme of Research, Development and Research Training in Human Reproduction. At present it involves scientists and institutions from 73 countries, of which 46 are developing and 27 developed countries. Through a network of collaborating centres and multinational studies, research is conducted on the safety of currently available birth-control methods, on the development of new methods, on infertility and on the service and psychosocial aspects of these problems. This allows the marshalling of the most appropriate disciplines and expertise from different countries, the division of labour and the accumulation of data in both large numbers and from varying populations. One of the Programme's achievements has been to bring into the mainstream of world effort the talents of many developing-country scientists. It has also strengthened many institutions in developing countries for research on fertility and sterility.

Another feature of the Programme is global co-ordination of research, not only by bringing together scientists, but also research policy making bodies, medical research councils, other funding agencies, non-governmental organizations, etc. This has led to joint planning of strategy and has served to disseminate information widely and avoid duplication of effort.

So much for what WHO can do. What can participants of the Congress do? The national societies of this Federation play an essential role in stimulating research on fertility and sterility and disseminating information through the meetings they convene and the journals they publish, as does the International Federation. What the

9

national societies are also in a particularly good position to do – and do well, given their sensitivity to local conditions – is to interact with two other groups; the national policy makers on the one hand and the general public on the other. These two audiences deserve the best possible information, which only the scientific community can provide. Maybe a still greater effort should go into this.

Many of the Congress participants are already collaborating with the WHO Programme. This collaboration is very valuable, is greatly appreciated and should continue. The Congress provided the welcome opportunity to discuss how it can be furthered and expanded in the future.

Part I

Main Themes of the Congress

Part I

Section 1

Neuroendocrinology – Reproductive Releasing Hormones

1
Mechanisms regulating LHRH release: implications for fertility regulation

A. NEGRO-VILAR

INTRODUCTION

Evidence accumulated during the last two decades indicates that a neural decapeptide, luteinizing hormone releasing hormone (LHRH), is the primary link between the brain and the pituitary–gonadal axis[1]. It is through this decapeptide that the brain transduces its neural signals into a chemical one (LHRH), ultimately resulting in the initiation, maintenance and modulation of normal gonadal function.

Large advances in our knowledge of the anatomy, physiology and pharmacology of LHRH were made possible by: (1) the combined use of immunohistochemical and microdissection techniques and sensitive and specific radioimmunoassays for LHRH; (2) the character-ization of specific receptors for the decapeptide in membranes from the anterior pituitary and gonads; and (3) the development of several peptidic analogues with agonistic and antagonistic properties. Both the synthetic decapeptide and its analogues have been found useful in the treatment of selected cases of infertility[2,3]. Moreover, the use of different agonistic analogues under a certain regimen has been shown to have paradoxical antifertility effects, and therefore those peptides may prove to be useful contraceptive agents[2,3]. It is evident, therefore, that an understanding of the intimate mechanisms used in

15

neural regulation of release and function of LHRH is of paramount importance for the effective use and application of LHRH as a prime regulator of fertility in animals and humans.

ANATOMY OF THE LHRH SYSTEM

Most of the decapeptide produced in neurons is stored in secretory granules in the axon terminals. The cell bodies of the LHRH neurons are widely distributed in the septal–preoptico-hypothalamic regions, with a small number of cells also distributed in extrahypothalamic areas[4-6]. The majority of the neurons projecting to the median eminence (ME) contain the largest concentration of LHRH in the brain. The LHRH terminals in the ME abut in the hypophysial portal vessels, where the peptide is released to be carried to the anterior pituitary *via* the portal circulation. LHRH has been demonstrated to be present in gonadal tissues from different species[3] and this raises the possibility that the peptide may also have direct gonadal effects which can contribute to the overall action of the peptide in the reproductive sphere.

PHYSIOLOGICAL MECHANISMS REGULATING LHRH RELEASE AND ACTION

As in other peptidergic neuronal systems, the regulation of LHRH release can be exerted at multiple anatomical and functional levels, involving factors such as synthesis, transport, degradation, release, target tissue sensitivity, etc. We will analyse below in detail some relevant aspects of these regulatory mechanisms.

Synthesis, transport and degradation of LHRH

Recent evidence indicates that LHRH biosynthesis is a multi-step process[7], with a precursor peptide of larger molecular weight being translated from ribosomes and undergoing post-translational modifications to produce the decapeptide[8,9]. Following synthesis of new peptide in the soma of the neurons, subsequent movement by axoplasmic transport occurs, with the resulting accumulation of LHRH in nerve terminals[10]. Degradation of LHRH by brain and pituitary tissues is initiated by endopeptidases that cleave the decapeptide between positions 5–6 or 6–7 or, in other instances, position 9–10[11]. The endopeptidases have been shown to be highly specific for the

16

amino acids at these positions. Most active analogues synthesized, therefore, have chemical substitutions on amino acids 6 and 7 (Gly-Leu) and amino acids 9 and 10 (Pro-Gly NH$_2$), resulting in reduced rates of degradation. It is obvious from the above that factors regulating LHRH function may do so by modulating the enzymatic processes involved in synthesis and/or degradation of the peptide, the latter occurring either at storage sites in the nerve terminal or at the active membrane sites in the target cells (gonadotrophs).

Role of central neurotransmitter systems in the release of LHRH

The central noradrenergic system plays a major role in the regulation of LHRH release, a concept supported by many reports entailing a variety of experimental approaches. Studies of both rodents and subhuman primates indicate that inhibition of norepinephrine (NE) synthesis, blockage of α-adrenergic receptors or interruption of noradrenergic pathways projecting to the hypothalamus results in inhibition of LH release in different experimental situations (see 1 for specific references).

Direct evidence for a stimulatory role of NE on LHRH release was first presented by Negro-Vilar et al.[12]. This study used microdissected ME fragments containing only nerve terminals, including those of LHRH neurons, which were incubated in medium with different concentrations of neurotransmitters. A concentration-related increase in LHRH release was observed after NE stimulation[12], and this effect was inhibited by phentolamine, an α-receptor blocker. This observation was later confirmed and further substantiated by additional studies indicating that the stimulation of α-receptors by NE, which resulted in enhanced LHRH release, was blocked in a concentration-dependent fashion by phentolamine, with an IC_{50} of 0.9×10^{-7} mol l^{-1} [13]. Propranolol, a β-receptor blocker was ineffective in blocking the release of LHRH induced by NE[13] as was pimozide, a dopamine receptor blocker[12,13]. Recent studies using clonidine, a mixed α-agonist, and specific α-1 (prazosin) and α-2 (yohimbine) receptor blockers indicate that the noradrenergic stimulatory input on the presynaptic LHRH terminal in the ME is mediated by an α-2 receptor (see reference 14). To further support the concept that NE is physiologically involved in the regulation of LHRH and LH release, we presented evidence that changes in NE-stimulated LHRH release from the ME occur during the oestrous cycle, and in particular around

17

the critical period that precedes the release of LHRH prior to the LH surge[15]. *In vivo* blockage of the preovulatory LH surge with barbiturates completely abolishes the release of LHRH induced by NE *in vitro*, suggesting that the ovulation-blocking effect of barbiturates is mediated, at least in part, by changes in ME responsiveness to NE[15].

Another catecholamine, epinephrine, has been reported to elicit mixed responses which seem to be dependent upon the experimental system in which the effects are tested. In intact males or ovariectomized females, epinephrine had no effect upon LHRH release[12,16], but in ovariectomized, oestrogen–progesterone primed animals epinephrine effectively enhanced release of LHRH from the ME[16]. From these observations we can conclude that presynaptic sensitivity of LHRH terminals to specific neurotransmitters can be enhanced or depressed by gonadal steroids, and this might represent one of the several modulatory actions through which steroids regulate the hypothalamic–pituitary–gonadal axis (see below). We have recently provided evidence that epinephrine is present in hypophysial portal blood in concentrations higher than those found in peripheral blood, and that a substantial amount of the amine is of central origin[17]. These findings, coupled with other reports indicating an involvement of epinephrine in the preovulatory release of LH[18–20], suggest that this amine may play an important physiological role in the regulation of gonadotrophin release.

Dopamine (DA) has also been shown to stimulate release of LHRH from the ME, an effect nullified by the addition of specific blockers of dopamine receptors[12]. Increases in dopamine turnover and metabolism have also been described in situations that call for an increased output of LHRH/LH, both in males and females[21,22].

Presynaptic receptors in LHRH neurons within the ME should, therefore, be considered as an important target upon which different catecholamines, other neurotransmitters and neuromodulators, and steroid hormones act to regulate LHRH release and, indirectly, gonadal function.

Role of intracellular messengers in the release of LHRH

Several reports indicate that both basal and stimulated release of LHRH *in vitro* from hypothalamic or ME fragments is Ca^{2+}–dependent[23–25]. In the absence of extracellular Ca^{2+} most secretagogues are ineffective in releasing LHRH. An exception to this is the action of prostaglandin E_2 (see below), which can still induce a moderate degree of stimulation in the absence of extracellular Ca^{2+}, perhaps by mobilizing calcium from an intracellular pool (Ojeda and Negro-Vilar, unpublished observations).

Arachidonic acid metabolites are involved in the release of LHRH. Arachidonic acid added to the incubation medium enhanced LHRH output from ME fragments *in vitro*[26]. Of the different metabolites of arachidonic acid tested, prostaglandin E_2 (PGE_2) was found to be the most potent releasor of LHRH[27]. Evidence accumulated over the past few years indicates that PGE_2 is a physiological intracellular regulator of LHRH release[28]. Nanomolar concentrations of PGE_2 are potent stimulators of LHRH release *in vitro*[27]. More significantly, our studies indicate that stimulation of PGE_2 release is an obligatory step in the effect of NE upon LHRH release. Blockage of the cyclo-oxygenase pathway with indomethacin, which essentially results in a complete suppression of PGE_2 release from the incubated ME fragments[27], is accompanied by: (1) a reduction in basal LHRH release; and (2) a complete suppression of the stimulatory effect of NE[27]. One conclusion from our studies is that NE stimulates PGE_2 production and release and PGE_2 in turn enhances LHRH output. These and other results from either *in vivo* or *in vitro* experiments[15,27,28] support our conclusion that PGE_2 is a physiologically important intracellular mediator of LHRH release[28].

Brain and pituitary effects of steroids to modulate LHRH release

Regulation of LHRH and gonadotrophin release by gonadal steroids is orchestrated by a highly complex series of negative and positive feedback mechanisms which operate both at central and peripheral sites. The activity of LHRH neurons is clearly modulated by gonadal steroids[1]. This modulatory activity of steroids (oestradiol, testosterone, progesterone) involves activation (nuclear translocation) of specific receptors in neurons located in certain brain regions, and interaction with other aminergic and peptidergic systems involved in regulation of LHRH release[1,22,29]. Gonadal steroids may also affect the release of LHRH by interacting with intracellular messengers such as PGE_2 which participate in the neurotransmitter–peptide interactions previously described[15].

Another important regulation site of LHRH activity is the pituitary gland itself where oestradiol and, to some extent, other gonadal steroids can exert profound influence on the response of gonadotroph cells to LHRH stimulation[30].

REGULATION OF PULSATILE LHRH/LH-FSH RELEASE

Early studies from Knobil's laboratory indicated that LH is secreted in an episodic or pulsatile fashion in the ovariectomized Rhesus monkey[31]. This observation was subsequently extended to other species, including the human, and it soon became clear that both gonadotrophins and, indeed, LHRH are secreted in an episodic fashion. Additional evidence presented by Knobil[31] indicated that pulsatile LHRH release was essential to obtain an effective and sustained stimulation of LH release and provided the experimental and rational basis for the therapeutic application of pulsatile LHRH substitution in the treatment of hypothalamic hypogonadism[32].

We have recently presented evidence indicating that each episode of LH release is preceded by the release of LHRH from the ME. Concomitant analysis of norepinephrine, dopamine and LHRH levels in three different preoptico-hypothalamic regions was performed and correlated with the LH secretory episode. To accomplish this, frequent (10 min) blood samples were obtained from chronically cannulated, freely moving, ovariectomized subjects during a 2-hour period. In this way, we were able to reconstruct in every case the relative position in the LH secretory episode at the time that all amine and peptide determinations were performed[33]. The results indicate that prior to the rising phase in each LH secretory episode, a concomitant drop in DA and LHRH levels in the ME occurs, suggesting that both DA and LHRH are released prior to, or in conjunction with, the initiation of the LH surge. Simultaneously with these changes, a parallel rise in NE levels in the suprachiasmatic-medial preoptic region was observed, which we interpreted as suggestive of increased noradrenergic activity in that area at the time of the LH surge.

From these observations and from additional data from our laboratory and from the literature, we can formulate the following comprehensive hypothesis to account for the sequence of events leading to pulsatile LH release: noradrenergic input originating in the midbrain and projecting to the suprachiasmatic–medial preoptic region activates LHRH perykaria located in that region, resulting in the transport of peptide to more caudal and basal hypothalamic areas.

This serves to provide a continuous replenishment of LHRH stores in the ME to replace the peptide that is periodically released from that region. Noradrenergic input to the basal hypothalamic areas may also play an additional role in LHRH release. Finally, dopamine neurons within the tuberoinfundibular system projecting to the ME stimulate LHRH release[33]. The oscillator that entrains the episodic release of LHRH is probably located in the suprachiasmatic nucleus receiving appropriate environmental cues[34].

CONCLUDING REMARKS

The last 20 years have witnessed a remarkable advance in our knowledge of reproductive physiology with the discovery, isolation and synthesis of LHRH. Further advancements in the areas of physiological regulatory mechanisms, particularly concerning the mode of secretion and mechanism of action; and in the development of potent and long-acting agonists and antagonists have opened a promisory area for the successful clinical application of LHRH and its analogues to different fertility disorders.

Acknowledgements

These studies were supported by NIH grant HD-09988. The editorial assistance of Mr Thomas Denham is gratefully acknowledged as is the secretarial assistance of Ms Jeanne Clark and Ms Anna Lee Howard.

References

1. Negro-Vilar, A. and Ojeda, S. R. (1981). Hypophysiotrophic hormones of the hypothalamus. In McCann, S. M. (ed.). *Endocrine Physiology III, International Review of Physiology*. Vol. **24**, pp. 97–156. (Baltimore: University Park Press)
2. Schally, A. V., Coy, D. H. and Meyers, C. A. (1978). Hypothalamic regulatory hormones. *Annu. Rev. Biochem.*, **47**, 89
3. Sandow, J. (1982). Gonadotropic and antigonadotropic actions of LHRH analogues. In Muller, E. E. and MacLeod, R. M. (eds.). *Neuroendocrine Perspectives*. Vol. **1**, pp. 339–95. (Amsterdam: Elsevier Biomedical Press)
4. Barry, J. (1977). Immunofluorescence study of LRF neurons in man. *Cell Tiss. Res.*, **181**, 1
5. Silverman, A. J., Krey, L. C. and Zimmerman, E. A. (1979). A comparative study of the luteinizing hormone-releasing hormone (LHRH) neuronal network in mammals. *Biol. Reprod.*, **20**, 98
6. Elde, R., Hokfelt, T., Johansson, O., Ljungdahl, A., Nilsson, G. and Jeffcoate, S. L. (1978). Immunohistochemical localization of peptides in the nervous system.

In Hughes, J. (ed.). *Centrally Acting Peptides*. pp. 1–35. (Baltimore: University Park Press)

7. McKelvy, J. F., Lin, C. J., Chan, L. *et al.* (1979). Biosynthesis of brain peptides. In Gotto, A. M. Jr., Peck, E. J. and Boyd, A. E. (eds.). *Brain Peptides: A New Endocrinology*. pp. 183–96. (Amsterdam: Elsevier)

8. Curtiss, A. and Fink, G. (1983). A high molecular weight precursor of luteinizing hormone-releasing hormone from rat hypothalamus. *Endocrinology*, **112**, 390.

9. Gautron, J. P., Pattou, E. and Kordon, C. (1981). Occurrence of higher molecular weight forms of LHRH in fractionated extracts from rat hypothalamus, cortex and placenta. *Mol. Cell. Endocrinol.*, **24**, 1

10. Barry, J. (1976). Immunohistochemical localization of hypothalamic hormones (especially LRF) at the light microscopy level. In Labrie, F., Meites, J. and Pelletier, G. (eds.). *Hypothalamus and Endocrine Functions*. pp. 451–73. (New York: Plenum Press)

11. Taubert, H. D. and Kuhl, H. (1977). The regulation of luteinizing hormone release by a hypothalamic and pituitary enzyme system. In Hubinont, P. O., L'Hermite, M. and Robyn, C. (eds.). *Progress in Reproductive Biology*. Vol. **2**, pp. 69–77. (Basel: Karger)

12. Negro-Vilar, A., Ojeda, S. R. and McCann, S. M. (1979). Catecholaminergic modulation of luteinizing hormone-releasing hormone release by median eminence terminals *in vitro*. *Endocrinology*, **104**, 1749

13. Ojeda, S. R., Negro-Vilar, A. and McCann, S. M. (1982). Evidence for involvement of α-adrenergic receptors in norepinephrine-induced prostaglandin E_2 and luteinizing hormone-releasing hormone release from the median eminence. *Endocrinology*, **110**, 409

14. Negro-Vilar, A. (1982). The median eminence as a model to study presynaptic regulation of neural peptide release. *Peptides*, **3**, 305

15. De Paolo, L., Ojeda, S. R., Negro-Vilar, A. and McCann, S. M. (1982). Alterations in responsiveness of median eminence luteinizing hormone-releasing hormone nerve terminals to norepinephrine and prostaglandin E_2 *in vitro* during the rat estrous cycle. *Endocrinology*, **110**, 1999

16. Negro-Vilar, A., Ojeda, S. R. and McCann, S. M. (1980). Hypothalamic control of LHRH and somatostatin: Role of central neurotransmitters and intracellular messengers. In Litwack, G. (ed.). *Biochemical Actions of Hormones*. Vol. **7**, pp. 245–85. (New York: Academic Press)

17. Johnston, C. A., Gibbs, D. M. and Negro-Vilar, A. (1983). High concentrations of epinephrine derived from a central source and of 5-hydroxy-indole-3-acetic acid in hypophysial portal plasma. *Endocrinology*, **113**, 819

18. Rubinstein, L. and Sawyer, C. H. (1970). Role of catecholamines in stimulating the release of pituitary ovulatory hormone(s) in rats. *Endocrinology*, **86**, 988

19. Crawley, W. R., Cass Terry, L. and Johnson, M. D. (1982). Evidence for the involvement of central epinephrine systems in the regulation of luteinizing hormone, prolactin and growth hormone release in female rats. *Endocrinology*, **110**, 1102

20. Kalra, S. P. and Crawley, W. R. (1982). Epinephrine synthesis inhibitors block naloxone-induced LH release. *Endocrinology*, **111**, 1403

21. Advis, J. P., McCann, S. M. and Negro-Vilar, A. (1980). Evidence that catecholaminergic and peptidergic (LHRH) neurons in suprachiasmatic, medial preoptic, medial basal hypothalamus and median eminence are involved in estrogen negative feedback. *Endocrinology*, **107**, 892

22. De Paolo, L., McCann, S. M. and Negro-Vilar, A. (1982). A sex difference in the activation of hypothalamic catecholaminergic and luteinizing hormone-releasing

hormone (LHRH) peptidergic neurons following acute castration. *Endocrinology*, **110,** 531

23. Bigdeli, H. and Snyder, P. J. (1978). Gonadotropin-releasing hormone release from the rat hypothalamus: dependence on membrane depolarization and calcium influx. *Endocrinology*, **103,** 281

24. Gallardo, E. and Ramirez, V. D. (1977). A method for the superfusion of rat hypothalami: secretion of luteinizing hormone-releasing hormone (LHRH). *Proc. Soc. Exp. Biol. Med.*, **155,** 79

25. Ojeda, S. R., Negro-Vilar, A. and McCann, S. M. (1980). On the role of Ca^{2+} in prostaglandin E_2 (PGE_2)-induced LHRH release by rat median eminence (ME). *Fed. Proc.*, **39,** 487

26. Capdevila, J., Chacos, N., Falck, J. R., Manna, S., Negro-Vilar, A. and Ojeda, S. R. (1983). Novel hypothalamic arachidonate products stimulate somatostatin release from the median eminence. *Endocrinology*, **113,** 421

27. Ojeda, S. R., Negro-Vilar, A. and McCann, S. M. (1982). Evidence for involvement of α-adrenergic receptors in norepinephrine-induced prostaglandin E_2 and luteinizing hormone-releasing hormone release from the median eminence. *Endocrinology*, **110,** 409

28. Ojeda, S. R., Naor, Z. and Negro-Vilar, A. (1979). The role of prostaglandins in the control of gonadotropin and prolactin secretion. *Prostaglandins Med.*, **5,** 249

29. Negro-Vilar, A. and De Paolo, L. (1981). Brain-gonad interactions in the regulation of gonadotropin and prolactin release. In Frajese, G., Hafez, E. S. E., Conti, C. and Fabbrini, A. (eds.). *Oligozoospermia: Recent Progress in Andrology.* pp. 323–36. (New York: Raven Press)

30. Negro-Vilar, A. (1973). Interaction between gonadal steroids and LH-releasing hormone to control gonadotropin secretion at the pituitary level. *Acta Physiol. Latinoamer.*, **23,** 494

31. Knobil, E. (1980). The neuroendocrine control of the menstrual cycle. *Rec• Progr. Horm. Res.*, **36,** 53

32. Crowley, W. F., Jr., and McArthur, J. W. (1980). Stimulation of the normal menstrual cycle in Kallman's syndrome by pulsatile administration of luteinizing hormone-releasing hormone (LHRH). *J. Clin. Endocrinol. Metab.*, **51,** 173

33. Negro-Vilar, A., Advis, J. P., Ojeda, S. R. and McCann, S. M. (1982). Pulsatile LH patterns in ovariectomized rats: Involvement of norepinephrine and dopamine in the release of LHRH and LH. *Endocrinology*, **111,** 932

34. Moore, R. Y. (1983). Organization and function of a central nervous system circadian oscillator: The suprachiasmatic hypothalamic nucleus. *Fed. Proc.*, **42,** 2783

2
Medical castration in men: the first clinical application of LHRH agonists

F. LABRIE, A. BÉLANGER, A. DUPONT and
R. ST-ARNAUD

INTRODUCTION

Discovery of LHRH[1,2] and the availability of its potent agonistic analogues has led to a rapid increase in our knowledge of the pituitary–gonadal axis and has offered new and exciting therapeutic approaches in reproductive endocrinology as well as in sex steroid-dependent diseases.

Although the pulsatile administration of LHRH is highly effective in the treatment of infertility, LHRH agonists are potent inhibitors of gonadal functions both in men and in women. This presentation will attempt to summarize the data describing the inhibition of testicular functions achieved by LHRH agonists in the male with special emphasis on the first clinical application of these peptides in the human, namely in prostatic cancer.

INHIBITION OF TESTICULAR STEROIDOGENESIS

Experimental animals

Stimulated by the unexplained lack of success of LHRH and its agonists in the treatment of infertility in men[3,4], we investigated in detail the effect of acute and chronic administration of these peptides on testicular functions in experimental animals. Somewhat unexpectedly, we then made the observation that short-term administration of the LHRH agonist [D-Leu[6], des-Gly-NH$_2$[10]]LHRH ethylamide, ([D-Leu[6]]LHRH-EA) to adult male rats led to a loss of testicular LH and prolactin receptors, as well as to decreased serum testosterone levels accompanied by inhibition of ventral prostate, seminal vesicle and testis weight[5,6]. It is now well recognized that treatment of adult male rats with LHRH and its agonists exerts marked inhibitory effects on Leydig cell function[7-17].

These inhibitory effects can, at least partly, be explained by LHRH agonist-induced endogenous LH release causing secondary gonadal desensitization[5-8]. LHRH agonists can also exert direct inhibitory effects at the testicular level in hypophysectomized rats *in vivo* as well as in testicular cells *in vitro*[18]. The direct gonadal site of action of LHRH agonists is supported by the finding of high-affinity LHRH binding sites in rat Leydig cells[8,19,20].

All *in vivo* studies on the direct gonadal site of action of LHRH agonists were first performed in hypophysectomized animals. Since hypophysectomy by itself has profound effects on gonadal functions, we have used another approach which minimizes hormonal disturbances, in order to assess the importance of the direct action of LHRH agonists, namely by using intact animals treated with an excess of equine antibovine LH serum. This study provided, for the first time, an assessment of the importance of the direct testicular site of action of LHRH agonists in their antifertility activity in intact rats.

It showed that while LHRH agonists can have direct inhibitory effects on Leydig cell function at high doses, their predominant effect, in short-term studies, is mediated by LHRH agonist-induced LH release rather than by a direct inhibitory action at the testicular level, at least in the rat[21,22]. Treatment with LHRH agonists is also known to decrease the gonadotrophin responsiveness to LHRH[10,13]. However, it is now clear that blockage of the steroidogenic pathway at the level of 17α-hydroxylase and 17,20-desmolase activities is responsible for at least most of the short-term inhibitory effects of LHRH agonists in the rat[8,13,16,17].

Man

It is of great interest that inhibitory effects on testosterone secretion similar to those first described in the rat[5,6] are exerted in the male hamster[23], rabbit and dog (Tremblay, Bélanger and Labrie, unpub-

26

lished observations). The only exception so far reported is the monkey where androgen biosynthesis is exceptionally resistant to treatment with LHRH agonists[24].

Among the species so far studied and for reasons that are only partially understood[8], man appears to be the most sensitive to the inhibitory effect of treatment with LHRH agonists on testicular steroidogenesis. In fact, while, in the rat, treatment with LHRH agonists increases 5α-reductase activity and formation of 3α-androstanediol and 5α-dihydrotestosterone which can partially counteract the inhibitory effect on testosterone production[16,17], no such effect is seen in man[8,25-28] where androgen biosynthesis can be completely inhibited and medical castration is thus achieved relatively easily.

Following our preliminary study showing that twice daily intranasal administration of [D-Ser(TBU)^6]LHRH-EA led to a 75% inhibition of serum testosterone concentration after 16 days[8], we then performed a long-term study of the effect of treatment with the same LHRH agonist by the intranasal and subcutaneous routes[28,29]. The effect of chronic treatment with [D-Ser(TBU)^6]LHRH-EA administered by nasal spray (200 or 500 μg, twice daily) or subcutaneously (50 μg daily) for periods up to 8 months was studied on serum sex steroid and LH levels in 18 patients with cancer of the prostate. Basal serum testosterone concentration decreased to 71.1 ± 18.3 (not significant) and $28.6 \pm 9.3\%$ ($p < 0.01$) of control in patients receiving the 200 and 500 μg doses by nasal spray, respectively. In patients treated subcutaneously at the 50 μg dose, a more rapid inhibition of serum testosterone levels to $19.6 \pm 6.4\%$ of control ($p < 0.01$) was observed[28]. A more complete and rapid inhibition of serum testosterone levels to 5–8% of control (castrated levels) is achieved with the daily 500 μg dose[26,27]. Elegant studies by Crowley et al.[30] have shown the potent antisteroidogenic activity of another LHRH agonist in patients with precocious puberty.

INHIBITION OF SPERMATOGENESIS

Since the marked loss of testis weight following treatment with the LHRH agonist[5,6] was probably due to some defect in spermatogenesis, it seemed important to investigate the cellular changes occurring in rat testis during chronic administration of [D-Ala^6]LHRH-EA.

When the LHRH agonist was administered at the dose of 1 μg every second day, degenerative changes were observed after 4 weeks in almost all seminiferous tubules. In about 20–30% of tubules, both germinal and Sertoli cells were almost completely absent.

Although long-term treatment with LHRH agonists in male rats causes degenerative changes in a large proportion of the seminiferous tubules with a complete loss of spermatozoa in most tubules, the inhibitory effects are never complete. This is probably due to the fact that, in this species, LHRH agonist treatment increases 5α-reductase activity[8,31] which, as mentioned earlier, counteracts the inhibitory effect resulting from the almost complete inhibition of testosterone production. Although the rat was the first species where the inhibitory effects of treatment with LHRH agonists were described on both androgen biosynthesis[5,6] and spermatogenesis[9] and studies in this species have been essential for understanding some of the mechanisms involved[7,8], it is not the best model for the human. In fact, in man, there is no stimulatory effect of LHRH agonist treatment on 5α-reductase activity and a parallel inhibitory effect is observed on both testosterone and 5α-dihydrotestosterone formation[8,25–28]. Our current studies in the dog indicate that this species is a more appropriate model for studying the antifertility effects of LHRH agonists. The pattern of serum steroid levels observed after LHRH agonist treatment in man and in dog is very similar. Histology of the testis after chronic treatment of dogs with [D-Ser(TBU)⁶]LHRH-EA shows a marked atrophy of the tubules and a complete inhibition of sperm formation (Tremblay, Bélanger and Labrie, unpublished observations). That treatment with LHRH agonists can inhibit spermatogenesis in men has been shown by the study of Linde et al.[32].

So far, the responsibility for fertility control has almost exclusively been limited to women. It is thus important that special efforts be made in order to develop a safe, acceptable, reliable and reversible method of fertility regulation in men. The current approaches in male contraception have serious limitations. While gossypol presents some toxicity problems[33,34], the combination of gestagens and androgens induces azoospermia in only approximately 70% of men while varying degrees of oligospermia are obtained in the remaining 30% of subjects[35,36]. Moreover, the development of immunological reactions in vasectomized men is of some concern.

An alternative approach is the combined use of an LHRH agonist and androgen replacement therapy. Now that reversibility of sperm formation has been observed in an experimental model, clinical studies in adult men receiving androgen replacement therapy should provide the required answers on the efficacy and acceptability of this approach.

CANCER OF THE PROSTATE

Cancer of the prostate is the second commonest cause of death due to cancer in man. The pioneering studies of Huggins and collaborators[37] have demonstrated the role of testicular androgens in prostatic cancer. In fact, significant improvement in the clinical condition follows castration or oestrogen administration in a large proportion of patients with far-advanced prostatic carcinoma[38]. Subsequently, during the last 40 years, the principal goal of hormonal therapy in the treatment of prostatic cancer has been the suppression of androgens of testicular origin.

Inhibition of testicular androgen secretion by oestrogen administration and removal of the source of testicular androgens by surgical orchidectomy have shown similar palliative effects in advanced prostatic carcinoma. In fact 60–70% of patients with prostatic carcinoma show a positive response to either of these two treatments as evidenced by objective and/or subjective parameters. These hormonal manipulations thus provide remission for various time intervals in a large proportion of patients. However, castration is not always well accepted by the patients while high doses of oestrogens have serious cardiovascular side-effects.

In agreement with all previous endocrine therapies which had shown that a positive response is observed in 60–70% of cases of prostatic cancer when serum testosterone levels are reduced to castration levels, it was observed, in a collaborative preliminary study, that a similar rate of response is found following treatment with LHRH agonists[29]. This has now been confirmed by a study of the Abbott group[39] as well as by ICI studies (unpublished observations).

However, treatment with LHRH agonists is accompanied, during the first 5–15 days of treatment, by increased serum androgen levels leading to a flare-up of the disease in some patients[29]. Moreover, androgens of adrenal origin could well play a role in the relapse which regularly follows standard hormonal therapy. We thus felt that the next logical step in the hormonal therapy of prostate cancer was the combined use of an LHRH agonist and a pure antiandrogen.

A major previous limitation to the use of pure antiandrogens in the treatment of prostate cancer has been the escape phenomenon due

29

to the neutralization of the inhibitory feedback action of androgens by the antiandrogen which led to a progressive increase of gonadotrophin and testosterone secretion. This readjustment of androgen secretion at higher levels requires progressively higher doses of the antiandrogen leading to toxicity problems as well as lack of efficient neutralization of the effect of androgens on the growth of the cancer. Since treatment with LHRH agonists causes a desensitization of the gonadotrophin response to LHRH as well as an inhibition of testicular androgen biosynthesis, a solution is thus found to the previous limitations of pure antiandrogens. We then found that daily administration for 5 months of a potent LHRH agonist in combination with a pure antiandrogen, RU 23908, causes an almost complete inhibition of ventral prostate and seminal vesicle weight[40].

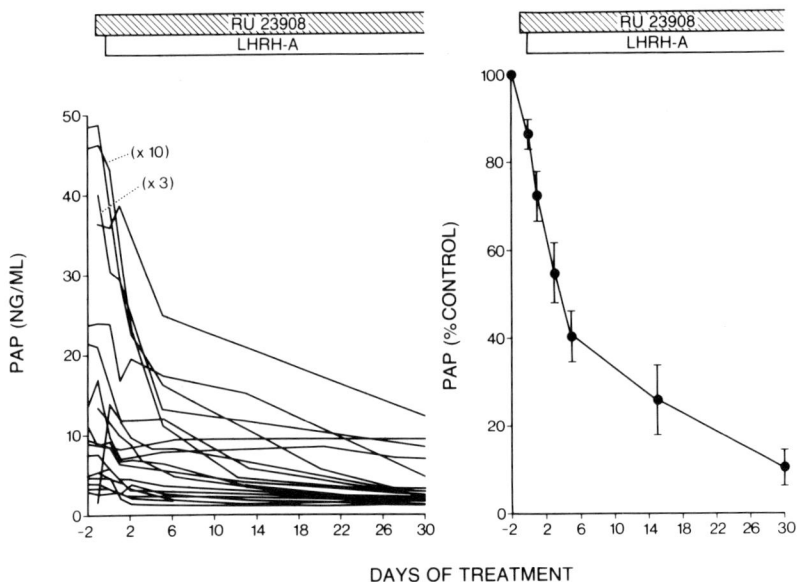

Figure 1 Effect of combined treatment with an LHRH agonist (HOE–766) and a pure antiandrogen (RU 23908) on serum PAP levels in previously untreated patients with advanced (stage C or D) prostatic cancer. Individual values are shown on the left panel while means ±SEM are illustrated on the right panel (27 patients). Reproduced with permission from reference 27

Following these encouraging results, we have performed a preliminary study using combination therapy with the same LHRH agonist and pure antiandrogen[26] in patients with advanced prostatic cancer. This preliminary study was originally performed in nine patients at stage D and in one patient at stage C of the disease. Objective remission as ascertained by bone scan, acid phosphatase levels and ultrasonography of the prostate was recorded in nine patients.

The present report is a continuation of this study with the combination therapy in 53 previously untreated as well as in 21 patients previously treated with diethylstilboestrol (DES)[27]. In ten previously untreated patients, the combination castration + antiandrogen was used. Comparison is also made with the effect of antiandrogen administration alone in 26 previously castrated patients. Drastic changes to the standard hormonal therapy in prostatic cancer are suggested.

Figure 1 shows that serum PAP levels were rapidly reduced to 40% of pretreatment values as early as 5 days after starting the combination therapy (LHRH agonist + antiandrogen) in previously untreated patients with a progressive decrease to normal values within 2 months in all except two patients. Although the number of patients was small, a comparable pattern was seen in the eight patients previously untreated who were surgically castrated (instead of LHRH agonist administration for inhibition of testicular androgens) and received the same dose of the antiandrogen (Table 1). Thus, after complete androgen removal in previously untreated patients, a decrease of serum PAP to normal values was obtained within 2 months of treatment in 47 out of 49 patients (96%).

A striking difference of change of serum PAP is, however, observed in patients previously treated with high doses of DES or castrated and showing relapse of the disease. In patients previously treated with DES and receiving the same combination therapy with the LHRH agonist and the antiandrogen, a decrease to normal was seen in only 46% of patients (Table 2). In patients previously castrated and receiving the antiandrogen, the mean serum PAP concentration returned to normal in only two out of 17 patients (12%).

As already shown in the first adult man treated with a high dose of an LHRH agonist[8], treatment with these peptides alone is always accompanied by a rise of serum testosterone (T) and dihydrotestosterone (DHT) which lasts for 5–15 days and is accompanied in a significant proportion of cases by a flare-up of the prostatic cancer[39]. It is thus of great interest to see in Figure 1 that a marked decrease of serum PAP ($p < 0.01$) is already observed during the first 2–5 days

31

Table 1 Objective response observed following combined hormonal treatment with an LHRH agonist (or surgical castration) (LHRH-A) and a pure antiandrogen (Anti-A) in advanced prostatic cancer

Previous treatment (RX)	Months of RX M (Limits)	Current RX	No. of Patients			% Positive objective response*		
			Stage C	Stage D	Total	PAP	Bone scan	Total
Nil	6.5 (1–15)	LHRH-A + Anti-A	19	34	53	95 (39/41)	90 (18/20)	95 (39/41)
Nil	4.4 (2–9)	Castration + Anti-A	1	9	10	100 (8/8)	–	100 (8/8)
DES	6.5 (2–14)	LHRH-A + Anti-A	4	17	21	46 (6/13)	70 (7/10)	50 (8/16)
Castrated	6.4 (4–14)	Anti-A	2	12	14	12.5 (1/8)	37.5 (3/8)	30 (3/10)
Castrated and oestrogens	5.2 (2–9)	Anti-A	1	11	12	11 (1/9)	43 (3/7)	27 (3/11)

DES = Diethylstilboestrol.
*Numbers of subjects given in parentheses.
PAP = Prostatic Acid Phosphatase.

of treatment with the LHRH agonist, at a time when serum androgen levels are increased by 100–200% ($p < 0.01$) (Figure 2).

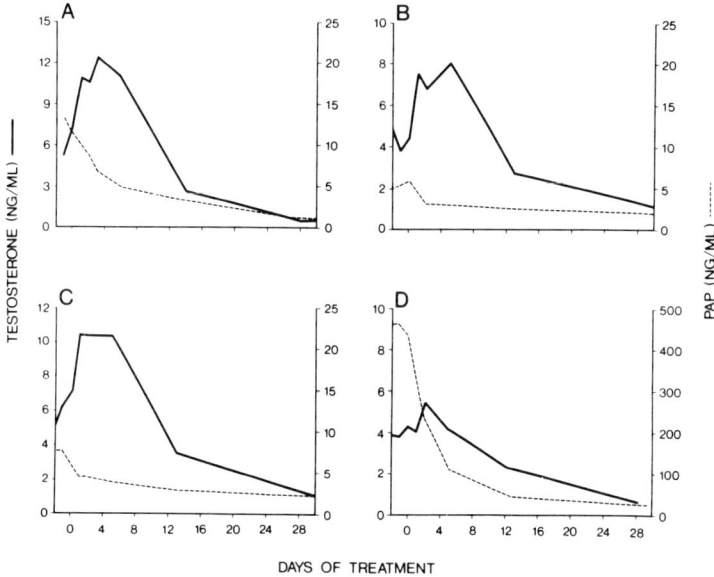

Figure 2 Changes of serum PAP and testosterone levels during the first month of treatment in four previously untreated patients having advanced prostatic cancer and receiving the combined treatment with the LHRH agonist HOE–766 and the pure antiandrogen RU 23908. Note the rapid and marked decrease in serum PAP in the presence of elevated serum T levels, thus indicating the efficiency of the antiandrogen at the dose used. Reproduced with permission from reference 27

Before treatment, except in patients treated with high doses of DES or castration, serum steroid values were within the normal range. Administration of HOE-766 in combination with RU 23908 led, after 2 months of treatment in previously untreated patients, to a decrease in testosterone, dehydroepiandrosterone sulphate and dehydroepian-drosterone levels to 2.5±0.03, 45±4.7 and 64±5% of control, respectively, while serum cortisol levels remained unchanged (Figure 3).

In the presence of a more than 95% inhibition of serum T and DHT levels, serum LH measured by RIA remains normal or is only slightly decreased. Since we had previously found a discrepancy between serum LH measured by RIA and bioassay in rhesus monkeys treated

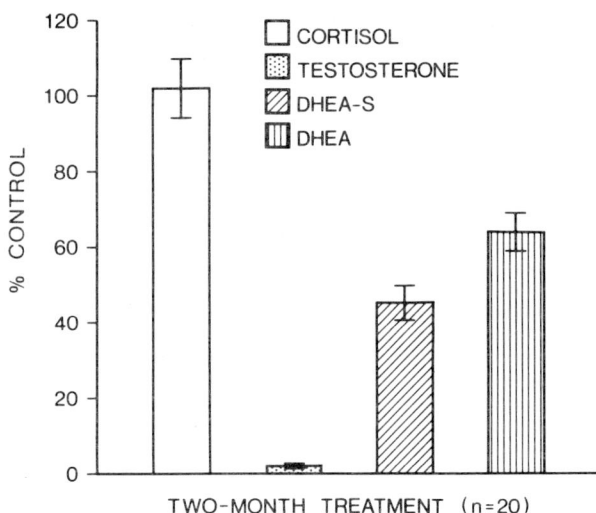

Figure 3 Effect of 2-month combined treatment with the LHRH agonist (HOE–766) and the antiandrogen RU 23908 on serum levels of cortisol (F), testosterone (T), dehydroepiandrosterone (DHEA) and dehydroepiandrosterone sulphate (DHEA-S) in 20 previously untreated patients having prostatic cancer. Mean ($\pm$SE) control levels of F, T, DHEA-S and DHEA were 156$\pm$6, 5.44$\pm$0.44, 834$\pm$147 and 1.9$\pm$0.3 ng ml^{-1} respectively. Reproduced with permission from reference 27

with a high dose of an LHRH agonist[24], we have performed a similar study in men. We found that while the values of serum LH measured by RIA and by bioassay (mouse Leydig cell assay) were parallel during the first 2 weeks of treatment, a progressive and marked loss of bioactivity was found at later time intervals. Thus, after 1 month of treatment, the LH bioactivity was reduced to approximately 5% of control while the radioimmunoassayable LH was reduced by only 40–50%[41] (Figure 4) (St-Arnaud *et al.*, unpublished observations). These data indicate that the loss of LH bioactivity, rather than testicular desensitization, is the major factor responsible for the almost complete inhibition of testicular steroidogenesis during chronic treatment with LHRH agonists in man.

Approximately 50% of patients receiving the combination therapy (LHRH agonist + antiandrogen or castration + antiandrogen) developed, to various degrees, climacteric-like vasomotor phenomena consisting of perspiration and hot flushes. Most patients complained of a decrease in libido and erectile potency after 2–3 weeks of treatment.

In six cases, libido and erectile potency were maintained despite complete androgen withdrawal. No other side-effects were observed which could not be related to hypoandrogenicity.

As revealed by a series of standard tests, treatment with the LHRH agonist and the antiandrogen had no detectable effect on any of the following parameters: complete (WBC, RBC, haemoglobin, haematocrit and platelets) and differential blood count, γ-glutamyl transaminase, glutamic oxaloacetic transaminase, glutamic pyruvic transaminase, lactic dehydrogenase, creatinine, total bilirubin and other parameters of blood biochemistry (SMA-12).

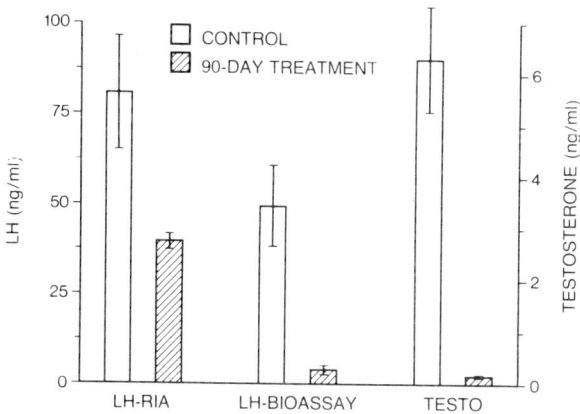

Figure 4   Effect of 1 months' treatment with the LHRH agonist Buserelin (500 μg daily, subcutaneously) and the pure antiandrogen RU 23908 (Anandron, 100 mg, three times daily, per os) on serum LH measured by RIA and by the mouse Leydig cell bioassay as well as on serum testosterone (TESTO) concentration in patients with advanced cancer of the prostate

Although they should still be considered as preliminary, the present data obtained in stages C and D prostate cancer suggest three highly consequent conclusions exclusively based on objective criteria:

(1)   Complete withdrawal of androgens achieved through the combined use of an LHRH agonist and an antiandrogen (or castration and an antiandrogen) causes a positive objective response in more than 95% of previously untreated patients. This percentage of positive objective response is clearly sup-

35

erior to the 60–70% objective and/or subjective response previously observed after partial withdrawal of androgens achieved by castration or the administration of high doses of oestrogens.

(2) A much lower rate of positive objective response (less than 50%) is observed in patients previously treated with oestrogens and receiving the same combination therapy. Administration of the antiandrogen to patients showing relapse after castration shows an even lower rate of positive response, at approximately 30%.

(3) The antiandrogen completely neutralizes the transient rise of circulating androgens which always accompanies the first days of treatment with the LHRH agonist. The antiandrogen thus completely eliminates the unacceptable and unethical flare-up of the disease previously observed in a significant proportion of patients treated with the LHRH agonist alone.

The aim of initial hormonal therapy in advanced prostate cancer during the last 40 years has been limited to the removal of testicular androgens. Standard approaches such as castration[42] and high doses of oestrogens leave a substantial amount (5–10%) of circulating androgens of adrenal origin[43,44]. Prostatic carcinomas are probably composed of an heterogeneous but androgen sensitive population of cells which differ in their requirement for androgens to perform vital cellular processes. The most androgen-dependent cells regress after partial androgen withdrawal such as achieved by castration or high doses of oestrogens, thus accounting for the 60–70% positive response previously reported. Complete withdrawal of androgens achieved with the present combined hormonal therapy does, however, cause regression in a much larger proportion of cases (up to at least 95%). Although adrenal androgens account for only 5–10% of total androgens under basal conditions, any increase of adrenocortical activity in response to various types of stress (pain, anxiety, concurrent disease) is likely to be accompanied by a parallel increase in the stimulatory action of adrenal androgens on the tumour.

References

1. Matsuo, H., Baba, Y., Nair, R. M. G., Arimura, A. and Schally, A. V. (1971). Structure of the porcine LH- and FSH-releasing hormone. I. The proposed amino acid sequence. *Biochem. Biophys. Res. Commun.*, **43**, 1334

2. Burgus, R., Butcher, M., Ling, N., et al. (1971). Structure moléculaire du facteur hypothalamique (LRF) d'origine ovine contrôlant la sécrétion de l'hormone gonadotrope hypophysaire. C. R. Acad. Sci. [D] (Paris), **273**, 1611

3. Schwartzstein, L. (1976). Diagnostic and therapeutic use of LHRH in the infertile man. In Labire, F., Meites, J. and Pelletier, G. (eds.). Hypothalamus and Endocrine Functions, pp. 73–91. (New York: Plenum Press)

4. Krabbe, S. and Shakkeback, N. E. (1977). Gonadotropin-releasing hormone (LHRH) and human chorionic gonadotropin in the treatment of two boys with hypogonadotrophic hypogonadism. Acta Paediatr. Scand., **66**, 361

5. Auclair, C., Kelly, P. A., Labrie, F., Coy, D. H. and Schally, A. V. (1977). Inhibition of testicular luteinizing hormone receptor levels by treatment with a potent luteinizing hormone-releasing hormone agonist or human chorionic gonadotropin. Biochem. Biophys. Res. Commun., **76**, 855

6. Auclair, C., Kelly, P. A., Coy, D. H., Schally, A. V. and Labrie, F. (1977). Potent inhibitory activity of [D-Leu[6], des-Gly-NH$_2$[10]]LHRH ethylamide on LH/hCG and PRL testicular receptor levels in the rat. Endocrinology, **101**, 1890

7. Labrie, F., Auclair, C., Cusan, L., Kelly, P. A., Pelletier, G. and Ferland, L. (1978). Inhibitory effects of LHRH and its agonists on testicular gonadotropin receptors and spermatogenesis in the rat. In Hansson, V. (ed.). Endocrine Approach to Male Contraception. Int. J. Androl. (Suppl.), **2**, 303

8. Labrie, F., Bélanger, A., Cusan, L., et al. (1980). Antifertility effects of LHRH agonists in the male. J. Androl., **1**, 209

9. Pelletier, G., Cusan, L., Auclair, C., Kelly, P. A., Désy, L. and Labrie, F. (1978). Inhibition of spermatogenesis in the rat by treatment with [D-Ala[6], des-Gly-NH$_2$[10]]LHRH ethylamide. Endocrinology, **103**, 641

10. Sandow, J., Von Rechenberg, W. V., Konig, W., Hahn, M., Jerzabek, G. and Fraser, H. (1978). Physiological studies with highly active analogue of LHRH. In Gupta, D. and Voelter, W. (eds.). Hypothalamic Hormones – Chemistry, Physiology and Clinical Applications, pp. 307–326. (Berlin: Verlag Chemie)

11. Tcholakian, R. K., De la Cruz, A., Chowdhury, M., Steinberger, A., Coy, D. H. and Schally, A. V. (1978). Unusual anti-reproductive properties of the analog [D-Leu[6], des-Gly-NH$_2$[10]]LHRH ethylamide in male rats. Fertil. Steril., **30**, 600

12. Rivier, C., Rivier, J. and Vale, W. (1979). Chronic effects of [D-Trp[6], Pro[9], NEt]LHRH on reproductive processes in the male rat. Endocrinology, **105**, 1191

13. Cusan, L., Auclair, C., Bélanger, A., et al. (1979). Inhibitory effects of long-term treatment with an LHRH agonist on the pituitary–gonadal axis in male and female rats. Endocrinology, **104**, 1369

14. Arimura, A., Serafini, P., Talbot, S. and Schally, A. V. (1979). Reduction of testicular luteinizing hormone/human chorionic gonadotropin receptors by [D-Trp[6]]luteinizing hormone-releasing hormone in hypophysectomized rats. Biochem. Biophys. Res. Commun., **90**, 687

15. Catt, K. J., Baukal, A. J., Davies, T. F. and Dufau, M. L. (1979). Luteinizing hormone-releasing hormone-induced regulation of gonadotropin and prolactin receptors in the rat testis. Endocrinology, **104**, 17

16. Bélanger, A., Auclair, C., Ferland, L., Caron, S. and Labrie, F. (1980). Time-course of the effect of treatment with a potent LHRH agonist on testicular steroidogenesis and gonadotropin receptor levels in the adult rat. J. Steroid Biochem., **13**, 191

17. Bélanger, A., Cusan, L., Auclair, C., Séguin, C., Caron, S. and Labrie, F. (1980). Effect of an LHRH agonist and hCG on testicular steroidogenesis in the adult rat. Biol. Reprod., **22**, 1094

18. Hsueh, A. J. W. and Erickson, G. F. (1979). Extrapituitary inhibition of testicular function by luteinizing hormone-releasing hormone. Nature (Lond.), **281**, 66

19. Lefebvre, F. A., Reeves, J. J., Séguin, C., Massicotte, J. and Labrie, F. (1980). Specific binding of a potent LHRH agonist in rat testis. *Mol. Cell. Endocrinol.*, **20**, 127

20. Perrin, N. H., Vaughan, J. M., Rivier, J. E. and Vale, W. W. (1980). High affinity GnRH binding to testicular membrane homogenates. *Life Sci.*, **26**, 2251

21. Séguin, C., Bélanger, A., Cusan, L., *et al.* (1981). Relative importance of the adenohypophyseal and gonadal sites of inhibitory action of LHRH agonists. *Biol. Reprod.*, **24**, 889

22. Séguin, C., Bélanger, A., Labrie, F. and Hansel, W. (1982). Study of the direct action of luteinizing hormone-releasing hormone agonists at the testicular level in intact rats treated with an antiluteinizing hormone serum. *Endocrinology*, **110**, 524

23. Sandow, J. and Hahn, M. (1978). Chronic treatment with LHRH in golden hamsters. *Acta Endocrinol.*, **88**, 601

24. Resko, J., Bélanger, A. and Labrie, F. (1982). Effects of chronic treatment with a potent LHRH agonist on serum LH and steroid levels in the male rhesus monkey. *Biol. Reprod.*, **26**, 378

25. Bélanger, A., Labrie, F., Lemay, A., Caron, S. and Raynaud, J. P. (1980). Inhibitory effects of a single intranasal administration of [D-ser(TBU)6, des-Gly-NH2^10]LHRH ethylamide on serum steroid levels in normal adult men. *J. Steroid Biochem.*, **13**, 113

26. Labrie, F., Dupont, A., Bélanger, A., *et al.* (1982). New hormonal therapy in prostatic carcinoma: combined treatment with an LHRH agonist and an antiandrogen. *J. Clin. Invest. Med.*, **5**, 267

27. Labrie, F., Dupont, A., Bélanger, A., *et al.* (1983). New approach in the treatment of prostate cancer: complete instead of only partial withdrawal of androgens. *Prostate* (In press)

28. Faure, N., Labrie, F., Lemay, A., *et al.* (1982). Inhibition of serum androgen levels by chronic intranasal and subcutaneous administration of a potent luteinizing hormone-releasing hormone (LH-RH) agonist in adult men. *Fertil. Steril.*, **37**, 416

29. Tolis, G., Ackman, D., Stellos, A., *et al.* (1982). Tumor growth inhibition in patients with prostatic carcinoma treated with agonists of LHRH. *Proc. Natl. Acad. Sci. USA*, **79**, 1658

30. Crowley, W. F., Jr., Comite, F., Vale, W., Rivier, J., Loriaux, D. L. and Cutler, G. B., Jr. (1981). Therapeutic use of pituitary desensitization with a long-acting LHRH agonist: a potential new treatment for idiopathic precocious puberty. *J. Clin. Endocrinol.*, **52**, 370

31. Carmichael, R., Bélanger, A., Cusan, L, Séguin, C., Caron, S. and Labrie, F. (1980). Increased testicular 5α-androstane-3α, 17β-diol formation induced by treatment with [D-Ser(TBU)6, des-Gly-NH2^10]LHRH ethylamide in the rat. *Steroids*, **36**, 383

32. Linde, R., Doelle, G., Alexander, N., *et al.* (1981). Reversible inhibition of testicular steroidogenesis and spermatogenesis by a potent gonadotropin-releasing hormone agonist in normal men. *N. Engl. J. Med.*, **305**, 663

33. National Coordinating Group on Male Antifertility Agents (1978). Gossypol – a new antifertility agent for males. *Clin. Med. J. (Engl.)*, **4**, 417

34. Djerasi, C. (1980). The politics of contraception. In Norton, W. W. (ed.). pp. 183–213. (New York)

35. Schearer, S. B., Alvarez-Sanchez, F., Anselmo, J., *et al.* (1978). Hormonal contraception for men. *Int. J. Androl. Suppl.*, **2**, 680

36. Lee, H. Y., Kim, S. I. and Kwon, E. H. (1979). Clinical trial of reversible male contraception with long-acting sex hormones. *Scand. J. Med.*, **20**, 1

37. Huggins, C. and Hodges, C. V. (1941). Studies of prostatic cancer. I. Effect of castration, estrogen and androgen injections on serum phosphatases in metastatic carcinoma of the prostate. *Cancer Res.*, **1**, 293

38. Bailer, J. C., Byar, D. P. and Veterans Administration Cooperative Urology Research Group (1970). Estrogen treatment for cancer of the prostate. *Cancer*, **26**, 257

39. Glode, L. M. (Abbott Prostatic Cancer Study) (1982). Leuprolide therapy of advanced prostatic cancer. *ASCO Proceedings*, Abstract, p. 110

40. Lefebvre, F. A., Séguin, C., Bélanger, A. *et al.* (1982). Combined long-term treatment with an LHRH agonist and a pure antiandrogen blocks androgenic influence in the rat. *Prostate*, **3**, 569

41. Kelly, S., Labrie, F. and Dupont, A. (1983). Loss of LH bioactivity in men treated with an LHRH agonist and an antiandrogen. *Proceedings of the 65th Annual Meeting of the Endocrinology Society*, p. 81

42. Sanford, E. J., Paulson, D. F., Rohner, T. J., *et al.* (1977). The effects of castration on adrenal testosterone secretion in men with prostatic carcinoma. *J. Urol.*, **118,** 1019

43. Bhanalaph, T., Varkarakis, M. J. and Murphy, G. P. (1974). Current status of bilateral adrenalectomy of advanced prostatic carcinoma. *Ann. Surg.*, **179,** 17

44. Geller, J., Albert, J., Loza, D., Geller, S., Stoeltzing, W. and De La Vega, D. (1978). DHT concentrations in human prostate cancer tissue. *J. Clin. Endocrinol. Metab.*, **46,** 440

3
Reproductive releasing hormones – the future

J. SANDOW

In the treatment of reproductive disorders, gonadotrophin preparations and steroid hormones have traditionally had an important role.
More recently, the therapeutic potential of synthetic hypothalamic
hormone analogues has been established in reproductive and non-
reproductive disorders. Due to the complexity of hypothalamic–pituitary–gonadal interactions, the transition from physiology
and pharmacology to clinical medicine has sometimes been difficult,
but a review of the current results indicates that we can look forward
to the future with confidence. The development of potent peptide
hormone analogues, new biomedical devices for pulsatile administration and sustained delivery, and sophisticated experimental methods
for the evaluation of hypothalamic–pituitary–gonadal function have
all contributed to a rapid application of the experimental concepts to
clinical reality.

PHYSIOLOGICAL REGULATION OF GONADOTROPHIN SECRETION

Hypothalamic secretory activity is indispensable for pituitary activation. Elucidation and synthesis of luteinizing hormone-releasing
hormone (LHRH, GnRH) in 1971 by the group of Schally[1] initiated a
fruitful development of physiological and clinical research. Reproductive releasing hormones now comprise synthetic LHRH used in a

41

variety of stimulatory applications, LHRH agonists explored in several promising clinical indications[2-4], and antagonist analogues under intense pharmacological investigation[1,5-8]. Both groups of LHRH-derived peptides have been eminently useful in the investigation of physiological problems related to pituitary activation. Pituitary function is sequentially activated by LHRH, at low frequency with regard to FSH during puberty, and at higher frequency for subsequent LH secretion. Pituitary secretion is frequency modulated by LHRH, with an additional amplitude modulation by gonadal steroids. The variable frequency and amplitude of LH pulses observed during the menstrual cycle is due to steroid conditioning in the presence of an unvarying LHRH pulsatility[9]. Active immunization against LHRH abolishes FSH and LH pulses, and passive transfer of an LHRH antiserum rapidly suppresses LH pulsatility[10]. *In vitro*, pulsatile pituitary activation can be demonstrated on dispersed pituitary cells suspended in suitable columns for superfusion experiments[11,12]. Regular LH pulses are elicited by short-lasting LHRH pulses, and desensitization is observed after continuous LHRH infusion or after agonist stimulation. Desensitization may have important therapeutic and pathophysiological implications.

PITUITARY DESENSITIZATION

Continuous exposure to a stimulatory concentration of LHRH reduces pituitary responsiveness, e.g. in the absence of gonadal steroids in postmenopausal women or women with premature ovarian failure. The direct inhibitory effect on responsiveness may be maintained for extended time periods, and is associated with a gradual decrease in LHRH receptors[13]. Under pathological conditions, increased plasma LHRH may block pituitary–gonadal function in patients with renal failure (due to the reduced inactivation and excretion rate), and in Klinefelter's syndrome because of progressive gonadal failure.

LHRH agonists rapidly induce pituitary desensitization when infused subcutaneously from osmotic minipumps[13-15], or by sustained release from suitable implant materials[16]. Desensitization is a dose-dependent phenomenon; it is transiently overcome by injection of a high stimulatory dose. During long-term infusion, agonists and antagonists have similar effects although operating through entirely different mechanisms. Whereas agonists induce desensitization *via* an initial short-lasting stimulation phase, the antagonists immediately block pituitary secretion by neutralizing the effect of endogenous or exogenous LHRH. Pituitary inhibition by continuous stimulation has been compared to a 'chemical hypophysectomy'. There is, however, an important difference to hypophysectomy, because the extent of gonadotrophin suppression can be adjusted by the intensity of the permanent stimulus.

During agonist infusions, a basal secretion rate of FSH and LH is preserved, even though the pituitary becomes refractory to endogenous LHRH stimulation. Hypothalamic secretory activity is not reduced by pituitary suppression. There is no change in hypothalamic LHRH content, and the urinary excretion of LHRH metabolites also does not decrease during prolonged agonist suppression in rats. Shortly after the end of a suppressive infusion, spontaneous pituitary and gonadal function are resumed. It is this inherent reversibility that makes treatment by sustained-release preparations of LHRH agonists clinically attractive.

Pituitary desensitization by LHRH antagonists is also highly effective, in particular because these peptides are highly resistant to degradation. The extent of suppression can be adjusted; at low doses FSH secretion is maintained in primates, whereas high doses reduce both FSH and LH secretion[5].

INHIBITION OF GONADAL STEROID SECRETION

High doses of agonist cause a transient deficiency in gonadotrophin utilization by a temporary loss of receptors (down-regulation). Numerous studies on gonadotrophin stimulation of ovarian/testicular function and on supraphysiological LHRH stimulation have confirmed the transient decrease of gonadotrophin receptors associated with qualitative changes in steroid biosynthesis[14]. These regulatory events are initiated by excessive LH stimulation. The extent of down-regulation of LH and FSH receptors depends on the initial quantum of LH released; it is associated with a concomitant decrease in prolactin receptors. Many of the currently investigated regimens for the treatment of hormone-dependent tumours (prostate and mammary carcinoma), endometriosis and precocious puberty depend on high-dose injections of agonists, to achieve maximal gonadotrophin receptor down-regulation. The ensuing block in steroid secretion has been described as a 'chemical castration', with gonadal steroids decreasing to post-gonadectomy levels. Once gonadal receptor inhibition has been achieved, smaller maintenance doses are sufficient for long-term reduction of gonadal steroid production. However, daily stimulation of the pituitary is essential to maintain suppression: infrequent injections every second or third day fail to achieve the same result[17]. The quantitative changes in androgen biosynthesis consist of a block in 17α-hydroxylase and 17,20-desmolase, with preferential accumulation of C21-androgen precursors of low androgenic activity.

DIFFERENTIAL SUPPRESSION OF FSH- AND LH SECRETION

There are marked species differences in the response of FSH and LH secretion to agonist suppression. In general, after daily injections LH release is more readily desensitized than FSH release. This is of particular relevance for endometriosis, where only a lasting reduction in serum FSH levels will result in arrest of follicular maturation with sufficiently low oestradiol secretion to ensure involution of the endometriosis lesions. Whereas FSH secretion is maintained to a significant extent during daily agonist injections, infusions are highly effective to reduce plasma oestradiol and induce endometrial atrophy. Antagonists may be of particular importance in achieving reduced FSH levels for prolonged time periods.

CLINICAL POTENTIAL OF LHRH AGONISTS

There are significant advantages in the use of peptide analogues for therapy. The hormonal effect on gonadotrophin release is highly specific, and all preclinical safety studies indicate an exceptionally favourable biological tolerance. During long-term administration, the inhibitory effects on gonadotrophins and gonadal steroids are specific, and other hormone systems are not affected[14]. There are also no side-effects on organ systems in general pharmacology. Metabolic inactivation of LHRH agonists is rapid, they are degraded by endo- and exopeptidases in liver and kidney, and the resulting peptide fragments are biologically inactive. The endocrine suppressive effects are rapidly reversible at the end of a treatment period, and long-term studies in primates have shown a selective inhibition of reproductive function[18].

A major problem for the long-term use of agonists and antagonists is the mode of administration. In the initial phase of therapy, high dose injections or infusions are required. Subsequently, self-administration by a nasal spray or vaginal suppository has been successfully used, but the effective doses are limited due to a lower rate of absorption. For nasal spray administration, the rate of absorption is 2.5% as compared with subcutaneous or intravenous injection. Oral activity is negligible, but may be better for antagonists. Long-term therapy would be facilitated by injectable sustained release formulations, or peptide implants. Preliminary reports on two agonists, D-Ser (Bu^t)[6], AzGly[10] (ICI 118,630) and [D-(naphthyl-2)Ala[6]] LHRH (nafarelin)[16] are encouraging. For monitoring of therapy, sensitive pharmacokinetic methods for the plasma level of agonists have been developed[19].

The therapeutic objective in all clinical indications is a transient or long-lasting suppression of gonadal steroid secretion. Different dose ranges and regimens have been investigated. With low suppressive doses, a reliable contraceptive effect can be obtained by an agonist administered daily throughout the follicular phase, to inhibit ovulation. During long-term inhibition with a nasal spray of D-Ser(Bu^t)[6]LHRH(1-9)nonapeptide-ethylamid (buserelin), different responses of plasma oestradiol and endometrial histology were observed[20]. The wide range of individual reactions was due to variable oestradiol secretion, and to the absence of luteal progesterone increases. To obtain a regular bleeding pattern, a cyclic contraceptive regimen was investigated, similarly to sequential steroid preparations[21]. During the first phase of the contraceptive cycle, the agonist is administered by nasal spray for 21 days. During the third week, an orally active progestagen is added to obtain secretory transformation of the endometrium. A more physiological transformation is achieved by administering the progestagen at lower doses for 7 days. This contraceptive regimen eliminates the problem of unopposed oestradiol secretion, and is in agreement with studies on progestagen substitution in postmenopausal women[22]. One advantage of using an agonist for inhibition of ovulation is a rapid reversibility of the contraceptive effect. The method is suitable in adolescence and in women at risk for oral contraceptives containing an oestrogen component.

The luteolytic activity of agonists has been confirmed in the human, but there are practical difficulties for a contraceptive, because the corpus luteum of early pregnancy is protected by chorionic gonadotrophin (hCG) from the luteolytic effect of agonists[2,23,24]. Currently, contraceptive regimens are being investigated that rely on suppression of FSH secretion during the early follicular phase to induce a deficiency in follicular maturation resulting in an inadequate luteal phase[2].

Suppression of ovarian function by high-dose agonist therapy may be a suitable approach to the temporary block of oestrogen secretion required for treatment of endometriosis[25]. At present, endometriosis is treated with steroidal compounds, prescribed at effective doses causing amenorrhoea. The therapeutic effect is associated with signs of oestrogen deficiency, and a characteristic symptom of full suppression are hot flushes as a symptom of pseudomenopause. A similar effect can be obtained with LHRH agonists at high doses. Suppression is fully reversible, but a clinically acceptable treatment may require sustained-release preparations. Endometriosis is a frequent cause of infertility[26], and a reversible suppression of ovarian function without general side-effects would be a major advance in its treatment.

A complex situation is found in hormone-dependent tumours. Suppression of testosterone secretion by daily agonist administration is effective in prostate cancer[27,28], but in oestrogen-responsive mammary carcinoma it would be necessary to suppress oestrogen secretion completely[29]. The therapeutic effect in this indication again depends on effective FSH suppression and may require sustained-release preparations of an agonist together with an antioestrogen to neutralize intermittent steroid increases as well as adrenal oestrogen production.

THERAPEUTIC POTENTIAL OF ANTAGONISTS

The absence of an initial stimulatory phase during pituitary suppression by antagonists warrants a more detailed investigation of their application. With enzyme-resistant highly active antagonists, the treatment intervals could be extended or sustained-release formulations could be developed. The extent of differential FSH and LH suppression can be adjusted by selecting an appropriate dose range[5], and preliminary clinical experience is encouraging[30]. In a rat prostate tumour model, recent studies with an antagonist have confirmed the effectiveness[6]. In rodent studies, both male and female reproductive function can be inhibited[7,8]. Clinical acceptance will depend on a suitable mode of administration by sustained-release preparations, or by orally active antagonists.

References

1. Schally, A. V., Arimura, A. and Coy, D. H. (1981). Recent approaches to fertility control based on derivatives of LH-RH. *Vitam. Horm.*, **38**, 257
2. Yen, S. S. C. (1983). Clinical applications of gonadotropin-releasing hormone and gonadotropin-releasing hormone analogs. *Fertil. Steril.*, **39**, 257
3. Swerdloff, R. S. and Heber, D. (1983). Superactive gonadotropin-releasing hormone agonists. *Ann. Rev. Med.*, **34**, 491
4. Sandow, J. (1983). Clinical applications of LHRH and its analogues. *Clin. Endocrinol.*, **18**, 571
5. Pineda, J. L., Lee, B. C., Spiliotis, B.E., *et al.* (1983). Effect of GnRH antagonist (Ac-delta³Pro¹,pFDPhe²,DTrp³,⁶)GnRH, on pulsatile gonadotropin secretion in the castrate male primate. *J. Clin. Endocrinol. Metab.*, **56**, 420
6. Redding, T. W., Coy, D. H. and Schally, A. V. (1982). Prostate carcinoma tumor size in rats decreases after administration of antagonists of luteinizing hormone-releasing hormone. *Proc. Natl. Acad. Sci. USA*, **79**, 1273
7. Rivier, C., Rivier, J. and Vale, W. (1979). Effect of the LRF-antagonist (D-pGlu¹,D-Phe²,D-Trp³,⁶)-LRF on pregnancy in the rat. *Contraception*, **19**, 185
8. Rivier, C., Rivier, J. and Vale, W. (1981). Antireproductive effects of a potent GnRH antagonist in the female rat. *Endocrinology*, **108**, 1425
9. Knobil, E. (1980). The neuroendocrine control of the menstrual cycle. *Recent Prog. Horm. Res.*, **36**, 53
10. Fraser, H. M., Sharpe, R. M., Lincoln, G. A. and Harmer, A. J. (1982). LHRH antibodies: Their use in the study of hypothalamic LHRH and testicular LHRH-like material, and possible contraceptive applications. In Jeffcoate, S. L. and Sandler, M. (eds.). *Progress Towards a Male Contraceptive*, pp. 41–78. (London: John Wiley and Sons)
11. Badger, T. M., Loughlin, J. S. and Naddaff, P. G. (1983). The luteinizing hormone-releasing hormone (LHRH)-desensitized rat pituitary: luteinizing hormone responsiveness to LHRH *in vitro*. *Endocrinology*, **112**, 793
12. Yeo, T., Grossman, A., Belchetz, P. and Besser, G. M. (1982). Response of luteinizing hormone from columns of dispersed rat pituitary cells to a highly potent analogue of luteinizing hormone releasing hormone. *J. Endocrinol.*, **91**, 33
13. Clayton, R. N. and Catt, K. J. (1981). Gonadotropin-releasing hormone receptors: characterization, physiological regulation, and relationship to reproductive function. *Endocrinol. Rev.*, **2**, 186
14. Sandow, J. (1982). Gonadotropic and antigonadotropic actions of LH-RH analogues. In Müller, E. E. and McLeod, R. M. (eds.). *Neuroendocrine Perspectives*. Vol. **1**, pp. 339–95. (Amsterdam: Elsevier Biomedical Press)
15. Bint Akhtar, F., Marshall, G. R., Wickings, J. and Nieschlag, E. (1983). Reversible induction of azoospermia in rhesus monkeys by constant infusion of a gonadotropin-releasing hormone agonist using osmotic minipumps. *J. Clin. Endocrinol. Metab.*, **56**, 534
16. Vickery, B. H. (1981). Physiology and antifertility effects of LHRH and agonistic analogs in male animals. In Zatuchni, G. I., Shelton, J. D. and Sciarra, J. J. (eds.). *LHRH Peptides as Female and Male Contraceptives*, pp. 275–90. (Philadelphia: Harper & Row)
17. Sandow, J. (1982). Inhibition of pituitary and testicular function by LHRH and analogues. In Jeffcoate, S. L. and Sandler, M. (eds.). *Progress Towards a Male Contraceptive*, pp. 19–39. (London: John Wiley and Sons)
18. Fraser, H. M. (1983). Effect of treatment for 1 year with a luteinizing hormone-releasing hormone agonist on ovarian, thyroidal, and adrenal function and menstruation in the stumptailed monkey (*Macaca arctoides*). *Endocrinology*, **112**, 245

19. Sandow, J., Jerabek-Sandow, G., Krauss, B. and Stoll, W. (1982). Metabolic and dispositional studies with LHRH analogs. In Zatuchni, G. I., Shelton, J. D. and Sciarra, J. J. (eds.). *LHRH Peptides as Female and Male Contraceptives*, pp. 321–36. (Philadelphia: Harper & Row)

20. Schmidt-Gollwitzer, M., Hardt, W., Schmidt-Gollwitzer, K. and von der Ohe, M. (1982). The contraceptive use of Buserelin, a potent LH-RH agonist: clinical and hormonal findings. In Zatuchni, G. I., Shelton, J. D. and Sciarra, J. J. (eds.). *LHRH Peptides as Female and Male Contraceptives*, pp. 199–215 (Philadelphia: Harper & Row)

21. Hardt, W., Schmidt-Gollwitzer, K., Nevinny-Stickel, J. and Schmidt-Gollwitzer, M. (1982). Fortschritte in der kontrazeptiven Anwendung des LHRH Agonisten Buserelin: Diskontinuierliche Medikation mit gestageninduzierter Abbruchblutung (Progress in contraceptive application of the LHRH agonist, buserelin: discontinuous medication with progestogen-induced withdrawal bleeding). *Gesburtsch. Frauenheilk.*, **42**, 874

22. Flowers, C. E., Wilborn, W. H. and Hyde, B. M. (1983). Mechanisms of uterine bleeding in postmenopausal patients receiving estrogen alone or with a progestin. *Obstet. Gynecol.*, **61**, 135

23. Casper, R. F., Sheehan, K. L. and Yen, S. S. C. (1980). Chorionic gonadotropin prevents LRF agonist-induced luteolysis in the human. *Contraception*, **21**, 471

24. Bergquist, C., Nillius, S. J. and Wide, L. (1980). Luteolysis induced by a luteinizing hormone-releasing hormone agonist is prevented by human chorionic gonadotropin. *Contraception*, **22**, 341

25. Meldrum, D. R., Chang, R. J., Lu, J., Vale, W., Rivier, J. and Judd, H. L. (1982). 'Medical oophorectomy' using a longacting GnRH agonist – a possible new approach to the treatment of endometriosis. *J. Clin. Endocrinol. Metab.*, **54**, 1081

26. Strathy, J. H., Molgaard, C. A., Coulam, C. B. and Melton, L. J. (1982). Endometriosis and infertility: a laparascopic study of endometriosis among fertile and infertile women. *Fertil. Steril.*, **38**, 667

27. Tolis, G., Ackermann, D., Stellos, A., *et al.* (1982). Tumor growth inhibition in patients with prostatic carcinoma treated with luteinizing hormone-releasing hormone agonists. *Proc. Natl. Acad. Sci. USA*, **79**, 1658

28. Borgmann, V., Hardt, W., Schmidt-Gollwitzer, M., Adenauer, H. and Nagel, R. (1982). Sustained suppression of testosterone production by the luteinizing hormone-releasing hormone agonist Buserelin in patients with advanced prostate carcinoma: a new therapeutic approach? *Lancet*, **1**, 1097

29. Klijn, J. G. M. and DeJong, F. H. (1982). Treatment with a luteinizing hormone-releasing hormone analogue (Buserelin) in pre-menopausal patients with metastatic breast cancer. *Lancet*, **1**, 1213

30. Cetel, N. S., Rivier, J., Vale, W. and Yen, S. S. C. (1983). The dynamics of gonadotropin inhibition in women induced by an antagonistic analogue of GnRH. *J. Clin. Endocrinol. Metab.* (In press)

Part I

Section 2

Prediction and Detection of Ovulation

4
The physiological basis of the fertile period

H. G. BURGER

INTRODUCTION AND DEFINITIONS

Definition of the fertile phase of the menstrual cycle is based on the probability that coitus during that period will result in pregnancy, or, alternatively, that coitus outside that period is very unlikely to be fertile. The most significant determinant of the location of the fertile phase within the cycle is the timing of ovulation[1]: because of the limited fertilizable life-span of the ovum, the fertile period ends shortly after ovulation, but begins a variable number of days before that event, depending on the fertilizing life-span of the spermatozoa. Ovarian oestradiol-17β (E_2) is the physiological basis of the onset and duration of the fertile period: it plays a central role in follicular development and oocyte maturation, is involved in ovum transport, and is responsible for endometrial proliferation and preparation for implantation, stimulation of the cervical mucus glands to secrete a fluid favourable to sperm survival and transport, and facilitation of the mid-cycle surge of luteinizing hormone (LH) which precipitates ovulation. It may enhance female receptivity to the male. The central role of E_2 is reflected in the extensive use that is made of oestrogen assays, and of observations of oestrogen-induced phenomena in the clinical delineation of the fertile period. The intervals between fertile periods are determined by corpus luteum function and by breast feeding.

OESTRADIOL AND FOLLICULAR DEVELOPMENT

Oestradiol enhances ovarian follicular responsiveness to pituitary gonadotrophins and is an important intra-ovarian regulator of follicular development. Evidence in the rat indicates that, although oestrogen enhances ovarian uptake of follicle stimulating hormone (FSH), this effect is not on the number of FSH receptors per granulosa cell, but on the total cell number[2]. Enhancement of granulosa cell responsiveness to FSH by oestrogen is a post-receptor phenomenon, and results in enhanced aromatase activity (with the further production of E_2, a form of positive feedback), as well as in the induction of LH receptors on the granulosa cell surface[2]. Increased secretion of E_2 from the ovary destined to be the site of ovulation is demonstrable in the rhesus monkey menstrual cycle 5–7 days before the mid-cycle gonadotrophin surge[3], and is a marker of the presence of the dominant follicle. The onset of asymmetrical E_2 production corresponds to the initiation of the progressive increase of E_2 secretion which characterizes the second half of the follicular phase of the menstrual cycle.

Evidence for the important intrafollicular role of E_2 also comes from the measurement of follicular fluid concentrations during laparoscopic oocyte collection and follicular fluid aspiration for the purposes of *in vitro* fertilization and embryo transfer (IVF and ET). We have found that E_2 levels were significantly higher in follicles giving rise to oocytes which were successfully fertilized and transferred than those in whom these procedures were unsuccessful[4].

Oestradiol and the endometrium

During the follicular phase of the cycle, cell division in the glands and stroma of the endometrium results from E_2 stimulation. The mechanisms are typical of those involved in steroid hormone effects on target cells, with diffusion of free E_2 into the cytoplasm, binding to the E_2 receptor, and translocation of the complex to the nucleus where it binds to DNA. Gene transcription is subsequently modulated, resulting in the synthesis of proteins which express the endpoints characteristic of oestrogen action. Although the human endometrial E_2 receptor has not been characterized fully, the calf uterine receptor has been shown to be a single polypeptide chain, of molecular weight 70 000 daltons, with high affinity (Kd 0.1 nmol l^{-1}) for E_2, and much lower affinities for oestrone and oestriol[5]. The total cell content of the receptors is high during the proliferative phase $(2.0 \, pmol \, (mg \, DNA)^{-1})$, and at mid-cycle the number of nuclear receptors doubles, from 0.4 to $0.9 \, pmol \, (mg \, DNA)^{-1}$, as a result of nuclear translocation from the cytoplasm[6]. At ovulation, it is estimated that there are about 8000 E_2 receptors per endometrial cell. Levels fall during the luteal phase. One of the proteins synthesized under the influence of E_2 is the endometrial progesterone receptor, which appears early in the follicular phase, long before the establishment of progesterone secretion by the corpus luteum. There is a preovulatory increase of these receptors to a concentration of about $3.0 \, pmol \, (mg \, DNA)^{-1}$, with about 12000 progesterone receptors per cell at mid-cycle. Peak levels are reached during the mid-luteal phase. These changes in endometrial receptors are consistent with the essential role of E_2 in preparing the endometrium for implantation and of progesterone in early pregnancy maintenence.

OESTRADIOL AND THE CERVIX

The other uterine target of oestrogen action is the cervical mucosa, responsible for mucus secretion. Based on a variety of techniques, three types of mucus are recognizable: G, L and S[7]. G-type mucus is secreted during the luteal phase and is thick, opaque and not receptive to sperm. L-type mucus consists of elliptical 'loafs' of a viscid gell, $0.3 \times 1 \times 3 \, mm$ in size, while S mucus consists of strings of a fluid gell, $100 \, \mu m$ in diameter and 2–3 cm long. Under the influence of rising E_2 concentrations, and in the absence of progesterone, G-type mucus disappears and L-type mucus is produced to reach a peak about 2 days before ovulation; its secretion then falls, while S-type mucus appears to reach its maximum on the day after ovulation, at a time when G-type mucus production has also begun to rise under the influence of progesterone. The ovulatory mucus is a mosaic of mucus strings and loafs, the S material making up 30% and the L 70%. The S mucus flows between the loafs orienting the mucin molecules to form long, thin aggregates, separated by the low-viscosity aqueous phase which permits rapid sperm transit, some passing directly into the uterus, others being conveyed to the S-secreting crypts from which they are released with an estimated half life of 15 hours. The loafs may capture low-quality sperm, allowing their expulsion from the cervix by bulk flow. The physical changes in mucus can be observed readily at the lower end of the vagina by the majority of women, allowing self-detection of the fertile period[8].

OESTRADIOL AND OVULATION

The major event leading to ovulation is the mid-cycle surge of LH, and it has been well established that the primary determinant of the cyclic pattern of gonadotrophin secretion is E_2[9]. The interrelationships of the ovary, hypothalamus and pituitary, resulting in the LH surge and ovulation, have been comprehensively reviewed[10]. Increasing E_2 secretion from the dominant follicle, commencing at about cycle day 7, leads to plasma levels sufficient to trigger the LH surge. In the human female, E_2 levels must exceed a threshold of about $600\,pmol\,l^{-1}$ and must be maintained for up to 50 hours to be effective. Study of circulating E_2 concentrations during cycles in which conception occurred indicated that such levels are attained for at least 3 days at mid-cycle[11].

Such rising E_2 levels lead to increased pituitary sensitivity to exogenously administered gonadotrophin-releasing hormone (GnRH or LHRH), an effect which can be demonstrated *in vitro* in dispersed, cultured pituitary cells[12], and which may therefore be mediated directly at the pituitary level, where E_2 receptors are demonstrable in the gonadotroph. One mechanism may involve an E_2 induced increase in the number of LHRH receptors.

Endogenous LHRH is synthesized and secreted by neurosecretory neurones which are widely distributed in the hypothalamus, though those located in the arcuate nucleus in the medial basal hypothalamus are specifically involved in the control of gonadotrophin secretion. The episodic pattern of peripheral LH levels, with pulses every 60–90 minutes during the follicular phase, and every 3–4 hours during the luteal phase of the cycle, has been presumed to reflect pulsatile secretion of LHRH. The development of a technique that allows simultaneous frequent blood sampling from the hypophyseal portal vessels and from the jugular vein in conscious, resting ovariectomized ewes has now provided direct evidence that pulses of LHRH in portal blood are followed by pulses of LH in peripheral blood, and that, in general, every pulse of LH is preceded by a pulse of LHRH[13]. The technique promises to provide a means of examining critically the site(s) of action of feedback factors, brain peptides and neurotransmitters that influence gonadotrophin secretion. An unresolved question is whether an increase in LHRH secretion (manifested as an increase in pulse amplitude and/or frequency) occurs under physiological circumstances to cause the LH surge, and whether such an increase represents an effect of E_2 at the hypothalamic level. Recent experience in my laboratory with subcutaneous pulsatile administration of LHRH to anovulatory women with hypothalamic amenorrhoea has shown that ovulation and pregnancy can occur despite an unvarying frequency of administration of a constant dose of LHRH (5–10 μg every 90 minutes), which leads to patterns of urinary excretion of oestrogen and pregnanediol characteristic of normal ovulatory cycles. These observations confirm results of pulsatile LHRH administration to rhesus monkeys with arcuate nucleus lesions[14], in which normal ovulatory menstrual cycles can be induced. Such experiments suggest that LHRH plays a permissive role, and that the mid-cycle surge of LH can be induced at the pituitary level, provided that there is LHRH input of appropriate frequency and amplitude, which may in turn be determined by E_2 in the absence of progesterone. A further aspect of the mid-cycle surge is the possibility that there may be a change in the properties of the secreted LH, with the production of a molecule with increased biological activity[15].

Periovulatory changes in ovarian progesterone secretion may also be of importance in the induction of the mid-cycle gonadotrophin surge. Increasing levels of progesterone can be detected in the ovarian vein of the ovary bearing the dominant follicle 24–48 hours before ovulation in the rhesus monkey[3], and circulating levels rise significantly on the day of the LH peak in the human cycle[16]. As it has been shown that progesterone can induce an LH surge in the presence of subthreshold levels of E_2, and can alter the timing and amplitude of the surge, it may augment the positive feedback action of E_2. Further, in the absence of administered progesterone, a mid-cycle type peak of FSH, which normally accompanies that of LH, did not occur in ovariectomized women on long-term E_2 replacement treated acutely with E_2–progesterone combinations[17]. Thus, the mid-cycle surge of LH and FSH depends on appropriate ovarian signals. The actual mechanisms of follicular rupture, and the stimulation of resumption of meiosis by the oocyte, involve actions of LH, with increased levels of cyclic AMP, increased progesterone secretion, increased distensibility of the follicle wall (resulting from collagen digestion) and increased levels of prostaglandin and protease activities[10].

The temporal relationships between the periovulatory hormonal events and ovulation have been established[16]. Thus E_2 rose significantly 82.5 hours (median) before ovulation, and peaked 24 hours before. Corresponding intervals were 32 and 16.5 hours for LH, 21.1 and 15 hours for FSH, and 7.8 hours (first significant rise) for progesterone.

OESTRADIOL AND SEXUAL BEHAVIOUR

Studies on the rhesus monkey strongly favour a role for E_2 in sexual behaviour in primates, consistent with its established role in lower species. Thus, in studies of the rhesus menstrual cycle, the highest number of ejaculations occurred 1 day after the E_2 peak, and this coincided with shorter times taken by females to gain access to males. Females have been noted to spend more time in proximity to males at this time of the cycle[18]. Such data indicate a further role for E_2 in determining the fertile period.

CHARACTERISTICS OF THE HUMAN FERTILE PERIOD

We have demonstrated that changes in cervical mucus which can be observed at the vulva correlate with periovulatory hormonal events: the first mucus change coincides with the first rise in urinary oestrogen excretion ($r = 0.89$[19]) and the last day on which the mucus is of low viscosity (resembling raw egg white), termed the 'peak day' (PD), is usually the day of ovulation, as estimated hormonally[8]. These observations provide the scientific basis for defining the fertile period as commencing with the first day of mucus secretion detectable at the vulva, and as ending on the fourth day after PD. In a study of 687 fertile women in five centres, during 6472 'normal' cycles (mean ($\pm$SD) length 28.5 $\pm$ 3.18 days), we observed that the mean length of the fertile period was 9.6 days (90% frequency interval 5.3–13.8). The probability of conception outside that period was 0.004 per cycle, supporting the concept that the fertile period can be defined as proposed. The probability was 0.024 on days of 'sticky' mucus 4 days or more before PD, and rose to 0.667 on PD (nine recorded coital acts, six pregnancies). It fell to 0.089 on PD+3[20].

CONCLUSIONS

Ovarian E_2 is the major physiological determinant of the onset and duration of the fertile period. The ability to define this period by simple clinical means, by hormonal assays and by imaging techniques provides the basis for current approaches both to the regulation of fertility and to the management of infertility. Further research should help to define our concepts of folliculogenesis and the mechanisms of E_2 action on its target tissues.

References

1. Ogino, K. (1930). Ovulationstermin und Konzeptionstermin. *Zentralblatt fur Gynakologie*, **54**, 464
2. Richards, J. S. (1980). Maturation of ovarian follicles: actions and interactions of pituitary and ovarian hormones on follicular cell differentiation. *Physiol. Rev*, **60**, 51
3. di Zerega, G. S., Marut, E. L., Turner, C. K. and Hodgen, G. D. (1980). Asymmetrical ovarian estradiol secretion during the follicular phase of the primate menstrual cycle. *J. Clin. Endocrinol. Metab.*, **51**, 698
4. Carson, R. S., Trounson, A. S. and Findlay, J. K. (1982). Successful fertilisation of human oocytes *in vitro*: concentration of estradiol-17β, progesterone and androstenedione in the antral fluid of donor follicles. *J. Clin. Endocrinol. Metab.*, **55**, 798
5. Pucca, G. A., Medici, M., Molinari, A. M., Moncharmont, B., Nola, E. and Sica, V. (1980). Estrogen receptor of calf uterus: an easy and fast purification procedure. *J. Steroid Biochem.*, **1**, 105
6. Bayard, F., Damilano, S., Robel, P. and Baulieu, E. E. (1978). Cytoplasmic and nuclear estradiol and progesterone receptors in human endometrium. *J. Clin. Endocrinol. Metab.*, **46**, 635
7. Odeblad, E., *et al.* (1983). The biophysical properties of the cervical–vaginal secretions. *Int. Rev. Nat. Family Planning*, **XII**, 1
8. Billings, E. L., Billings, J. J., Brown, J. B. and Burger, H. G. (1972). Symptoms and hormonal changes accompanying ovulation. *Lancet*, **1**, 282
9. Knobil, E. (1974). The control of gonadotropin secretion in the rhesus monkey. *Rec. Progr. Hormone Res.*, **30**, 1
10. Fritz, M. A. and Speroff, F. (1982). The endocrinology of the menstrual cycle: the interaction of folliculogenesis and neuroendocrine mechanisms. *Fertil. Steril.*, **38**, 509
11. Lenton, E. A., Sulaiman, R., Sobowale, O. and Cooke, I. D. (1982). The human menstrual cycle: plasma concentrations of prolactin, LH, FSH, oestradiol and progesterone in conceiving and non-conceiving women. *J. Reprod. Fertil.*, **65**, 131
12. Drouin, J., Lagace, L. and Labrie, F. (1976). Estradiol-induced increase of the LH responsiveness to LH releasing hormone (LHRH) in rat anterior pituitary cells in culture. *Endocrinology*, **99**, 1477
13. Clarke, I. J. and Cummins, J. T. (1982). The temporal relationship between gonadotropin releasing hormone (GnRH) and luteinizing hormone (LH) secretion in ovariectomized ewes. *Endocrinology*, **111**, 1737
14. Knobil, E., Plant, T. M., Wildt, L., Belchetz, P. E. and Marshall, G. (1980). Control of the rhesus monkey menstrual cycle: permissive role of hypothalamic gonadotropin-releasing hormone. *Science*, **207**, 1371
15. Marut, E. L., Williams, R. F., Cowan, B. D., Lynch, A., Lerner, S. P. and Hodgen, G. D. (1981). Pulsatile pituitary gonadotropin secretion during maturation of the dominant follicle in monkeys: estrogen positive feedback enhances the biological activity of LH. *Endocrinology*, **109**, 2270

16. World Health Organization Task Force Investigators (1980). Temporal relationships between ovulation and defined changes in the concentration of plasma, estradiol-17β, luteinizing hormone, follicle stimulating hormone and progesterone. *Am. J. Obstet. Gynaecol.*, **138**, 383
17. March, C. N., Goebelsmann, U., Nakimura, R. N. and Mishell, D. R. (1979). Roles of estradiol and progesterone in eliciting the mid-cycle luteinizing hormone and follicle stimulating hormone surges. *J. Clin. Endocrinol. Metab.*, **49**, 507
18. Michael, R. P. and Bonsall, R. W. (1979). Hormones and the sexual behaviour of rhesus monkeys. In Beyer, C. (ed.). *Endocrine Control of Sexual Behaviour*, pp. 279–302. (New York: Raven Press)
19. Brown, J. B., Harrisson, P., Smith, M. A. and Burger, H. G. (1981). *Correlations between the Mucus Symptoms and the Hormonal Markers of Fertility throughout Reproductive Life*. (Melbourne: Advocate Press Pty)
20. World Health Organization Task Force on Methods for the Determination of the Fertile Period (1983). A prospective multicentre study of the ovulation method of natural family planning. III. Characteristics of the menstrual cycle and of the fertile phase. *Fertil. Steril.* (In press.)

5
Biochemical methods for predicting ovulation

W. P. COLLINS, H. N. SALLAM, L. E. M. SCHIPHORST
and P. ROYSTON

INTRODUCTION

The measurement of oestradiol, LH and progesterone (or their metabolites) in various body fluids can provide probabilistic information about the occurrence of ovulation and the time of potential fertility during each menstrual cycle. The results obtained may be used in the practice of reproductive medicine to help achieve or avoid a pregnancy. Numerous tests have been developed to identify the limits of the fertile period (FP), the time of maximum potential fertility, and the presence of a mature oocyte[1,2]. The aims of the present report are to indicate the range of alternative methods that are available for specific applications, and to illustrate how the results from a single oestrogen test may be processed to provide signals of value in the practice of family planning (by periodic abstinence, or the limited use of barrier methods) and the management of infertility (by indicating the optimum time for coitus or artificial insemination).

REFERENCE POINTS

The following reference points have been used:
- (1) Day 1 of menstruation.
- (2) Day of LH peak in early morning urine (EMU).
- (3) Day of maximum follicular diameter (MFD).

It is well known that the first day of menstruation is a poor reference point for the study of ovarian function because it signals the end of a cycle, and the process may occur in the presence of different levels of circulating hormones. Nevertheless, it is usually an easily recognizable event and serves as a starting point for the application of chemical and other tests. The day of the LH peak in early morning urine, between days 5 and 25 of the menstrual cycle, can be determined retrospectively and used as a reference point for ovulation. In practice, the peak occurs on the day of MFD in about 50% of menstrual cycles, and 24 hours later in 30% of cases. A defined rise in the concentration of LH in serial samples of peripheral plasma, or 2–4 hourly collections of urine under well-controlled conditions, may be used for the immediate prediction of ovulation[3]. The time of MFD, or the time when the follicle has definitely ruptured, can serve as alternative reference points for ovulation[2].

Presently, there is not a definitive index of ovulation (other than pregnancy), and the precision with which changes in associated variables can be determined is dependent upon the frequency of the observations. Nevertheless, a peak of urinary LH has been observed in all of 118 apparently normal ovarian or menstrual cycles and although the hormonal reference point usually occurred on the same day as the MFD, the time interval between the two events could be 2 days. In addition, follicular rupture does not necessarily confirm that ovulation has occurred, and in our experience acoustic changes in the mature follicle can only be seen with confidence in about 85% of women.

DEFINITIONS

Ovulation is the release of a secondary oocyte from a mature ovarian follicle, and to date all tests to predict or detect the event are presumptive. The FP is essentially a statistical or probabilistic concept and is defined as the time during each menstrual cycle when intercourse might lead to pregnancy. In order to evaluate the potential usefulness of chemical tests, before they are assessed in clinical practice, we have used a mathematical model of conception risks[4] to estimate the time of the probable fertile period in relation to the two reference points for ovulation. The first definition of the probable FP is the time from the day of the LH peak minus 3 to day plus 2 inclusive, and the second is the time from the day of MFD minus 2 to day plus

3. Both definitions should allow for the life-span and motility of the gametes in the female reproductive tract in over 90% of cases. The first definition should on average provide better warning of the start of the FP and the second more cover at the end. The duration of the FP is usually quoted in calendar days, although 24-hour periods or hours are more accurate, depending on the times when the tests were performed.

CHEMICAL TESTS

In order to develop a practical chemical test for use in reproductive medicine it is necessary to identify marker compounds in readily accessible body fluids, and the main approaches that have been

Table 1 Chemical indices for predicting and detecting ovulation and identifying the probable limits of the fertile period

Analyte	Fluid
Detection of ovulation:	
Peak LH	P,U
Peak FSH	P
Rise progesterone	P,S
Rise Pd-3α-G	U
Identification of the fertile period:	
Rise day 1 E_1-3-G to peak day plus 4	U
Rise day 1 ratio E_1-3-G/Pd-3α-G to peak	
day plus 5	U
Rise day oestradiol to peak day plus 4	S
Immediate prediction of ovulation:	
Rise LH	P,U
Rise FSH	P
Rise or threshold oestradiol	P,S
Rise 2 E_1-3-G	U

P = plasma; U = urine; S = saliva.

studied are listed in Table 1. The time intervals between changes in the concentration of various hormones in peripheral plasma are used as reference values[5] for the development of simpler techniques. Frequent samples of saliva may be obtained and direct methods are now available for measuring the relatively low concentrations of progesterone (from 5 to $100 \, pg \, ml^{-1}$) and oestradiol (from 1 to $5 \, pg \, ml^{-1}$) throughout the menstrual cycle, and algorithms are being developed to optimize the predictive usefulness of each test. Various enzymes and other analytes may be measured in cervical mucus, but it is still difficult to obtain appropriate samples at all stages of the menstrual cycle. Most information, to date, has been obtained from the measurement of various steroid glucuronides in daily samples of urine – either pooled 24-hour collections, or EMUs with and without correction factors applied for the volume and duration of each collection. It has been established that oestrone-3-glucuronide (E_1-3-G) is a major urinary metabolite of plasma oestradiol, and pregnanediol-3α-glucuronide (Pd-3α-G) is the principal product of plasma progesterone. Tests based upon changes in the concentration of E_1-3-G or the derived concentration ratio E_1-3-G/Pd-3α-G have been developed and evaluated[6]. The results from the E_1-3-G may be processed to provide prospective information about the limits of the FP and the time of maximum potential fertility.

OESTRONE GLUCURONIDE

The structure of E_1-3-G is shown in Figure 1. The compound is very hydrophilic and contains a carboxyl group at carbon 1 of the

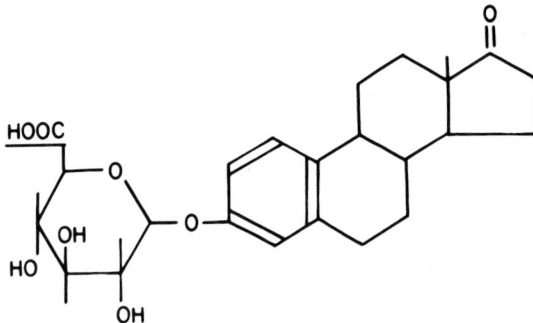

Figure 1 The structure of oestrone-3-glucuronide

glucuronyl residue, which may be attached to a protein in order to raise antibodies, and to various non-isotopic labels for use in immunoassays. High-titre monoclonal antibodies are now available for the measurement of both compounds, and methods with colorimetric[7] or luminescent end-points have been devised and evaluated[8].

The mean excretion pattern of E_1-3-G as determined by both radioimmunoassay (RIA) and chemiluminescence immunoassaay

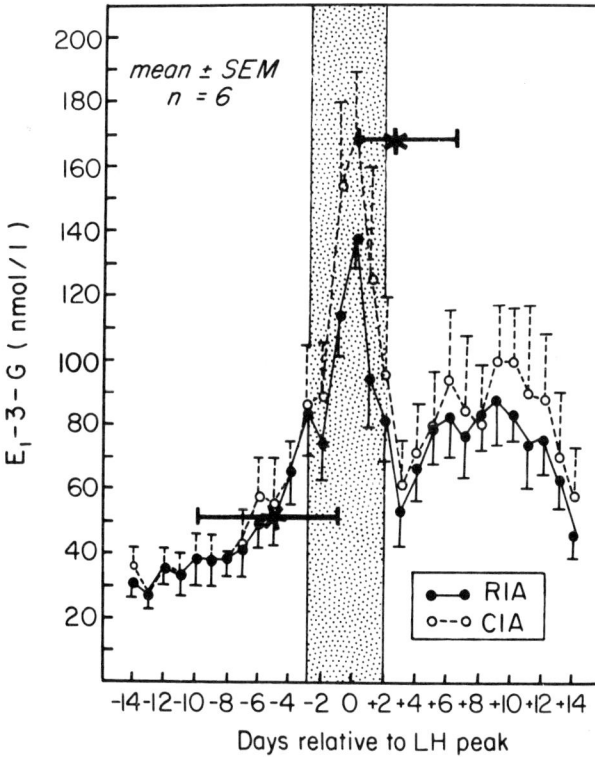

Figure 2 The mean concentrations of oestrone-3-glucuronide in EMU relative to the day of the LH peak and the limits of the fertile period

(CIA) is shown in Figure 2. The values in $nmol\,l^{-1}$ are plotted relative to the day of the LH peak, and the shaded area represents the defined FP. In order to predict the onset of potential fertility it is necessary to identify a rise in the concentration of E_1-3-G above a variable background, and the start of the infertile period can be calculated from the peak value. Accordingly, algorithms have been developed to identify the rise and peak day prospectively, and hence indicate the duration of the probable FP. The mean times and 90% limits for the start and end signals during the six menstrual cycles are also shown in the figure. The time of higher or maximum potential fertility may also be predicted from a second defined rise in the concentration of E_1-3-G.

The rise days are determined by a CUSUM test, which precedes

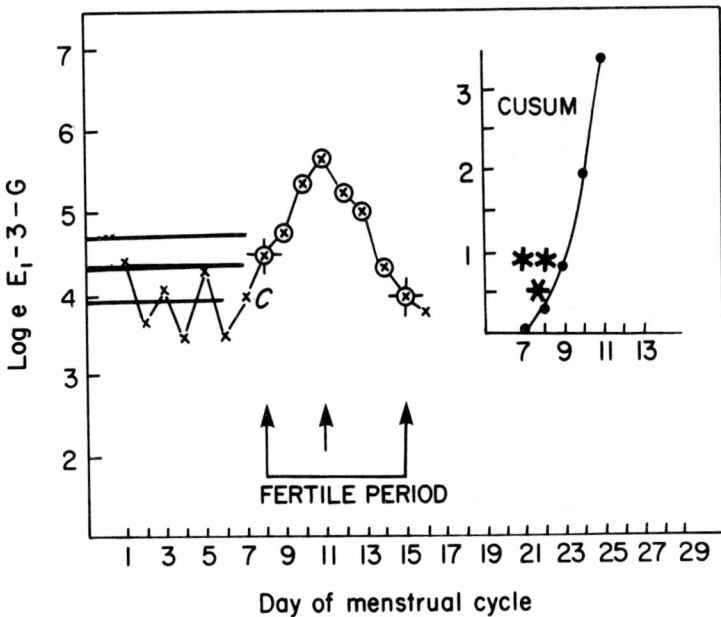

Figure 3 Application of the CUSUM test and peak selecting algorithm to data from the first menstrual cycle.
* First day of rise (R1); ** day of significant rise (R2)

the peak selecting algorithm. The method is illustrated in Figure 3 by application to the first of a series of 118 menstrual cycles. The days of the menstrual cycle are shown on the x axis. The daily concentrations of E_1-3-G are converted to log_e units, and a mean baseline value is calculated for days 1–6. A reference level is obtained by adding the value for 1SD of the whole baseline population, in log_e units, to the individual mean baseline value. A decision level for the CUSUM test is calculated as 2SDs in log_e units. The value for the reference level is then subtracted from each successive daily value and the amount added to the current CUSUM. The day of the defined first rise (R1, used to indicate the start of the fertile period) is the day on which the data first exceeded the reference level in the run leading to a significant CUSUM. The day (R2) on which the CUSUM reached a decision level may be used to indicate the time of maximum potential fertility. The peak day (used to calculate the end of the potential fertility) is determined by starting with the rise day (R1) plus 1 and taking the day with the highest value that is followed by four consecutive lower amounts.

A simpler graphical method based on the same data is illustrated

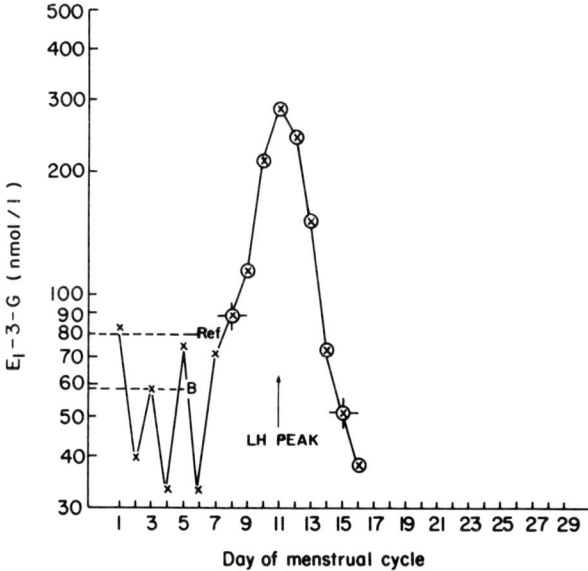

Figure 4 Application of the graphical method to data from the first menstrual cycle

in Figure 4. The data for the first 5 days of the menstrual cycle are plotted, and the median (i.e. the middle) value is identified and used as the baseline. The reference level is obtained by multiplying the median value by 1.35 which is the antilog of the value for 1SD as used in the CUSUM test. The daily values are plotted and the rise and peak days identified by eye.

The E_1-3-G test to identify the limits of the fertile period was applied initially to data from 58 menstrual cycles, and the results compared with the biological indices used in natural family planning[6]. The mean times of the signals, and 90% limits, relative to the day of the LH peak and the FP were compared. It was observed that there was a progressive reduction in mean times from the day of the shortest cycle length minus 18, the first day of cervical mucus detectable at the vulva, the day of rise in ratio, the day of rise in the concentration of E_1-3-G, to the day of the first slippery type mucus.

65

The mean time of the end signal from the four methods to the LH peak was similar, but there were some apparent false-positive signals. Frequency distribution curves for the days on which the start or end signals occurred for the two immunochemical tests are shown relative

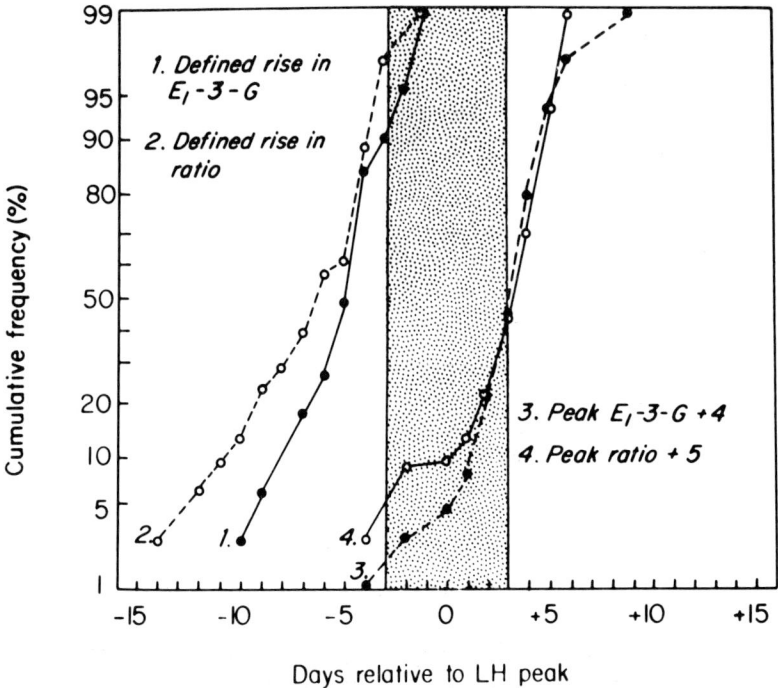

Figure 5 The cumulative frequency (%) of days on which signals from two immunochemical tests occurred relative to the day of the LH peak and the limits of the fertile period

to the day of the LH peak and the defined FP in Figure 5. The median time interval was −6.5 days for the ratio test, −4.9 days for the E_1-3-G test and −6.6 days for the mucus test. It may be seen that about 5% of the start signals probably occur too late, and similarly there may be up to 20% of false-positive signals for the start of the infertile period. Both immunochemical tests successfully delineated the FP in about 85% of the menstrual cycles. If the results from the E_1-3-G test were used in conjunction with those obtained from the cervical mucus method (i.e. the start of the FP is the earliest of rise day in E_1-3-G or first day of mucus, and the end of the FP is the latest of peak E_1-3-G plus 4 days, or peak mucus plus 4 days) then the defined FP was circumscribed in all menstrual cycles[2].

Our most recent results on the application of the E_1-3-G test to

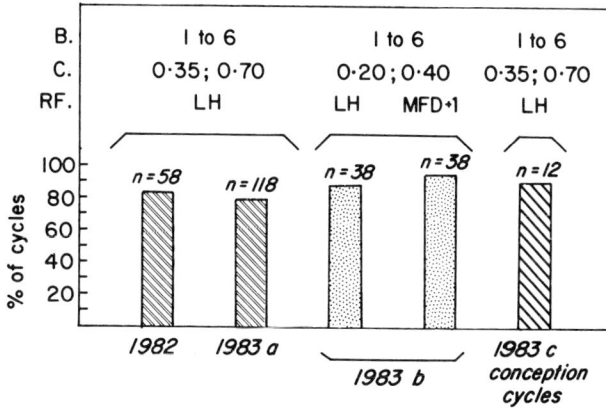

Figure 6 The days of baseline (B) and CUSUM parameters (C) and the success of the oestrone test to delineate the fertile period according to different reference points (RF) for ovulation

delineate the FP are illustrated in Figure 6. For the first study, which was completed in 1982, the baseline for the CUSUM was calculated from the values on days 1 to 6, the constants required to calculate the reference and decision levels were 0.35 and 0.70 $\log_e$ units respectively and the reference point for ovulation was the peak day of urinary LH in EMU. Under these conditions the success rate of the test to delineate the FP completely was 84%. Subsequently data were accumulated from an additional 60 menstrual cycles and the success rate of the test dropped to 79%. Thirty-eight of the 118 cycles were also monitored with ultrasound, and the apparent success rate of the test using optimized constants or the CUSUM was 84% with the day of LH peak as the reference point and 95% using the day of MFD. Conception occurred during 12 cycles and the test successfully delineated the FP in 10 (i.e. 83%) and an additional rise in concentration during the mid-luteal phase indicated the possible time of implantation in all cases using the measurement of LH/HCG as the reference points[9].

Rise day 2 has also been calculated during the 38 cycles monitored with ultrasound and the mean time from the signal to the time of MFD, with 24-hour sampling, was 43 hours. 81% of the signals occurred within the period −48 hours to +24 hours from the time of MFP[10].

DISCUSSION

We believe that defined changes in the concentration of E_1-3-G in daily samples of EMU may be used to identify the limits of a probable fertile period in 85–95% of menstrual cycles. In addition, the test may possibly be used to indicate the time of maximum potential fertility in about 81% of cycles. Attempts are being made to simplify the methods for clinical trials and eventual home use. In addition, the same statistical analysis is being applied to the concentration of oestradiol in more frequent samples of saliva. It is apparent, however, that more information is derived if the results from chemical tests are interpreted in conjunction with the signals from biological indices, and from the appearance of the reproductive system as observed with ultrasound.

Acknowledgements

This investigation received financial support from the Special Programme of Research, Development and Research Training in Human Reproduction, World Health Organization.

References

1. Collins, W. P. (1982). Ovulation prediction and detection. *IPPF Med. Bull.*, **16**, 1
2. Collins, W. P. (1983). Biochemical approaches to ovulation prediction and detection and the location of the fertile period in women. In Jeffcoate, S. (ed.). *Ovulation Prediction and Detection*. (Chichester: John Wiley and Sons)
3. Edwards, R. G., Anderson, G., Pickering, J. and Purdy, J. M. (1982). Rapid assay of urinary LH in women using a simplified method of Hi-gonavis. In Edwards, R. G. and Purdy, J. M. (eds.). *Human Conception In Vitro*, pp. 19–34. (London: Academic Press)
4. Royston, J. P. (1982). Basal body temperature, ovulation and the risk of conception with special reference to the lifetimes of sperm and egg. *Biometrics*, **38**, 397
5. World Health Organization Task Force on Methods for the Determination of the Fertile Period (1980). Temporal relationships between ovulation and defined changes in the concentrations of plasma estradiol-17β, luteinizing hormone, follicle stimulating hormone and progesterone. 1. Probit analysis. *Am. J. Obstet. Gynecol.*, **138**, 383
6. World Health Organization Task Force on Methods for the Determination of the

Fertile Period (1983). Temporal relationships between indices of the fertile period. *Fertil. Steril.*, **39,** 647

7. Shah, H. P. and Joshi, U. M. (1982). A simple, rapid and reliable enzyme-linked immunosorbent assay (ELISA) for measuring estrone-3-glucuronide in urine. *J. Steroid. Biochem.*, **16,** 283

8. Weerasekera, D. A., Kim, J. B., Barnard, G. J., Collins, W. P., Kohen, F. and Lindner, H. R. (1982). Monitoring ovarian function by a solid-phase chemiluminescence immunoassay. *Acta Endocrinol.*, **101,** 254

9. Branch, C., Collins, P. O., Kilpatrick, M. J. and Collins, W. P. (1980). The effect of conception on the concentration of oestrone-3-glucuronide, LH/HCG and pregnanediol-3α-glucuronide. *Acta Endocrinol.*, **93,** 228

10. Schiphorst, L. E. M., Sallam, H. N., Adekunle, Y., Collins, W. P. and Royston, P. (1984). The optimization of an immunological test to locate the fertile period in women. Presented at the XIth World Congress on Fertility and Sterility, June 1983, Dublin.

6
Ultrasound and follicular development

S. NITSCHKE-DABELSTEIN

Ultrasound monitoring of ovarian structural changes has become a widely accepted method for the evaluation of ovarian function. The non-stimulated ovary of the early follicular phase shows a relatively homogeneous structure partly interrupted by small areas of 'thinning' (Figure 1). Regardless of whether ovulation is spontaneous or induced, the beginning follicular reaction is signalled by the appearance of small cystic-like structures, not yet persistently demonstrable from one day to the next (Figure 2). This *discontinuous* follicular reaction is paralleled by widely varying 17β-oestradiol concentrations and corresponds to the latent follicular phase defined by Insler and Lunenfeld[1]. Data from nine conception cycles in gonadotrophin-treated women showed this phase to last 5–7 days, with a mean $\pm$ SE of 6.1 $\pm$ 0.26 days. It is followed by the phase of *continuous* follicular growth, which is to be expected as soon as one follicle has reached a size greater than 13 mm. (For a definition of size, see below.) This phase resembles the active follicular phase[1] and lasted 4–7 days in the gonadotrophin-treated women, with a mean $\pm$SE of 5.2 $\pm$ 0.32 days. Growth rates for the follicle are described ranging between 2.1 and 3.0 mm[2-4].

Uni-, bi- and multifollicular development cannot be differentiated before the phase of continuous follicular growth. This active phase includes a progressive increase in 17β-oestradiol values lasting until shortly before ovulation.

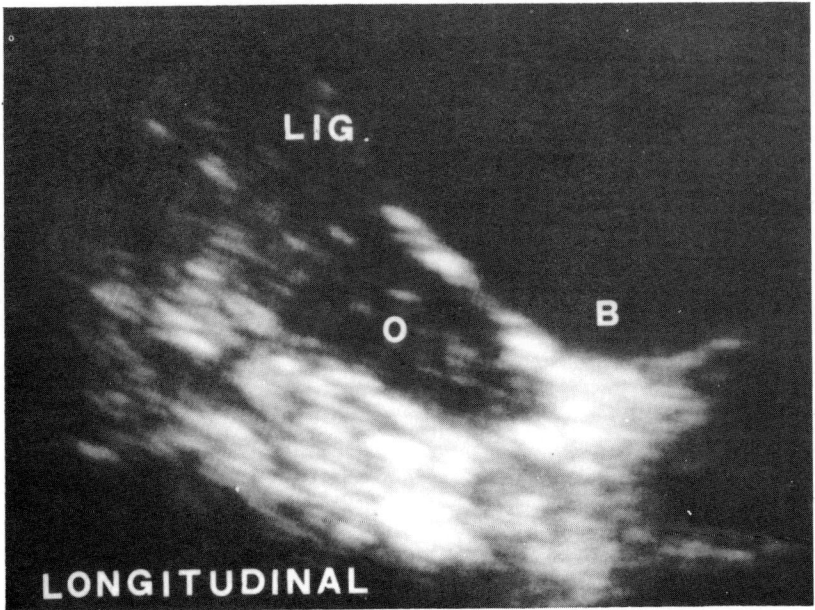

Figure 1 Non-stimulated ovary of the early follicular phase[2]. Lig = Infundibulopelvic ligament; O = ovary; B = full urinary bladder. Longitudinal scan

The size of the graafian follicle is the most commonly discussed ultrasound parameter. Published data differ widely for spontaneous ovulatory cycles, for example between 19.3 and 27.0 mm[3,5–13]. Since no standard technique of follicular measurement, however, has so far been agreed, comparative discussions are of minor value. In regard to the ovoid shape of the follicle we have defined follicular size as the mean derived from the maximal transversal, sagittal and longitudinal diameter. O'Herlihy, who used the same technique, could show a highly significant correlation of follicular fluid content aspirated during laparoscopy[10]. Table 1 shows the mean follicular

Table 1 Mean (±SE) follicular sizes (in mm) of 55 unifollicular and 20 multifollicular cycles on the last 4 days before ovulation

Day of cycle:	−3	−2	−1	0
Unifollicular cycle	15.9 ± 0.6	17.3 ± 0.5	19.5 ± 0.4	21.7 ± 0.4
Multifollicular cycle	14.3 ± 0.8	17.8 ± 0.7	20.5 ± 0.7	22.3 ± 0.5

Table 2 Mean (±SE) follicular sizes (in mm) in 12 conception cycles on the 4 days before ovulation

Day of Cycle	−3	−2	−1	0
Unifollicular cycle (n = 6)	15.2 ± 1.7	17.7 ± 1.5	20.7 ± 0.6	22.7 ± 0.6
Multifollicular cycle (n = 6)	13.8 ± 1.4	15.8 ± 0.5	18.7 ± 0.7	22.0 ± 0.3

sizes derived from 55 unifollicular and 20 multifollicular cycles of spontaneous ovulation as well as of epimestrol-, clomiphene- and gonadotrophin-induced ovulation.

Table 2 lists the mean value for 12 conception cycles out of this group. Growth rates as well as the sizes of the graafian follicles are not significantly different between the cycles. The smallest graafian follicle observed in a conception cycle measured 20.9 mm. Regarding the whole group of 75 cycles the graafian follicle was observed in the

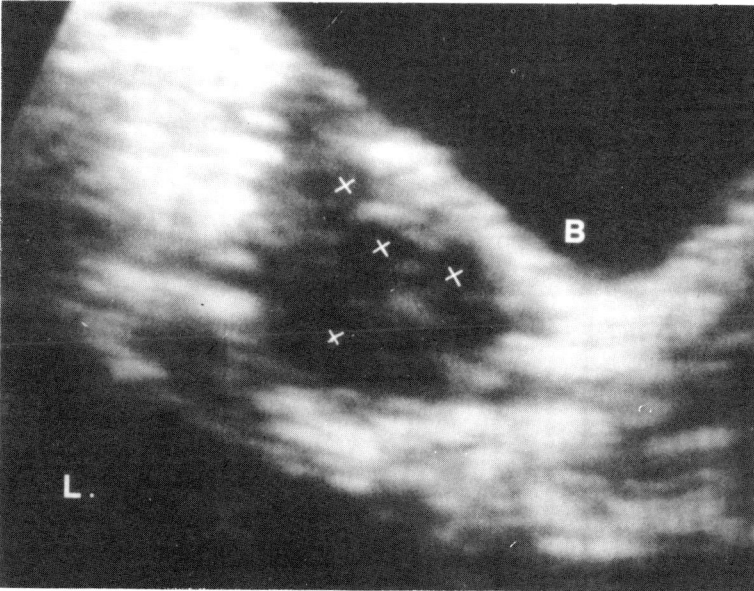

Figure 2 Discontinuous follicular reaction – latent follicular phase (1). + = Follicular structures under 13 mm; B = full urinary bladder; L = longitudinal scan

right ovary in 58.7%, in the left ovary in 32.0% and in both (multi-follicular development) in 13.3% of the cycles.

A linear regression of 17β-oestradiol values and follicular size has been proved by several authors; coefficients of correlation range between 0.52 and 0.77 for unifollicular cycles[5,7,13–15]. Significant correlations for both parameters were also seen when data were compared for every preovulatory day during continuous follicular growth. The highest coefficient was determined for the day of 17β-oestradiol maximum, which means 2 days before ovulatory structural changes were observed by ultrasonography. For multifollicular reaction correlation of follicular sizes and 17β-oestradiol are discussed controversially.

Critical evaluation of progesterone and ultrasound data of the follicle are published by Kerin *et al.*[7] and our group[16]. Mature graafian follicles with progesterone concentrations of the preovulatory state range between 18 and 30 mm with a mean of 23.6 mm[7]. Unifollicular cycles showed varying preovulatory progesterone levels between 0.84 and 1.99 ng ml^{-1} depending chiefly on whether ovulation was spontaneous or induced by epimestrol, clomiphene or gonadotrophin. The different values paralleled, as 17β-oestradiol, the differences in follicular size. Correlation of both data for each day during the active follicular phase proved an increasing dependency towards ovulation with a coefficient of correlation of 0.43 on the day prior to the observation of ovulatory changes in ultrasound. Preovulatory progesterone levels above 'normal' were measured in multifollicular cycles. Conception did not occur above a progesterone value of 4.5 ng ml^{-1}.

For ultrasonic evaluation of the ovulatory cycle the demonstration of early ovulatory changes of the follicle is of great importance. Different structural changes signalling ovulation are described:

(1) Disappearance of the follicle with an indistinguishable corpus luteum[11,12].
(2) Collapse of the follicle with gradual replacement by a cystic corpus luteum[2,11].
(3) Irregular cyst gradually decreasing in size or a slight partial collapse of the follicle[4,17,18].
(4) Opacification, which means an increase of echoes within the cystic follicular structure[4,19].
(5) Invasion of solid echoes from the wall or 'filling in' partly

74

without decrease in size[11,12,19,20]. In our experience this is rather a sign of impaired ovulation, especially when this cycle shows a short luteal phase[17] and a cystic enlargement of the follicle.

FINAL REMARKS

In consensus with other authors we think that ultrasound monitoring of ovarian cyclic changes gives an adequate information on follicular development by follicular size, follicular growth rate, and length of continuous follicular growth. For the management of ovulation induction it is as effective as any hormonal monitoring. However, for prediction of ovulation ultrasound parameters are not sufficiently precise. Investigation of more exact signs of follicular maturity, such as possibly opacification and demonstrable cumulus oophorus, has to be undertaken.

References

1. Insler, V. and Lunenfeld, B. (1977). Human gonadotropins. In Phillip, E., Barnes, J. and Newton, M. (eds.) *Scientific Foundations of Obstetrics and Gynecology*, p. 629. (London: Heinemann Medical Books)
2. Nitschke-Dabelstein, S. (1983). Monitoring of follicular development using ultrasonography. In Insler, V. and Lunenfeld, B. (eds.) *Infertility – Male and Female*. (In press). (London: Churchill-Livingstone)
3. Renaud, R. L., Macler, J., Dervain, I., *et al.* (1980). Echographic study of follicular maturation and ovulation during the normal menstrual cycle. *Fertil. Steril., 33*, 272
4. Ylöstalo, O., Lindgren, P. G. and Nillius, S. J. (1981). Ultrasonic measurement of ovarian follicles, ovarian and uterine size during induction of ovulation with human gonadotrophins. *Acta Endocrinol., 98*, 592
5. Bryce, R. L., Shuter, B., Sinosich, M. J., Stiel, J. N., Picker, R. H. and Saunders, D. M. (1982). The value of ultrasound, gonadotropin, and estradiol measurements for precise ovulation prediction. *Fertil. Steril., 37*, 42
6. Hackelöer, B. J., Dörfler, R., Nitschke, S. and Buchholz, R. (1980). Ultraschalldarstellung des Follikelwachstums und Basaltemperaturmessung. *Ultraschall, 1*, 133
7. Kerin, J. F., Edmonds, D. K., Warnes, G. M., *et al.* (1981). Morphological and functional relations of graafian follicle growth to ovulation in women using ultrasonic, laparoscopic and biochemical measurements. *Br. J. Obstet. Gynaecol., 88*, 81
8. Nilsson, L., Wikland, M. and Hamberger, L. (1982). Recruitment of an ovulatory follicle in the human following follicle-ectomy and lute-ectomy. *Fertil. Steril., 37*, 30
9. Nitschke-Dabelstein, S., Sturm, G. and Buchholz, R. (1981). Plasmaprogesterone und Follikelgröße als Gradmesser follikulärer Reife. *Geburtsh. u. Frauenheilk., 41*, 591
10. O'Herlihy, C., De Crespigny, L., Lopata, A., Johnston, I., Hoult, I. and Robinson, H. (1980). Preovulatory follicular size: a comparison of ultrasound and laparoscopic measurements. *Fertil. Steril., 34*, 24

11. Queenan, J. T., O'Brian, G. D., Bains, L. M., Aimpson, J., Collins, W. P. and Campbell, S. (1980). Ultrasound scanning of ovaries to detect ovulation in women. *Fertil. Steril.*, **34**, 99
12. Robertson, R. D., Picker, R. H., Wilson, P. C. and Saunders, D. M. (1979). Assessment of ovulation by ultrasound and plasma estradiol determinations. *Obstet. Gynecol.*, **54**, 686
13. Smith, D. H., Picker, R. H., Sinosich, M. and Saunders, D. M. (1980). Assessment of ovulation by ultrasound and estradiol levels during spontaneous and induced cycles. *Fertil. Steril.*, **33**, 387
14. Hackelöer, B. J., Fleming, R., Robinson, H. P., Adam, A. H. and Coutts, J. R. T. (1979). Correlation of ultrasonic and endocrinological assessment of human follicular development. *Am. J. Obstet. Gynecol.*, **135**, 122
15. Nitschke-Dabelstein, S., Sturm, G., Hackelöer, B. J., Daume, E. and Buchholz, R. (1980). Welchen Stellenwert besitzt die endokrinologische Überwachung in der Gonadotropinstimulierung anovulatorischer Patientinnen. *Geburtsh. u. Frauenh.*, **40**, 702
16. Nitschke-Dabelstein, S., Sturm, G., Prinz, H. and Buchholz, R. (1981). Plasma-17β-estradiol and plasma progesterone as indicators of cyclic changes in the follicle-bearing ovary. In Insler, V. and Bettendorf, G. (eds.) *Advances in Diagnosis and Treatment of Infertility*, p. 57. (Amsterdam: Elsevier)
17. Nitschke-Dabelstein, S., Hackelöer, B. J. and Sturm, G. (1981). Ovulation and corpus luteum formation observed by ultrasonography. *Ultrasound Med. Biol.*, **7**, 33
18. Terinde, R., Distler, W., Freundl, G. and Herberger, J. (1979). Hormonelle und ultrasonographische Kontrolle der spontanen Ovulation bei Patientinnen mit primärer und sekundärer Sterilität. *Arch. Gynecol.*, **228**, 168
19. Hackelöer, B. J. and Robinson, H. P. (1978). Ultraschalldarstellung des wachsenden Follikels und Corpus luteum im normalen physiologischen Zyklus. *Geburtsh. u. Frauenh.*, **38**, 163
20. de Crespigny, L.Ch., O'Herlihy, C. and Robinson, H. P. (1981). Ultrasonic observation of the mechanism of human ovulation. *Am. J. Obstet. Gynecol.*, **139**, 636

7
Biological methods of identifying the fertile period

J. BONNAR

INTRODUCTION

Despite the advances in the understanding of the menstrual cycle and the ovulatory process direct proof that ovulation has taken place still rests on occurrence of pregnancy or the recovery of an ovum from the Fallopian tubes. The actual fertile period in women exists when a viable ovum is present and the survival time of the ovum is calculated to be less than 48 hours[1]. In gynaecological practice a number of methods are available which provide presumptive evidence that ovulation may be about to occur or may have occurred:

(1) *Medical:*
  (a) Endometrial histology and vaginal cytology;
  (b) Plasma progesterone and urinary pregnanediol;
  (c) Urinary LH;
  (d) Ultrasonography;
  (e) Physicochemical changes in cervical mucus;
  (f) Composition of saliva.

(2) *Biological:*
  (a) Calculation or calendar method;
  (b) Basal body temperature;
  (c) Changes in cervical mucus and morphology;
  (d) Mittelschmerz (intermenstrual pain);
  (e) Menstrual cycle molimina.

These medical methods have important applications in the investigation and management of infertility but they all require appropriate technology and their repeated use is both expensive and inconvenient to the woman. This chapter will review certain recognizable biological effects that occur due to the major changes in the circulating blood levels of oestrogen and progesterone and discuss the on-going use of these biological signals for the self-detection of ovulation and the fertile phase of the cycle. These biological changes include the basal body temperature (BBT), changes in the cervix and its mucus secretion, Mittelschmerz and the menstrual cycle molimina.

BIOLOGICAL METHODS OF IDENTIFYING THE FERTILE PERIOD

Calculation or calendar method

The calculation or calendar method is the oldest technique for determining the fertile period and followed the work of Ogino[2] and Knaus[3] in the 1930s. The fertile phase of the cycle was identified from the records of the previous 6–12 menstrual cycles. The potential fertile period was then calculated on the following basis:

(1) Define the shortest and longest menstrual cycle over the preceding six and preferably 12 cycles.
(2) The first day of the potentially fertile period is the shortest cycle minus 19/20 days.
(3) The last day of the potentially fertile phase is the longest cycle minus 11 days.

For a woman whose menstrual cycles have varied between 26 and 31 days the potential fertile period would be day 8–20 of the cycle.

The greatest weakness of the calendar calculation is that it depends on a prediction, based on the menstrual history, of what is likely to occur and not on what is actually taking place. The same objection, however, applies to the calculation of a woman's expected date of confinement which is often accorded in obstetric practice a precision that is not only biologically unsound but also somewhat hazardous in that it is often used as the sole basis for induction of labour.

Basal body temperature method

A relationship between the timing of ovulation and the change in the BBT was first suggested in 1905 by the Dutch gynaecologist van de Velde[4]. For extensive reviews of the temperature patterns of the menstrual cycle the reader is referred to the work ·of Marshall[5], Vollman[6] and Zuspan and Zuspan[7]. The rise in the temperature around the time of ovulation is due to the thermogenic effect of progesterone. Moghissi et al.[8] found that the BBT rose soon after the luteinizing hormone surge and that the significant rise in BBT coincided with the rise of plasma progesterone level to a mean value of $4\,\text{ng ml}^{-1}$ and urinary pregnanediol to greater than $1.8\,\text{mg}\,(24\,\text{h})^{-1}$. The BBT remained elevated until the progesterone level fell below these concentrations.

The shift in temperature is small – between 0.2 and 0.5 °C (0.4 and 1.0 °F) – and usually occurs abruptly over 24 hours and is sometimes preceded by a small dip in the temperature. A significant temperature shift is defined as one that occurs in 48 hours or less and in which three consecutive daily temperatures are at least 0.2 °C higher than in the last six daily temperatures prior to the start of the shift. Marshall[9] from a detailed study of thermal changes in 1088 menstrual cycles with biphasic temperature patterns concluded that an acute rise with an elevation of at least 0.2 °C between 2 consecutive days occurred in 80% of cycles.

In this study only 10% of the cycles had a dip preceding the temperature rise. In a more recent study which included hormonal measurements to provide an estimate of the time of ovulation, Hilgers and Bailey[10] observed the temperature dip in only 10 of 66 hormonally normal cycles. The temperature rise associated with ovulation may also be gradual or step-like in pattern over several days. If fertilization of the ovum occurs the temperature remains at the higher level. Since it is a shift in BBT rather than the temperature itself which is important, the readings should be taken daily usually in the morning immediately on wakening and before rising. This is to ensure that physiological conditions are as close to basal as possible. A method of correcting temperatures for differing wakening times has been proposed recently by Royston et al.[11].

Special 'ovulation' thermometers with expanded scales and charts which facilitate the identification of the temperature shift have been developed. Records of BBT taken by clinical thermometers and recorded on ordinary clinical temperature charts are of little value. The temperature can be taken in the mouth, axilla, vagina or rectum, providing the same procedure is always used. More important is the scale of the graph paper or chart used for recording the temperature. A scale in which the space covered by 2 days on the horizontal axis is equal to the space of 0.1 °C on the vertical axis facilitates the identification of the shift. A 'coverline' method identifies the day of the temperature shift by drawing a line from left to right across the temperature chart just above the pre-ovulatory readings (Figure 1).

Vollman[6] has made an outstanding contribution to knowledge of the menstrual cycle and has analysed BBT recordings of 20 672 cycles in 621 women. In short menstrual cycles of less than 17 days, monophasic temperature curves occurred in 57.1%. The incidence of monophasic curves decreased with an increase in length of the menstrual cycles and dropped to 5.8% at cycles of 24 days. In cycles of 25–32 days the incidence of monophasic curves was lowest at 1.8–4.8%. With increasing length of the menstrual cycle beyond 33 days, the rate of monophasic BBT curves steadily increased, reaching 41.3% in cycles of 60 days or longer. Monophasic charts also showed, as expected, an age-dependent distribution. In the year of menarche, monophasic BBT curves were observed in 55.7% of menstrual cycles and the incidence decreased sharply during adolescence. In mature women the rate of monophasic curves was around 2% and was as low as 1.2% between 23 and 29 years. In the pre-menopausal years, the incidence of monophasic cycles rose to 34%.

Other workers have confirmed the low frequency of monophasic temperature charts during the cycles of mature ovulating women. Magyar et al.[12] reported a 2% incidence and Hilgers and Bailey[10] reported a 3% incidence. Moghissi[13] claimed that in approximately 20% of ovulatory cycles the BBT failed to demonstrate ovulation, but his observations seem to be at variance with the experience of others[14]. The reliability of temperature charting is greatly influenced by the quality of the instruction in temperature recording and the keeping of the temperature records.

The temporal relationship between the shift of BBT and ovulation has been extensively investigated and the relationship appears to be variable. In a detailed study of peri-ovulatory basal temperature changes and ovulation Hilgers and Bailey[10] examined the relationship of the temperature dip, the temperature nadir, the first day of the temperature rise and the 'coverline' end-point, to the estimated

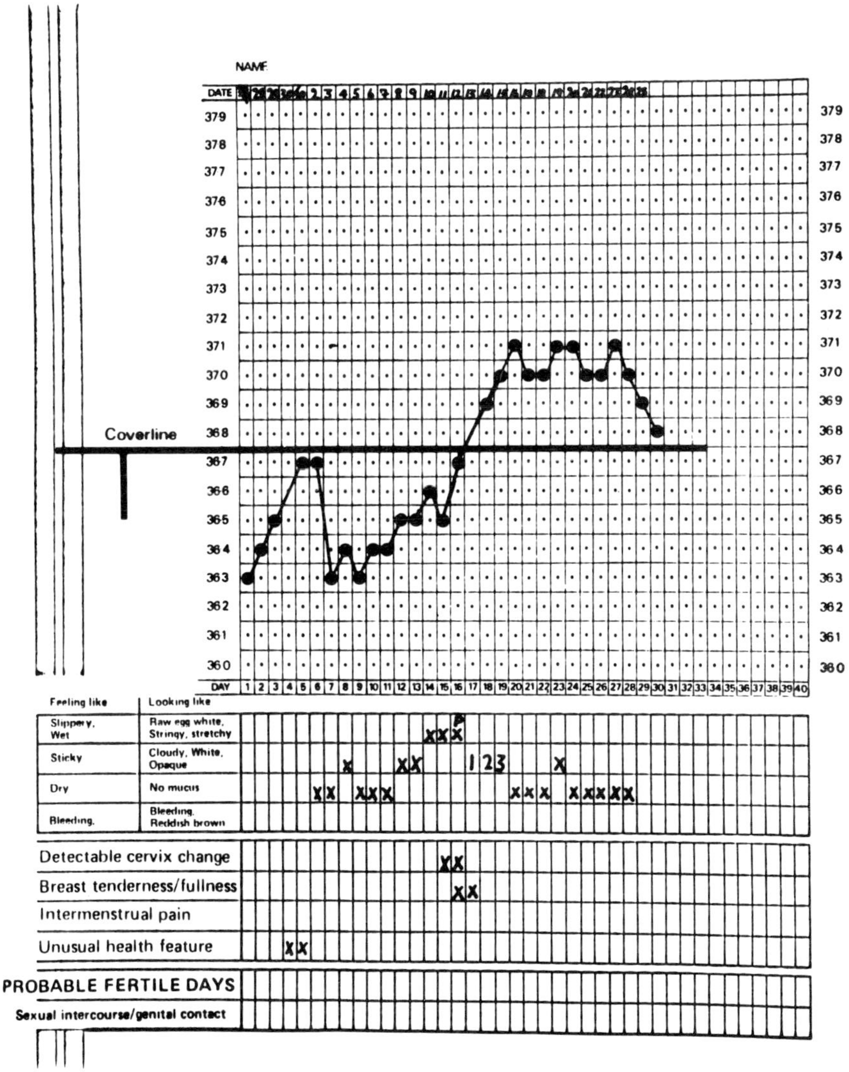

Figure 1 Symptothermal chart. The scale of the temperature chart facilitates the detection of the temperature shift during the menstrual cycle. Produced by the World Health Organization Special Programme for Research in Human Reproduction

time of ovulation. The estimated time of ovulation was calculated from the early rise in plasma progesterone level. They concluded that none of the temperature end-points which they tested was precise enough to indicate the day of ovulation and had a range of ±2 days. A similar conclusion was reached by Lenton et al.[15].

Very rapid electronic thermometers are now available which offer considerable advantages over the clinical thermometer. The daily taking and charting of the BBT is the simplest and most widely used method for detecting ovulation. In infertility clinics the instruction of the woman should not be rushed and is best done by a nurse.

Poor charts usually reflect poor quality of teaching. The temperature chart identifies the ovulatory cycle and the duration of the follicular and luteal phase. The timing of plasma progesterone or urinary pregnanediol is best guided by the temperature record. In any particular cycle, however, the temperature chart will not indicate the optimal time for intercourse for the couple who are trying to conceive.

Changes in cervical mucus (ovulation method)

To overcome the drawbacks of the calendar method and the BBT method for identifying the fertile period, John and Evelyn Billings of Melbourne in the early 1970s developed the ovulation method[16]. Billings, Brown and Burger[17] reported that cervical mucus symptoms appeared at a mean of 6.2 days before ovulation, which was defined as occurring the day after the mid-cycle peak of luteinizing hormone. This was confirmed by Flynn and Lynch[18] who investigated the hormonal parameters of ovulation and mucus symptoms and found that the mucus first appeared at a mean of 5.2 days before the day of the luteinizing hormone peak. The changes in the cervical mucus are of vital importance to sperm transport and survival within the female reproductive tract.

The changes in cervical mucus are shown in Figure 2 and are briefly as follows. In the early follicular phase when the oestrogen levels are low the cervix secretes only a small amount of highly viscous mucus. The hydrogel glycoprotein content of the mucus forms a complex network of fibrils which prevent sperm penetration. As the ovarian follicle develops, the rising oestrogen level stimulates the cervical glands to secrete a cascade of clear watery mucus of low viscosity and high threadability (spinnbarkeit). This 'fertile' mucus is highly receptive to sperm. The glycoprotein fibrils in the fertile mucus form a micellar structure orientated along the direction of the cervical canal. Sperms are directed along channels between the micelles towards the uterine cavity and into the crypts of the endocervix where sperms are stored. As the oestrogen level falls and the progesterone level rises following ovulation the mucus secretion from the cervix sharply decreases and returns to the highly viscous type of the early part of the cycle.

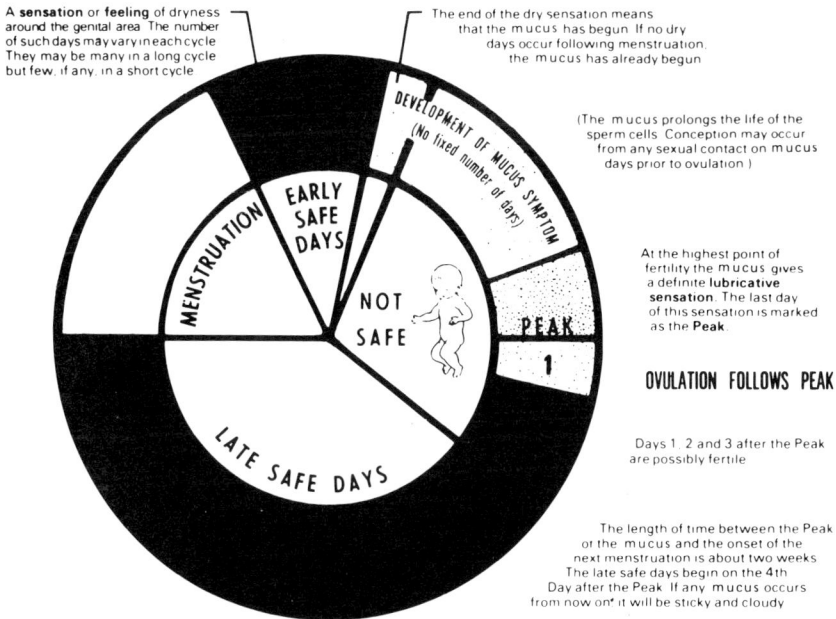

Figure 2   The ovulation method of fertility regulation. The mucus patterns of fertility and infertility. Reproduced from reference 16, with permission

Moghissi et al.[8] reported that maximal values for sperm penetration, pH and ferning and minimal values for viscosity and cell content for the cervical mucus occurred on the day of the rise in serum LH level. The greatest amount of mucus and the maximum spinnbarkeit occurred one day before the LH peak and on the day of peak urinary excretion of total oestrogens. Moghissi and colleagues[8] concluded that the changes in cervical mucus were an excellent guide to hormonal events during the menstrual cycle and therefore of value in fertility investigations. The appearance of abundant clear mucus of low viscosity and high spinnbarkeit, however, will not indicate ovulation. These mucus changes reflect optimal levels of circulating oestrogen which can occur without ovulation.

A cervical score of the mucus characteristics was designed by Insler et al.[19] who found it to be a reliable method for detecting ovulatory cycles. This technique was to be used by the gynaecologist when examining the cervix. The major advance of the Billings method was to teach women themselves to recognize the changes in the cervical mucus. This method enables a woman to recognize the infertile and fertile days of her cycle and by timing intercourse accordingly can either avoid pregnancy or enhance the possibility of pregnancy. The mucus symptom is assessed not at the cervix but at the vulva. The woman is asked to observe her sensations and the presence of mucus symptoms especially before and after micturition using either toilet tissue or her fingers. The observations should only take a few seconds. The sensation produced by the cervical mucus is more important than the quantity or the appearance of the mucus. Women are taught:

(1) Menstrual bleeding is followed by a variable number of 'dry' days when no mucus secretion is present and the genital area feels 'dry' (infertile).

(2) The end of the dry sensation indicates that the production of mucus has started. The type of mucus rather than the quantity is important. Infertile-type mucus is opaque and is described as tacky, sticky, crumbly and may be white or yellow.

(3) The immediate pre-ovulatory phase is characterized by the appearance of clear, thin, glistening, lubricative mucus having the physical characteristics of raw white of egg. The last day of the highly fertile lubricative mucus is called the 'peak' day which indicates the day of maximal fertility in the cycle.

(4) After ovulation the mucus becomes thick, tacky, opaque and less in quantity. The duration of this mucus symptom is variable and is followed by days when no vaginal loss is observed. The fertile period of the cycle is considered to commence with the onset of fertile mucus symptoms and end on the evening of the fourth day after the 'peak'.

The question of whether the woman's observations of the vulva are an accurate index of the status of cervical mucus at the site of secretion, the endocervix, was investigated by Hilgers and Prebil[20] who found that the fertility indices in the cervical mucus correlated well with the vulval observations.

Self-recognition of cervical mucus symptoms provides the woman with a simple means of detecting the fertile phase of her cycle and the likely time of ovulation.

Morphological changes in the cervix

In addition to effects on cervical mucus, oestrogen also changes the morphology of the cervix. The pre-ovulatory rise in oestrogen softens the tissues of the cervix and opens the cervical os. The softened cervix and gaping os with a cascade of clear mucus is a sign of optimal oestrogen response and of imminent ovulation. After ovulation the os closes, cervical tissues become firm and the cervix returns to a lower position. Daily self-palpation of the cervix to assess the patency of the os and condition of the cervix was advocated by Keefe[21] as a method of ovulation detection.

INTERNATIONAL STUDIES ON THE OVULATION METHOD

In 1977 the World Health Organization set up a multi-centre study of the ovulation method to determine the percentage of women in different cultures and social groups who could be taught to recognize cervical mucus changes and to investigate the effectiveness of this approach to family planning[22-24]. Women were recruited from five countries: New Zealand, India, Ireland, Phillippines and El Salvador. All were of proved fertility with no previous training in the ovulation method, representing various cultures and socioeconomic levels and ranging in educational status from illiteracy to postgraduate education. The most striking finding of the study was that in the first cycle following instruction 93% of the women were able to recognize and record their mucus symptoms which allowed self-recognition of the fertile period. A previous study in British women who were instructed by correspondence showed that 75% of the subjects observed mucus symptoms in every cycle[25]. In the WHO study self-recognition of cervical mucus was achieved regardless of the educational level, 94% of the women in El Salvador produced an interpretable mucus

85

pattern although 92.5% had less than 6 years schooling and 47.8% were illiterate. The subjects' understanding of the method was assessed as excellent or good in 91% after the first cycle increasing to 95% and 97% after the second and third cycles. The WHO study tended to suggest that women of low socioeconomic status and education in developing countries could learn the self-recognition of the fertile period by the mucus symptom more readily than highly educated women in developed countries. Another surprise finding was that a history of vaginal discharge did not affect the ability of the women to recognize the mucus symptom.

The WHO study provided a substantial amount of information on the characteristics of the normal menstrual cycle of a large number of women of proved fertility in the age group 18–39 years, whose cycles were not influenced by the use of hormonal or other methods of contraception. Each subject recorded her data on charts provided by the WHO. Before retiring for the night the woman made an assessment of the previous 24 hours' experience and summarized this by the use of coloured stickers, one for each day. A red sticker indicated bleeding, a green sticker an absence of blood or mucus (a dry day), a white sticker indicated mucus. She also made a written note on the nature of the mucus or if illiterate she used a symbol to show the type of mucus she had experienced. The mucus was classified into two types: the infertile type mucus which was thick, sticky, tacky and/or cloudy and the fertile type mucus which was raw egg white and was clear stretchy, slippery and/or lubricative. The last day in which fertile type mucus was noticed, or one on which a wet or lubricative sensation was felt at the vulva was designated as the peak day, which was marked by a cross superimposed upon the white stamp.

The fertile phase during which couples were advised to abstain from intercourse commenced on the first day of any recognizable mucus at the vulva whether a fertile type or infertile type and ended on the fourth day past the peak day.

Length of cycles

A total of 6472 cycles were analysed from the five centres, as shown in Table 1. The mean (±SD) length of the 6472 normal cycles was 28.5 ± 3.18 days; the median was 27.7 days. With increasing age, there was a significant trend towards shorter cycles.

Phases of the cycle

The mean length of the various phases of the menstrual cycle is shown in Table 2. The mean length of bleeding was 5.0 days for all cycles, but this varied between 4.3 days in Manila and 5.9 days in Dublin; the two centres with the longest bleeding period were in the developed countries, Dublin and Auckland. The mean length of pre-ovulatory dry days was 3.5 days for all cycles but this varied between 1.5 days in Dublin and 5.1 days in Manila. The mean duration of sticky (infertile type mucus) was 3.3 days varying from 2.3 days in San Miguel to 4.1 days in Dublin. The mean duration of slippery

Table 1 Characteristics of normal ovulatory menstrual cycles

Study	No. of cycles	Median (days)	Mean (days)
Dublin	1663	27.4	28.2
Bangalore	1996	27.8	28.7
Auckland	738	27.6	28.6
San Miguel	984	27.6	28.1
Manila	1091	28.2	28.9
Total	6472	27.7	28.5

(fertile type) mucus was 3.3 days and the centres ranged from 1.9 days in San Miguel to 4.3 days in Auckland. The length of the cycle was divided into two major phases, the follicular and the luteal phase. The last day of the slippery mucus was defined as the peak day and marked the close of the follicular phase. The mean length of the follicular phase was 15 days and the 90% frequency interval was 10.5–19.0 days. The remainder of the cycle after the 'peak day' was defined as the luteal phase and the mean length was 13.5 days.

Table 2 Phases of normal ovulatory menstrual cycles (6472 cycles in five countries)

Days	Mean	(SD)
Bleeding	5.0	(1.3)
Dry days	3.5	(2.5)
Sticky mucus (infertile type)	3.3	(2.2)
Slippery mucus (fertile type)	3.6	(1.8)

The fertile period was defined as those days on which any mucus, sticky or slippery was detected and the first 3 days after the peak day. The mean length of this fertile period was 9.6 days.

Probability of pregnancy by phase of cycle

In the WHO study, the day of every act of intercourse during the fertile phase was recorded. The available data enabled a calculation of the risk of pregnancy for each day relative to the peak day and

Table 3 Chance of pregnancy by phase of cycle

Phase	Days to peak day	Probability of pregnancy	
Sticky mucus	PD−4+	2.4	0.24
	PD−3 to −1	5.0	0.50
Slippery mucus	PD−4+	35.3	0.35
	PD−3 to −1	54.6	0.546
Peak day	PD 0	66.7	0.667
	PD 1	44.4	0.444
	PD 2	20.5	0.205
	PD 3	8.9	0.089
Outside fertile phase		0.4	0.004

PD=Peak day.

separately for both infertile and fertile types of mucus (Table 3). The risk of pregnancy in the presence of sticky (infertile type) mucus was 0.24 on peak day minus 4 or earlier but rose to 0.50 on peak day minus 3 to peak day minus 1. In the presence of slippery (fertile type) mucus, the risk was 0.353 on peak day minus 4 or earlier and rose to 0.546 on peak day minus 3 to peak day minus 1. There were nine acts recorded on the peak day out of the 7514 cycles which resulted in six pregnancies giving a pregnancy risk of 0.667. In the post-peak period, the risk declined from 0.444 on peak day plus 1 to 0.205 on peak day plus 2, and to 0.089 on peak day plus 3. Outside the fertile phase, the probability of pregnancy was 0.004. Barrett and Marshall[26], using the day of the rise in BBT as an index of ovulation, found a maximum probability on the day of the rise minus 2 of 0.30 where the conceptus had to survive 6 weeks to be included in the study. Schwartz et al.[27] had a maximum daily probability of fertilization of 0.65 and a maximum probability of conception of 0.34. Schwartz and colleagues estimated that only 0.5 of the fertilized eggs were alive after 6 weeks. The WHO study did not allow for a separate estimation of fertilization and conception rates but conception rates are so high that the loss of fertilized ova is very much lower than that reported by Schwartz.

The probability of pregnancy correlates therefore very well with the self-identification of the peak day. The interval which includes the days of mucus before the peak day and the 3 post-peak days adequately defines a fertile and an infertile phase of the menstrual cycle. This has important implications in the diagnosis and management of the infertile couple.

Outcome of pregnancies in the ovulation method

In the WHO study, data were available on the outcome of 160 pregnancies. The rates for spontaneous abortion (10%) and for congenital malformation (1.25%) were not significantly different from those reported in other series[28]. Spontaneous abortion and congenital malformation were not related to the time interval between coitus and ovulation. Likewise, timing of coitus in relation to the likely day of ovulation had no effect on the sex of the child. The study does not therefore support the suggestion that the sex of the child can be influenced by the timing of intercourse with specific relation to the estimated time of ovulation.

MITTELSCHMERZ (Intermenstrual pain)

Lower abdominal pain in one or other iliac fossa near the time of ovulation is a frequent occurrence in women during their fertile years. Volman[6] described this intermenstrual pain as acute and peristaltic in nature. In a recent study[29] incorporating ultrasound observations of the ovary and plasma LH measurements, the occurrence of mittelschmerz was investigated in a group of 96 women with regular ovulation and lower abdominal pain was noted by 34 women (35%) usually lasting 6–12 hours during the mid-cycle period. In 27 subjects the discomfort was localized to one or other iliac fossa and in all but two subjects, this corresponded with the side of the developing follicle. In the other seven subjects, the pain was central and supra-pubic. Pain occurred on the day of the LH peak in 25 (77%) of the 34 subjects. Pain occurred from 24–48 hours before the ultrasonically determined time of ovulation. The mean diameter of the follicle on the day of the pain was 19.3 ± 2.2 mm. Ovulation was confirmed in each cycle by the luteal phase urinary pregnanediol level being greater than

$6.2\,\mu\mathrm{mol}\,l^{-1}$ $(2\,\mathrm{mg}\,(24\,\mathrm{h})^{-1})$. This study shows that mittelschmerz clearly precedes ovulation and that the cause of the pain is not the rupture of the follicle. These new data suggest that the woman with a history of intermenstrual pain is having an ovulatory cycle.

Menstrual cycle molimina, pre-menstrual abdominal fullness, breast tenderness, headache, mood changes and dysmenorrhoea are grouped together as a symptom complex under the designation of pre-menstrual molimina. These symptoms occur along with the exclusively ovulatory cycles[12]. In many women, however, similar symptoms occur around the time of ovulation.

CONCLUSION

Despite the major advances in hormone assays and the development of new technology such as ultrasound, the BBT recording is still the only available device for home use which can be used to detect ovulation. Simple chemical tests or kits for predicting ovulation are being developed. At present, the subjective self-observation of the cervical mucus changes is the only method which can be used by the woman herself to predict ovulation and identify the fertile phase. Used on its own or in conjunction with temperature charting (sympto-thermal method), cervical mucus symptoms are the basis of natural family planning. These methods are of major value in the investigation and management of the infertile couple. Apart from providing evidence about the ovulatory process on a day-to-day basis these methods also provide the couple with information on the optimum timing for intercourse to achieve pregnancy. The ovulation method or symptothermal method charts are also of help in timing blood or urine collections for hormone analysis as well as interpreting the significance of the hormone results.

ACKNOWLEDGEMENTS

Most of the recent work referred to in this chapter was carried out by the World Health Organization Task Force on Methods for the Determination of the Fertile Period, Special Programme of Research, Development and Research Training in Human Reproduction.

References

1. Royston, J. P. (1982). Basal body temperature, ovulation and the risk of conception with special reference to the lifetimes of sperm and egg. *Biometrics*, **38**, 397

2. Ogino, K. (1930). Ovulationstermin und Konzeptionstermin. *Zentralbl. Gynaekol.*, **54**, 464

3. Knaus, H. (1933). Die Periodische Frucht – und Unfruchtbarkeit des Eribes. *Zentralbl. Gynaekol.*, **57**, 24

4. Van de Velde, T. H. (1905). *Uber den Zusammenhang zwischen Ovarialfunction Wellenbewegung und Mebstualblutung und Uber die Enstenhung des Sogenannten Mittelschmerzes.* (On the relationship between ovarian function, periodicity and menstrual flow, and on the origins of the so-called Mittelschmerz.), p. 39. (Bonn: Haarlem F.)

5. Marshall, J. (1965). *Planning for a Family: An Atlas of Temperature Charts*, p. 159. (London: Faber and Faber)

6. Vollman, R. F. (1977). *The Menstrual Cycle. Major Problems in Obstetrics and Gynaecology*, Vol. **7**. (Philadelphia: W. B. Saunders)

7. Zuspan, K. J. and Zuspan, F. P. (1979). Basal body temperature. In Hafex, E.S.N. (ed.) *Human Ovulation.* pp. 291–9 (Amsterdam: North Holland)

8. Moghissi, K. S., Syner, F. N. and Evans, T. (1972). A composite picture of the menstrual cycle. *Am. J. Obstet. Gynecol.*, **114**, 405

9. Marshall, J. (1963). Thermal changes in the normal menstrual cycle. *Br. Med. J.*, **1**, 102

10 Hilgers, T. W. and Bailey, A. J. (1980). Natural family planning. II. Basal body temperature and estimated time of ovulation. *Obstet. Gynecol.*, **55**, 333

11. Royston, J. P., Abrams, R. M., Higgins, M. P. and Flynn, A. (1980). The adjustment of basal body temperature measurements to allow for time of waking. *Br. J. Obstet Gynaecol.*, **87**, 1123

12. Maygar, D. M., Boyers, S. P., Marshall, J. R. and Abraham, G. E. (1978). Regular menstrual cycles and premenstrual molimina as indications of ovulation. *Obstet. Gynecol.*, **53**, 411

13. Moghissi, K. S. (1976). Accuracy of basal body temperature for ovulation detection. *Fertil. Steril.*, **27**, 1415

14. France, J. T. and Boyer, K. G. (1975). The detection of ovulation in humans and its application on contraception. *J. Reprod. Fertil. Suppl.*, **22**, 107

15. Lenton, E. A., Weston, G. A. and Cooke, I. D. (1977). Problems in using basal body temperature recordings in an infertility clinic. *Br. Med. J.*, **1**, 803

16. Billings, E. L., Billings, J. J. and Catarinich, M. (1977). *Atlas of the Ovulation Method. The Mucus Pattern of Fertility and Infertility*, 3rd edn. (Melbourne: Advocate Press)

17. Billings, E. L., Billings, J. J., Brown, J. B. and Burger, H. G. (1972). Symptoms and hormonal changes accompanying ovulation. *Lancet*, **1**, 282

18. Flynn, A. M. and Lynch, S. S. (1976). Cervical mucus and identification of the fertile phase of the menstrual cycle. *Br. J. Obstet. Gynaecol.*, **83**, 656

19. Insler, V., Melmed, H., Eden, E., Serr, D. and Lunenfeld, B. (1970). In Bettendorf, G. and Insler, V. (eds.) *Clinical Application of Human Gonadotrophins. Proceedings of a Workshop Conference, Hamburg*, p. 87. (Stuttgart: Georg Thieme Verlag)

20. Hilgers, T. W. and Prebil, A. M. (1979). The ovulation method – vulvar observations as an index of fertility/infertility. *Obstet. Gynecol.*, **53**, 12

21. Keefe, E. F. (1962). Self observation of the cervix to distinguish days of possible fertility. *Bull. Sloane Hosp. Women*, **VIII**, 129

22. World Health Organization (1981). Task Force on Methods for the Determination of the Fertile Period, Special Programme of Research, Development and Research Training in Human Reproduction. A prospective multicentre trial of the ovulation method of natural family planning. I. The Teaching Phase. *Fertil. Steril.*, **36**, 152

23. World Health Organization (1981). Task Force on Methods for the Determination of the Fertile Period, Special Programme of Research, Development and Research

91

Training in Human Reproduction. A prospective multicentre trial of the ovulation method of natural family planning. II. The Effectiveness Phase. *Fertil. Steril.*, **36**, 591

24. World Health Organization (1984). Task Force on Methods for the Determination of the Fertile Period, Special Programme of Research, Development, and Research Training in Human Reproduction. A prospective multicentre study of the ovulation method of natural family planning. III. Characteristics of the menstrual cycle and of the fertile phase. *Fertil Steril.* (In press)

25. Marshall, J. (1975). The prevalence of mucus discharge as a symptom of ovulation. *J. Bio. Sci.*, **7**, 49

26. Barrett, J. C. and Marshall, J. (1969). The risk of conception on different days of the menstrual cycle. *Pop. Stud.*, **23**, 455

27. Schwartz, D., McDonald, P. D. M. and Heuchel, V. (1980). Fecundability coital frequency and viability of ova. *Pop. Stud.*, **34**, 397

28. Huggins, G., Vessey, M., Flabel, R., Yeates, D. and McPherson, K. (1982). Vagina spermicides. Outcome of pregnancy: Findings in a large cohort study. *Contraception*, **25**, 219

29. O'Herlihy, C., Robinson, H. P. and De Crespigny, L. J. Ch. (1980). Mittelschmerz is a preovulatory symptom. *Br. Med. J.*, **280**, 986

8
A critical review of natural family planning studies

J. M. SPIELER

Periodic abstinence, rhythm and natural family planning are terms often used synonymously to describe fertility regulating methods based on the cyclic pattern of fertile and infertile phases during the menstrual cycle. Rhythm traditionally refers to the use of calendar calculations, developed by Ogino and Knaus, based on the lengths of previous menstrual cycles to estimate the days of the fertile phase. Although many couples continue to rely *solely* on such calculations they do so either because they have been found to be useful in their own situations or because they or their instructors are not aware of the newer methods based on periodic abstinence. It should be noted, however, that the calendar rhythm method has never been subjected to prospective clinical study using a well-developed protocol and subject selection criteria which minimize the chance of method failures resulting from very wide intra-woman variations in the cycle lengths. For example, using the selection criteria established for the WHO multicentre study of the ovulation method[1,2] it would not be surprising to find a theoretical effectiveness rate for the calendar method of 90–95%

General use of the term NFP began around 1971 just prior to a Research Conference on Natural Family Planning sponsored by the Human Life Foundation and the Center for Population Research, National Institute of Child Health and Human Development convened at Airlie House, Warrenton, Virginia in January 1972[3].

93

Recently there have been several reviews of methods based on periodic abstinence prepared by the Population Information Program, The Johns Hopkins University[4], the Population Crisis Committee[5], Dr H. Klaus[6] and by the International Planned Parenthood Federation (IPPF)[7]. The preface to the booklet prepared by IPPF states that 'the term "natural family planning" will not be found in this booklet ... it is not considered that these methods are entirely natural, as they require abstinence from sexual intercourse for varying times during the menstrual cycle, sometimes for more than half the cycle days'. I find this embargo on the term NFP somewhat inaccurate for two reasons. First, although slowly disappearing, sexual abstinence within marriage is still traditional and widespread in many cultures, especially during the post-partum period. Second, the 'natural' in NFP does not refer to sexual behaviour but to the monitoring of *natural* physiological signs and symptoms of the fertile phase.

Methods based on periodic abstinence appeal to persons who wish to capitalize on knowledge of the fertile and infertile phases of the menstrual cycle for their approach to family planning, or to those who do not wish to use drugs or devices either because they are concerned about their side-effects or for religious or other reasons. In addition, these methods can be used to help both avoid or achieve pregnancy by timing intercourse in relation to the infertile or fertile phase of the menstrual cycle, respectively.

Currently there are three main methods of NFP that are being promoted – the basal body temperature method (BBT); the cervical mucus method (CM), e.g. the Billings ovulation method; and the symptothermal method (S-TM). Although the BBT method alone is relatively effective if intercourse is confined to the post-ovulatory phase of the menstrual cycle the degree of abstinence required, especially during long or anovulatory cycles (for example, in post-partum or premenopausal women), detracts from its use and acceptability. The cervical mucus method is based on changes during the menstrual cycle in the quality and quantity of cervical mucus which may be subjectively assessed by women. The symptothermal method relies on a variety of indications of ovulation including cervical mucus changes, mittelschmerz, calendar calculations, etc., combined with BBT measurements. In certain circumstances the symptothermal method may be more suitable for a given woman than the cervical mucus method alone, e.g. when difficulty in assessing the changing characteristics of the mucus is experienced. On the other hand, for women using the symptothermal method who find that the mucus symptom and BBT end-points that signal the beginning of the post-ovulatory infertile phase coincide perhaps the somewhat tedious task of temperature taking and recording can be abandoned.

The physiological basis of the currently promoted NFP methods has been studied by numerous investigators, is presented in Chapter 1 and was reviewed by myself at the Tenth World Congress in Fertility and Sterility held in Madrid in July 1980[8].

Since there is controversy over the use and cost-effectiveness of NFP methods, even when a considerable effort is made in motivation and teaching, family planning administrators have hesitated to include them in national programmes despite their apparent advantages in terms of lack of side-effects, non-physician delivery and educational value. Nevertheless, there does appear to be a renewed scientific and political interest in NFP.

It is noteworthy that in June 1974 Population Reports produced their first issue on *Periodic Abstinence – Birth Control without Contraceptives*[9]; the bibliography included 126 references. In September 1981, Population Reports produced *Periodic Abstinence – How Well Do New Approaches Work?*[4]. 578 references were cited; 431 were dated between 1975 and 1981. Furthermore, during recent years the governments of several countries have enacted legislation related to family planning that specifically mentions the inclusion of NFP (e.g. Argentina, Brazil, Chile, Ireland, USA and Zambia). Numerous other governments are providing national funds to support work on NFP (e.g. Australia, Canada, France, Kiribati, Mauritius, Papua–New Guinea, Rwanda and the UK). In addition, major national and international agencies and organizations supporting family planning research and services include activities related to NFP (e.g. The Agency for International Development (AID), the Population Council, Family Health International, the Program for Applied Research on Fertility Regulation, National Institutes for Health, United Nations Fund for Population Activities and the World Health Organization). In fact, in 1981 the United States Foreign Assistance Act was amended to ensure that information and services relating to NFP methods be included among the population activities supported by AID[10].

While many family planning providers recognize the importance of NFP, those who are opposed to this approach usually do not accept that all women (couples) can use these methods, that the high theoretical effectiveness has any validity in terms of real-life

95

situations, that sexual abstinence cannot be perceived in positive terms and they believe that methods requiring daily motivation on the part of both partners are doomed to failure. Furthermore, they question the cost-effectiveness of providing NFP (which requires a labour-intensive educational delivery system and considerable follow-up) and whether the very limited demand for these methods warrants the expenditure of anything other than token support.

RESEARCH

During the past 10 or so years there have been more than 50 studies undertaken on the effectiveness of NFP. Most of these studies have been reviewed and reported in several recent publications[4-7,11]. It is not necessary to review all of this work but I will make some comments on the design of NFP studies, discuss a couple of specific trials and draw some general conclusions.

As a guest scholar at the Brookings Institute, Washington, DC in 1978-79, Paul Gross prepared a report on NFP as an appropriate health technology[12]. Amongst other things he undertook an assessment of past research on NFP. In his opinion the major weaknesses of many of the studies were the lack of multivariate data analysis and the lack of formal theory of relationships between key variables. He decided to exclude several studies from detailed analysis because: 'there were nonexistent or nonstandard protocol definitions and procedures, or inadequate study supervision, or inadequate follow-up of subjects; an inadequate number of cycles were studied; the basic demographic characteristics of the study sample were not reported; the analytical methods were deficient; there was no indication of the number of exposure cycles for different types of subjects (e.g. lactating, premenopausal); and there was exclusion ex-post of certain respondents from the final calculation of use-effectiveness without adequate justification'.

In addition to the usual question of the value of retrospective studies versus prospective studies, the 'exclusion criteria' of Gross fairly well summarize the problems associated with drawing valid conclusions from many of the clinical trials conducted on NFP. Furthermore, some of the advocates of NFP are unwilling to accept the yardsticks currently used by family planning investigators to measure effectiveness and continuation of use of contraceptive methods. Specifically, they raise the point that NFP is uniquely different from all other methods because it can be used as an aid to both prevent or achieve pregnancy. If the major rules of NFP (i.e. those governing abstinence) are broken the use of the method automatically shifts from avoiding to achieving pregnancy or vice versa. For this reason some NFP researchers classify pregnancies into two categories – planned and unplanned. The unplanned pregnancies are further classified, for example by Brennan and Klaus[13] into 'method-related' (those that occur despite correct application of the rules), 'informed choice' (those that result from a conscious decision to have intercourse on fertile days without previous indication of planning a pregnancy), 'teaching-related' (those that occur from an error in the application of the rules, whether due to incorrect teaching or to not learning correctly), and 'unresolved' pregnancies that cannot be categorized because of insufficient data. Using these categories Brennan and Klaus[13] have reviewed four NFP studies and report method effectiveness rates ranging from 98.5 to 100% and informed-choice pregnancy rates up to 23% (life table rate).

In the WHO prospective multicentre trial of the Billings ovulation method[2] the unplanned pregnancies were classified as method-related, inadequate teaching, inaccurate application of instructions, conscious departure from the rules and uncertain. Using these categories the pregnancy rates reported for the 725 subjects who learned the method and entered a 13-cycle effectiveness cycle study were 2.8, 0.4, 3.5, 15.4, and 0.5 pregnancies per 100 woman-years (modified Pearl index), respectively. However, the important point for family planning programme administrators is that the use-effectiveness, regardless of sub-classifications, in some quite good studies have shown a range of about 5–40 pregnancies per 100 woman-years[4]. These studies also emphasize that the effectiveness of NFP appears to depend greatly upon the motivation of the couple, the couple's family planning intention, the quality of the instruction provided and to a lesser extent the regularity of the phenomena monitored to identify the fertile period.

A study that is particularly noteworthy was conducted by Hilgers et al.[14] in Nebraska and Missouri between 1977 and 1980. The 559 subjects (couples) in the study were provided with high-quality instruction in the Billings ovulation method using a 'new picture dictionary' and follow-up forms that permitted the standardization of the teaching and of recording mucus observations. In the introductory session the couples were taught that there was no such thing as 'taking a chance' in the use of the method. The couples were taught that to have intercourse on the days of fertility was to use the method as a means of achieving pregnancy and that if the method was to be used to avoid pregnancy, intercourse must be confined to the infertile days of the cycle. Pregnancies occurring during the study were to be classified as 'achieving-related', 'avoiding-related' and 'unresolved'.

The investigators stated that the major justification for the study appears to be the fact that 'without exception, (previous) studies have ignored the uniqueness of NFP' and that the study would assess 'the effectiveness of the ovulation method as a means of achieving as well as avoiding pregnancy'. In this respect, it is important to note that of the 1012 women who attended the introductory session, 204 (20.2%) were excluded from the study because they entered as *infertility patients*, 113 (11.2%) decided not to use the ovulation method, 10 (0.9%) were already pregnant and 126 (12.5%) were not 'genitally active'. The remaining 559 patients (55.2%) formed the basis of the study.

Of the 559 subjects, 44% had 'regular cycles' at entry; the remaining 56% included women with long cycles, breast-feeding women, post-pill women and premenopausal women. Contrary to what Gross[12] suggests the further analysis of the data is not stratified by different reproductive categories of the volunteers.

The cumulative adjusted pregnancy rate at 12 months was 26.5% (total) – 21.3% 'achieving-related' and 5.2% 'avoiding-related'. The method and use-effectiveness rates at 12 months in couples choosing to avoid pregnancy were 99.6% and 94.8%, respectively (based on 4957 couple-months of use). The discontinuation rate at 12 months was 47.8% – 21.3% 'planned pregnancies', 5.2% 'unplanned pregnancies', 13.4% 'discontinuers' (7% switched to an 'artificial' method, 3.4% discontinued for 'personal reasons', 1.1% switched to another NFP method and 0.9% had difficulty with abstinence) and 7.7% were lost to follow-up. The continuation rate for those using the method to avoid pregnancy was 52.2%.

Perhaps the most noteworthy facet of this study was the fact that the so-called achieving-related adjusted pregnancy rates at 12 and 18 months were *only* 21.3% and 26.8%, respectively, especially since infertile couples were not admitted into the study. It appears that couples were placed in the category of using the method to achieve pregnancy by the project staff if they had intercourse on fertile days, which is consistent with the way the method is taught by the investigators. If these couples were actually trying to achieve pregnancy you would expect that at least 25% would become pregnant in the first month[1]. Furthermore, 36.5% of the so-called achievers stated that the pregnancy was unplanned. The authors explain this paradox by stating that pregnancy 'achieving-related behaviour and achieving-related intention do not always coincide'.

The authors have used an interesting study design which they believe is more appropriate for the evaluation of NFP methods. However, the results do not differ much from the first trial of the ovulation method[15] where it was decided not to include in the calculation of use-effectiveness the 50 pregnancies in women who 'took a chance'. Couples are free to exercise their right to abstain or not during the fertile period and thus the effectiveness of NFP is directly proportional to the motivation of the couple to avoid pregnancy. This is one of the reasons why family planning programmes that are interested in having an impact on demographic statistics are somewhat hesitant to promote the use of methods that are coitus-related, especially those methods like NFP which require continued motivation on the part of *both* partners.

In order to avoid the problem of distinguishing between unplanned and planned pregnancies in research studies, WHO[1,2] adopted the convention of asking women at each follow-up interview if they wished to continue to use the method to avoid pregnancy in the next cycle. If the reply was affirmative then all pregnancies occurring in the next cycle were considered as unplanned. This system is recognized as inappropriate for use in family planning service delivery programmes but in a research study aimed at assessing the effectiveness of NFP it was considered essential.

It is worthwhile to mention some of the results of NFP studies conducted in India.

Dorairaj[16] developed a modified mucus method of family planning to simplify and 'improve the acceptability of NFP in couples of high fertility who are illiterate with a low motivation to control fertility and high pro-child values'. Preliminary results showed that in 1977 acceptors there were 65 drop-outs of which five were due to unplanned pregnancy. A Pearl index failure rate was calculated for 15 052 months of use at 0.39 pregnancies per 100 woman-years. The effectiveness rate calculated with a life table method was reported to be 0.992 with a standard error of 0.19. The modified mucus method was studied in five Indian cities with a total of 3758 women contributing

33 210 months of use resulting in a failure rate of 1.59 pregnancies per 100 woman-years (range between centres 0.39–17.2). These results are indeed surprising and it is unfortunate that few details are available on the actual study design, admission criteria, follow-up procedure, data collection forms, etc.

The Indo-German Social Service Society in New Delhi prepared an All India Documentation and Evaluation Report (AIDER) on NFP in India[17]. The conclusions are summarized in Section V of the report with the preface that 'the limitations and all possible inaccuracies of the data collected from the diocesan half-yearly progress reports are realized'. Some of the information provided in the conclusion of the report is quoted below:

(1) '182 districts including 3062 villages and 333 towns are covered by the NFP Programme.'

(2) 'There are 2427 NFP Centres functioning and 1920 workers (81% lay and 19% religious) working mostly part-time.'

(3) 'Over the period from January 1978 to December 1980, as many as 96 641 NFP user-couples have been recruited and are being followed-up in 61 dioceses.'

(4) 'Hindu and other religion user-couples constitute 68% and Christians are 32%, which reveals that NFP is accepted widely by all user-couples irrespective of religion.'

(5) 'Nearly two-thirds of the user-couples are either illiterates or have studied up to primary school level.'

(6) 'The continuation rate after 36 months of NFP use was 92.5%.'

(7) 'The overall average cost for recruiting and following-up one NFP user-couple works out to Rs.42 (about $4.00) over an average period of 2 years. The overall staff-to-user couples ratio comes to 1 : 50.'

(8) 'A total 2478 pregnancies have been reported of which 1718 were planned pregnancies and 760 were unplanned ones. Taking the total number of user-couples as 96 641, of whom 760 couples had pregnancies against their wish, it can be considered that the NFP Programme has been effective to the extent of 99.2% during the period covered by the report.'

Unfortunately, without details of all aspects of the study these 'service program' results can only be considered interesting but not necessarily valid.

In terms of the ability of women to learn the ovulation method, the

WHO-supported studies did show that 94% of women representing a wide range of cultural, educational and socioeconomic characteristics were able to recognize and record the cervical mucus symptom which allows self-recognition of the fertile period[1,2].

Some advocates of the Billings ovulation method claim that the method can be used to pre-select the sex of the baby. According to this theory intercourse on days when the cervical mucus begins to thin out, becomes stretchy and produces a lubricative, slippery feeling tends to result in a girl. Intercourse confined to the day of 'peak fertility' (i.e. the last day of raw egg-white-type mucus) tends to result in a boy. The only study cited by Dr Billings in her book entitled *The Billings Method*[18] confirming this theory took place in Nigeria. Quoting from the book, 'success in pre-selection of a boy was achieved by 310 couples. Failure in pre-selection of a boy occurred in four couples. Success in pre-selection of a girl was achieved in 90 couples. Failure in pre-selection of a girl occurred in two couples.' That is, 310 out of 314 couples (98.7%) were successful in conceiving a boy and 90 out of 92 couples (97.8%) in conceiving a girl. These findings are incredible but unsubstantiated. In fact, they could not be corroborated in the WHO multicentre study of the ovulation method[19]. Among the 140 live births where the sex of the child was known, there were 81 males and 59 females (58% males). Among children conceived 2–5 days before the day of 'peak fertility' there were 14 males and nine females (61% males). For those conceived 2–4 days after the day of 'peak fertility' there were 18 males and nine females (67% males) and among those conceived within 1 day of the 'peak', 27 males and 22 females (55% males). For the method failures (intercourse apparently occurring outside the fertile period as defined by the cervical mucus symptoms) there were six males and seven females (46% males). The WHO study concludes that meaningful differences were not observed in the sex ratios of offspring conceived on different days in relation to the presumed day of ovulation. However, it was noteworthy that the lowest proportion of male births was seen among method failures, where it would be expected that the coital act leading to conception would be relatively far removed from the day of 'peak fertility'.

In order to improve the effectiveness of NFP one can either try to improve the existing methods (through, for example, modifications of the methods or improvement of their service delivery) or develop entirely new methods. It is not the intention of this paper to deal

101

with this subject in depth but, again, some of the recent WHO findings are particularly worthy of mention. The WHO efforts in this field have been described during the past few years in the Annual Reports of the Special Program of Research, Development and Research Training in Human Reproduction[20]. Work on the rationale for the development of simple chemical tests to identify the start and duration of the fertile period based on measuring conjugated metabolites of oestrogen and progesterone in early-morning urine samples was reported by the WHO Task Force on Methods for the Determination of the Fertile Period[21]. A prospective study of the time intervals between indices used in NFP to locate the probable fertile period and those obtained from the application of non-invasive, immunochemicals tests was conducted by the WHO Task Force[22]. For this study the probable fertile period was defined as the day of the urinary LH peak −3 to the day of the LH peak +2.

Some of the main findings included:

(1) The symptothermal method gave the highest mean value for the apparent duration of the fertile period (13.4 days; range 9–21) and entirely covered the whole of the probable fertile period in all but 2% of cycles. An examination of the data showed that the calendar calculation for the start of the fertile period (shortest cycle length −18) was used in 32 cycles (55%), the first day of cervical mucus secretion in 15 cycles (26%) and in 11 cycles (19%) the signal from both variables occurred in the same day. In contrast, the day of the peak mucus +4 was used to signal the last day of the fertile period in 28 cycles (48%), the BBT shift +3 in 16 cycles (28%) and in 14 cycles (24%) both signals occurred in the same day.

(2) The mean duration of the fertile period using the ovulation method only was slightly shorter (11.9 days, range 5–29) than the symptothermal method. However, this was associated with a corresponding increase in the number of cycles (9%) where the fertile period was not completely covered by the method.

(3) The mean duration of the fertile period using a calendar calculation (shortest cycle length −18) to identify the start and the BBT shift +3 to determine the end of the fertile period was 11.8 days (range 6–21). The number of cycles where the defined fertile period was incompletely covered increased to 10%,

mainly caused by the end-signal occurring during the probable fertile period.

(4) The immunochemical test based on concentration changes of urinary oestrone-3-glucuronide (day of defined rise to peak level +4) gave a mean fertile period duration of only 9.3 days but the proportion of possible failures rose to 17%.

(5) The duration of the fertile period using an immunochemical test based on the ratio of urinary oestrone-3-glucuronide to pregnanediol-3α-glucuronide (day of defined rise to peak ratio day +5) was 10.7 days with 16% of the fertile periods not covered by the method.

In summary, because of the imprecision of the NFP methods the duration of the fertile period is somewhat longer than for the immuno-chemical tests, but the NFP methods better circumscribe a defined period of maximum fertility. The predictive value of the two immuno-chemical tests may render them more suitable for use in the infertility clinic than as aids for NFP.

CONCLUSION

As with research on all methods of family planning there are well-designed and poorly designed studies. Perhaps there are a greater proportion of 'non-studies' of NFP reported in the literature compared with other methods. The reason for this, I believe, relates to the fact that NFP is not a commercial product and there is, relatively speaking, almost no money going into this field. The majority of NFP investigators are still working at the grass-roots level and have not experienced the luxury of available funds for hiring research staff, purchasing or subcontracting computer facilities, conducting sophisticated research studies and promoting the use of NFP; *contraception is a big business, NFP is not*. Nevertheless, it appears that:

(1) When the rules of the methods, particularly those pertaining to sexual abstinence, are adhered to NFP is highly effective in preventing pregnancy.

(2) Knowledge of the fertile period and the practice of NFP can be an extremely useful aid in helping subfertile and normal couples achieve pregnancy.

(3) NFP requires an educational delivery system with access to medical facilities. Its cost-effectiveness will be relatively low

at first but over the long run it should be high, especially if services continue to be provided primarily by non-physician volunteers.

(4) NFP, like all other available methods, surely is not suitable for everybody. However, about half of the women who entered the WHO five-country study of the Billings ovulation method completed the project in a non-pregnant state[2]. They had found a method that suited their needs and behaviour. One of the challenges before us is to ensure that couples who may be suited to NFP have access to high-quality and efficient services, especially from among those who have found the currently available so-called artificial methods unacceptable and are therefore not practising contraception.

References

1. WHO Task Force on Methods for the Determination of the Fertile Period (1981). A prospective multicentre trial of the ovulation method. I. The teaching phase. *Fertil. Steril.*, **36,** 152
2. WHO Task Force on Methods for the Determination of the Fertile Period (1981). A prospective multicentre trial of the ovulation method. II. The effectiveness phase. *Fertil. Steril.*, **36,** 591
3. Uricchio, W. and Williams, M. K. (1973). *Proceedings of a Research Conference on Natural Family Planning.* (Washington, D.C.: The Human Life Foundation)
4. Liskin, L. (1981). Periodic abstinence: How well do new approaches work? *Pop. Rep.*, Series I, No. 3
5. Population Crisis Committee (1981). Natural family planning: Periodic abstinence as a method of fertility control. *Population,* **11**
6. Klaus, H. (1982). Natural family planning: A review. *Obstet. Gynecol. Survey,* **37** (Suppl.), 128
7. Kleinman, R. (1983). *Periodic Abstinence for Family planning.* (London: IPPF medical publications)
8. Spieler, J. (1981). Self-detection of ovulation and the fertile period. In Cortes-Prieto, J., Campos de Paz, A. and Neves-e-Castro, M. (eds.) *Research on Fertility and Sterility,* pp. 35–51. (Lancaster: MTP Press)
9. Ross, C. and Piotrow, P. (1974). Birth control without contraceptives. *Pop. Rep.,* Series I, No. 1
10. Bureau for Program and Policy Coordination (1982). *A.I.D. policy paper: Population Assistance,* p. 7. (U.S. Agency for International Development)
11. Department of Health, Dublin, Ireland (1979). *International Seminar on Natural Family Planning.* (Dublin: Cahill Printers)
12. Gross, P. (1979). NFP as an appropriate health technology: Towards an agenda for global research and development. *Int. Rev. Nat. Fam. Plann.,* **3,** 279
13. Brennan, J. and Klaus, H. (1982). Terminology and core curricula in natural family planning. *Fertil. Steril.,* **38,** 117
14. Hilgers, T., Prebil, A. and Daly, K. (1980). The effectiveness of the ovulation method as a means of achieving and avoiding pregnancy. Presented at the

Education Phase III, Continuing Education Conference for Natural Family Planning Practitioners, July 24, Omaha

15. Weissman, M., Foliaki, L., Billings, E. and Billings, J. (1972). A trial of the ovulation method of family planning in Tonga. *Lancet,* **2,** 813
16. Dorairaj, K. (1981). The modified mucus method of family planning. *Bul. Nat. Fam. Plann. Assoc. India,* **4,** 1
17. All India Documentation and Evaluation Report (1981). *Natural Family Planning in India.* (New Delhi: Indo-German Social Service Society)
18. Billings, E. and Westmore, A. (1980). *The Billings Method,* p. 70. (Victoria, Australia: Anne O'Donovan Pty)
19. WHO Task Force on Methods for the Determination of the Fertile Period (1983). A prospective multicentre trial of the ovulation method. IV. The outcome of pregnancies with particular reference to the sex of offspring and the occurrence of spontaneous abortions and congenital malformations. *Fertil. Steril.* (In press)
20. World Health Organization (1975–1982). *Fourth–Eleventh Annual Reports, Special Programme of Research, Development and Research Training in Human Reproduction.* (Geneva: WHO)
21. WHO Task Force on Methods for the Determination of the Fertile Period (1982). The measurement of urinary steroid glucuronides as indices of the fertile period in women. *J. Steroid Biochem.,* **17,** 695
22. WHO Task Force on Methods for the Determination of the Fertile Period (1983). Temporal relationships between indices of the fertile period. *Fertil. Steril.,* **39,** 647

105

Part I

Section 3

Fertilization *in Vitro* and *in Vivo*

9
Current status of human *in vitro* fertilization

R. G. EDWARDS

The situation today concerning human fertilization *in vitro* has been transformed beyond recognition. From the early, challenging ideas of 1965[1] the clinical opportunities of the method were first demonstrated in 1977, when the first embryo implanted after replacement in the uterus; unfortunately, this turned out to be an ectopic pregnancy[2]. Two years later, the birth of the first children conceived through *in vitro* fertilization ushered in the beginnings of this new form of clinical medicine for the alleviation of infertility and, perhaps, for the avoidance of inherited disorders by identifying embryos which were afflicted with genetic disorders. Today, the potential of *in vitro* fertilization as the cure for infertility has been amply proved, as I hope to show in this chapter.

Several steps in the procedure had to be solved before it became a clinical treatment. Most aspects of the work are now under a large measure of control today. There is no difficulty in persuading one or more follicles to grow in the ovary, by the use of treatments such as clomiphene, human menopausal gonadotrophin (HMG), tamoxifen or combinations of these methods. Indeed, several oocytes have been collected from ovaries since 1970, when mild forms of superovulation in cyclic women were introduced[3]. Different clinics now use various methods most suited to their own requirements, and have developed monitoring systems enabling them to assess follicular growth by ultrasound or by endocrine measurements. It is not difficult to induce the growth of several follicles in a patient, and many will ovulate in response to an endogenous LH surge or to an injection of human chorionic gonadotrophin (HCG). Moreover, simpler methods of aspirating oocytes are being introduced. This was first suggested by Lentz and Lauritsen in 1982[4], and by Wikland and his associates[5], and excellent progress in the ultrasonic aspiration of oocytes has been reported recently by several groups of workers[6]. This method promises to avoid the need for general anaesthesia for many patients, to simplify the whole procedure for aspirating oocytes and to open up new non-invasive methods of examining follicles and other internal organs. Laparoscopy is still the most widely used method for collecting oocytes, with very high levels of success. Some indication of the incidence of success with these methods is provided in a recent series of 150 patients in Bourn Hall; one or more preovulatory oocytes were collected from 96% of them, and the proportion of oocytes from individual follicles approached 90%. Other clinics have reported similar success rates, and it is clear that the endocrine and surgical methods for aspirating oocytes are becoming simplified and routine.

There is, however, at least one reservation about these treatments used to stimulate ovulation. We do not know enough about the nature of growth of individual follicles, especially under conditions of heavy superovulation. The only measure to assess growth is by ultrasound, which measures the size of a follicle, but this is not enough. The largest follicle is not necessarily the most advanced, and smaller follicles may be preovulatory[3,7]. It was clear some years ago that there was some variation in the degree of maturation amongst the several follicles responding to human menopausal gonadotrophins[8], implying that some follicles are more mature than others. This observation was based on the varying steroid concentrations in different follicles. Perhaps such variations are unimportant endocrinologically, because the dominant or leading follicles may be able to sustain an adequate luteal phase and a pregnancy. On the other hand, it is possible that the luteinization of several follicles, resulting in high levels of plasma progesterone in the luteal phase, may lead to disorders in uterine development, and this point has not been satisfactorily established in any clinic as far as I am aware.

Another, perhaps more important consideration arises from the growth of several follicles. Since follicles vary in their developmental maturation, the oocytes may also vary in their potential. An arbitrarily timed injection of HCG could induce some oocytes to mature before they were fully competent to do so, e.g. before they had fully completed their preovulatory synthesis of proteins. The incidence of fertilization, the growth of embryos *in vitro*, and – most important – the incidence of implantation could therefore vary among oocytes collected from follicles in different stages of growth, and this may be reflected in poor performance results for *in vitro* fertilization as a whole. There is, indeed, clear evidence from our own work that the occurrence of a natural LH surge after treatment with clomiphene gives higher rates of pregnancy than does treatment with clomiphene

Table 1 Clinical pregnancies in relation to the treatment and the number of embryos replaced*

No. of embryos replaced	Natural Cycle		Clomiphene/ LH surge		Clomiphene/HCG		Other stimulants	
	No. of patients	No. (%) pregnant	No. of patients	No. (%) pregnant	No. of patients	No. (%) pregnant	No. of patients	No. (%) pregnant
One	250	38 (15.2)	228	37 (16.2)	109	13 (11.9)	31	4 (12.8)
Two	7	1 (14.3)	111	34 (30.6)	111	25 (22.5)	10	3 (30.0)
Three			8	3 (37.5)	15	2 (13.3)	10	2 (20.0)
Four					1	1		

*The binomial expansion for clomiphene/LH surge, where a = 0.16, predicts 33 pregnancies when two embryos are replaced, and 3.3 after replacing three. With clomiphene/HCG, where a = 0.12, 24.9 pregnancies would be expected with two embryos and 4.8 with three. Reproduced from reference 9, with permission.

and injection of HCG (Table 1). The reason could well be that the dominant follicle causes the LH surge and also produces an embryo which is capable of implanting more successfully than are oocytes produced in response to HCG. The HCG is administered at a convenient time to perform subsequent laparoscopy, and not because of any clear indication that follicles are ready to ovulate; its use in such an arbitrary manner may be 'paid for' by a lower rate of implantation. We therefore make great efforts to permit the LH surge to occur, and to monitor it very carefully; HCG is given only when oestrogen levels are very high, large (> 2.0 cm) follicles are present, and the LH surge has not begun. Laparoscopy for oocyte recovery is then carried out 26 hours after the first rising assay for urinary LH, or 34–36 hours after an injection of HCG.

There can also be little doubt that fertilization and embryonic growth *in vitro* are under a high degree of control in many clinics. In

our experience, the rates of fertilization are very high – over 90% –
provided the samples of semen contain progressively motile spermatozoa, and are free of antibodies, inflammatory cells or debris (Table
2). Under such circumstances, more than 90% of oocytes are fertilized,

Table 2 Incidence of fertilization *in vitro**

	Total no. of patients	No. (%) with one oocyte fertilized	% Oocytes fertilized
Influence of various conditions in semen			
Spermatozoa:			
Satisfactory	95	87 (92)	85
Head clumps, viscous			
seminal plasma	11	10 (90)	95
Some cells/debris	25	20 (80)	70
Many immotile,			
sluggish/erratic	20	12 (60)	50
Massive clumping	10	5 (50)	45
Tail agglutination,			
many immotile	12	5 (41)	41
Massive cells/debris	7	2 (30)	30
Results with various groups of patients			
Tubal	95	87 (92)	85
Oligospermic†	31	23 (74)	65
'Idiopathic'	10	9 (90)	80

*Reproduced from reference 10, with permission.
†Fertilization rates depend on the presence of agglutination, inflammatory cells, etc.
in the semen.

and more than 95% of the subsequent embryos are replaced in the
mother. Such levels of success are so high that rare variations in
spermatozoa such as ultrastructural or biochemical defects, or the
aspiration of a few incompletely matured oocytes, could explain the
failure rate. The medium used is very simple: Earle's solution with
pyruvate, penicillin and the patient's own inactivated serum. It would
be difficult to find a simpler medium, yet it sustains the growth of
embryos until blastocysts[1]. Some clearly obvious conditions in semen
reduce fertilization rates drastically: antibodies causing clumping
of the spermatozoa, inflammatory damage resulting in numerous
leukocytes and other cells in the semen, large amounts of debris of
unknown origin, and inadequate forward movement of spermatozoa.
These problems offer a major area for research at the present time in
order to improve success rates for patients with these afflictions. We

believe that studies on the male could result in the alleviation of a great deal of infertility and stress for those couples.

Many unusual observations have been made on fertilization and embryonic growth *in vitro*. Increasingly, it is becoming apparent that the final stages of oocyte maturation can be completed *in vitro*, and that many pregnancies can result. In Bourn Hall, we must sometimes advance the timing of laparoscopy because the beginning of the LH surge indicates oocyte recovery at some impossibly early hour in the morning. Under such circumstances, the oocytes are collected in late evening and are matured overnight in a mixture of follicular fluid and culture medium. The procedure was introduced some years ago when delays arose during the collection of sperm by individual men. Even when insemination is delayed, many oocytes retain an excellent morphology *in vitro*. They can be fertilized, will cleave normally, and produce pregnancies. Much more information is needed on the degree of success with such treatments, in comparison with the use of oocytes which are fully mature when aspirated from their follicle and inseminated immediately and such data will accumulate over the coming years. One clinic has reported that two oocytes matured *in vitro* for longer periods developed into live births[12]. Obviously, the successful maturation of oocytes *in vitro* would relieve many of the pressures on the timing of operations for oocyte collection. If, for example, oocytes could be collected at, say 15–20 hours after the LH surge, matured *in vitro*, fertilized and developed into embryos, and then implanted at rates similar to those collected later, then the clinical convenience could be considerable.

There is also much evidence to show that fertilization can be delayed for some time, without precluding the chance of pregnancy. In two of our patients at least, fertilization was delayed by many hours – perhaps up to 20 hours – after the oocytes were aspirated from their follicles (Table 3). Yet the embryos developed *in vitro*, and some appeared to cleave more quickly and normally as if they were 'catching up' on the developmental programme, and two healthy children were born. We would not counsel that insemination is routinely delayed after oocyte aspiration, but it is comforting to know that delays in the collection of spermatozoa, or some other unforeseen difficulty leading to a delayed insemination, do not necessarily prevent a successful outcome to the treatment. This evidence is also fascinating in showing that delayed fertilization can lead to normal diploid development in man, because it is associated with polyspermy and digyny in animal eggs[14]. Perhaps the human oocyte can retain its block to polyspermy for long periods under the conditions

Table 3 Timing of embryonic development *in vitro* in two cases of prolonged delay in insemination*

Hours after begin- ning of LH surge	Hours after oocyte recovery	Stage of development	Development of freshly insemi- nated embryost
		Patient 1	
34	8	Insemination	–
56	30	1-cell (no pronu- clei)	
59	33	1-cell (additional sperm added)	
84	58	? syngamy	4-cell
87	61	3-cell	
108	81	6-cell	8/16-cell
110	83	6-cell embryo re- placed into mother	
		Patient 2	
42	19	Insemination	
58	35	1-cell	
83	60	4-cell	4-cell
92	69	8-cell	4-cell
94	71	8-cell embryo re- placed into mother	

*Reproduced from reference 13, with permission.
†Reproduced from reference 11, with permission.

used for culture, and it is even possible that their storage in a mixture of culture media and follicular fluid is preferable to conditions in the oviduct, which may predispose to polyspermy.

The greatest problem concerning *in vitro* fertilization still remains the induction of implantation, a difficulty that has faced us since 1970. The rates of implantation are still depressingly low in some clinics, and it is obvious that standards of quality control at all stages of follicular growth, ovulation, laparoscopy, fertilization and cleavage *in vitro* and embryo replacement are essential if satisfactory success is to be obtained through *in vitro* fertilization. The first problem to solve undoubtedly concerns the method of replacement of embryos. We have developed a catheter, called the Wallace catheter, which is simple, non-toxic, and very easy to use. With skill, it can be passed simply and easily through the cervical canal, adapting its shape to the canal as it moves forward. It can be given some support if needed by a stiffer movable outer catheter. The whole procedure of replacing embryos, from the loading of embryos into the catheter to the final check to make sure the embryos have left it, can take less than 1 minute. The procedure is non-traumatic, performed without anaesthesia, but very skilful, and the latter factor is perhaps instrumental in gaining high rates of success. In our work in Bourn Hall, success

Table 4 Analysis of the incidence of pregnancy and abortion following embryo replacement*

Date	No. of patients replaced	No. with clinical pregnancies (%)	Incidence of abortion (%)
Oct. 1980 – 5 Mar. 1982	515†	85 (16.5)	24 (28.2)
6 Mar. 1982 – 18 Sept. 1982	316‡	52 (16.5)	18 (34.6)
19 Sept. 1982 – 31 Dec. 1982	162	38 (23.5)	10 (26.3)
1 Jan. 1983 – 28 Feb. 1983	82	24 (29.2)	
1 Mar. 1983 – 30 Apr. 1983	125	36 (28.1)	

*Reproduced from reference 9, with permission.
†'Biochemical' pregnancies identified in 15 of these patients; ‡'Biochemical' pregnancies identified in >20 of these patients – these have not been included as clinical pregnancies.

rates have exceeded 30% in 1983 (Table 4), which is a wonderful tribute to the skill of the people working in embryo growth and replacement.

Some detailed evidence is now indicating the nature of some of the factors which may be involved in the implantation of embryos. There is no doubt that replacing two or more embryos is more successful than replacing one. Indeed, it is only this observation which has led us to abandon the natural menstrual cycle and use stimulated cycles. However, the incidence of pregnancy in our hands using the natural cycle is much higher than in other clinics using stimulated cycles and replacing two or more embryos. The rate of implantation when clomiphene is combined with an LH surge is approximately 16% with one embryo, 31% with two embryos, and 38% with three, which reflects a binomial progression in the rate of implantation (Table 1). The results are obviously highly encouraging. These data were obtained until the end of 1982; recently, success rates have increased even more.

A slightly lower result is obtained from our patients given clomiphene and HCG to induce ovulation (Table 1). In them, the rates of implantation were lower with one, two or three embryos, even though the same embryologists were using the same methods on both groups of patients. This observation is most interesting. Embryos arising

Table 5 Effect of age on implantation (until 31 December 1982)

	Natural cycle		Clomiphene/LH surge		Clomiphene/HCG	
Age of patients	Total No.	No. with clinical pregnancies (%)	Total No.	No. with clinical pregnancies (%)	Total No.	No. with clinical pregnancies (%)
20–24	3	0	4	0	1	0
25–29	42	7 (16.7)	49	10 (20.4)	32	7 (21.9)
30–34	116	19 (16.4)	158	42 (26.6)	101	18 (17.8)
35–39	89	12 (13.5)	136	22 (23.5)	102	16 (15.7)
40+	6	0 (0)	29	1 (3.4)	14	1 (7.1)
20–39	250	38 (15.2)	347	74 (21.3)	236	41 (17.4)

Table 6 Maternal age and abortion*

	All stimulated cycles		Natural cycle		
Age and no. of embryos replaced	No. pregnant	No. aborted	No. pregnant	No. aborted	Overall (%)
25–29:					
Single	5	2	7	0	16.7
Multiple	12	3			25
30–34:					
Single	30	6	19	7	26.5
Multiple	35	11			31.4
35–39:					
Single	19	4	12	7	35.5
Multiple	22	10			45.5
40+:					
Single	2	1			50
Multiple	2	2			100

*Overall data: single replacements in stimulated cycles, 23.2%; single replacements in natural cycle, 36.8%; multiple replacements in stimulated cycles, 36.6%.

from clomiphene/HCG might be slightly less viable than those obtained after clomiphene and an LH surge as discussed earlier. On the other hand, poorer endocrine conditions in the mother might arise after the use of HCG as compared with an LH surge, which would not be surprising to physiologists. There are, at present, no studies on the endometrium to find out if these two forms of treatment result in differing uterine responses. It is possible to develop statistical models based on our observations which explain why success with clomiphene/HCG is far less successful than with clomiphene/LH surge, especially when three or more embryos are replaced. It is, indeed, highly essential to develop such models, and to develop parameters to estimate the success on embryonic growth, maternal capacity to implant one or more embryos and individual variations in response to treatments. Success can be influenced by various factors, e.g. maternal age (Tables 5 and 6). Such knowledge would enable us to produce the most effective treatment for individual patients, which must be the primary target for all of us. At present, we would recommend clomiphene with an LH surge as preferable treatment, followed by clomiphene combined with HMG and an LH surge. This is again the reason why we believe it is essential to monitor closely the follicular phase of our patients within the Clinic, and so increase the chances of implantation.

An obvious benefit arises from the replacement of two or more embryos or the occurrence of some multipregnancies. We have had many twins and rare triplet pregnancies, especially with clomiphene/

Table 7 Incidence of multipregnancy

No. of embryos replaced	Clomiphene/LH surge		Clomiphene/HCG	
	Single	Twin	Single	Twin
2	9	3	11	8
3		1		

HCG (Table 7). How curious that the incidence of implantation is greater with clomiphene/LH, but the incidence of multipregnancy is greater with clomiphene/HCG. Obviously, the birth of twins is helpful to many mothers, enabling them to establish their family at one attempt, and this must be an important factor in our calculations of the success of *in vitro* fertilization.

Why, then, do more twins arise with clomiphene/HCG which is less successful if one embryo is replaced? Once again, it is essential to try to understand the factors involved, and to produce statistical models which enable us to predict the best interests of each patient.

117

At present, we can explain theoretically the high incidence of twins with clomiphene/HCG, and the lower incidence of implantation with this treatment through the poorer ability of mothers to implant their embryos[9]. Clearly, studies on implantation – on its endocrinology, physiology and statistics – are now urgently needed because success rates through embryo replacement might even surpass those attained following conception *in vivo* during the natural menstrual cycle. Many commentators have predicted that the success of *in vitro* fertilization will maximize at approximately 25% of replacements, i.e. the rate during natural conception. I have always disagreed with this pessimistic outlook on the success of *in vitro* fertilization.

By now, more than 110 babies have been born from work in Bourn Hall, and another three from the earlier work in Oldham, and more than 300 pregnancies have been established. We believe that these figures represent approximately one-half of the world's total. None of the children has any serious physical anomaly, hence we can conclude that *in vitro* fertilization does not appear to be associated with any teratological damage to the child. Follow-up studies on the children are needed, and are being carried out in Bourn Hall, and no overt problems have arisen with the growth of these children up to the age of 5 years. There is a slight excess of girls among the children, whereas a slight excess of boys occurs after conception *in vivo*; we have insufficient information to decide if this difference is significant.

There is no doubt now that *in vitro* fertilization is an acceptable and desirable treatment of infertility, becoming widely practised, and simpler with increasing experience. Further increase in success rates will result in it becoming the primary treatment of female infertility and some forms of male infertility. Such indices of success imply that new clinical treatments may soon be introduced: e.g. the identification of embryos with genetic defects. Already, DNA probes are being introduced which can identify characteristics in a few cells, e.g. probes for the Y chromosome in mice[13], and other Y probes, may be effective with human tissues. Identifying the sex of an embryo through the sex-determining genes on the Y chromosome would be a beginning for such a genetic programme, and would indicate its potential by showing that heterozygous (carrier) embryos can be identified. Perhaps too, the study of embryos *in vitro* until slightly later stages of growth – now increasingly accepted by many authorities pronouncing on the ethics of *in vitro* fertilization – would yield stem cells capable of repairing haemopoietic, neural, myocardial and other tissues in children and adults. These exciting possibilities are becoming closer as the advantages of *in vitro* fertilization become apparent.

The introduction of *in vitro* fertilization into clinical practice on a wide scale has also led to many fundamental studies on human reproduction. So many studies have begun or are impending: e.g. endocrinological studies on the astonishing diurnal rhythm in the timing of the LH surge and, inevitably, of ovulation in women, the close relationship between the daily LH rhythm and the daily cortisol rhythm, and the analysis of inhibin and other factors in follicular fluid. Studies on gametes include the karyotyping of human oocytes to find out the causes of chromosomal imbalance, the identification of defective spermatozoa at the ultrastructural level and the use of probes to find out deficient elemental components. Embryonic studies include the factors leading to polyspermy in eggs, the conditions necessary for the growth of embryos to blastocysts and their hatching from the zona pellucida and the differentiation of embryonic stem cells. These are opportunities offering the widest scope for research. I have commented on these elsewhere, and would merely like to draw attention to them in this chapter.

In vitro fertilization has now come of age. It has proved successful, acceptable, simple and capable of being adopted on a wide scale. It will be fascinating to discuss developments at the next meeting of the International Federation of Fertility Societies, and we can predict that considerable progress will be made on many areas of medical and scientific research by then.

Acknowledgements

I wish to thank my colleagues at Bourn Hall for their sustained support during this work, especially Patrick Steptoe, Simon Fishel, Jean Purdy and John Webster.

References

1. Edwards, R. G. (1965). *Nature*, **208**, 349 and *Lancet*, **2**, 926
2. Steptoe, P. C. and Edwards, R. G. (1978). *Lancet*, **2**, 366
3. Steptoe, P. C. and Edwards, R. G. (1970). *Lancet*, **1**, 683
4. Lenz, S. and Lauritsen, J. G. (1982). *Fertil. Steril.*, **38**, 673
5. Wikland, M., Nilsson, L., Hansson, R., Hamberger, L. and Janson, P. O. (1983). *Fertil Steril.*, **39**, 602

6. Feichtinger, W. and Kemeter, P. (1983). Paper presented at the *Conference on the In Vitro Fertilization of the Human Egg*, Vienna.
7. Edwards, R. G. and Steptoe, P. C. (1975). *J. Reprod. Fertil., Suppl.*, **22**, 121
8. Fowler, R. E., Edwards, R. G., Walters, D. E., Chan, S. T. H. and Steptoe, P. C. (1978). *J. Endocrinol.*, **77**, 161
9. Edwards, R. G. and Steptoe, P. C. (1983). (In preparation.)
10. Fishel, S. B. and Edwards, R. G. (1982). *Human Conception in Vitro*. (London: Academic Press)
11. Edwards, R. G., Purdy, J. M., Steptoe, P. C. and Walters, D. E. (1981). *Am. J. Obstet. Gynecol.*, **141**, 408
12. Veeck, L. L., Wortham, J. W. E., Witmyer, J., *et al.* (1983). *Fertil. Steril.*, **39**, 594
13. Fishel, S. B., Edwards, R. G. and Purdy, J. M. (1983). (In preparation)
14. Austin, C. R. (1961). *The Mammalian Egg*. (Oxford: Blackwell)
15. Singh, L. and Jones, K. W. (1982). *Cell*, **28**, 205

10
Events leading to fertilization in mammals

P. TALBOT

THE GAMETES

Mammalian fertilization occurs in the ampulla of the oviduct. In most eutherians, the oocyte at fertilization is surrounded by three investing coats: the zona pellucida, corona radiata and cumulus layer (Figure 1). An extracellular matrix (ECM) containing hyaluronic acid and residual follicular fluid separates cells of the corona radiata and cumulus.

The zona pellucida is a 6–8 μm thick acellular layer, normally penetrable only by sperm of the same species. The cells of the corona radiata and cumulus are 7–12.5 μm in diameter. In hamsters, distances between corona cells average 14 μm while distances between cumulus cells average 50±20 μm[1]. Thus fertilizing sperm must penetrate the ECM of the cumulus and corona radiata and the zona pellucida before crossing the perivitelline space and fusing with the oolemma. Structural features of the oocyte–cumulus complex (OCC) suggest that these layers become more difficult to penetrate as the sperm gets closer to the oocyte[1].

Mammalian sperm are well designed for penetrating these investments. They are thin, streamlined, motile cells possessing an acrosome at their leading edge[2]. The acrosome is a membrane-bound vesicle, which contains several hydrolytic enzymes including hyaluronidase and acrosin[3]. Sperm develop their streamlined form in the

121

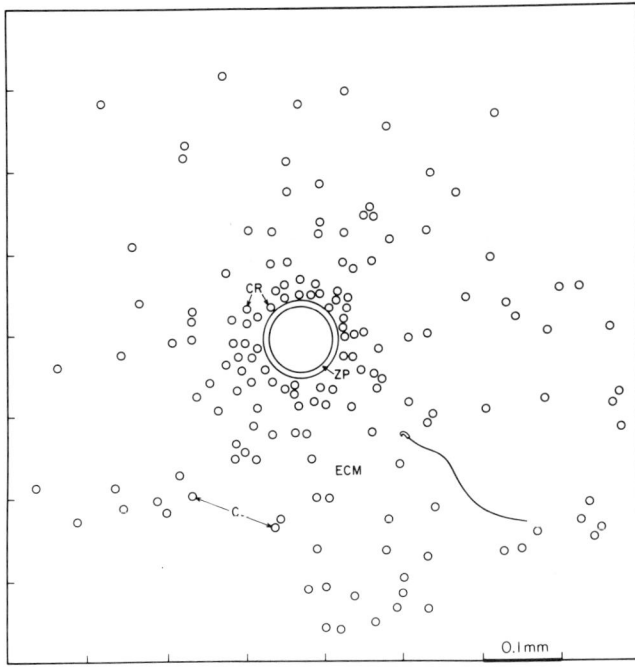

Figure 1 A diagram of the oocyte–cumulus complex being penetrated by a hamster sperm. ZP = Zona pellucida; CR = corona radiata cell; C = cumulus cell; ECM = extracellular matrix

testis during spermiogenesis, but do not actually become capable of fertilizing an oocyte until they have passed into the cauda epididymis[4,5]. During epididymal passage, subtle modifications occur in the sperm endowing it with the potential to fertilize an oocyte should appropriate conditions later develop.

PREPARATION OF THE SPERM FOR FERTILIZATION

Because sperm have completed their anatomical differentiation by the time they reach the cauda epididymis, it is tempting to consider them mature, static cells, ready to fertilize. Indeed, this is not the case. It is known from the classic experiments of Austin[6,7] and Chang[8] that fresh epididymal sperm are unable to fertilize oocytes when first mixed with them. This is because sperm are dynamic, changing cells which must undergo a series of morphological and physiological

122

alterations before they acquire the 'capacity to fertilize'. These changes begin to occur after sperm have left the cauda epididymis or vas deferens, and they can be successfully completed either in the female reproductive tract or the appropriate *in vitro* culture conditions. The length of time required to prepare a sperm to fertilize varies for each species; in the mouse it may be as short as 30–60 minutes, whereas in rabbits it requires 10–14 hours.

Two of the early events in fertilization, capacitation and the acrosome reaction, have been the subject of much recent research, and will be the focus in the remainder of this report. I will give a brief overview of these events, emphasizing some of the recent work done in my laboratory. There are several excellent reviews which may be consulted for more detail[3,9].

SPERM CAPACITATION

The term 'capacitation' is an operational definition. In current usage, it refers to the changes sperm undergo *in vitro* or in the female reproductive tract prior to the acrosome reaction. Capacitation is required in all mammalian species which have been examined, including man. As sperm become capacitated, they exhibit a wide amplitude flagellar beat[10,11], which has been termed 'hyperactivation'[3]. Recently, Yanagimachi[3] has summarized changes that are known to occur in sperm during the capacitation interval. Examples include loss of surface-absorbed molecules, loss or redistribution of lectin binding sites, reduction in net negative surface charge, rearrangement of intrinsic plasma membrane proteins, increased permeability to calcium, and changes in cAMP. It is difficult to show that any of these changes are essential in achieving a state of capacitation. At this point in our understanding of the process, it is fair to state the capacitation is required for fertilization and includes reorganization or restructuring of the sperm surface.

We have found that changes in the capacitated sperm surface can be detected using plant lectins. Lectins, which are multivalent glycoproteins capable of recognizing specific carbohydrate residues, will bind to living sperm and cause them to agglutinate. Sperm cells are particularly well suited for agglutination studies for two reasons. First, because they are motile, there is extensive interaction or colliding among cells; this appears to aid in promoting agglutination and setting up sharp agglutination patterns. Also, because the sperm is a highly polarized cell, precise information can be gained regarding the location of lectin receptors by examining agglutination patterns. For example, some lectins produce all head-to-head agglutination.

We have probed changes occurring in living guinea-pig sperm surface using a variety of lectins. Soybean agglutinin (SBA) binds to N-acetyl-galactosamine residues and has been particularly useful in our studies. Relatively high concentrations (120 μg ml^{-1}) of SBA are required to produce detectable agglutination of uncapacitated guinea-pig sperm. However, during capacitation and before the acrosome reaction, the guinea-pig sperm surface is modified in such a way that much less SBA (1–10 μg ml^{-1}) will produce agglutination[12,13]. Moreover, the pattern of agglutination changes from predominantly head-to-head before capacitation to tail-to-tail following capacitation

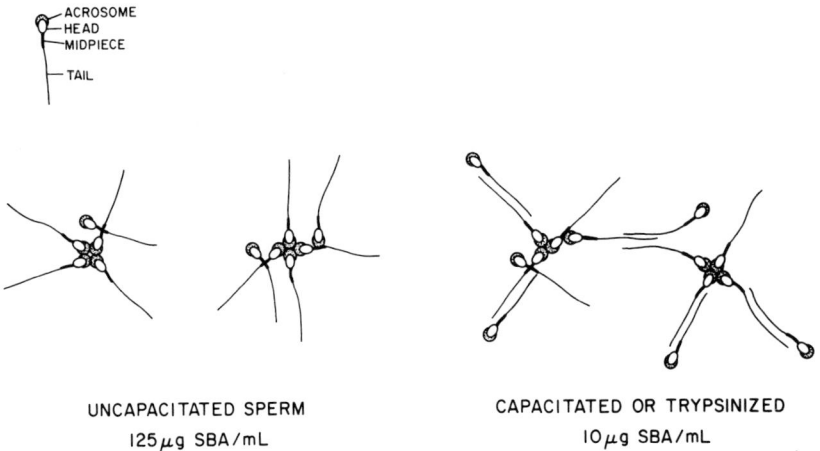

UNCAPACITATED SPERM
125 μg SBA/mL

CAPACITATED OR TRYPSINIZED
10 μg SBA/mL

Figure 2 Agglutination patterns of guinea-pig sperm incubated in soybean agglutinin. Uncapacitated sperm would require 125 μg SBA ml^{-1} or more to produce agglutination. The pattern is primarily head-to-head with occasional head-to-midpiece or midpiece-to-midpiece. Sperm which are either trypsinized briefly or capacitated will agglutinate in 1–10 μg SBA ml^{-1} and the pattern is now characterized by a significant increase in tail-to-tail agglutination

(Figure 2). Brief trypsinization of uncapacitated sperm will make them as agglutinable by SBA as capacitated sperm[14]. This suggests that removal of surface coating molecules results in this increase in lectin-induced agglutinability, perhaps by exposing a new array of sugar groups and/or by releasing constraints on the mobility of intrinsic membrane proteins (IMP). In some systems, an increase in the planar mobility of IMP correlates well with increased agglutinability by lectins[15].

The observation that trypsin alters the sperm surface in a manner similar to normal *in vitro* capacitation could indicate that a trypsin-like enzyme functions in capacitation. We are currently looking for evidence of this. It is intriguing that similar changes occur in cell surfaces during otherwise unrelated processes. For example, transformed cells are more agglutinable by lectins than their untransformed counterparts, and untransformed cells can be made highly agglutinable by trypsinization[16,17].

The concept that the modification of the sperm surface is an essential component of capacitation is supported by recent work done by my graduate student, Johannah Corselli. Freshly ovulated hamster OCCs were placed in flat, optically clear capillary tubes and challenged with either uncapacitated or capacitated (acrosome intact) hamster sperm. The interaction of the sperm and the OCCs was videotaped then analysed. Uncapacitated sperm bind to cumulus cells on the periphery of the OCC and do not penetrate it. However, capacitated sperm, which have not yet undergone an acrosome reaction, do not bind to cumulus cells or corona radiata cells and are able to penetrate up to the zona pellucida in a matter of 2–10 min. We interpret these data to mean that changes that occur in the sperm surface during capacitation are necessary for sperm penetration of the OCC up to the zona pellucida and that capacitated hamster sperm can penetrate to the zona without undergoing an acrosome reaction.

THE ACROSOME REACTION

The acrosome reaction occurs after capacitation. During the reaction, the plasma membrane overlying the acrosomal cap and the outer acrosomal membrane fuse together at multiple sites to form many small vesicles[18]. At the level of the equatorial segment of the acrosome, the plasma membrane and acrosomal membrane fuse to maintain a continuous membrane limiting the sperm. As a consequence of the reaction, the membrane vesicles and contents of the acrosome are lost from the cell. A sperm that has reacted is capable of completing two essential events in fertilization. These are (1) penetration of the zona pellucida; and (2) fusion with the oolemma. Since unreacted sperm are unable to do either, we may conclude that the acrosome reaction is a necessary event that sperm must undergo to fertilize an oocyte.

The factors that regulate occurrence of the reaction have been studied in several laboratories. Extracellular calcium and its influx into the sperm are necessary for acrosome reactions[11,19,20]. Catecholamines, such as epinephrine, have been shown by Meizel[21] and his colleagues to stimulate reactions in hamsters. Soluble components of the OCC[22,23] and a zona pellucida glycoprotein[24] have been implicated as stimulators of reactions in several systems. Yanagimachi[3] has recently reviewed some current models of the reaction in mammals.

The biological significance of the acrosome reaction is currently controversial. For many years, the reaction was thought to allow release of acrosomal enzymes which in turn aid sperm in penetrating the cumulus and corona radiata. This idea, which makes good biological sense, is supported by many observations[25-28]. However, it is currently being subjected to closer examination as it does not fit all data[29-32]. An alternative view is that either no enzyme or a hydrolase(s) on the sperm's plasma membrane aids in penetration of the cumulus and corona radiata layers; the sperm then binds to the zona pellucida where it undergoes the acrosome reaction. In this model, acrosomal hydrolases would be released onto the zona pellucida, which may be the most impenetrable layer the sperm encounters, and these hydrolases may assist in zona penetration. The zona pellucida does contain hyaluronic acid which is removed by testicular hyaluronidase[33], and acrosin, in concert with other hydrolases, can dissolve the remainder of the zona pellucida[3]. However, hydrolysis of the zona or dispersion of the cumulus and corona radiata cells by a particular acrosomal enzyme(s) does not constitute proof of its function. At this point, we should be cautious about the role of the acrosomal enzymes and the biological significance of the reaction. At best, we can say that the fertilizing sperm must undergo an acrosome reaction, and this reaction occurs before penetration of the zona pellucida.

After penetrating the zona pellucida, the sperm enters the perivitelline space, binds to the oolemma, then the sperm plasma membrane and oolemma fuse. In all mammals examined to date, only acrosome-reacted sperm can fuse with the oolemma[3] and only a small region of the sperm's plasma membrane is capable of fusion. This region is comprised of the plasma membrane overlying the equatorial segment of the acrosome and anterior portion of the postacrosomal region[34-38]. Because sperm acquire this ability to fuse after the acrosome reaction, it is sometimes said that one function of the reaction is to alter the plasma membrane so it can fuse[3]. However, it has not yet been shown experimentally that these events are causally related (and indeed it is difficult to do so) nor is it known why such a restricted region of the sperm's membrane becomes fusable.

RELEVANCE TO HUMAN FERTILIZATION

Observations on fertilization in non-human species have made it clear that sperm are not static cells. During fertilization, sperm undergo morphological, biochemical and physiological changes, several of which have been identified as essential to fertilization. This knowledge can be viewed from two perspectives with respect to humans.

First, in controlling fertility, there are numerous opportunities to prevent fertilization (only several have been discussed in this review). Blocking fertilization by preventing a necessary event, such as capacitation or the acrosome reaction, is certainly a possibility. At this time, such an approach seems rather sophisticated, but a more thorough understanding of fertilization through continued basic research may eventually lead to breakthroughs in this area. There are currently no contraceptive methods which are ideal, and continued improvement in controlling unwanted fertilization will surely develop as our understanding of the process increases.

Perhaps more relevant to current interests is the need to alleviate certain types of infertility using newly developed *in vitro* fertilization techniques for humans. Infertility has multiple causes, many of which have probably not yet been identified. Quite likely, some failures of human oocytes to be fertilized *in vivo* or *in vitro* are due to a breakdown in the sequence of changes occurring in sperm. For example, sperm from some individuals may not be able to undergo capacitation or the acrosome reaction or zona pellucida penetration. There is a precedent for this in hamsters. Cummins[39] has shown that hamster sperm taken from the caput or corpa epididymis are unable to undergo acrosome reactions and accordingly would be infertile. Epididymal dysfunction in humans could produce similar subtle forms of infertility, not detected in a routine semen analysis.

Fortunately several assays are in development which may provide the clinician with valuable information regarding causes of male infertility. The ability of sperm to penetrate cervical mucus[40] seems

127

to correlate well with fertility. A commercial kit, Penetrak, is available from Syva to perform this test. Positive results are probably a measure of successful progressive movement by sperm. While there is not yet a direct test to monitor human sperm capacitation, the lectin agglutination assay developed with guinea-pigs[13] could probably be adapted to humans. It has the advantages of being inexpensive and easy to perform. Acrosome reactions can now be scored in human sperm using a triple staining technique which permits a distinction to be made between normal acrosome reactions and false reactions occurring during sperm death[41,42]. The ability of human sperm to penetrate the zona pellucida can be tested on salt-stored human oocytes[43] or on frozen then thawed oocytes recovered from human cadavers[44]. In these assays, the vitellus is dead but the zona pellucida is thought to present a realistic challenge to human sperm. Finally, the zona-free hamster assay provides a means for testing the ability of human sperm to fuse with the plasma membrane of a hamster oocyte[45]. This assay has been evaluated more thoroughly than the others, and most data indicate a good correlation between infertility and failure to penetrate.

It is important to realize that each of these assays measures a different aspect of a sperm's ability to fertilize, thus all assays are important and should be developed and tested. It is likely that new types of male infertility will be identified as data acquired with these tests increases. With the plethora of new *in vitro* human fertilization laboratories opening world-wide, we have an excellent opportunity to evaluate these assays using human volunteers. Caution should be used in interpreting data, and large data bases will need to be collected at multiple laboratories before meaningful correlations can be made. All of this will take time, but the opportunity certainly exists to begin collection of data on the subtle forms of infertility. I hope research scientists and clinicians will work together to accomplish these goals.

Acknowledgements

Work from my laboratory was funded by grants from NIH and the Academic Senate of the University of California, Riverside.

References

1. Talbot, P. and DiCarlantonio, G. (1983). Architecture of the hamster oocyte–cumulus complex. *Gam. Res.* (In press.)
2. Fawcett, D. W. (1975). The mammalian spermatozoa. *Dev. Biol.*, **44**, 394
3. Yanagimachi, R. (1981). Mechanisms of fertilization in mammals. In Mastrianni, L. and Biggers, J. (eds.). *Fertilization and Embryonic Development in vitro*, pp. 81–82. (London: Plenum)
4. Bedford, J. M., Calvin, H. and Cooper, G. W. (1973). The maturation of spermatozoa in the human epididymis. *J. Reprod. Fertil. Suppl.*, **18**, 199
5. Orgebin-Crist, M. C. (1967). Maturation of spermatozoa in the rabbit epididymis: fertilizing ability and embryonic mortality in does inseminated with epididymal spermatozoa. *Ann. Biol. Anim. Biochem. Biophys.*, **7**, 373
6. Austin, C. R. (1951). Observations on the penetration of the sperm into the mammalian egg. *Austr. J. Sci. Res. Ser. B.*, **4**, 581
7. Austin, C. R. (1952). The 'capacitation' of mammalian sperm. *Nature (Lond.)*, **170**, 326
8. Chang, M. C. (1951). Fertilizing capacity of spermatozoa deposited into fallopian tubes. *Nature (Lond.)*, **168**, 697
9. Meizel, S. (1978). The mammalian sperm acrosome reaction, a biochemical approach. In Johnson, M. H. (ed.). *Development in Mammals*, Vol. 3, pp.1–64. (New York: North-Holland)
10. Yanagimachi, R. (1970). The movement of golden hamster spermatozoa before and after capacitation. *J. Reprod. Fertil.*, **23**, 193
11. Yanagimachi, R. and Usui, N. (1974). Calcium dependence of the acrosome reaction and activation of the guinea pig spermatozoa. *Exp. Cell Res.*, **89**, 161
12. Talbot, P. and Franklin, L. E. (1978). Surface modification of guinea pig sperm during *in vitro* capacitation: an assessment using lectin-induced agglutination of living sperm. *J. Exp. Zool.*, **201**, 1
13. Talbot, P. and Chacon, R. (1981). Detection of modifications in the tail of capacitated guinea pig sperm using lectins. *J. Exp. Zool.*, **216**, 435
14. Talbot, P. and Franklin, L. E. (1978). Trypsinization increases lectin-induced agglutinability of uncapacitated guinea pig sperm. *J. Exp. Zool.*, **204**, 291
15. Nicolson, G. L. (1971). Differences in topology of normal and tumor cell membranes shown by different surface distributions of ferritin conjugated concanavalin A. *Nature (Lond.)*, **233**, 244
16. Burger, M. M. (1969). A difference in the architecture of the surface membrane of normal and virally transformed cells. *Proc. Natl. Acad. Sci. USA.*, **62**, 994
17. Nicolson, G. L. (1976). Transmembrane control of the receptors on normal and tumor cells. II. Surface changes associated with tranformation and malignancy. *Biochem. Biophys. Acta*, **458**, 1
18. Barros, C., Bedford, J., Franklin, L. and Austin, C. (1976). Membrane visualization as a feature of the mammalian acrosome reaction. *J. Cell Biol.*, **34**, C1
19. Talbot, P., Summers, R. G., Hylander, B., Keough, K. M. and Franklin, L. E. (1976). The role of calcium in the acrosome reaction: an analysis using ionophore A23187. *J. Exp. Zool.*, **198**, 383
20. Singh, J. P., Babcock, D. and Lardy, H. A. (1978). Increased Ca^{2+} influx is a component of sperm capacitation. *Biochem. J.*, **172**, 549
21. Meizel, S. (1981). Stimulation of sperm fertility *in vitro* by exogenous molecules. In Edwards, R. G. and Steptoe, P. (eds.). *Proceedings of the 4th World Congress on Fertility and Sterility*. (Lancaster: MTP Press)
22. Bavister, B. (1982). Evidence for a role of post-ovulatory cumulus components in supporting fertilizing ability of hamster spermatozoa. *J. Androl.*, **3**, 365

23. Lenz, R. W., Ax, R. L., Grimek, H. J. and First, N. L. (1982). Proteoglycan from bovine follicular fluid enhances an acrosome reaction in bovine spermatozoa. *Biochem. Biophys. Res. Comm.,* **106,** 1092

24. Bliel, J. and Wasserman, P. (1980). Mammalian sperm–egg interaction: identification of a glycoprotein in mouse egg zonae pellucidae possessing receptor activity for sperm. *Cell,* **20,** 873

25. Bedford, J. M. (1968). Ultrastructural changes in the sperm head during fertilization in the rabbit. *Am. J. Anat.,* **123,** 329

26. Talbot, P. and Franklin, L. E. (1974). The release of hyaluronidase from guinea pig sperm during the course of the normal acrosome reaction *in vitro. J. Reprod. Fertil.,* **39,** 429

27. Huang, T., Fleming, A., and Yanagimachi, R. (1981). Only acrosome-reacted spermatozoa can bind to the zona pellucida: a study using the guinea pig. *J. Exp. Zool.,* **217,** 287

28. Cummins, J. and Yanagimachi, R. (1982). Sperm–egg ratios and the site of the acrosome reaction during *in vivo* fertilization in the hamster. *Gam. Res.,* **5,** 239

29. Gwatkin, R. B. L., Carter, W. H. and Patterson, H. (1976). Association of mammalian sperm with the cumulus cells and the zona pellucida studied by scanning electron microscopy. In Johari, H. and Becker, R. P. (eds.). *Scanning Electron Microscopy,* Vol. **2,** pp. 379–384. (Chicago: ITT Research Institute)

30. Phillips, D. M. and Shalgi, R. (1980). Surface properties of the zona pellucida. *J. Ultrastruct. Res.,* **213,** 1

31. Saling, P., Sowinski, J. and Storey, B. T. (1979). An ultrastructural study of epididymal mouse spermatozoa binding to zonae pellucidae *in vitro:* sequential relationships to the acrosome reaction. *J. Exp. Zool.,* **209,** 229

32. Florman, H. M. and Storey, B. (1982). Mouse gamete interactions: the zona pellucida is the site of the acrosome reaction leading to fertilization *in vitro. Dev. Biol.,* **91,** 121

33. Talbot, P. (1983). Hyaluronidase dissolves a component of the hamster zona pellucida. *J. Exp. Zool.* (In press)

34. Piko, L. and Tyler, A. (1964). Fine structural studies of sperm penetration in the rat. Proceedings of the 5th International Congress on Animal Reproduction. *Trento,* **2,** 372

35. Barros, C. and Franklin, L. E. (1968). Behavior of the gamete membranes during sperm entry into the mammalian egg. *J. Cell Biol.,* **37,** C13

36. Yanagimachi, R. and Noda, Y. D. (1970). Electron microscopic studies of sperm incorporation into golden hamster eggs. *Am. J. Anat.,* **128,** 429

37. Bedford, J. M. and Cooper, G. W. (1978). Membrane fusion events in fertilization of vertebrate eggs. In Poste, G. and Nicholson, G. (eds.). *Cell Surface Reviews,* Vol. **5,** pp. 65–125. (Amsterdam: North-Holland)

38. Talbot, P. and Chacon, R. (1982). Ultrastructural observations on binding and membrane fusion between human sperm and zona pellucida-free hamster oocytes. *Fertil. Steril.,* **37,** 240

39. Cummins, J. M. (1976). Effects of epididymal occlusion on sperm maturation in the hamster. *J. Exp. Zool.,* **197,** 187

40. Alexander, N. J. (1981). Evaluation of male infertility with an *in vitro* cervical mucus penetration test. *Fertil. Steril.,* **36,** 201

41. Talbot, P. and Chacon, R. (1981). A triple-stain technique for evaluating normal acrosome reactions of human sperm. *J. Exp. Zool.,* **215,** 201

42. Talbot, P. and Dudenhausen, E. (1981). Factors affecting triple staining of human sperm. *Stain Technol.,* **56,** 307

43. Yanagimachi, R., Lopata, A., Odom, C., *et al.* (1979). Retention of biological characteristics of zona pellucida in highly concentrated salt solutions: the use of

salt-stored eggs for assessing the fertilizing capacity of spermatozoa. *Fertil. Steril.*, **31**, 562

44. Overstreet, J., Yanagimachi, R., Katz, D., Hayashi, K. and Hanson, F. (1980). Penetration of human spermatozoa into the human zona pellucida and the zona-free hamster egg: a study of fertile and infertile patients. *Fertil. Steril.*, **33**, 534

45. Yanagimachi, R., Yanagimachi, H. and Rogers, B. J. (1976). The use of zona-free animal ova as a test system for the assessment of fertilizing capacity of human spermatozoa. *Biol. Reprod.*, **15**, 471

11
Early human embryology

R. O'RAHILLY and F. MÜLLER

It is little exaggeration to state that human embryology was founded 100 years ago by Wilhelm His, senior, who published his *Anatomie menschlicher Embryonen* between 1880 and 1885[1]. This first systematic study was followed by another important landmark, the *Manual of Human Embryology* by Keibel and Mall, which was published in 1910 and 1912, simultaneously in English and German[2]. It was, in the words of its editors, the first attempt to provide 'an account of the development of the human body, based throughout on human material'. The influence of His on both Keibel and Mall extended to the foundation of the Carnegie Collection by Mall in 1914[3]. Ever since, this Collection has served as an embryological Bureau of Standards. Although a monograph on the early (stage 6) human embryo had been published by Peters in 1899[4], the details of early human development had to await investigations based on the Carnegie Collection. The addition of very early examples by Hertig and Rock in the 1940s and 1950s laid the foundation on which a systematic account of the first 3 weeks could be based[5].

Prenatal life may be divided conveniently into (1) the embryonic period proper, comprising the first 8 postovulatory weeks (i.e. timed from the last ovulation); and (2) the fetal period, which extends to birth. The embryonic period has been studied, and is still being investigated, in much greater detail because, during the first 8 weeks, the vast majority of the thousands of named structures of the body make their appearance. Furthermore, most, although not all, congenital anomalies become manifest during this time. Finally, the early

133

part of this period is of particular concern in regard to human conception *in vitro*.

At the end of the embryonic period, the embryo measures approximately 30 mm in sitting height (crown–rump length) and weighs between 2 and 3 g.

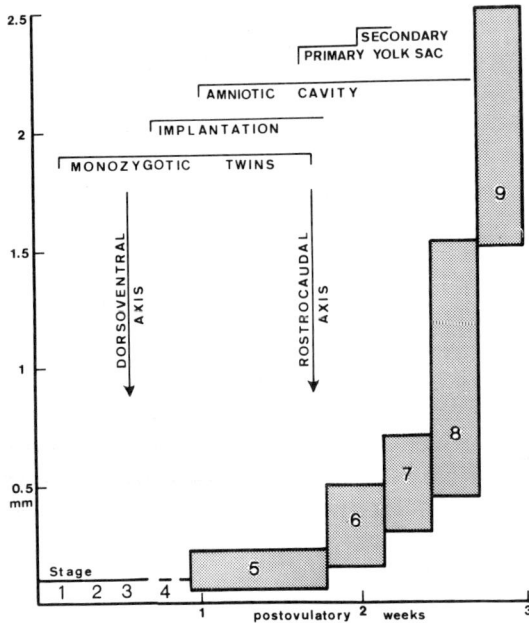

Figure 1 Graph of stages 1–9, showing the relationships of Carnegie stage (rectangles), embryonic length (ordinate), and postovulatory age (abscissa)

Just as postnatally neither age nor height is a satisfactory guide to maturity, in a similar way prenatally neither the presumed age nor the crown–rump length is an adequate indication of developmental status. Hence, a staging system based on the morphological level of development is employed. The idea was first introduced into human embryology by Mall in 1914. The present, internationally accepted arrangement is the Carnegie system, based on the investigations of Streeter and of O'Rahilly[5]. This system enables precise studies to be made on the timing and sequence of developmental events. Recent examples concern the reproductive and endocrine systems[6,7].

134

The importance of embryonic staging has been stressed repeatedly and it has been pointed out that the term stage should be used only in its technical, embryological sense. Such expressions as 'at the 3 mm stage' should, in the event that the stage is not known, be replaced by 'at 3 mm'.

The embryonic period proper is divided into 23 morphological stages. Stages 1–9, which comprise the first 3 weeks, may be regarded as an early sub-period, at the end of which the first organ systems (nervous and cardiovascular) have begun to appear. The following summary of these stages (Figure 1) is based largely on observations of serial sections of 80 early embryos in the Carnegie Collection, from some of which both solid and graphic reconstructions have been made. Detailed descriptions, photomicrographs and drawings are available elsewhere[5].

Stage 1– Fertilization of the oocyte initiates stage 1, which is unicellular and includes the formation of the pronuclei and the beginning of the first mitotic division. (It should be noted that the term ovum for oocyte is incorrect, and the translation egg is inappropriate.)

Stage 2– During stage 2 (about 2 days) the two-cell embryo continues to divide. Although, when 12–16 cells are present, the embryo is commonly referred to as a morula, this term is not appropriate in mammals because, unlike amphibians, non-embryonic structures (such as the chorion and amnion) are also derived from the initial mass of cells. Before differentiation of the trophoblast, separation of blastomeres could result in monozygotic twins with separate choria and amnia.

Stage 3 – As soon as a blastocyst cavity appears (at about 3 days), the embryo is assigned to stage 3. The zona pellucida then disappears. Trophoblast, epiblast and even some hypoblast may be distinguishable by the time that the embryo is composed of 100 cells. The embryo now possesses a dorsoventral axis. Before differentiation of the amnion, duplication of the inner cell mass could result in monozygotic twins with a common chorion but with separate amnia. Many embryos of the first three stages have been cultured *in vitro*[8].

Stage 4 – The previously free blastocyst becomes attached to the

135

endometrium at stage 4, a convincing example of which has not yet been recorded in the human.

Stage 5 – The embryo is now 1 week old and measures approximately 0.1 mm. Stage 5 exhibits varying degrees of implantation, although chorionic villi are not yet present. The amniotic cavity is developing[9] and the embryonic disc is bilaminar, being composed of epiblast and hypoblast. The hypoblast spreads (as extraembryonic endoderm) to form the primary yolk sac. The cytotrophoblast gives origin to syncytiotrophoblast, which is at first solid but soon develops lacunae (the future intervillous space) that communicate with the endometrial vessels. Extraembryonic mesoblast makes its appearance, although the mode of origin[10] is still under discussion. Before the appearance of axial features, complete duplication of the embryonic disc could result in monozygotic twins with a common chorion and amnion.

Stage 6 – The embryo is now 2 weeks old and is less than 0.5 mm in length. Chorionic villi appear in stage 6 and begin to branch almost at once. Axial features, especially the primitive streak, can be noted, at least in the more advanced examples. Hence, bilateral symmetry becomes manifest and the embryo thereby acquires rostral and caudal ends, and right and left sides. Blood islands are visible on the yolk sac. The primary becomes converted into the secondary yolk sac, probably by collapse of the former ('the result of pinching off of a portion of the larger primary yolk sac'[10]). The umbilical stalk begins to develop. Sex chromatin may be found in the trophoblast. From this stage onwards, partial duplication of the embryonic disc could result in conjoint twins.

Stage 7 – A further median elaboration, the notochordal process, characterizes stage 7. An allantoic diverticulum is now more readily distinguishable. The embryonic disc is becoming trilaminar and may then be said to be composed of ectoderm, mesoderm, and endoderm. The general region of the neural plate can be identified adjacent to the notochordal process. Primordial germ cells have been identified in the allantoic endoderm and in the stalk mesoderm at this and the next stage. Sex chromatin may be found in the wall of the yolk sac.

Stage 8 – Further median elaborations (such as the primitive pit) appear at stage 8. Sex chromatin may be found in the future notochordal region. In one-quarter of embryos of stage 8 the neural groove is identifiable rostrally, so that the initial development of the brain is distinguishable[11].

Stage 9 – When the somites begin to appear, the embryo has reached stage 9. The neural groove is considerably deeper and the forebrain, midbrain, and hindbrain become distinguishable before the neural tube has formed. The heart appears. In the more advanced examples, it consists of a myocardial mantle, cardiac jelly, and endocardium; moreover, atrial, ventricular and conal regions become distinguishable. It is believed that the heart begins to beat at either this or the next stage. An indication of the otic disc is found.

In conclusion, it is clear that great advances in knowledge of early human development have been made during the past half-century, chiefly from investigations based on the Carnegie Collection[5] and, more recently, from studies of embryos *in vitro*[8,12] although much more remains to be elucidated.

Acknowledgements

This work was supported by research grant No. HD-16702, Institute of Child Health and Human Development, National Institutes of Health, USA.

References

1. His, W. (1880–1885). *Anatomie menschlicher Embryonen* (three volumes). (Leipzig: Vogel)
2. Keibel, F., and Mall, F. P (1910, 1912). *Manual of Human Embryology* (two volumes). (Philadelphia: Lippincott)
3. O'Rahilly, R. (1979). Early human development and the chief sources of information on staged human embryos. *Eur. J. Obstet. Gynecol. Reprod. Biol.*, **9**, 273
4. Peters, H. (1899). *Über die Einbettung des menschlichen Eies und das früheste bisher bekannte menschliche Placentationsstadium.* (Leipzig: Deuticke)
5. O'Rahilly, R. (1973). *Developmental Stages in Human Embryos. Part A: Embryos of the First Three Weeks (Stages 1 to 9).* (Washington, D.C.: Carnegie Institution)
6. O'Rahilly, R. (1983). The timing and sequence of events in the development of the human reproductive system during the embryonic period proper. *Anat. Embryol.*, **166**, 247
7. O'Rahilly, R. (1983). The timing and sequence of events in the development of the human endocrine system during the embryonic period proper. *Anat. Embryol.*, **166**, 439

8. Edwards, R. G., and Purdy, J. M. (eds.). (1982). *Human Conception* in vitro. (London: Academic Press)

9. Luckett, W. P. (1975). The development of primordial and definitive amniotic cavities in early rhesus monkey and human embryos. *Am. J. Anat.*, **144,** 149

10. Luckett, W. P. (1978). Origin and differentiation of the yolk sac and extraembryonic mesoderm in presomite human and rhesus monkey embryos. *Am. J. Anat.*, **152,** 59

11. O'Rahilly, R. and Müller, F. (1981). The first appearance of the human nervous system at stage 8. *Anat. Embryol.*, **163,** 1

12. Edwards, R. G. (1980). *Conception in the Human Female.* (London: Academic Press)

12
Organization of an *in vitro* fertilization programme

A. A. ACOSTA, J. E. GARCIA, G. S. JONES, L. VEECK,
B. SANDOW and H. W. JONES

Any *in vitro* fertilization programme requires a very complex structure regardless of whether the programme is mainly or solely devoted to patient's services or whether it is also involved in research development and training. In either of these situations, a very strict quality control at all levels is mandatory; otherwise the programme is doomed to failure. Careful planning in each area should be done.

Figure 1 tries to depict some of the multiple aspects involved in such a programme based on the organizational chart of the Norfolk project as it stands in 1983. There are aspects of the programme mainly related to patient management, aspects of the programme mainly related to laboratory work including laboratories directly involved and support laboratories and finally aspects related to research, training, and data collection and processing. In the short time we have been assigned, we will try to cover very briefly each one of them.

The patient population, which is either self-referred or physician-referred has to be carefully screened by an experienced physician and this is a time consuming part of the programme because, besides the medical aspects, there are educational problems involved in order for the patient to be able to understand the procedure and to sign a valid informed consent. Once the patient is admitted, she is assigned to one of the main categories: namely tubal factors, male factors which is certainly not restricted to oligospermia, endometriosis, and other groups including the unexplained infertility and multi-factorial infertility, in which several aetiologic factors are involved. Ovulation stimulation can be achieved using several different protocols: clomiphene; clomiphene/hCG; clomiphene/hMG/hCG; hMG/hCG; etc. Regardless of the type of ovulation stimulation selected, which in our programme is almost exclusively restricted to hMG/hCG or FSH/hMG/hCG, oocyte retrieval is the next step.

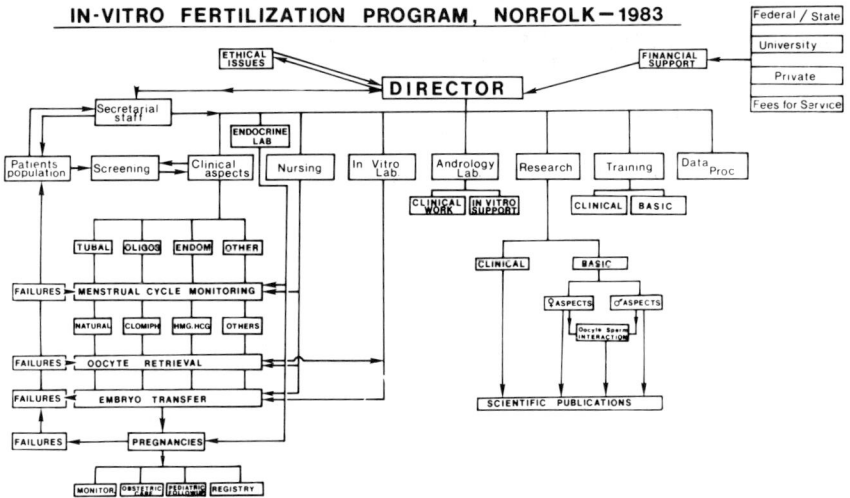

Figure 1 Organizational chart of the *in vitro* fertilization programme. Norfolk, 1983

Although a regular operating room can be used, there are specific aspects involved concerning this type of project which makes the surgical environment very special and in a certain way sophisticated. All the steps taking place at the time of retrieval need to be carefully recorded and in order to do that, a member of the laboratory team is always present in the operating room; besides the procedure is taped for medical reasons and for research purposes.

The *in vitro* laboratory, in our opinion, should be immediately adjacent to the operating room and properly equipped to search, identify, diagnose, and report findings on the material sent from the operating room; this is a very important part of the system. Rapid identification and classification of the oocytes and granulosa cells complement the work of the surgical team.

The process of pre-incubation, insemination, and embryo culture takes place in the *in vitro* laboratory, until embryo transfer is performed in the same environment in which the laparoscopy is done, here again very close to the laboratory.

After embryo transfer, careful monitoring takes place until pregnancy is proved or disproved, and if pregnancy is established monitoring proceeds according to each centre protocol and after that routine obstetrical care takes place. It is important to consider the possibility of having a neonatal and paediatric follow-up to evaluate the development of these children from a physical and mental point of view. It has been proposed that a registry of pregnancies and children born through this technique be kept at local, national or international levels in order to make the available population accessible for evaluation.

Failures at any level, abnormal results in ovulation induction, failure at oocyte retrieval, patients who are not transferred or that have an unsuccessful transfer and in whom pregnancies are not established, go back to the population that will return for repeat procedures and they will be added to the new incoming population requiring treatment. A balance between repeat procedures and new patients should be maintained.

At the time of menstrual cycle monitoring, and when pregnancies are established, a special endocrine laboratory is necessary which has to be able to do rapid hormone assays during these steps.

A well trained team of nurses is also required to carry out cycle monitoring under supervision and to assist during oocyte retrieval and embryo transfer. Needless to say, they should be very well aware of the different approaches to quality control, to be able to detect problems in anyone of the several steps involved in these two aspects of *in vitro* fertilization.

An important part of our programme is devoted to the male factor. The andrology laboratory is a very important part and arm of the programme, both in clinical work and in our project as a support laboratory. A mouse *in vivo* and *in vitro* fertilization experimental model or system has been established in order to test all the steps of the procedure and to answer any questions that may arise in regard to quality control.

If the programme decides to also do research, it could be involved in either clinical research, basic research, or both. Tremendous advances have been made, from a clinical point of view, in the knowledge of the natural process of ovulation and also in the knowledge of stimulated cycles in normal ovulating females. Basic research has contributed tremendously in the fields of male and female gametes and gamete interaction, and we have in front of us the unknown and unexplored aspect of human implantation. The result of these activities has brought an overwhelming amount of scientific publications in all aspects of reproduction profiting from the *in vitro* fertilization programmes.

It is also clear, at least to me, that if new programmes are going to start, as they are starting now all over the world, training in this aspect of reproductive biology needs to be available, both at the clinical level and basic laboratory level. In that particular regard, our programme offers a 3 month course for people with background and experience in reproductive laboratory techniques and regular 1 and 2 year fellowships for people interested mainly in the clinical aspects of reproductive endocrinology including *in vitro* fertilization and embryo transfer.

The amount of clinical and laboratory information produced by this kind of programme is of such magnitude, that Norfolk has designed a special computerized data base which besides patient identification information, is able to keep, retrieve, and analyse data on different aspects of the programme, including cycle monitoring and hormone values, follicular fluid and oocyte information, as well as data on incubation, insemination, embryo development, embryo transfer and results. This kind of computer program specially designed to fit our needs has provided an invaluable amount of information, that can be rapidly generated and which would be impossible to analyse otherwise.

There are other important issues related to such programmes that need to be considered carefully.

In the United States, federal and state funds are not available for such work. It has been our impression that this kind of programme should be mainly under university sponsorship for several different reasons, therefore, in our country most programmes have to rely on university funds, private donations, and fees for services, to support themselves. Few insurance companies cover the cost of such treatment and therefore, at least for the time being, the patient needs to be able to afford these costs.

Important ethical issues are at stake in any programme of *in vitro* fertilization; they need to be discussed thoroughly and clearly in such a way that straight guidelines, protocols, and consent forms are developed in each centre according to their own views, needs, and resources. The participation of Hospitals' and Medical Schools' Committees on Ethics and Human Experimentation and physician interaction with them is of utmost importance. There is a very touchy subject to consider at this point. Guidelines and minimal requirements should perhaps be developed and be made available for the groups that are planning to enter into the field. Only impeccable medical and ethical standards will prevent the method from falling into disrepute.

Devotion, expertise, tireless quality control efforts, adequate unified physical facilities and permanent review of performance and results are key factors to the success of *in vitro* fertilization and embryo transfer. Improvement of results is the immediate goal; better understanding of fertilization has resulted and will continue to improve; medicine in general. Obstetrics and gynaecology and reproductive physiology in particular have been extraordinarily benefited and advanced by these programmes since their inception.

We all involved in these programmes are deeply indebted to our British colleagues for developing a method, which has brought into the field such a tremendous advance in technology, knowledge, medical resources, and overall, treatment capabilities.

13
Clinical experiences with *in vitro* fertilization and embryo transfer programmes

W. FEICHTINGER and P. KEMETER

Our programme of *in vitro* fertilization (IVF) and embryo transfer (ET) has been successful since November 1981. Since then it was our aim to develop a uniform schedule for clinical use. Instigating further modifications and changes resulted in an increased pregnancy rate. Many procedures were simplified for routine work, and a schedule was established which was described previously as the 'Vienna IVF and ET program'[1]. Our clinical experiences are based on different types of *in vitro* fertilization centres which will be described below.

SYSTEMS AND METHODS
System I (Figure 1)

We started our work in a large hospital, i.e. a university clinic. Laparoscopic oocyte recovery was performed in the operating theatre with the IVF laboratory adjacent to it, monitoring of cycles and hormone assays were performed in the sterility out-patient office, ultrasonic department or hormone laboratory, respectively. The team consisted of an endocrinologist, a gynaecologist and a biologist who was in fact a specially trained gynaecologist. The IVF team was completed by well-trained technicians and nurses being responsible for the hormone assays and the organization of the monitoring of patients.

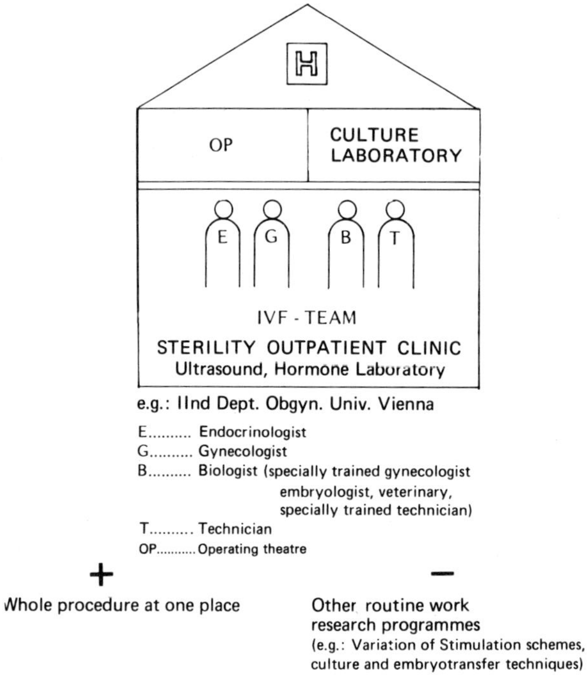

Figure 1 System I

System II (Figure 2)

Monitoring of cycles, hormone laboratory (haemagglutination tests for E_2 and LH) and ultrasonic examinations were performed in a gynaecological private office, with the IVF laboratory in the office; laparoscopic oocyte recoveries were performed in a hospital, and the recovered eggs were transported in follicular fluid at 37°C in a Thermos flask to the laboratory. ET was performed as an office procedure 24–28 hours after insemination (bed rest after ET was reduced to a maximum of 30 minutes).

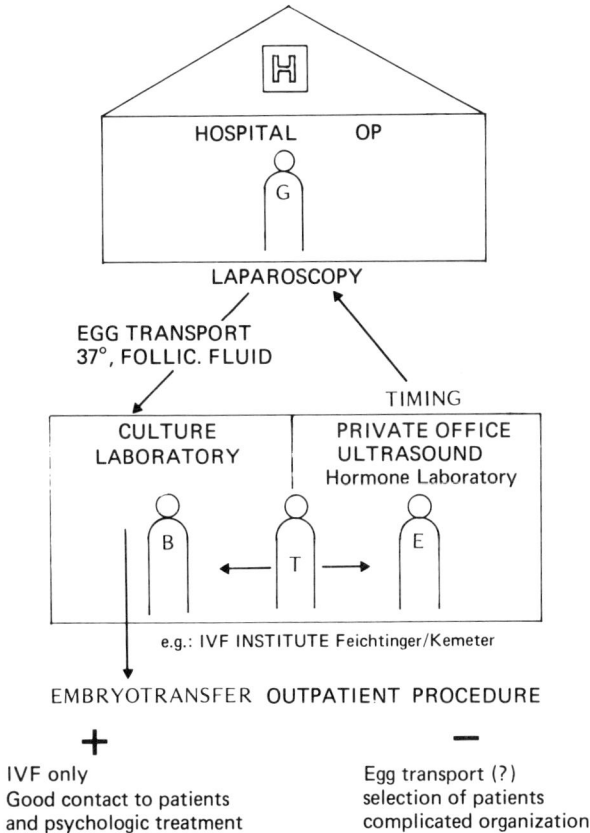

Figure 2 System II. For abbreviations, see legend to Figure 1

System III (Figure 3)

The idea of creating system III was that different gynaecologists and hospitals should co-operate with one specialized IVF laboratory. It was initiated with one large hospital and one gynaecologist in Vienna in 1982, but stopped after a few months since the results were not satisfactory.

Monitoring of the stimulated cycles as well as laparoscopic oocyte recoveries were performed in those places and eggs were transported to our laboratory at 37°C in follicular fluid, where insemination and culture was performed. Some embryos were replaced in our

147

laboratory, some of them were returned placed inside a ready-for-use transfer-catheter, sealed and kept under culture conditions for transport and ET which was performed by collaborating colleagues.

Methods of stimulation, oocyte recovery, egg insemination, embryo culture, ET, etc. were the same in all three systems and according to the technique published by us previously[1]. The only exception was that embryos were replaced earlier (1 day after insemination instead of 2 days) in system II. We continued system II in 1983 except that we introduced the technique of ultrasonically guided follicle aspiration under local anaesthesia according to the techniques of Lenz *et al.*[2], and Wikland *et al.*[3], making oocyte recovery, *in vitro* fertilization and embryo transfer a complete office and out-patient procedure[4].

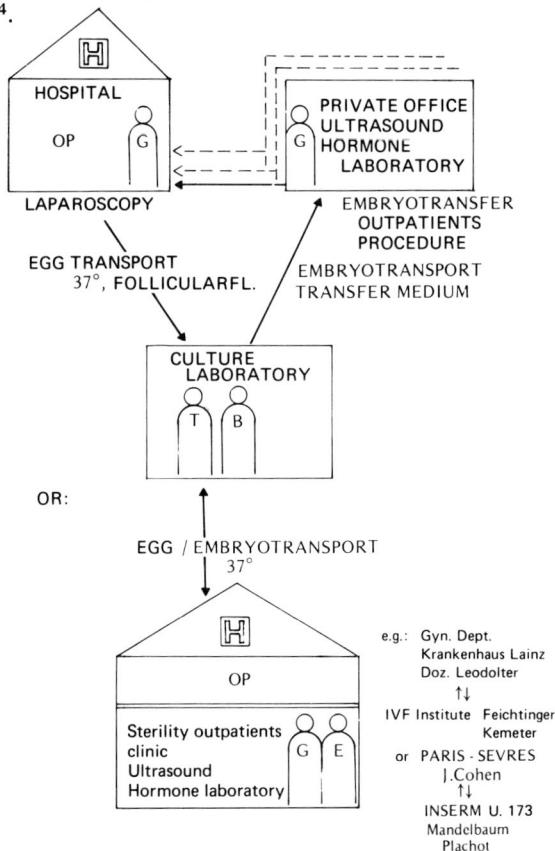

Figure 3 System III. For abbreviations, see legend to Figure 1

Technique of ultrasonically guided follicle aspiration

The equipment utilized is a sector scanner (Combison 100, Kretz, Austria). Before puncture 10 ml diazepam (Valium 10, Roche) and pentazocine (Fortral, Winthrop), are administered intravenously. Prophylactic antibiotic treatment is given by a mixture of mezlocillin and oxacillin (2:1) (Optocillin, Bayer) i.v. The follicular puncture is performed by use of a steering device provided by the Kretz company. The puncturing angle at which the needle enters the sound-field is pre-fixed, and marked on the monitor with a dotted line to indicate the needle direction. We use exactly the same needle and aspiration device as reported for laparoscopic oocyte recovery[5] (outer diameter of 1.4 mm). The transducer is placed in a sterile plastic bag, the puncture is always performed through a (spontaneously) filled bladder. The follicle to be punctured is located on the monitor where the dotted line, as mentioned above, indicates the needle direction. This line must pass through the maximal diameter of the follicle. Care has to be taken not to aspirate urine into the collecting system. This is prevented by the use of an electronically directed sucking-pump which builds up and declines the suction pressure immediately if necessary (Mikro-Makro Sauger, Labotect, Germany).

Computerized analysis of IVF results

A computerized analysis of all IVF data from system I and II was carried out on 233 treatment cycles of 170 patients (total number treated in 1982). The numbers of follicles, recovered eggs, fertilization and pregnancy rates were compared on both systems and in relation to the ages of the patients and different age groups. Another computer analysis was terminated in September 1982, and assayed technical and morphological data influencing the success of ET (number of embryos replaced, speed of embryo cleavage, quality of ET, different types of catheters) on 79 ETs. Those results have been already published by us[6]. All statistical analyses were carried out by means of standardized computer programs[7].

RESULTS

System I (Table 1) — 204 oocyte recoveries were carried out in 148 patients. At least one mature egg was recovered in 171 cases (84% of all laparoscopies), 336 eggs (86%) were recovered from 391 punctured

149

follicles, 75% were fertilized successfully. ET was performed in 119 cases (i.e. 58% of all laparoscopies or 70% of all laparoscopies when

Table 1   Results of system I*

No. of laparoscopies	204		
No. of patients	148		
No follicle/no egg	33		
Patients with mature eggs	171	84%	
No. of follicles punctured	391		
Recovered eggs	336	86%	
Fertilized eggs	252	75%	
Embryo transfers	119	58%	(70%)
Pregnancies	20	10%	(17%)
Abortions	5		
Ectopic pregnancies	2		

*Obtained in the second Department of Obstetrics and Gynaecology, University of Vienna, 1982.

at least one egg was found). Pregnancy resulted in 20 cases, i.e. a pregnancy rate of 10% of all treatment cycles or 17% of all ETs. Five patients aborted within the 6–14 weeks gestation and two had an ectopic pregnancy.

Table 2   Results of system II*

No. of laparoscopies	29		
No. of patients	22		
No follicle/no egg	5		
Patients with mature eggs	24	83%	
No. of follicles punctured	48		
Recovered eggs	36	75%	
Fertilized eggs	23	64%	
Embryo transfers	16	55%	(66%)
Pregnancies	3	10%	/L
		19%	/ET
Abortions	0		

*Obtained in the IVF Institute, 1982

System II (Table 2) — Twenty-nine laparoscopies were performed in 22 patients and at least one mature egg was recovered in 24 cases (83%). Thirty-six eggs were recovered from 48 follicles; 64% of them were fertilized. 16 ETs were performed (i.e. 55% of all treatment cycles or 66% of all laparoscopies where eggs were found). Three resulted in normal pregnancies and births of healthy normal babies. The ages of those patients were 36, 38 and 41 years. System II has

150

been continued in 1983 with a similar success rate (four normal pregnancies out of 47 treatment cycles, January–June 1983). There was no statistical difference in the number of follicles and recovered eggs and the pregnancy rates between system I and II, although the fertilization rate was slightly lower (statistically not significant) in system II.

Table 3 Results of system III*

No. of laparoscopies	20		
No follicle/no egg	4		
Patients with mature eggs	16	80%	
No. of follicles punctured	33		
Recovered eggs	24	73%	
Fertilized eggs	11	46%	
Embryo transfers	10	50%	(62%)
Pregnancies	–		

*Obtained in Vienna, 1982.

System III (Table 3) — Oocyte recovery rates were slightly lower than in systems I and II. The fertilization rate was remarkably lower at only 46%. No pregnancy resulted from 10 ETs in 1982. Before system III was abandoned, two pregnancies were achieved in 1983 from 26 treatment cycles, both of which aborted during the 6th and 11th week of gestation, respectively.

Table 4 Egg recovery. *In vitro* fertilization. Embryo transfer. Office procedure results. (Institute Feichtinger/Kemeter, May/June 1983)

Ultrasonically guided follicle puncture	10
No. of patients	9
No. of follicles punctured	22
Recovered eggs	20
Fertilized eggs	9
Embryo transfers	5
Pregnancies	1

First results of ultrasonically guided follicle aspiration (Table 4) — Our first attempts at ultrasonically guided follicle aspiration resulted in one normal on-going pregnancy out of 5 ETs. 20 eggs were recovered from 22 follicles, but only nine of them were fertilized.

Results of the computer analysis — The age range of all patients was

20–44 years. The mean (±SE) number of follicles found at laparoscopy was 1.9±1 in the age group ≤25 years (*n* = 34), 2.0±1 in the age group 26–35 years (*n* = 162), and 1.9±1 in the age group of >35 years. The recovery rate of mature eggs was 84.3±32 in the first age group, 83.9±29 in the second and 88.7±27 in the third age group. The fertilization rates were 65.5±42% in the age group ≤25 years, 62.4±43% in the age group 26–33 years, and 74.2±37% in the age group ≥35 years). So there were no significant differences in follicle numbers, recovered eggs, fertilization and pregnancy rates between the age groups, nor any significant correlation of the age of the patients with the variables mentioned above. The age distribution of

```
            NOT PREGNANT                        PREGNANT
AGE         ..............................+......................
MIDPOINTS
   48.000)
   46.500)
   45.000)
   43.500)**
   42.000)
   40.500)***                                  *
   39.000)********
   37.500)************                         *
   36.000)*********
   34.500)**********************************   ***
   33.000)*******************                  **
   31.500)**************************************  ****
   30.000)*******************                  N
   28.500)*****************************         *
   27.000)***********                          ****
   25.500)****************************          ******
   24.000)****
   22.500)**************
   21.000)*
   19.500)*                                    *
   18.000)
   16.500)
   15.000)
```

```
MEAN            30.757              29.565        YEARS
STD.DEV.         4.776               4.747
R.E.S.D.         4.881               5.102
S. E. M.         0.330               0.990        NOT SIGNIFICANT
MAXIMUM         44.000              40.000
MINIMUM         20.000              20.000
SAMPLE SIZE      210                   23
```

Figure 4 Age distribution of pregnant and non-pregnant women in our IVF-programme systems I and II. Results of a computerized analysis on 233 treatment cycles

all pregnant and non-pregnant cases is seen from Figure 4: the mean age was 30.75±4.7 years in the non-pregnant group and 29.56±4.7 years in the pregnant patients.

DISCUSSION

Based on a successful clinical IVF programme in a large university department (i.e. system I) simplifications and different organization systems of this technique were evaluated by us during the past year. The aim of our study was to find out if IVF and ET could be successful out-patient or even gynaecological office procedures in the near future. Besides this, the need for establishing system II was given by the pressure of other routine work as well as personal encumbrances and restrictions at the university department. Care was taken not to diminish the success rate at each step of simplification. Those steps were, for example, establishing a routine protocol for the whole procedure, egg recovery by laparoscopy during the routine operating-theatre programme, simplified egg and embryo culture using a pre-prepared commercially available culture medium (B_2 INRA-Menezo) and a simpler gassing system[1] and reducing the bed-rest time after ET. Later, during system II, laparoscopy was carried out under general anaesthesia in a hospital but with same-day discharge of the patient, embryos were replaced 1 day earlier (24–28 hours after insemination) as an office procedure and bed-rest time after ET was reduced to a maximum of 30 minutes.

When creating system II we had to use the idea of transporting eggs from the hospital to the laboratory inside a Thermos flask, a system which had already been successfully applied in Paris[8,9]. In fact, soon after we began to use this system (May 1983) the same success rate was obtained as at the university department although the fertilization rate was slightly lower in system II. This could be due to a potential adverse effect of the transport for the oocytes. However, the selection of the patients has also to be taken into consideration since many of the couples treated in system II were not accepted for the IVF programme at the university clinic because of their age, slight endocrine disorders, bad spermiograms, etc. Concerning age in fact it could be shown by our data that age seemed not to influence IVF and the success rates after ovarian stimulation therapy.

Based on our good experience with system II it seemed likely that such a system could also work in collaboration with different hospitals and gynaecologists (system III). Although others reported good experience with such a concept[8,9] we had to abandon it because the results were not satisfying. In our particular case, we believe that this was due to some complicated connections between the teams and therefore lack of close co-operation.

Anyway, an operating room adjacent to the IVF laboratory should be the optimum, thus allowing oocytes to be placed in optimal culture conditions within a few minutes following recovery[10]. Ultrasonically guided follicle aspiration offered us the opportunity to perform oocyte recoveries in our laboratory since this technique has been shown to be a suitable, convenient and harmless method for oocyte recovery for IVF[2,3]. Our first results were encouraging although we had some fertilization problems possibly due to our beginner's difficulties, e.g., aspiration of urine with follicular fluid. However, one normal on-going pregnancy was obtained from our first cases treated, and hence we have demonstrated for the first time that treatment of sterility by oocyte recovery, IVF and ET can be performed successfully as an office procedure.

However, we have to stress that our work was based on years of clinical experience in this field. Oocyte handling, fertilization and culture should in our opinion always be restricted to a specially trained staff. IVF is therefore still a long way from becoming a widespread routine office procedure.

References

1. Feichtinger, W., Kemeter, P. and Szalay, S. (1983). The Vienna program of *in vitro* fertilization and embryo transfer – a successful clinical treatment. *Eur. J. Obstet. Gynaecol. Reprod. Biol.*, **15**, 205
2. Lenz, S., Lauritsen, J. G. and Kjellow, M. (1981). Collection of human oocytes for *in vitro* fertilization by ultrasonically guided follicular puncture. *Lancet*, **1**, 1163
3. Wikland, M., Nilsson, L., Hansson, R., Hamberger, L. and Janson, P. O. (1983). Collection of human oocytes by the use of sonography. *Fertil. Steril.*, **39**, 603
4. Feichtinger, W. and Kemeter, P. (1983). *In vitro* fertilization and embryo transfer – an outpatient/office procedure. In Feichtinger, W. and Kemeter, P. (eds.). *Recent Progress in Human In Vitro Fertilisation*. (Palermo: Cofese) (In press)
5. Feichtinger, W., Szalay, S., Beck, A., Kemeter, P. and Janisch, H. (1981). Results of laparoscopic recovery of preovulatory human oocytes from non-stimulated ovaries in an ongoing *in vitro* fertilization program. *Fertil. Steril.*, **36**, 707
6. Feichtinger, W., Kemeter, P. and Szalay, S. (1983). Facteurs morphologiques, endocrines et techniques en relation avec le resultat du transfer d'embryons humains dans l'uterus. *Gynecol. Obstet. Biol. Reprod. (Paris)* (In press)
7. BMDP (1979). *Biomedical Computer Programs*. (University of California Press)
8. Cohen, J. (1982). Follicular aspiration: Methods of each group. In Edwards, R. G. and Purdy, G. M. (eds.). *Human Conception In Vitro*, p. 406. (London: Academic Press)
9. Plachot, M., Mandelbaum, J., Cohen, J., Salat-Baroux, J. and Junca, A. M. (1983). Organization of human IVF centres on the basis of egg and embryo transportation. In Feichtinger, W. and Kemeter, P. (eds.). *Recent Progress in Human In Vitro Fertilisation*. (Palermo: Cofese) (In press)
10. Edwards, R. G. (1983). Discussion remark at the congress, *Recent Progress in Human In Vitro Fertilization*, June 22–24, Vienna

Part I

Section 4

Tubal Factors in Reproduction

14
Physiology of tubal function

E. M. COUTINHO

The importance of the Fallopian tubes in reproduction cannot be overemphasized. It is in the tube that fertilization occurs. It is also in the tube that, following the fusion of the gametes, the fertilized ovum divides itself and rapidly becomes a morula. This process of cell multiplication or cleavage requires an appropriate environment which is provided by fluid secreted by the tube.

In addition to providing the perfect environment for the meeting of the gametes, fertilization, and early development of the zygote, the tube must provide the safe transport of the ovum to the uterus, where implantation occurs[1-3]. To accomplish all these functions the tube is endowed with two or more layers of smooth musculature which contract and relax continuously, a ciliated epithelium, and numerous secretory cells which secrete tubal fluid.

Four segments, which apparently have different functions, may be distinguished in the tube. The infundibulum with its fimbria sweeps over the ovary to collect the egg at the time of ovulation. The transport of the egg from the ovarian surface to the ampulla is accomplished mainly through the activity of the infundibular epithelium which is very rich in ciliated cells. The ampulla has well-developed muscular layers and its epithelium has both ciliated and non-ciliated cells. The non-ciliated cells have secretory activity and contribute with their secretions to the formation of tubal fluid. In the ampulla, the ovum is detained for many hours or several days. It is here that fertilization takes place. Early development of the zygote also occurs in the ampulla. Ovum transport from the ampulla and through the isthmus is accomplished mainly through muscular activity. The isthmus has thick muscular layers and its lumen is very narrow. The epithelium has non-ciliated cells but very few ciliated cells. At the isthmoampullar junction a block to further transport of the ovum seems to be established at the time of ovulation. The block is apparently caused by activation of the isthmic musculature and may last several days. This ability to control the interval of permanence of the ovum in the tube through activation of its musculature seems to be the most important function of that portion of the oviduct. The isthmus ends at the uterotubal junction or junctura. This portion of the tube has the most complex musculature in view of the fusion of the muscle fibres from the uterus with those of the tubes[4]. The thickness and the arrangement of the muscular layers vary with the species. In man, the autochthonous musculature of the uterus that forms the inner layer of the uterine wall consists of four bundles. This arrangement enables a constrictor effect to be placed upon the larger part of the intramural tube and leaves this portion of the oviduct under myometrial control.

The musculature of the oviduct consists of longitudinal and circular muscle layers. In women, there are three layers: an inner longitudinal, an intermediary circular, and an outer longitudinal layer. The musculature layers are covered by a serosal layer composed of mesothelium continuous with that of the peritorium and connective tissue[5]. This layer is well vascularized. Smooth muscle fibres are found subperitoneally and around the blood vessels. Muscle cells are also believed to exist in the mucosa which is the innermost layer of the oviductal wall. Innervation of the oviduct is predominantly adrenergic. The adrenergic nerves supply both the musculature and the blood vessels. The amount of the musculature innervation in the ampulla and the isthmus is moderate but at the ampullary junction the innervation is very dense.

Although autonomic innervation is not essential to the function of the tube, there is ample evidence indicating that tubal motility is under adrenergic control. The tubes are in almost continuous motion. These movements result not only from the spontaneous activity of its smooth musculature but also from the activity of associated structures such as the mesosalpinx and other membranes. The changes in intratubal pressure resulting from the activity of tubal musculature reveal, on the other hand, patterns of motility which are typical of the tube[6]. These patterns are characterized by small contractions of

5–10 mmHg interspersed at regular intervals by outbursts of increased activity when intratubal pressure exceeds 20 mmHg. Periods of quiescence lasting several minutes usually follow an outburst[7].

The occurrence of periodic outbursts of increased activity are probably the most typical feature of tubal activity and may be associated with the local release of norepinephrine by the adrenergic nerve endings which are so abundant therein. In women the outbursts of increased activity occur with greatest frequency at the time of menstruation and the early proliferative phase of the cycle. During the preovulatory and ovulatory phases the overall activity of the tube increases. The outbursts become less conspicuous and are not followed by long lasting periods of quiescence as they usually are during the preceding phases. After ovulation tubal activity is depressed. The contractions are less frequent, outbursts decrease their intensity and duration. It should be noted, however, that unlike the uterus which may be quite quiescent under the inhibitory influence of the corpus luteum, the tube is never completely quiescent. This ability of the tube to remain active under the inhibitory effect of the corpus luteum seems to be necessary to assure the transport of the fertilized ovum to the quiescent uterus.

The resistance of the tube to the inhibitory effect of the luteal hormones is emphasized during pregnancy. While the uterus is kept quiescent throughout the period of gestation the tubes remain quite active. Despite this relative lack of sensitivity towards the hormones of the corpus luteum the tube is affected not only by the ovarian steroids but also by several other hormones and smooth muscle activators.

Oestrogens activate whereas progestins depress tubal motility. Under the influence of oestrogen the tube appears to become also more sensitive to the stimulatory effects of norepinephrine, epinephrine and oxytocin. Progestins on the other hand depress tubal response to these tubal stimulants. This ability of the ovarian steroids to change the excitability of tubal musculature seems to be essential for the control of tubal function. The isthmic block which prevents the ovum from passing into the uterus too early and which retains the ovum in the tube for approximately 3 days is induced by oestrogen and suppressed by progesterone.

The stimulatory effects of oxytocin released by reflex following the stimulation of the breasts are also more marked and lasting when the tube is under oestrogen domination. The greater sensitivity of tubes under oestrogen may be of importance therefore in the mechanism of ovum pick-up by the tube. Stimulation of the breasts during intercourse may induce the release of oxytocin which by stimulating the tube will cause its fimbriated end to 'massage' the ovary facilitating thereby follicle rupture.

After ovulation the egg is propelled through the ampulla which is by now full of tubal fluid but no further progress is possible because of the oestrogen-induced isthmic block. This block should be released under the increasing influence of progestin but tubal relaxants like prostaglandin E_2 which is present in semen may induce a transient relaxation which allows spermatozoa penetration.

Although most available evidence points to the progestational hormones as the agents of oestrogen block release on the tubal isthmus, recent studies show that relaxation of the oestrogen-dominated Fallopian tube may be induced by other hormones.

Human chorionic gonadotrophin (hCG) and human placental lactogen (HPL) inhibit tubal activity in the human, whereas prolactin has been shown to relax oestrogen-induced cervical and isthmic contraction in the rat. Another powerful isthmic relaxant is prostaglandin E_2, which appears to act as an α-adrenergic blocker on the tube[8,9].

The relaxing effects of gonadotrophins and E prostaglandins are more prompt than those of progesterone and seem to be mediated through cyclic AMP. The cyclic nucleotide itself is a powerful inhibitor of tubal motility. Whatever the mechanism of release of oestrogen-induced tubal block, it certainly plays an important role in the regulation of ovum transport. The existence of such a mechanism in women is indicated by the long time taken by the ovum to reach the uterus after ovulation.

Tubal quiescence may also be important in allowing negotiation by the spermatozoa of the tubal isthmus during the preovulatory and ovulatory phases, when the tube is under oestrogen domination. We have proposed that PGE_2 present in human semen provides the necessary relaxing effect. Whether this occurs *in vivo* remains to be shown.

Because PGE_2 acts as an α-adrenergic blocker, its inhibitory effects are more dramatic in those portions of the tube that are more densely innervated. Although the relaxing effects of PGE_2 are apparently associated with an increase in cyclic AMP concentration, attempts to prolong its relaxing action by the administration of aminophylline were not successful. However, in studies carried out *in vitro*, tubal contractility has been markedly depressed by aminophylline.

The inhibitory effect of aminophylline is not suppressed by pretreatment with propranolol and is potentiated by cyclic AMP. Dibutyryl cyclic AMP itself inhibits tubal motility; dibutyryl cyclic AMP and aminophylline reduce the activating effects of prostaglandin $F_{2\alpha}$ and norepinephrine. Compounds such as imidazole which stimulate phosphodiesterase, the enzyme which inactivates cyclic AMP, are stimulants to the tube. The activating effect of imidazole on tubal contractility is obviated by aminophylline pretreatment or by removal of CA^{2+} from the bath[10].

The relaxant effects of β-adrenergic activators such as ritrodrine or isoproterenol may be enhanced by aminophylline pretreatment, whereas the effects of tubal stimulants such as the α-adrenergic compounds are potentiated by imidazole.

These observations suggest that cyclic AMP indeed plays an important role in the regulation of tubal contractility. It has been suggested that the effects of cyclic AMP are counteracted within the cell by the nucleotide cyclic GMP. In *in vitro* preparations, 8-bromo cyclic GMP (dibutyryl cyclic AMP and 8-bromo cyclic GMP cross cell membranes more easily and resist enzymatic degradation longer than the parent nucleotides) has only a weak stimulatory action on the tube but it does reduce the inhibitory effect of cyclic AMP. Evaluation of the effects of cyclic AMP and GMP may give equivocal results, since the penetration of these nucleotides into the cell varies considerably[11].

The response of the mesosalpinx to several tubal active compounds is also influenced by blood oestrogen and progesterone concentrations. Activation of the mesosalpinx by oxytocin, norepinephrine and prostaglandin $F_{2\alpha}$ appears to be maximal during mid-cycle, at the peak of oestrogen domination. The mesosalpinx also responds to ergonovine with long-lasting contractions.

The presence of specific receptors for oestradiol and progesterone in the oviduct was reported in human and rabbit oviducts. Cyclic changes in steroid receptor concentrations were also observed. These receptors selectively bind oestradiol and progesterone and transport the steroids into the nucleus, whereupon RNA synthesis, RNA polymerase activity and chromatin template activity are rapidly increased. These events are followed by the appearance of a new species of nuclear RNA. The link between these early molecular events and changes in muscular activity is not yet worked out. Both oestrogen and progesterone have variable effect on tubal motility in humans. Plain progesterone seems to activate the tube, but this effect is not shared by other progestins such as megestrol acetate, which has a relaxing effect on human mesosalpinx *in vivo*.

Acknowledgment

This study was supported by the World Health Organization.

References

1. Hamner, E. and Fox, S. B. (1969). Biochemistry of oviductal secretion. In Hafez, E. S. E. and Blandau, R. (eds.). *The Mammalian Oviduct* (University of Chicago Press)
2. Coutinho, E. M. (1971). Physiologic and pharmacologic studies of the human oviduct. *Fertil. Steril.*, **22**, 807
3. Coutinho, E. M. (1973). Hormonal control of tubal musculature. In Segal, S., Crozier, R., Corfman, P. and Condliffe, P. (eds.). *The Regulation of Human Reproduction*. (Springfield: Charles C. Thomas)
4. Nilsson, O. and Reinins, S. (1969). Light and electron microscopic structure of the oviduct. In Hafez, E. S. E. and Blandau, R. (eds.). *The Mammalian Oviduct* (University of Chicago Press)
5. Hafez, E. S. E. and Block, D. L. (1969). The mammalian utero-tubal junction. In Hafez, E. S. E. and Blandau, R. (eds.). *The Mammalian Oviduct* (University of Chicago Press)
6. Maia, H. and Coutinho, E. M. (1968) A new technique for recording human tubal activity *in vivo*. *Am. J. Obstet. Gynecol.*, **102**, 1043
7. Coutinho, E. M. and Maia, H., Jr. (1979). Advances in uterine and tubal physiology research. In Talwar, G. P. (ed.). *Recent Advances in Reproduction and Regulation of Fertility* (Amsterdam: Elsevier North Holland)
8. Coutinho, E. M. (1974). Motility of the human fallopian tube. In Persianinov, L. S., Chervakova, T. V. and Presl. J. (eds.). *Recent Progress in Obstetrics and Gynecology*. (Amsterdam: Excerpta Medica)
9. Coutinho, E. M. and Maia, H., Jr. (1979). Fallopian tube. In Scarpelli, E. M. and Cosmi, E. V. (eds.). *Reviews in Perinatal Medicine*, Vol. **3**. (New York: Raven Press)
10. Takeda, T., Tsutsumi, Y., Satoshi, H. and Motoyasu, I. (1978). Effects of prostaglandin $F_{2\alpha}$ on egg transport and *in vivo* egg recovery from the vaginas of rabbits. *Fertil. Steril.*, **30**, 79
11. Maia, H., Jr., Barbosa, I. C., Hodgson, B., Harper, M. J. K. and Pauerstein, C. J. (1977). Effects of ovulation and hormonal treatment on the *in vitro* response of the rabbit oviduct to prostaglandins. *Fertil. Steril.*, **28**, 97

15
The epidemiology of salpingitis

W. THOMPSON

INTRODUCTION

Infection of the Fallopian tubes, termed salpingitis, can result in tubal damage and is an aetiological factor in 30–40% of cases of infertility[1]. It is also claimed to be responsible for 40–50% of ectopic pregnancies. The great majority of such infections are caused by ascending spread of an infection in the lower genital tract[2].

The incidence of salpingitis continues to increase on a world-wide scale and consequently so does the prevalence of women with post-infective tubal damage. The increasing number of tubal infections is clearly linked to the current epidemic of sexually transmitted diseases[3]. A large proportion of salpingitis is caused by organisms that are transmitted by sexual intercourse.

AETIOLOGY

From the aetiological viewpoint salpingitis can be considered in the following four broad categories.

Post-partum and post-operative

These causes are closely related in that they involve genital tract trauma. Puerperal sepsis is now uncommon in developed countries but may still be a relatively important cause of salpingitis in areas of the world where obstetric services are lacking.

Pelvic infections, whose primary origin is outside the genital tract, may contribute to tubal damage and future fertility. The most frequent example is delayed operative treatment of appendicitis resulting in pelvic adhesions. In all such cases subsequently presenting with infertility and a relevant history the diagnosis must be confirmed by laparoscopy as peritubal adhesions are difficult to detect with a hysterosalpingogram.

Post-operative infections may occasionally follow even minor operative procedures such as a hysterosalpingogram. Physicians should be alert to this possibility in patients with obvious pre-existing pelvic pathology.

Post-abortal

There has been a world-wide revolution in both the availability and utilization of therapeutic abortion. This may have had a favourable result in that many unwanted pregnancies have been eliminated and the incidence of illegal abortions in most countries has fallen.

Unfortunately, there is an infective morbidity in some of these patients undergoing such procedures and this will influence the future childbearing potential of those affected women.

The risk of infection at pregnancy termination procedures increases with greater gestation. Tietze and Lewit[4] reported a pelvic infection rate of 0.9 per 1000 cases at 8 weeks' gestation but by 13 weeks' gestation the incidence had risen to 1.6 per 1000; a two-fold increase.

A recent report from the United Kingdom suggested an incidence as high as 5%[5]. If this is true then at least 8000 women per year will be affected when we consider the present high rates of termination of pregnancy in that country[6]. An additional factor is the method used to effect the termination; suction curettage appears to have lower sepsis rates than dilatation and curettage.

Genital tuberculosis

The incidence of genital tuberculosis in most Western countries continues to decline[7]. However, it still must be considered a significant cause of tubal damage in some developing countries. Mukerjee[8] found histological evidence of endometrial tuberculosis in over 14% of cases of primary sterility in India.

Because of the insidious nature of the disease and the high incidence of severe tubal damage it is important to identify at-risk patients such as those with a family history of tuberculosis and in such cases employ appropriate diagnostic procedures. The timely diagnosis may be vital in view of the reports, admittedly rare, of successful pregnancies after treatment. Schaefer[9] in a critical review of the subject noted that the prognosis as regards curing the patient from genital tuberculosis had greatly improved since the advent of effective chemotherapy but the chance of a successful pregnancy remains very low. In his review of 7357 patients with treated tuberculosis there were 115 full-term pregnancies, 67 abortions and 125 ectopic pregnancies. The successful outcome was therefore only 0.02%; concern has naturally been expressed at the high incidence of ectopic pregnancies since the introduction of antituberculosis therapy.

Both tubes are involved in the pathological process and it is therefore not surprising that one ectopic pregnancy may later be followed by a second in the contralateral tube.

Sexually transmitted pathogens

By far the most common cause of salpingitis is that due to sexually transmitted pathogens; coincident with the increase in such diseases during the past two decades has been an increase in the incidence of related salpingitis[10]. According to the World Health Organization gonorrhoea has reached epidemic proportions with more than 100 million cases per year[11]. A more realistic figure is probably 250 million as a large proportion of cases remain unreported to official agencies. Salpingitis from such causes is now one of the most common acute gynaecological problems, responsible for 10–20% of admissions to hospitals in the United States – an estimated 250000 cases per year[12].

The factors responsible for such trends must be identified for they have a direct bearing on the incidence of salpingitis. The last decade has witnessed a dramatic upsurge in liberal sexual behaviour and society's tolerance of casual sex[13]. The emancipation of women throughout most of the world has also had an important influence on behavioural patterns and has facilitated sexual contact. For example, in Singapore the percentage of economically active women in the 15–44 age group has risen from 21% in 1957 to 42% in 1975[14]. Air travellers have replaced seamen as one of the most important groups at risk of sexually transmitted diseases. Prostitutes play a less significant role in the spread of such diseases but remain important as core transmitters in the large city areas[15]. Rapid industrialization and urbanization in many countries has led to migration of labour, disruption of family life and promiscuity. This social disorganization has played an important part in Africa where the transition of tribal life to urban life combined with poverty and lack of medical facilities is a major factor responsible for the high incidence of gonorrhœa in these parts of the world[16]. A further important change is the marked increase in sexually transmitted diseases reported in young girls.

Age-specific case rates in Western countries show a disproportionately higher increase or continually high rates among 20–24 year olds[10]. When we consider that a smaller proportion of females in the younger age groups are sexually active then the risk of infection in those exposed is even greater than older women. In Sweden the risk of infection in a sexually active 15 year old is estimated to be 1 in 8 and this decreases rapidly to 1 in 80 in females 24 years and older[1]. There is now an increasing recognition of women who are symptomless carriers of sexually transmitted pathogens; the rate is probably over 55%[17]. Such individuals are not only responsible for the dissemination of disease in the community but will continue to remain at risk of developing salpingitis. This is much more likely to occur at or immediately after menstruation.

The infecting agents responsible for sexually transmitted salpingitis can be divided into gonoccocal and non-gonoccocal types. This division is based on the recovery of Neisseria gonorrhoeae from the endocervices of patients with salpingitis. Recovery rates vary between 33 and 45%[2]. The presence of pathogenic bacteria in the endocervix is not absolute proof that such organisms are responsible for upper genital tract infection. Utilization of culdocentesis, laparoscopy and laparotomy for obtaining culture specimens from peritoneal fluid and tubal exudate has shown a poor correlation between the cervical and intra-abdominal cultures; recovery rates vary between 6 and 70%[3]. An explanation for this finding is that the gonococcus may be important only in initiating the infective process and paving the way for other pathogenic bacteria of the cervical and vaginal flora to gain access to the upper genital tract. The recovery of Neisseria gonorrhoeae appears to depend on the time of sampling in relationship to the onset of tubal infection. Lip and Borgoyne[18] isolated the gonococcus from cul-de-sac aspirates in 70% of patients within 2 days of the onset of symptoms but very rarely if symptoms were present for 7 or more days. Another explanation for the low recovery rates of gonoccocus from the peritoneum may be the ability of the organism to attach to the epithelial cell. Studdiford *et al.*[19] were able to isolate *Neisseria gonorrhoeae* from tubal tissue in 67% of patients.

When considering the gonococcus as an infecting agent there are two recent developments pertaining to its control and treatment. In the first place the organism has become increasingly resistant to penicillin. In 1950, shortly after the widespread introduction of anti- biotics, all gonococci were sensitive to mean inhibitory concentra- tions of benzyl penicillin of $0.015 \mu g$ ml^{-1} but by 1969 it was necessary to use concentrations of $0.125 \mu g$ ml^{-1} to obtain the same response[20,21]. Increasing resistance continues to cause concern throughout the world but more so in developing countries, where the widespread abuse of antibiotics is rampant[22].

The most significant and alarming development since the discovery of penicillin has been the emergence of β-lactamase producing gonoc- occi totally resistant to penicillin[23]. The original outbreak in the United Kingdom in 1976 was effectively isolated and controlled[24]. However, since 1977 further cases have been reported all over the United Kingdom usually imported from Africa and Asia. More re- cently there has been a steep increase in the proportion of cases contracted from consorts themselves infected in the United Kingdom; therefore, for the first time endemic transmission is occurring[25].

Furthermore, there are now reports of gonococci with multiple antibiotic resistance. The WHO regards this matter as a very serious threat to public health[26]. Early effective treatment of gonococcal infections is most important in reducing the incidence of salpingitis and in the established disease, damage to the Fallopian tubes. The aforementioned trends will undoubtedly make this task more difficult to achieve. The UK can boast one of the most comprehensive services in the world for the diagnosis, treatment and control of sexually transmitted diseases – if it has failed to limit the spread of the newer strains of gonococci then one can only be alarmed by the damage they will cause in those areas of the world with less developed medical services.

The exact aetiology of non-gonococcal salpingitis is still the subject of controversy. However, the D to K strains of *Chlamydia trachomatis* have been incriminated in a high percentage of cases[27]. *Chlamydia trachomatis* has been isolated from tubal material and has produced salpingitis in the experimental animal[28]. Serological tests suggest that 66–80% of salpingitis is chlamydial in origin[29]. More direct clinical evidence is available from studies in Sweden which report a 30% incidence of *Chlamydia trachomatis* isolated from the Fallopian tubes of patients with salpingitis confirmed by laparoscopy[27].

Although mycoplasmas and related ureaplasmas have been frequently recovered from the lower genital tract in women with salpingitis[30], no difference exists between the rates of isolation from the cervix of those patients and in sexually active controls. Moreover, mycoplasmas have been recovered infrequently from the peritoneal cavity or Fallopian tube of patients with salpingitis. Mardh and Westrom[31] detected mycoplasmas in 8% of patients with salpingitis, none of whom had gonococcal infections. Somomon *et al.*[32] grew pure cultures of mycoplasma from pelvic abscesses. However, Taylor-Robinson and Carney[33] showed that genital strains of mycoplasma were capable of growing on human Fallopian tube organ cultures but did not produce any demonstrable tissue damage. The evidence regarding the role of genital tract mycoplasmas and salpingitis remains unclear. The same could be said of bacteroides; in spite of extensive studies the exact cause and effect relationship has not been proven as regards salpingitis[34].

Since the advent of bacteriological studies of the peritoneum in patients with salpingitis many workers have remarked on the wide range of organisms that can be isolated on culture; both anaerobic and aerobic[35]. The term polymicrobial pelvic infection has been used to described this condition[36]. Except for *Neisseria gonorrhoeae* and *Chylamydia trachomatis* there is no conclusive evidence to suggest that other bacteria have a primary role in causing infection of normal Fallopian tubes. As noted previously, once the integrity of the tube has been breached mixed infection occurs. Support for this thesis comes from the study by Holmes *et al.*[37] who reported a significantly lower number of gonococcal infections in women with recurrent salpingitis, in whom presumably the tubes were already damaged.

The only data relating to the incidence of PID in the UK comes from hospital inpatient statistics[11], which undoubtedly underestimated the incidence of the disease because many patients will not have been treated in hospital. These data show that the incidence of the condition has more than doubled in the last 20 years; from 5850 cases in 1960 to 12450 in 1979. Recent trends in sexually transmitted diseases show a fall in the incidence of gonorrhoea and a marked increase in non-specific genital infection in women. This suggests that there is an ever-increasing proportion of cases of PID caused by non-specific genital infection.

CONTRACEPTIVE METHODS AND SALPINGITIS

The revolution of contraceptive techniques in the 1960s leading to the widespread use of oral contraceptives and intrauterine contraceptive devices have played a significant role in the prevalence of salpingitis. In the first place they replaced the more traditional occlusive forms of contraception namely the condom and diaphragm. This in turn eliminated whatever protective action such methods provided in the prevention of the spread of genital infections.

Most epidemiological studies throughout the world have shown that IUD users have an increased risk of salpingitis; a factor of from 1.9 to 9.3[38–41]. Initially it was proposed that if there was any association between the IUD and salpingitis, it existed only immediately after insertion of the device. Infection occurring 2 months post-insertion was considered to be unrelated to the IUD. This belief was based on a study by Mishell and Moyer[42] who reported that positive endometrial bacterial cultures were found in all women within 24 hours of insertion and no positive cultures were obtained if the IUD has been in place longer than 45 days. It may be true that bacteria do not persist in the endometrial cavity but they are encouraged to be re-introduced usually at the time of menstruation or coitus. The presence of an IUD may alter in some way the local host defence mechanisms, and the tail of the device undoubtedly assists bacterial ascent through the cervix.

Some of these earlier studies were criticized because controls had used other methods of contraception which are known to reduce the risk of salpingitis[39]. Furthermore, except for Westrom's study[40] the diagnosis of salpingitis was not documented by direct means. There is a pre-conceived bias since patients presenting with some of the symptoms of salpingitis and an IUD *in situ* may be more likely to be diagnosed as having active infection. More recent studies have been designed to eliminate these objections and have still convincingly proved that IUD users have an increased risk of acute salpingitis.

Furthermore, it is possible to identify certain groups of patients at greatly increased risk, namely those with a previous history of salpingitis, women with multiple sexual partners and adolescents. Several studies have demonstrated that women under 30 years of age are at increased risk of developing salpingitis as compared with those over 30 years[38]. Nulliparous users have a greater risk than multiparous users. It is recommended that doctors should use these risk factors and counsel such women against IUD use. This is important when we consider that the number of women using IUDs in the UK rose by 31% between 1976 and 1980[11].

The introduction of copper-containing devices might have been expected to reduce the incidence of salpingitis[44] for studies have shown that copper ions have a lethal effect on the gonococcus. However, Westrom et al.[40] have shown that the rate of salpingitis was similar in patients matched for cervical gonorrhoea with plastic and copper-containing devices.

In contrast to the those fitted with an IUD, women using oral contraceptives appear to be at no increased risk of salpingitis[40]. In fact some reports suggest that the incidence is reduced. The change in cervical mucus and the scant short menstrual loss constitute a relative protection against ascending genital infections.

SALPINGITIS AND SUBSEQUENT FERTILITY

As noted previously, pregnancy rates following tuberculous salpingitis are very poor, and such patients have an alarmingly high incidence of ectopic pregnancy.

Non-gonococcal salpingitis is associated with higher infertility rates than gonococcal salpingitis[45]. The explanation for this is that gonococcal salpingitis tends to present with more classically described signs and symptoms and thus such patients are more likely to be diagnosed and treated with antibiotics. Most antibiotic regimens are aimed at the irradication of the gonococcus and do not take into account the polymicrobial aetiology of the disease. There is no doubt that the effectiveness of therapy depends upon the interval between the onset of the symptoms and the start of treatment. Viberg[46] reported that none of his patients treated within 2 days of the onset of symptoms had involuntary infertility. However, if treatment was delayed beyond 7 days only 70% had tubal patency. The use of steroids has been advocated to reduce tubal damage. Falk[47] in a prospective study reported that steroids produced no difference in the end results as judged by HSG and fertility rates.

The study by Westrom[45] has provided a most reliable assessment of the effects of acute non-tuberculous salpingitis on subsequent fertility in that the diagnosis was confirmed by laparoscopy. The series of 415 cases collected between 1960 and 1967 had a 21% involuntary infertility rate after one episode of salpingitis – matched controls had an incidence of only 3%. The most significant factor as regards prognosis is recurrent infection. Tubal occlusions were diagnosed in 12.8% of patients following one infection, 35.5% after two and after three or more infections it was 75%. The ratio between ectopic pregnancy and intrauterine pregnancy was one in 24, a six-fold increase over controls. Ectopic pregnancy is associated with pathological changes of salpingitis in over 50% of cases.

References

1. Westrom, L. (1980). Incidence, prevalence and trends of acute pelvic inflammatory disease and its consequences in industrialized countries. *Am. J. Obstet. Gynecol.*, **138**, 880
2. Eschenbach, D. A. and Holmes, K. K. (1975). Acute pelvic inflammatory disease; current concepts of pathogenesis, etiology and management. *Clin. Obstet. Gynecol.*, **18**, 35
3. Sweet, R. L. (1977). Diagnosis and treatment of acute salpingitis. *J. Reprod. Med.*, **19**, 21
4. Tietze, C. and Lewit, S. (1971). Use effectiveness of oral and intrauterine contraception. *Fertil Steril.*, **22**, 508
5. Ridgway, G. L., Mumtaz, G., Stevens, R. A. and Oriel, J. S. (1983). Therapeutic abortion and chlamydial infection. *Br. Med. J.*, **286**, 1478
6. Mills, A. (1983). Therapeutic abortion and chlamydial infection. *Br. Med. J.*, **286**, 1649
7. Sutherland, A. M. (1979). Gynaecological tuberculosis. *Br. J. Hosp. Med.*, **22**, 569
8. Mukerjee, K., Wagh, K. V. and Agarwal, S. (1967). Tuberculous endometritis in primary sterility. *J. Obstet. Gynaecol. India*, **17**, 619.
9. Schaefer, G. (1967). Diagnosis and treatment of female genital tuberculosis. *Int. Surg.*, 48, 240
10. Robinson, N., Beral, V. and Ashley, J. S. A. (1981). Trends in pelvic inflammatory disease in England and Wales. *J. Epidemiol. Commun. Med.*, 36, 265
11. *British Medical Journal* (1983). Sexually transmitted disease surveillance 1981. *Br. Med. J.*, **286**, 1500
12. Shafer, M. A., Irwin, C. E. and Sweet, R. L. (1982). Acute salpingitis in the adolescent female. *J. Pediatr.*, **100**, 339
13. O'Brien, E. T. (1976). Hibernian mores; hypocrisy of reality. *Br. Med. J.*, **i**, 145
14. Rajan, V. S. (1978). Sexually transmitted diseases on a tropical island. *Br. J. Ven. Dis.*, **54**, 141
15. Kolata, G. B. (1976). Gonorrhoea – more of a problem but less of a mystery. *Science*, **192**, 244
16. Verhagen, A. R. and Gemert, W. (1972). Social and epidemiological determinants of gonorrhoea in an East African country. *Br. J. Ven. Dis.*, **48**, 277
17. Catterall, R. D. (1970). The problem of gonorrhoea. *Br. J. Hosp. Med.*, **3**, 55
18. Lip, J. and Borgoyne, X. (1966). Cervical and peritoneal bacterial flora associated with salpingitis. *Obstet. Gynecol.*, **28**, 561

19. Studdiford, W. E., Casper, W. A. and Scadron, E. N. (1938). The persistance of gonococcal infections in the adnexae. *Surg. Gynecol. Obstet.*, **67**, 176
20. Gocke, T. M., Wilcox, C. and Finland, M. (1950). Antibiotic spectrum of gonococcus. *Am. J. Syph.*, **34**, 265
21. Keys, T. F., Halverson, C. W. and Clarke, E. J. (1969). Single dose treatment of gonorrhoea with selected antibiotic agents. *J. Am. Med. Assoc.*, **210**, 857
22. Arya, O. P., Osoba, A. O. and Bennett, F. J. (1980). *Tropical Venereology*. (Edinburgh: Churchill-Livingstone)
23. World Health Organization (1976). Neisseria gonorrhoeae producing penicilliniase. *Weekly Epidemiol. Rec.*, **38**, 293
24. Percival, A., Rowlands, J., Arya, O. P., *et al.* (1976). Penicilliniase-producing gonococci in Liverpool. *Lancet*, **2**, 1379
25. McCutchan, J. A., Adler, M. W. and Berrie, J. R. M. (1982). Penicilliniase-producing *Neisseria gonorrhoeae* in Great Britain 1977–81: Alarming increase in incidence and recent development of endemic transmission. *Br. Med. J.*, **285**, 337
26. World Health Organization (1977). A new complication in the fight against gonorrhoea. *WHO Chronicle*, **31**, 38
27. Mardh, P-A., Ripa, T., Svensson, L. and Westrom, L. (1977). Chlamydia trachomatis infection in patients with acute salpingitis. *N. Engl. J. Med.*, **296**, 1377
28. Ripa, K. T., Moller, B. R., Mardh, P-A., Freudt, F. A. and Melsen, F. (1979). Experimental acute salpingitis in grivet monkeys provoked by Chlamydia trachomatis. *Acta Pathol. Microbiol. Scand. (B)*, **87**, 65
29. Treharne, J. D., Ripa, T., Mardh, P-A., Svensson, L., Westrom, L. and Darougar, S. (1979). Antibodies to *Chlamydia trachomatis* in acute salpingitis. *Br. J. Ven. Dis.*, **55**, 26
30. Osborne, N. G. (1977). The significance of mycoplasma in pelvic infection. *J. Reprod. Med.*, **19**, 39
31. Mardh, P-A. and Westrom, L. (1970). Tubal and cervical cultures in acute salpingitis with special reference to mycoplasma hominis and T-stain mycoplasmas. *Br. J. Ven. Dis.*, **46**, 179
32. Solomon, F., Sompolinsky, D., Caspi, E. *et al.* (1970). Isolation and identification of mycoplasma from clinical material in Israel. *Isr. J. Med. Sci.*, **6**, 605
33. Taylor-Robinson, D. and Carney, F. E. (1974). Growth and effect of mycoplasmas in Fallopian tube organ cultures. *Br. J. Ven. Dis.*, **50**, 212
34. Cunningham, F. G., Hauth, J. C., Gilstrop, L. C., Herbert, W. N. P. and Kappus, S. S. (1978). The bacterial pathogenesis of acute pelvic inflammatory disease. *Obstet. Gynecol.*, **52**, 161
35. Sweet, R. L., Mills, J., Hadley, W. R. *et al.* (1979). Use of laparoscopy to determine the microbial etiology of acute salpingitis. *Am. J. Obstet. Gynecol.*, **134**, 68
36. Swenson, R. M., Michaelson, T. C., Daly, M. J. *et al.* (1973). Anaerobic bacterial infections of the female genital tract. *Obstet. Gynecol.*, **42**, 538
37. Holmes, K. K., Eschenback, D. A. and Knapp, J. S. (1980). Salpingitis: overview of etiology and epidemiology. *Am. J. Obstet. Gynecol.*, **138**, 893
38. Ory, H. W. (1978). A review of the association between intrauterine devices and acute pelvic inflammatory disease. *J. Reprod. Med.*, **20**, 200
39. Flesh, G., Weiner, J. M., Corlett, R. C., Boice, C., Mishell, D. R. and Wolf, R. M. (1979). The intrauterine contraceptive device and acute salpingitis. *Am. J. Obstet. Gynecol.*, **135**, 402
40. Westrom, L., Bengtsson, L. P. and Mardh, P-A. (1976). The risk of pelvic inflammatory disease in women using intrauterine contraceptive devices as compared to non-users. *Lancet*, **2**, 221
41. Lippes, J. (1975). Infection and the IUD; a preliminary report. *Contraception*, **12**, 103

42. Mishell, D. E. and Moyer, D. L. (1969). Association of pelvic inflammatory disease with the intrauterine device. *Clin. Obstet. Gynecol.*, **12**, 179
43. Jennings, J. (1974). Report of Safety and Efficacy of the Dalkon Shield and other IUDs. Prepared by the ad hoc Obstetric-Gynecology Advisory Committee to the US Food and Drug Administration
44. Fiscina, B., Oster, G. K., Oster, G. and Swanson, J. (1973). Gonococcidal action of copper *in vitro*. *Am. J. Obstet. Gynecol.*, **116**, 86
45. Westrom, L. (1975). Effect of acute pelvic inflammatory disease on fertility. *Am. J. Obstet. Gynecol.*, **121**, 707
46. Viberg, L. (1964). Acute inflammatory conditions of the uterine adnexa; clinical, radiological and isotopic investigations of non-gonococcal adnexitis. *Acta Obstet. Gynecol. Scand.*, **43**, (Suppl. 4), 1
47. Falk, V. (1965). Treatment of acute non-tuberculous salpingitis with antibiotics alone and in combination with glucocorticoids. *Acta Obstet. Gynecol. Scand.*, **44**, (Suppl. 6), 3

16
Pelviscopic therapy for tubal disease

K. SEMM

INFECTION

As long as only laparotomy was applied for the inspection of the Fallopian tubes acute and chronic adnexitis did not represent an indication for laporotomy. Pelviscopy – a far less aggressive procedure than laparotomy – heralded a change in operative procedures. Adnexitis was earlier often treated for weeks or months, by antibiotics and physical therapy without the possibility of establishing a bacteriogram. Nowadays, pelviscopy enables an early, exact diagnosis and the detection of responsible bacteria and mycoplasmas. This quick diagnosis of infection-causing organisms is of great importance. The longer the infection lasts, the more irreversible is the damage by bacteria to the cilia of the endosalpinx. A diminution of cilia to under $500 \, mm^{-2}$ reduces the chance of conception to zero.

The diagnosis of an infection is not only very important for the conservation of fertility; once a specific bacteriogram is obtained specific antibiotics can be given. The quick diagnosis of an infection in the minor pelvis also leads to a remarkable shortening of hospitalization time and avoids chronic infections and abdominal pain. The results of pelviscopy therefore not only shorten the time of illness, but also preserve fertility by a high degree.

TUBAL AND ECTOPIC PREGNANCY

Pelviscopy has led to a change in operative techniques in conditions other than adnexitis. Earlier, it was necessary during laparotomy to cure a tubal pregnancy by tubectomy. This classic procedure was justified as one did not perform a laparotomy in a second ectopic pregnancy or similar occurrence. The possibility of repeating a pelviscopy because of its minor physical danger permits the conservative treatment of tubal pregnancy. In a tubal pregnancy early diagnostic pelviscopy is preceded by palpation alone or by ultrasound. This diagnostic pelviscopy can immediately be followed by an operative pelviscopy. Hence tubal pregnancy is treated under optimal conditions. First, the blood is sucked from the minor pelvis, for which the Aqua-purator (Figure 1) and monofile-bivalent aspiration tube

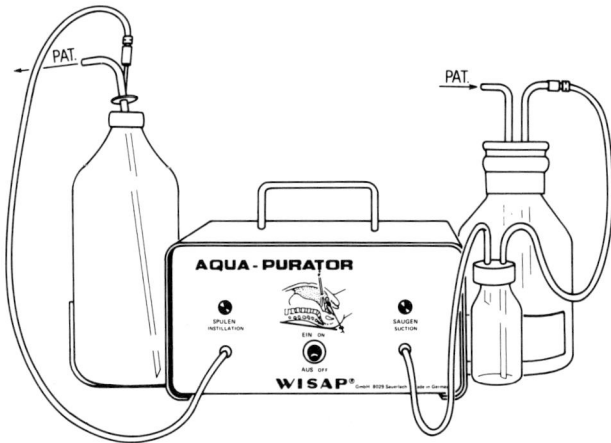

Figure 1 The Aqua-purator used for removing blood from the minor pelvis. PAT = Patient

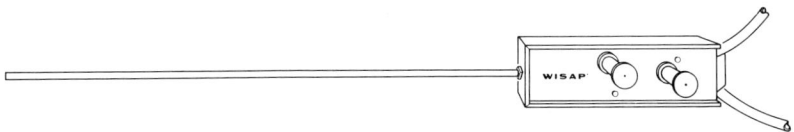

Figure 2 Monofile-bivalent aspiration tube

(Figure 2) are useful. With the point-coagulator (Figure 3 (a)), the anti-mesosalpinx is coagulated for 2–5 cm using the endocoagulation procedure. The endocoagulator (Figure 4) produces a temperature of 100° C, necessary for the protein coagulation. The human body thereby does not come into contact with the electric current. The tube is incised longitudinally (Figure 3 (b)) and the pregnancy product is taken out with a small spoon (Figure 3 (c)). After a careful rinsing of the minor pelvis, the wound is sutured by an endosuture with extracorporeal knotting (Figure 3 (d)).

The physical stress for the patient can be compared with that experienced during a sterilization procedure or curettage. 8 months after this operation, hardly any cicatrix can be seen in the tube. The tube may also be examined by ascending chromosalpingoscopy and is patent for consecutive tube pertubation.

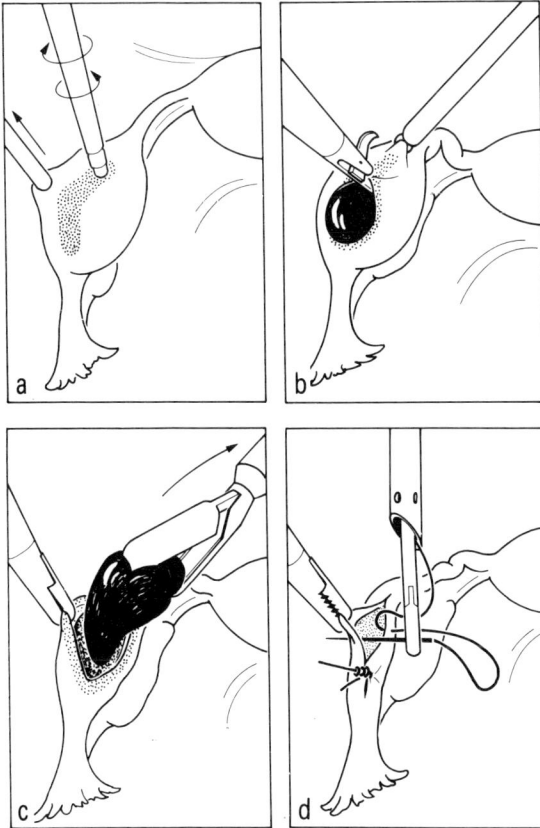

Figure 3 Operative procedure for ectopic pregnancy using pelviscopy

In summary, it can be said that endoscopic intra-abdominal surgery conserves fertility in 80% of ectopic pregnancies. So even in recurrent ectopic pregnancy, tubectomy is not justified. In one case after tubectomy in the first pregnancy and after two conserving operations of the tube on the contralateral side in a patient with recurrent ectopic pregnancy, a successful intrauterine pregnancy went to term.

In cases, however, of an ectopic pregnancy in an older person whose child bearing is concluded, endoscopic tubectomy is used in the much simpler procedure of tube-conserving therapy. We use our three-ligature technique. First, the small pelvis is washed with the Aqua-purator in order to free it from the sight-obstructing quantities

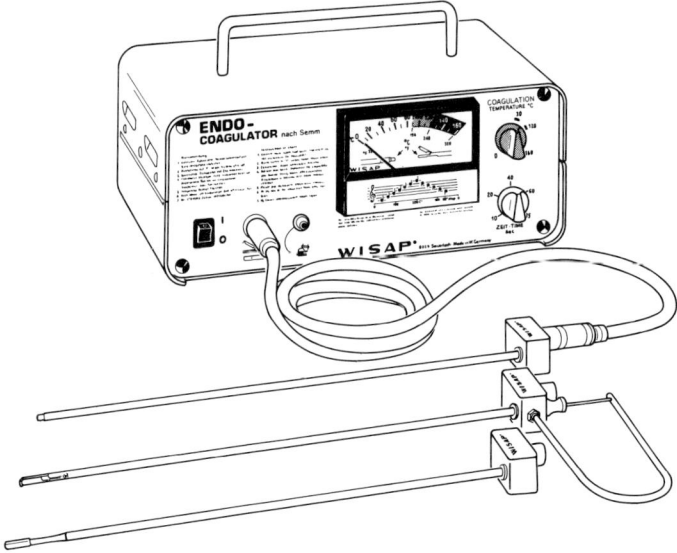

Figure 4 Endocoagulator for operative pelviscopy

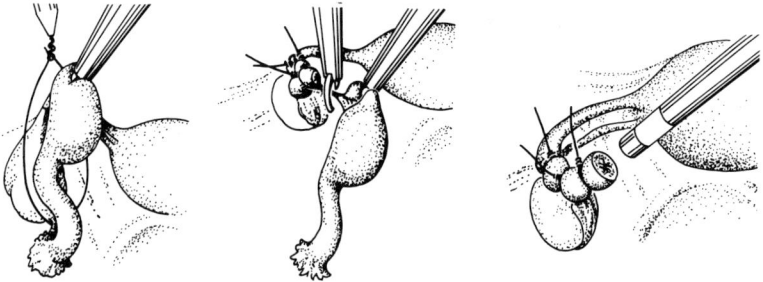

Figure 5 Placing of three Roeder loops around product of ectopic pregnancy in endoscopic tubectomy

of blood. Three Roeder loops (Figure 5) are put around the pregnancy product, partially ligating the tube. After dissection of the tube, the

178

fetus and the corresponding chorionic tissue are taken out after careful rinsing of the whole minor pelvis with saline solution at 37° C. The postoperative situs is topographically normal.

In the case of a pure ectopic pregnancy where the blastocyst nidates in an endometriotic focus in the pouch of Douglas, the pregnancy is terminated by curettage with a small spoon-forceps. After repeated rinsing of the minor pelvis, a normal genital situs should remain.

INFERTILITY SURGERY

Endoscopic abdominal surgery is specifically indicated for the correction of peripheral tubal occlusions and intense abdominal adhesions. While pelviscopy used to be exclusively a diagnostic procedure to indicate whether a laparotomy was necessary, it is nowadays used mainly for surgical therapy.

I shall not discuss the technical advances of instruments and apparatus that were necessary for the development of endoscopic intra-abdominal surgery (Figure 6). With the help of these new

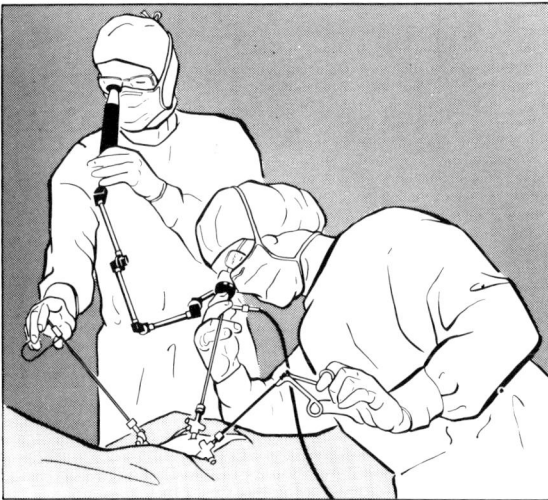

Figure 6 Instruments used in endoscopic intra-abdominal surgery and positions of surgeon and assistant

instruments, in cases of sterility the following endoscopic surgical procedures are possible:

(1) General adhesiolysis with omentum and bowel-preparation

179

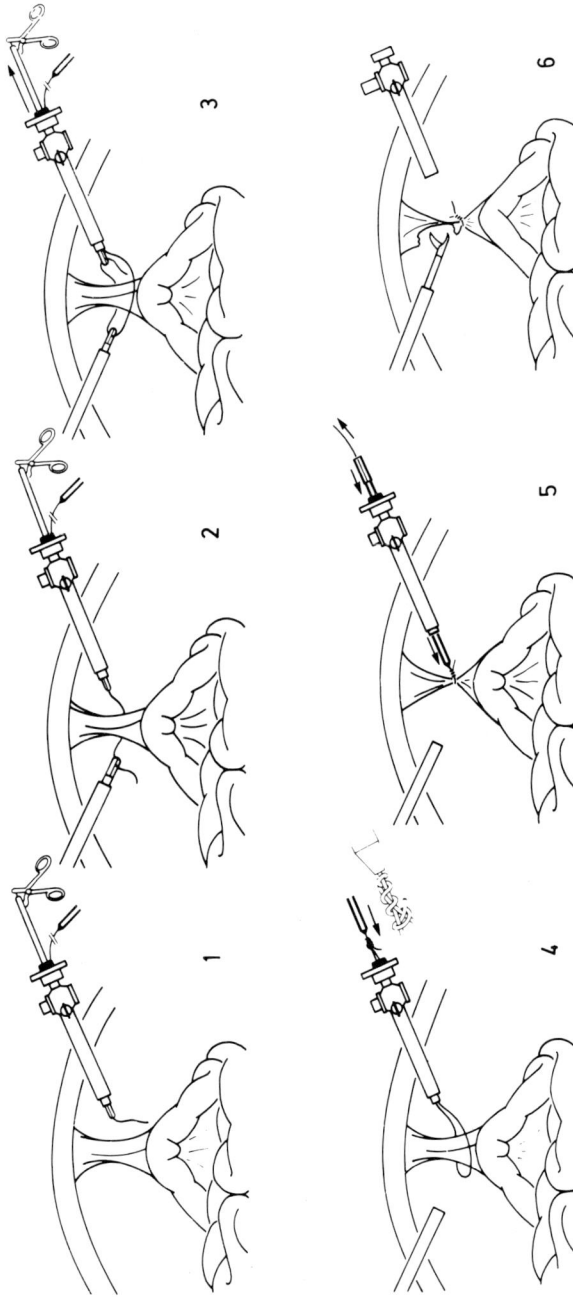

Figure 7 Application of endoligatures and sutures in pelviscopic treatment of omentum adhesions

in the entire abdomen. This may be important especially after previous laparotomies.

(2) Careful salpingolysis which after infectious processes in the minor pelvis presents the baseline for an operation on the ampullar ends of the tubes.

(3) An ovariolysis.

(4) A fimbrioplasty.

(5) A salpingostomy.

Massive adhesions are often found at the beginning of pelviscopy. Applying endoligatures and sutures (Figure 7) enables us to free massive omental adhesions without bleeding. In operations on the omentum and intestines, I no longer advise using coagulation to stop bleeding. Near the intestines and with the omentum, ligatures and sutures should be the only devices used – in the same way as in laparotomy.

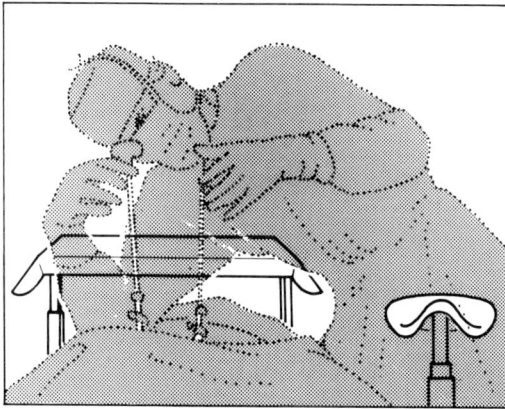

Figure 8 Position of surgeon performing endoscopy

In salpingolysis, the crocodile forceps (Figure 4) are used for haemostasis. Coagulated tissue remains without adhesions. Cases of broad adhesions are treated with a myoma-enucleator (Figure 4) to achieve a bloodless adhesiolysis. Also, in cases of ovariolysis, the application of the myoma-enucleator is advised, as with its help – using an atraumatic forceps – the ovary can be separated from its adhesions without any bleeding.

I would like to stress the following points: the endoscopic surgeon

181

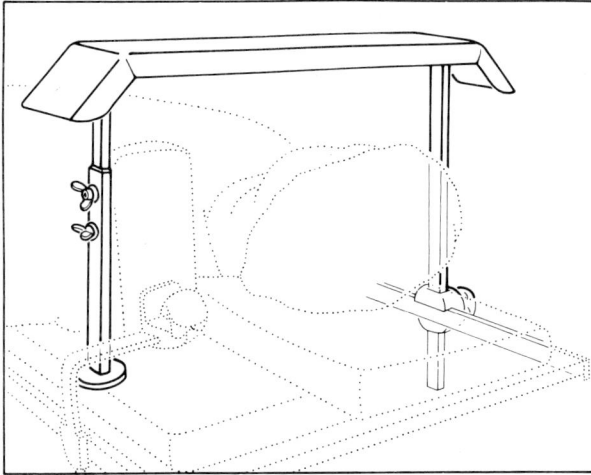

Figure 9   Shoulder support for surgeon during endoscopy (supine position)

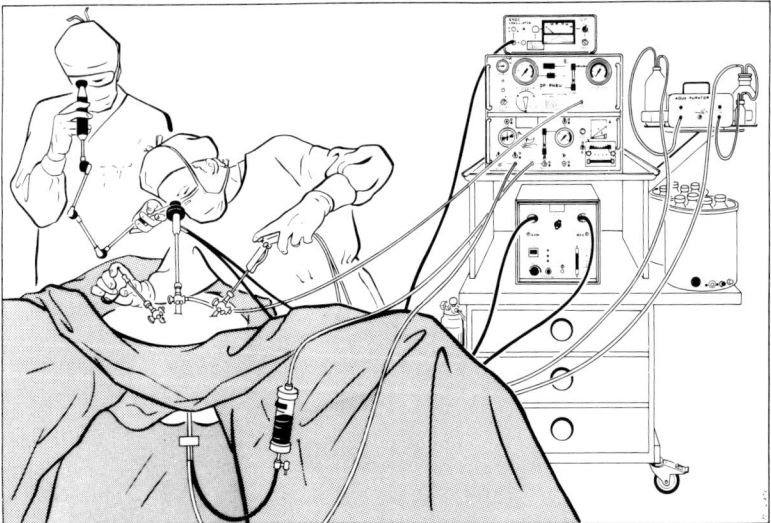

Figure 10   Operating theatre lay-out for endoscopy

182

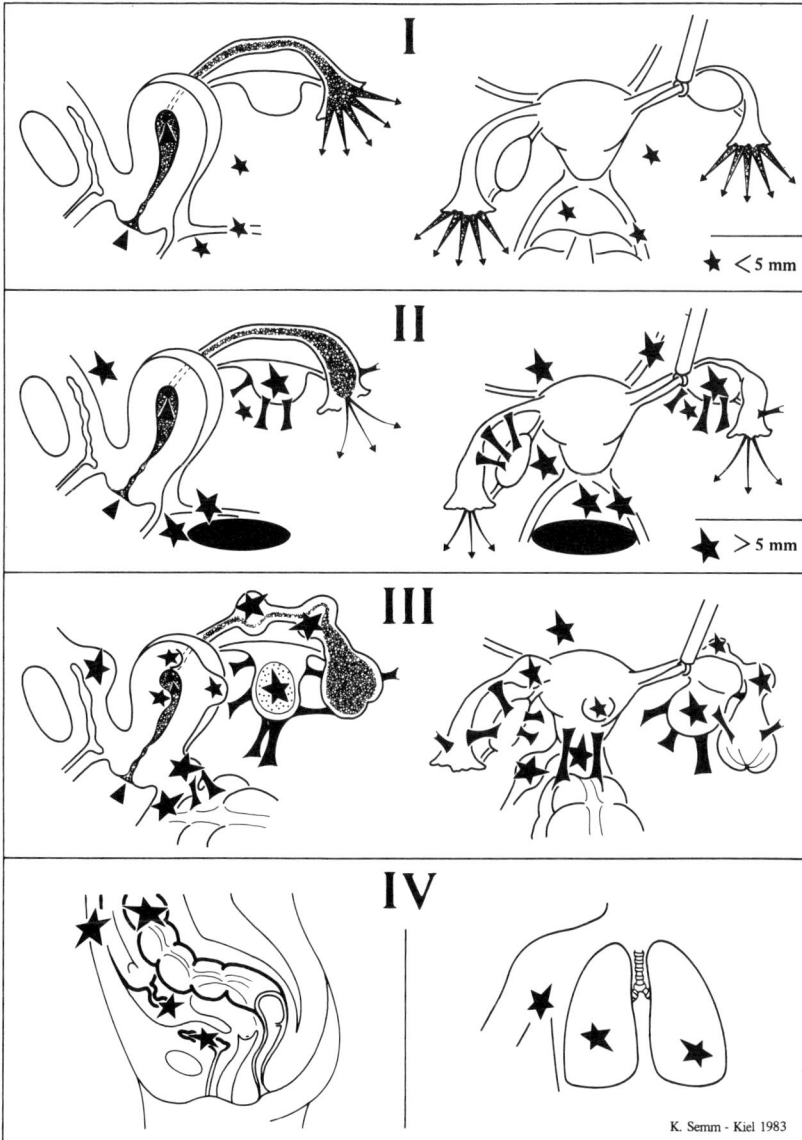

Figure 11   Endoscopic endometriosis classification (for details, see text)

has to sit (Figure 8), his shoulder has to be supported (Figure 9) and he must work with two hands with the aid of one assistant. Standing or one-handed endoscopic surgical procedures are not possible (Figure 10).

For statistical evaluation of our operative procedures, especially in fimbrioplasty and salpingostomy, we should discern between infectious tubal occlusions and occlusions originating from genital endometriosis. For the classification of endometriosis we know so far on the one hand the classification of the American Fertility Society and on the other hand the one according to ACOSTA. Both systems deal with the descriptive divisions, which can be co-ordinated with endoscopic pictures only with difficulty. Therefore in Kiel, we have tried to combine both classifications in a graphic picture according to endoscopic guidelines. A clear survey (Figure 11) is easily identified with endoscopic observations. A new classification is easily possible. Group I comprises exclusively small foci (smaller than 5 mm) spread over the peritoneum and into the pouch of Douglas. If, however, we see larger foci, such as on the roof of the bladder and behind the ovaries, together with small adhesions, we classify this as belonging to Group II. If in addition to all this there are chocolate cysts or bladder-roof foci or retrocervical knots larger than 5 mm in diameter this is classified as Group III. Group IV results if we find endometriotic foci outside of the inner genitals.

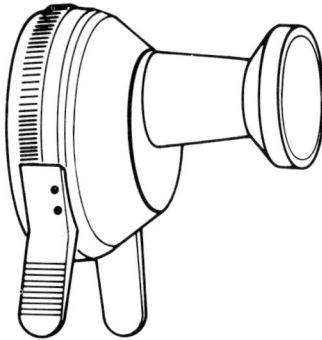

Figure 12   Loop used for endoscopic fimbrioplasty

We think that this endoscopic endometriosis classification provides a simple key for the endoscopists to estimate the grade of endometriosis enabling him to yield statistically comparable results.

Extensive discussion of endoscopic microsurgery on the Fallopian tubes would not be germane to this chapter. I shall mention only two examples. Applying a loop (Figure 12) on the endoscope facilitates the performance of a fimbrioplasty with controlled ascending chromo-

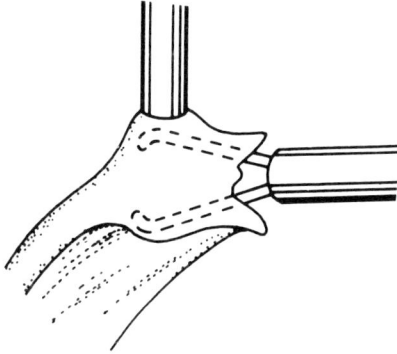

Figure 13 Atraumatic forceps in position for opening ampulla tubae

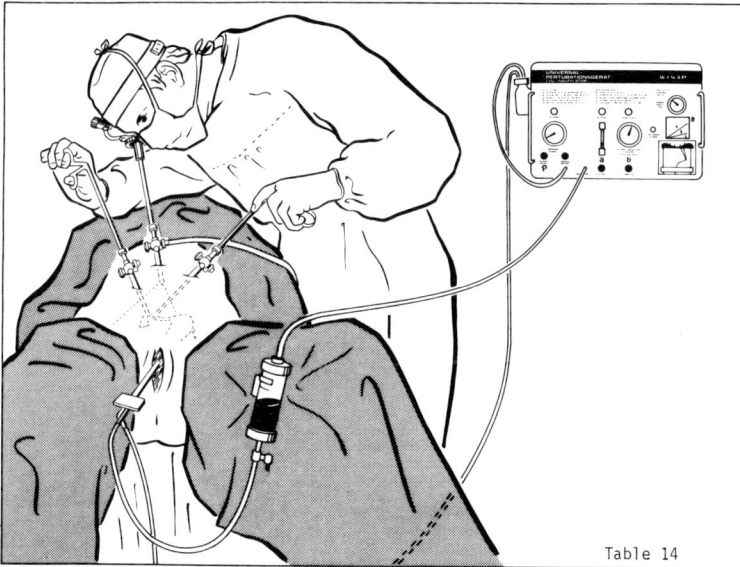

Figure 14 Operative lay-out for consecutive tubal patency test

salpingoscopy. Under a pressure of 200 mmHg, the tube presents itself as a tightly filled heel. With the help of two atraumatic forceps the drawn-in and hardly cicatrized old ampullary end is sought and a stump dilatation performed. In order to open the old ampullary end wholly, a closed atraumatic forceps is placed 2–3 cm deep in the ampulla tubae and then withdrawn in an opened position (Figure 13). This procedure is repeated frequently and the old ostium always bluntly dilated. The consecutive tubal patency test (Figure 14) shows a tubal patency of Grade I according to Fikentscher and Semm.

During salpingostomy (Figure 15), the ampullary end is distended with 200 mm Hg and blue solution and then coagulated with a point-coagulator (Figure 15 (a)) for 2–3 cm; the fimbrial end is then incised with micro-scissors (Figure 15 (b)) and the blue solution expelled.

Afterwards, using two atraumatic forceps (Figure 15 (c)), the old ampullary end is everted in a typical manner. The ampullary edge is fixed with resorbable endosuture material four times to the tubal serosa (Figure 15 (d)). The sutures (Figure 15 (e)) are applied under 4–6 times augmentation. Afterwards (Figure 15 (f)) the tube is patent for ascending chromopertubation solution and CO_2 gas and represents, according to Fikentscher and Semm a tubal patency of Grade I. Our pregnancy rates have, thanks to the application of microsurgical

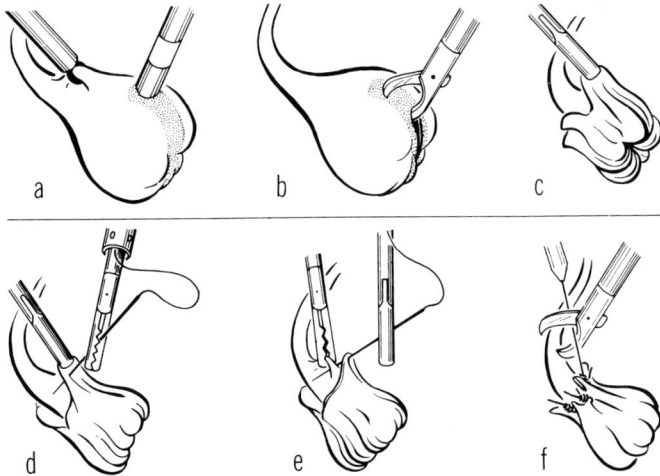

Figure 15 Operative procedure for salpingostomy

endoscopic methods, greatly increased in the last few years. If the cause of tubal occlusions was exclusively infectious ($n = 857$), we obtained a pregnancy rate of 21% with fimbrioplasty and salpingostomy. If we had to apply a fimbrioplasty and salpingostomy together with genital endometriosis, we proceeded according to our three-step technique. The first step comprised surgical treatment of endometriosis; the second step comprised treatment with antigonadotrophins (e.g. Danazol or Gestrinon); and in the third step – if tubal endometriosis was at Grade II or higher – the tubal damage was corrected.

Use of this three-step therapy in 771 patients yielded a pregnancy rate of 48%.

Endoscopic intra-abdominal surgery is only possible with the development of new instruments, for example:

(1) Endocoagulator (Figure 4).
(2) Aqua-purator (Figure 1).
(3) Lying and sitting positions for the surgeon (Figures 8 and 9).
(4) Optic (Figure 16) for the operation assistant.

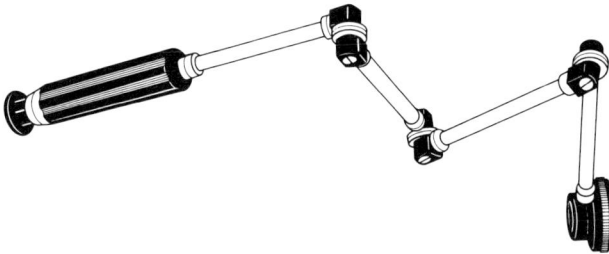

Figure 16 Optic for assisted endoscopic operation

(5) Microsurgical instruments including suture material for loop-ligatures (Figure 17), endoligatures (Figure 7) with extracorporeal knotting and endosuture (Figure 18) with endocorporeal knotting, e.g. for appendectomy and bowel-sutures.
(6) The attachable loop for enlarging the endoscopic picture (Figure 12).

Operative correction of tubal occlusions is increasingly performed by operative pelviscopy rather than laparotomy with microsurgery. Altogether, diagnosis and treatment of tubal functions is performed more easily than could ever be achieved with laparotomy.

Bibliography

Semm, K. (1983). *Operationslehre für Endoskopische Abdominal-Chirurgie.* (Stuttgart: Schattauer Verlag)

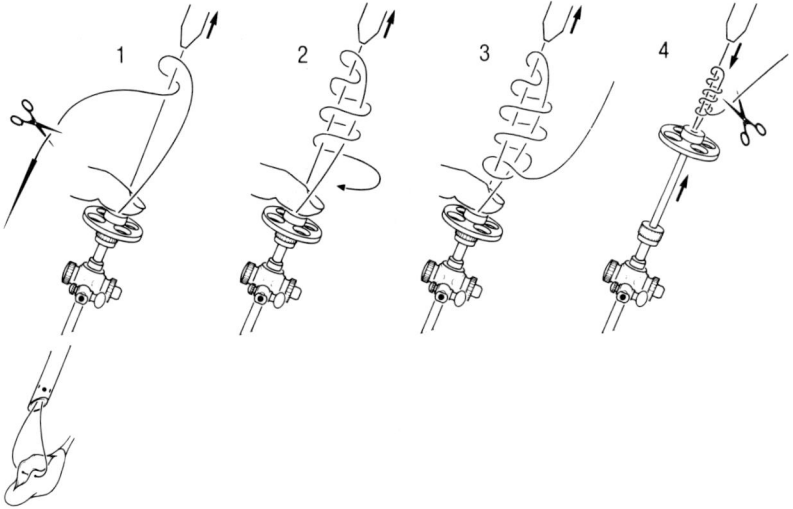

Figure 17 Suture material for performing loop ligatures

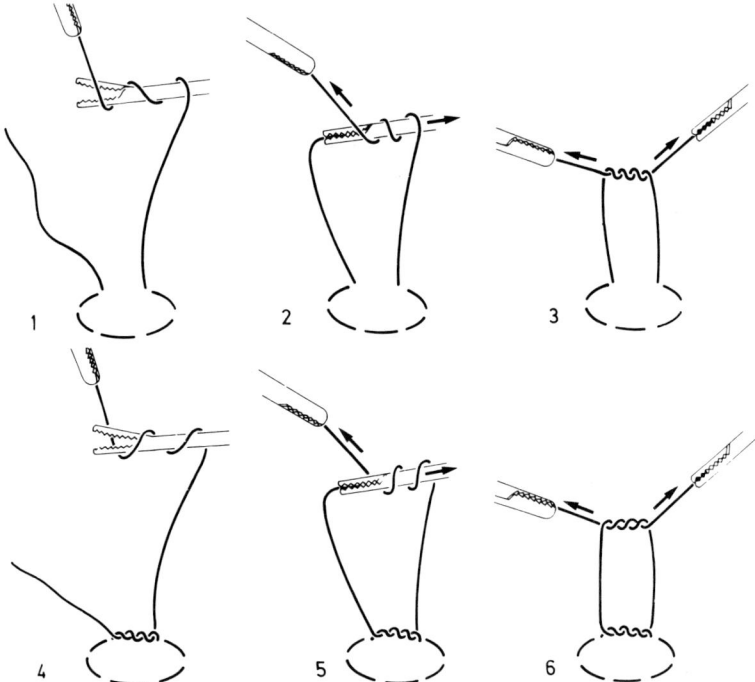

Figure 18 Extracorporeal knotting and endosutures in pelviscopy

17
Prevention of postoperative adhesions

W. H. UTIAN

INTRODUCTION

I had hoped to say 'Eureka! I have got it!' in referring to an effective and safe adjuvant for the prevention of postoperative adhesions. Regrettably and truthfully this is not the case. Indeed, I would have been wiser to have entitled this presentation 'The Practical and Logistical Problems Encountered in Testing Adjuvants for Prevention of Postoperative Adhesions'. I will expand on this aspect shortly in relation to my own experience with the high molecular weight dextrans.

The specific purpose of my presentation is to consider the possibilities for prevention of adhesion formation following surgical repair. Infertility can of course be directly due to adnexal adhesions and these have assumed a growing importance in surgical treatment. It is, however, the problem of post-tuboplasty adhesions that can be the cause of most frustration and disappointment to both patient and physician. In addressing this issue, it is pertinent to review three aspects of the problem, namely: (1) its magnitude, that is, the incidence of adhesions following tuboplasty; (2) the pathogenesis of postoperative adhesions; and (3) an overall evaluation of commonly used adjuvants for prevention of postoperative adhesions.

189

MAGNITUDE OF THE PROBLEM

Outside the reversal of sterilization, surgical repair of the Fallopian tubes remains less successful than hoped for. Despite improvements that have been reported in postoperative pregnancy rates using the new microsurgical techniques, these results have not been universally duplicated by others and some scepticism still remains concerning microsurgery[1]. For example, in a highly detailed recent review of the surgical treatment for distal tubal occlusion, Verhoeven and co-workers were only able to report an overall livebirth rate of 15.8%, not far removed from our recent expectations with *in vitro* fertilization[2].

Failure has been ascribed to numerous causes, including: (1) the type and extent of the pre-existing pathology; (2) the criteria for selection of patients for operation; (3) poor surgical technique; (4) damage to the endosalpinx by intratubal stents left *in situ* after repair; and (5) adhesion formation after the surgical repair itself.

Unfortunately, little reliable data exist on the incidence of adhesion formation after tuboplasty and the effect of such adhesions on subsequent fertility rates. Currently available data suggest that the problem of post-tuboplasty adhesions may be immense.

Swolin reviewed the literature before 1977 and reported postoperative adhesions to be present in as many as 70–95% of cases[3]. The increasing popularity of the second-look laparoscopy for adhesiolysis after recent tuboplasty has allowed a little more insight into the incidence of the problem[4]. Daniell and Pittaway found mild adhesions in 19 and severe adhesions in five of 25 patients undergoing short-interval second-look laparoscopy[5]. Verhoeven *et al.*, on the other hand, while reporting adhesiolysis to sometimes be more difficult and dangerous than the tubal repair itself, report a less than 30% incidence of adhesions after second-look laparoscopy. However, they only performed this procedure in less than 25% of their total population group[2].

Prevention is obviously better than cure, and in this instance would at least reduce the need for repeat laparoscopy. Moreover, the problem of adhesions does not only apply to tuboplasty. Any laparotomy, and certainly any form of pelvic operation, could be responsible for adhesion formation that later results in infertility. For example, Weinstein and Polishuk[6] reviewed 57 patients who had undergone ovarian wedge resections and noted significant periadnexal adhesions in eight out of 19 patients who failed to conceive[7].

190

THE PATHOGENESIS OF POSTOPERATIVE ADHESIONS

The process of reperitonization after surface peritoneal injury and the actual development of adhesions have been investigated in depth. These subjects have been well reviewed by several authors[8-10]. The present discussion will be limited to an outline of these processes in order to highlight the rationale usually presented for the use of certain substances as adhesive preventives.

In brief, peritoneum does not heal in the same manner as skin. Whereas a skin defect heals by cell growth from the edge of the wound, peritoneal repair depends on a series of cell proliferations. The new peritoneum appears to arise by metaplasia of subperitoneal cells to mature fibroblasts. There are several possible explanations for the origin of new mesothelium[8,11,12]:

(1)   Direct development from primitive mesenchymal cells present in the perivascular connective tissue.
(2)   Indirect development from primitive mesenchymal cells via fibroblasts.
(3)   Indirect development from subperitoneal fibroblasts which in turn arise from differentiated but quiescent fibroblasts in the perivascular connective tissue.

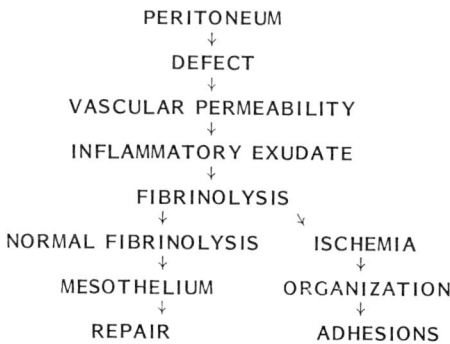

```
                      PERITONEUM
                          ↓
                        DEFECT
                          ↓
                VASCULAR PERMEABILITY
                          ↓
                INFLAMMATORY EXUDATE
                          ↓
                     FIBRINOLYSIS
                     ↓          ↘
      NORMAL FIBRINOLYSIS        ISCHEMIA
              ↓                     ↓
         MESOTHELIUM           ORGANIZATION
              ↓                     ↓
           REPAIR                ADHESIONS
```

Figure 1   Peritonization

The process of peritonization is summarized in Figure 1. As a result of trauma or some inflammatory process – either infective or non-infective as with, for example, endometriosis – a defect develops in the peritoneum. Increased vascular permeability accelerated by

191

histamine from mast cells results in an inflammatory exudate of monocytes, histiocytes, polymorphs and plasma cells in a fibrin matrix. Plasminogen activator activity, normally present in the mesothelium and submesothelial blood vessels of peritoneum, results in the spontaneous lysis of fibrinous attachments within 72–96 hours of development[13]. Concomitant with the resolution of fibrin the process of fibroblast proliferation occurs as previously described with transformation into mesothelium and subsequent full surface repair.

However, under certain circumstances the above normal process may not occur. These adverse factors include, not necessarily in order of importance:

(1) Excessive serosal injury.
(2) Marked surface denudation.
(3) Residual blood or active haemorrhage.
(4) Prolonged tissue drying.
(5) Foreign bodies, e. g. reactive suture material, talc.
(6) Infection.

In this event, there may be suppressed fibrinolytic activity with persistence of fibrin, organization of fibrin matrix involving cellular growth, vascularization and ultimately adhesion formation.

The key to normal healing is good vascularization. Ischaemia is a potent cause of failure of fibrinolytic activity with adhesions[13].

COMMONLY USED ADJUVANTS FOR PREVENTION OF POSTOPERATIVE ADHESIONS

In the constant search for adjuvants against adhesion formation, efforts have been directed towards preventing or counteracting all of the above-mentioned adverse factors. Unfortunately, virtually all of the more fashionable therapeutic methods for prevention of postoperative adhesion formation have been used on an essentially empirical basis. Most lack good supportive data, particularly in the area of comparative controlled prospective studies in women after tubal surgery.

The principles in adhesion prophylaxis have been well summarized by Levinson and Swolin[10] and are as follows:

(1) Minimize trauma.
(2) Minimize the initial inflammatory reaction.
(3) Promote dissolution and early removal of the fibrinous clot.

(4) Appose injured tissue precisely.

(5) Avoid the presence of blood at the injury site.

(6) Avoid prolonged drying of tissues.

(7) Delay fibroblast organization and collagen formation.

Many of the above principles can be satisfactorily complied with by observing the modern principles of microsurgery and I will not labour this point other than to emphasize the need for gentle tissue handling, excision of all diseased tissue, good tissue approximation, the use of appropriate lavage media and suture material, and the selective application of second-look laparoscopy[10]. Use of the laser may also be advantageous[14].

It is pertinent, however, to survey some of the more frequently used pharmacological agents for adhesion prevention. Holtz listed

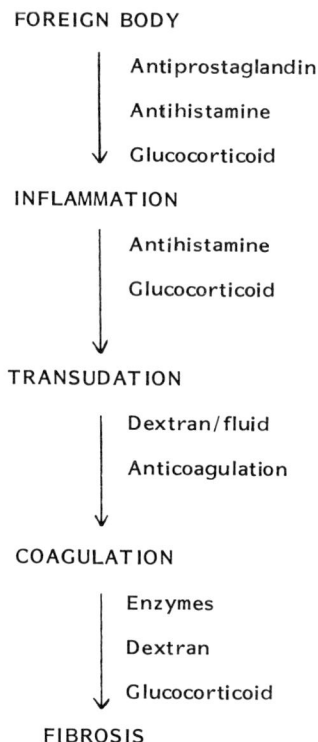

FOREIGN BODY

    Antiprostaglandin

    Antihistamine

↓   Glucocorticoid

INFLAMMATION

    Antihistamine

    Glucocorticoid

↓

TRANSUDATION

    Dextran/fluid

    Anticoagulation

↓

COAGULATION

    Enzymes

    Dextran

↓   Glucocorticoid

FIBROSIS

Figure 2 Role of agents used for adhesion prevention in the inflammatory cascade

over 50 agents in a recent review[9]. Unfortunately, only a few even begin to warrant consideration.

The place of each substance as a potential agent or antidote in the inflammatory cascade is illustrated in Figure 2. The following agents continue to have some rationale for use, but without exception have not been substantiated in the literature by any prospective randomized double-blind clinical study.

Antiprostaglandins

Early reports have suggested some role for the use of non-steroidal anti-inflammatory agents such as ibuprofen[6,15]. However, equally good data exists to refute this effect when used alone[16], or compared with dexamethazone[17].

Antihistamines

Despite the theoretical value of antihistamines to limit the transudation of fibrin-containing fluid and thus the matrix for adhesion formation, these agents have never been tested alone for their effectiveness in post-surgical adhesion formation in humans[8].

Antibiotics

The same criticism as above applies to antibiotics. The fear of infection, however, is great, and many surgeons choose to use these agents on an empirical basis for infection prophylaxis.

Glucocorticoids

Glucocorticoids have long been recommended as adhesive preventives because of their anti-inflammatory effect[8]. None the less, most recent studies have tended to refute this value[18].Moreover, DiZerega and Hodgen reported a combination of promethazine, dexamethasone and ampicillin to be completely ineffective in preventing tubal adhesions in rhesus monkeys[19]. Granat et al. reported steroid therapy to have no inhibiting effect on fibroblast proliferation, but to suppress the immune response of patients during the early postoperative phase, a potentially adverse effect[20].

Heparin

Prevention of coagulation of exudates and fibrin formation at the time of surgery has a sound theoretical basis. There are no satisfactory controlled studies in relation to results after tuboplasty.

The one constant feature of each of the above-mentioned modalities has been the lack of proper drug evaluation for efficacy. This has not been for want of trying. There are, however, many problems in attempting to evaluate properly any drug for its clinical use in adhesion prevention. These problems include:

(1) Non-predictability of animal-to-human model.
(2) Size of sample.
(3) Classification/standardization of pathology.
(4) Randomization of cases.
(5) Standardization of surgical technique.
(6) Selection of controls.
(7) Excluding *post hoc ergo propter hoc*.
(8) Problems in follow-up.

The investigations into the use of high molecular weight dextran serve as an excellent example of these practical difficulties, and my own personal involvement in its evaluation over the last few years allow me to expand on this aspect in greater detail.

AN IN-DEPTH EVALUATION OF HIGH MOLECULAR WEIGHT DEXTRAN

The early studies on use of dextrans in adhesion prophylaxis related to dextran-40. The theoretical rationale includes a possible mechanical effect, so-called 'hydroflotation', a 'siliconizing effect', or altered surface polarity[21]. Dextran-70 has replaced dextran-40 because it is resorbed far more slowly.

Following an early positive study by Neuwirth and Khalaf with a 32% dextran-70/dextrose solution in rabbits undergoing uterine trauma[22], a specific study was designed by myself and co-workers, Goldfarb and Starks, to determine whether adhesions could be prevented in New Zealand white rabbits undergoing tubal transection and microsurgical anastomosis. These results were reported to the American Fertility Society in 1978 and published in 1979[23]. There were two important observations. First, use of 32% dextran-70 reduced adhesion scores and enhanced the fertility rates. Secondly, many animals died in the dextran-70 group as a result of dehydration

195

brought on by fluid transfer from the vascular compartment to the peritoneal cavity[23].

Confirmation of adhesion prevention was reported at the American Fertility Society meeting in 1979 by DiZerega and Hodgen in a study conducted on 20 rhesus monkeys[19]. Histological examination of fimbrial biopsy specimens suggested that adhesion prevention was due to a coating effect of the 32% dextran-70 which was present in the peritoneal cavity for at least 5 days.

At about that time I had designed a randomized prospective double-blind clinical study comparing the effect of normal saline versus 32% dextran-70 in the prevention of adhesions at the time of surgical treatment for distal tubal occlusion. By mutual agreement this study was expanded into a multicentre national study in the United States in an effort to increase the number of cases, with myself and DiZerega as principle co-investigators, the study under the auspices of the National Institutes of Health in Washington, and funded by Pharmacia in Sweden.

I would like to briefly refer to the outcome of the study in which virtually all of the previously listed problems eventuated. I would emphasize that these problems are related to the nature of such a study and do not reflect on the investigators, all of whom are individuals of the highest integrity working at some of the best units in the United States.

The study design is illustrated in Figure 3.

A specific grading protocol was utilized to measure the extent of adhesions both at the time of initial surgery and again at the second-look laparoscopy. Adhesions were measured at several sites, namely both ovaries, both tubes, omentum, small bowel, colon, pelvic side wall, cul-de-sac and total pelvic adhesions.

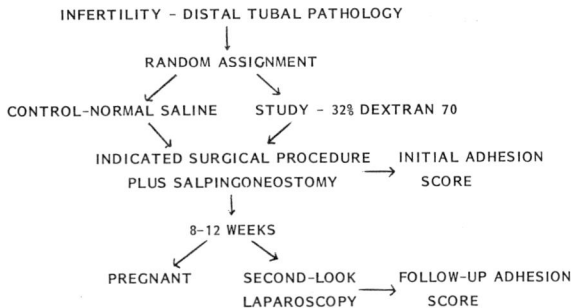

INFERTILITY – DISTAL TUBAL PATHOLOGY
↓
RANDOM ASSIGNMENT
↙   ↘
CONTROL-NORMAL SALINE   STUDY – 32% DEXTRAN 70
↘   ↙
INDICATED SURGICAL PROCEDURE → INITIAL ADHESION
PLUS SALPINGONEOSTOMY   SCORE
↓
8-12 WEEKS
↙   ↘
PREGNANT   SECOND-LOOK → FOLLOW-UP ADHESION
             LAPAROSCOPY   SCORE

Figure 3 Study design

196

The number of cases and participating study centres, listed in Table 1, the pathology at initial laparotomy, listed in Table 2, and the use or exclusion of magnification, listed in Table 3 make immediately

Table 1 Number of cases and participating centres

Study Centres	No. of Cases	
	NaCl	Dextran
Duke	12	11
Yale	7	9
Baylor	7	3
USC	4	4
Vanderbilt	4	4
Washington	3	5
Indiana	4	3
Navy	1	3
Massachusetts	0	3
Total	42	45

Table 2 Pathology at initial laparotomy

Pathology	Group	
	NaCl	Dextran
PID, hydrosalpinx	13	18
PID, no hydrosalpinx	16	24
Endometriosis	6	8
Idiopathic	4	3
Other	3	2
Total	42	45

Table 3 Operative magnification

	Group	
	NaCl	Dextran
None	18	24
Loupes	14	14
Microscope	10	7
Total	42	45

apparent the marked diversity in case selection and possibilities for variation in surgical skill and technique. This variability affects the size of the sample, so that when pure distal tubal disease is analysed, the number of cases becomes small. The results up to April 30, 1983 are in press[24].

Even if we are to accept the total group as homogeneous and the surgical technique as similar, the results are not clear cut. The most pertinent sites are of course the ovaries and fimbria. Both areas were carefully scrutinized at laparotomy and second-look laparoscopy by a specific adnexal adhesion score. While a significant improvement was achieved by the corrective surgery in both groups, there was no significant improvement in adhesion prophylaxis with dextran usage as compared with the saline control group (Table 4). Despite this disappointing aspect, it should be noted that a significant reduction of general pelvic adhesions, particularly involving the colon and cul-de-sac, was achieved by use of dextran.

Table 4 Examination of ovaries and fimbria in treatment groups

| | Group | | |
Parameter	NaCl	Dextran	Significance
No. completed	42	45	
No. pregnant < 12 weeks	7	4	
No. of 2nd look laparoscopies	35	41	
Total adnexal score:			
1st evaluation	7.64±1.55	7.16±1.32	NS
2nd evaluation	4.63±0.86	3.70±0.69	NS
Significance	$p<0.01$	$p<0.01$	

NS = not significant.

It is my own personal opinion that the overall results of the study, while promising, are inconclusive as the definitive proof needed to justify the broad use of dextrans after all pelvic surgery. Moreover, dextrans are not without risk[25]. Recurrent anaphylactic reactions to intraperitoneal dextran have been reported[26], (Stangel, unpublished observations). It should be emphasized that this indication for the use of dextrans has not been approved by the Food and Drug Administration in the United States.

CONCLUSION

Almost no satisfactory prospective controlled clinical trials exist in relation to adhesion prevention for the simple reason that such studies are difficult to complete. One important plea can therefore be made, and that is for satisfactory classification, description and documentation of pelvic adhesions at every opportunity. Only if this is done will it be possible to evaluate causative and therapeutic agents for such adhesions. This is one area of medical research where collective experience will be invaluable[21].

Despite this obvious void in the infertility literature, it should be emphasized that adhesion recurrence can be reduced by observation of all the principles of modern infertility microsurgery, including avoidance of foreign bodies and infection, maintenance of vascular integrity, and perhaps the judicious, but empirical usage of some of the adjuvants discussed above. At this time, it would still seem that the two most important determinants for adhesion recurrence are the nature and severity of the pre-existing pathology and the skill of the surgeon.

References

1. Goldfarb, J. M., Utian, W. H. and Weiss, R. (1983). Microscopic versus macroscopic tubal anastomosis in rabbit fallopian tubes. *Fertil. Steril.* (In press)
2. Verhoeven, H. C., Berry, H., Frantzen, C. and Schlosser, H. (1983). Surgical treatment for distal tubal occlusion. A review of 167 cases. *J. Reprod. Med.*, **28**, 293
3. Swolin, K. (1977). Laparoscopy as an operative tool in female sterility. *J. Reprod. Med.*, **19**, 167
4. DiZerega, G. and Utian, W. H. (1982). Efficacy of 32% dextran-70 in the prevention of peritoneal adhesions, and the utility of the second-look laparoscopy in infertility surgery. *Fertil. Steril.*, **37**, 291
5. Daniell, J. F. and Pittaway, D. E. (1983). Short-interval second-look laparoscopy after infertility surgery. *J. Reprod. Med.*, **28**, 281
6. Bateman, B. G., Nunley, W. C. and Kitchin, J. D. (1982). Prevention of postoperative peritoneal adhesions with ibuprofen. *Fertil. Steril.*, **38**, 107
7. Weinstein, D. and Polishuk, W. Z. (1975). The role of wedge resection of the ovary as a cause for mechanical sterility. *Surg. Gynecol. Obstet.*, **141**, 417
8. DiZerega, G. S. (1980). *The Cause and Prevention of Postsurgical Adhesions.* (National Institutes of Health, Bethesda, MD: Pregnancy Research Branch)
9. Holtz, G. (1980). Prevention of postoperative adhesions. *J. Reprod. Med.*, **24**, 141
10. Levinson, C. J. and Swolin, K. (1980). Postoperative adhesions: etiology, prevention and therapy. *Clin. Obstet. Gynecol.*, **23**, 1213
11. Eskeland, G. (1964). Regeneration of parietal peritoneum. *Acta Path. Microbiol. Scand.*, **62**, 459
12. Rafferty, A. T. (1967). Regeneration of parietal and visceral peritoneum: An enzyme histochemical study. *J. Anat.*, **121**, 589
13. Buckman, R. F., Buckman, P. D., Hufnagel, H. V., *et al.* (1976). A physiologic basis for the adhesion-free healing of deperitonealized surfaces. *J. Surg. Res.*, **21**, 67
14. Choe, J. K., Dawood, Y. and Andrews, A. H. (1983). Conventional versus laser reanastomosis of rabbit ligated uterine horns. *Obstet. Gynecol.*, **61**, 689
15. Siegler, A. M., Kontopolous, V. and Wang, C. F. (1980). Prevention of postoperative

adhesions in rabbits with ibuprofen, a non-steroidal anti-inflammatory agent. *Fertil. Steril.*, **34,** 46

16. Holtz, G. D. (1982). Failure of a non-steroidal anti-inflammatory agent (Ibuprofen) to inhibit peritoneal adhesion formation after lysis. *Fertil. Steril.*, **37,** 582

17. O'Brien, W. F., Drake, T. S. and Bibro, M. C. (1982). The use of ibuprofen and dexamethasone in the prevention of postoperative adhesion formation. *Obstet. Gynecol.*, **60,** 373

18. Seitz, H. M., Schenker, J. G. *et al.* (1973). Postoperative intraperitoneal adhesions: A double-blind assessment of their prevention in the monkey. *Fertil. Steril.*, **24,** 935

19. DiZerega, G. S. and Hodgen, G. D. (1980). Prevention of postsurgical tubal adhesions: Comparative study of commonly used agents. *Am. J. Obstet. Gynecol.*, **136,** 173

20. Granat, M., Schencker, J. G., *et al.* (1938). Effects of dexamethasone on proliferation of autologous fibroblasts and on the immune profile in women undergoing pelvic surgery for infertility. *Fertil. Steril.*, **39,** 180

21. Utian, W. H. (1980). Prevention of adhesions after tubal surgery by use of dextran-70. *S. Afr. Med. J.*, **58,** 204

22. Neuwirth, R. S. and Khalaf, S. M. (1975). Effect of thirty-two percent dextran 70 on peritoneal adhesion formation. *Am. J. Obstet. Gynecol.*, **121,** 420

23. Utian, W. H., Goldfarb, J. M. and Starks, G. C. (1979). Role of dextran 70 in microtubal surgery. *Fertil. Steril.*, **31,** 79

24. The Adhesion Study Group (1983). Reduction of postoperative pelvic adhesions with intraperitoneal dextran-70: A prospective, randomized study. *Fertil. Steril.* (In press)

25. Bernstein, J., Mattox, J. H. *et al.* (1982). The potential for bacterial growth with dextran. *J. Reprod. Med.*, **27,** 77

26. Borten, M., Seibert, C. P. and Taymor, M. D. (1983). Recurrent anaphylactic reaction to intraperitoneal dextran 75 used for prevention of postsurgical adhesions. *Obstet. Gynecol.*, **61,** 755

Part I

Section 5

Immunology and Reproduction

18
Immunological aspects of implantation

K. TSUBATA, H. NAKAMURA, Y. TSUKAHARA,
E. KAWAGUCHI, T. K. FUJII and S. TAKAGI

INTRODUCTION

This project was designed to investigate the process of trophoblastic invasion of cells from the villous cell column into maternal tissues, the functions and antigenicity of these 'invasive' trophoblasts, and the immuno-response of the maternal tissues to these cells of fetal origin. To paraphrase, the trophoblasts distal to the cell column migrate into the endometrial interstitia, proliferate and form lacunae. These migrating cells intrude into the lumen of blood vessels of the interstitia and replace the endothelial linings and act as the vanguard for the formation of the intervillous spaces. The maternal tissues, in order to suppress unlimited infiltration by fetal elements which might lead to uncontrolled destruction of the host, respond with an active immuno-defense. These various reactions are of importance to the understanding of nidation and maintenance of pregnancy. However, as it is difficult to obtain clinically adequate specimens at the time of implantation, this investigation was performed on specimens obtained at surgery performed during early pregnancy.

MATERIALS AND METHODS

Twenty specimens were obtained at hysterectomy for myoma uteri complicated with pregnancy of 7–12 weeks duration. The nidation sites were excised and a portion cryoprocessed followed by 95% ethanol:acetone fixation. These specimens were immunohistochemically evaluated with mouse monoclonal antibodies to HLA-ABC (Cappel Labs. & Bethesda Res. Labs.), OK T_3, T_4, T_8, Ia1, (Ortho), and IgG, IgM, C_3C, C_1q (Behring Labs.). Another portion of the specimens were fixed in formalin, Zamboni and 95% ethanol and embedded in paraffin. These specimens were immunohistochemically evaluated with antisera to hCG, its subunits and fibrinogen (Teikoku Zoki), hPL (Mochida Co.), SP_1 (Behring Labs.) and Aromatase (NIH).

A third portion was fixed in 0.25% gluteraldehyde, cryoprocessed, sliced, and stained with antisera to progesterone previously adsorbed with steroid extracted placental powder.

A fourth portion was evaluated by TEM.

RESULTS

We observed cytotrophoblasts from the distal portion of the cell column which had migrated into maternal tissues where a portion of them were destroyed by the maternal defence mechanisms to form Nitabuch's fibrinoid layer. Other trophoblasts found deep to Nitabuch's layer were apparently unaffected by the maternal defences.

Trophoblasts in the cell column and the zone of trophoblastic degeneration showed no reaction to antisera to hCG and its subunits, hPL, SP_1, aromatase, progesterone or oestradiol, whereas viable trophoblasts found deep to this zone showed positive reactions to all of the above.

Decidual cells in close approximation to viable trophoblasts were observed secreting a moderately electron dense, finely granular material.

The syncytial and cell column trophoblasts show no reaction to HLA-ABC, a strong reaction in the zone of degenerating trophoblasts, and either a positive or negative reaction in viable trophoblasts found deep to the fibrinoid layer.

Reactions to C_1q and IgG were found in the fibrinoid layer and diffusely in the capillary walls of the decidua.

A profusion of neutrophils and macrophages with some lymphocytes and Ia positive cells were seen in the fibrinoid layer and immediately deep to it; in contrast, deep in the decidua and myometrium, only plasma cells and OKT_3 responsive lymphocytes were seen.

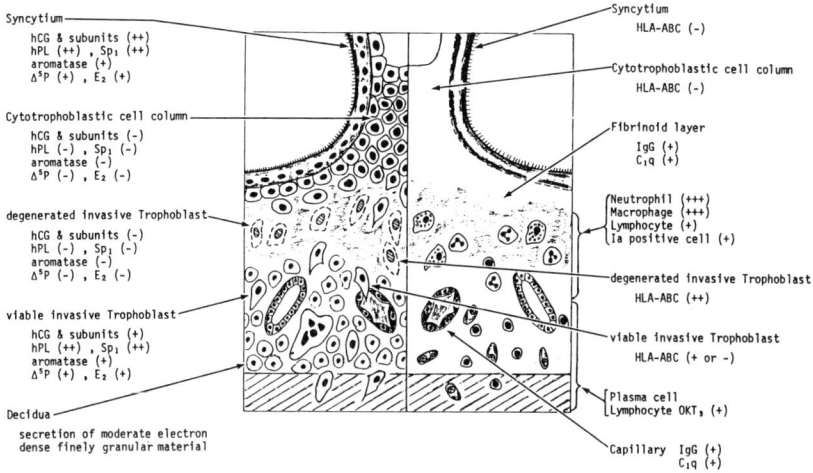

Syncytium
    hCG & subunits (++)
    hPL (++) , Sp₁ (++)
    aromatase (+)
    $\Delta^5 P$ (+) , E_2 (+)

Cytotrophoblastic cell column
    hCG & subunits (-)
    hPL (-) , Sp₁ (-)
    aromatase (-)
    $\Delta^5 P$ (-) , E_2 (-)

degenerated invasive Trophoblast
    hCG & subunits (-)
    hPL (-) , Sp₁ (-)
    aromatase (-)
    $\Delta^5 P$ (-) , E_2 (-)

viable invasive Trophoblast
    hCG & subunits (+)
    hPL (++) , Sp₁ (++)
    aromatase (+)
    $\Delta^5 P$ (+) , E_2 (+)

Decidua
    secretion of moderate electron
    dense finely granular material

Syncytium
    HLA-ABC (-)

Cytotrophoblastic cell column
    HLA-ABC (-)

Fibrinoid layer
    IgG (+)
    C₁q (+)

Neutrophil (+++)
Macrophage (+++)
Lymphocyte (+)
Ia positive cell (+)

degenerated invasive Trophoblast
    HLA-ABC (++)

viable invasive Trophoblast
    HLA-ABC (+ or -)

Plasma cell
Lymphocyte OKT₈ (+)

Capillary IgG (+)
           C₁q (+)

Figure 1

A schematic representation of our findings is shown in Figure 1.

DISCUSSION

The present status of the various hypotheses concerning the non-rejection of the allogenic fetoplacental unit include the masking effect of various surface substances of the chorionic villi, the hormonal effects, the immunosuppressive effect of the various substances secreted by the villi, blocking antibodies, early pregnancy factor, etc. – a very complex mixture of somewhat conflicting opinions. Our approach was to study the various events occurring at the fetomaternal junction.

We saw active invasion of trophoblasts from the cytotrophoblastic cell column into maternal tissues. These trophoblasts develop a progressively complex organelle system with an accompanying filamentous structure, thought to be closely associated with the mobility of these cells. These invading trophoblasts progressively gain HLA antigenicity, in the presence of destruction of some of these cells, by mechanisms in which macrophages, neutrophils, and lymphocytes are intimately involved.

Nitabuch's fibrinoid layer is said to be comprised of degenerated trophoblasts, cell debris, fibrin, and material excreted from the decidua.

This formation of Nitabuch's layer may be in actuality the resultant aftermath of the events in the 'Battle Zone'.

Trophoblasts which do not undergo degeneration are of great interest, although the mechanisms by which they avoid destruction are unclear. Perhaps the lPL, hCG, SP_1, oestrogen and progesterone act to suppress immunologic responses. Perhaps the steroids secreted by these cells stimulate the endometrial interstitia to undergo decidual change, which in turn secrete material which coat the invading trophoblasts and protects them from destruction. A further possibility is the timing with which these trophoblasts develop antigenicity in relation to their gaining the ability to synthesize immunosuppressive defences.

In any event, the fetal components represented by the placental elements which actively invade maternal tissues to effect implantation are balanced by the defensive maternal mechanisms to establish a homeostatic environment for the maintenance of the gravid state.

Acknowledgements

We wish to express our gratitude to Dr Osawa, Medical Foundation Buffalo, N.Y., for antisera to aromatase.

19
The nature of the placental immunological barrier

T. G. WEGMANN

INTRODUCTION

Many hypotheses have been proferred to explain the survival of the mammalian fetal allograft to term without maternal rejection. Currently, these explanations fall into two major categories. The first is that active suppression of some form or other acts systemically on the maternal immune response to prevent either recognition of or reactivity to paternal alloantigens. The second is that the placenta serves as a barrier to the entry of maternal antibodies and cells into the fetus. While these explanations are not mutually exclusive, most current evidence supports the latter type of explanation and contradicts the former (reviewed in references 1 and 2). I will therefore focus this article on the nature of the placental barrier to maternal antibodies and cells.

Perhaps the most convincing demonstration that the trophoblastic derivatives of the placenta are crucial for fetal survival comes from the experiments of Rossant and her colleagues, using interspecies chimeras[3,4]. They have shown that whereas Mus caroli embryos are rejected between 10 and 13 days when implanted into a Mus musculus pseudopregnant female, chimeras made with a Mus caroli inner cell mass and Mus musculus trophoblast survive into adulthood. Reverse chimeras, with a Mus caroli trophoblast and a Mus musculus inner cell mass, are rejected by the Mus musculus host female. Circumstantial and correlative evidence suggests that the rejection is immunological in nature. Given the apparently crucial role played by the trophoblastic components of the placenta, I shall now discuss how this barrier works.

THE PLACENTA AS A BARRIER TO MATERNAL ANTIPATERNAL MHC ANTIBODIES

As early as 1970, Swinburne proposed that the placenta could serve as an immunoadsorbent barrier for maternal antipaternal MHC antibodies that are made during allopregnancy[5], for which there is much evidence[2]. A number of laboratories thereafter produced circumstantial evidence that this might be the case[1]. More recent experiments using radiolabelled monoclonal antifetal MHC antibodies indicate that this is clearly the case[6-8]. If pregnant female mice are injected *intravenously* on day 13 of gestation with anti-Class I monoclonal antibodies (or their F (ab)'$_2$ derivatives) directed against the fetus, one sees an increased uptake in the placenta, compared with females in which the fetus does not bear the target antigen. In the latter type of pregnancy, the fetuses show higher counts than in the pregnancies in which the fetus contains the target antigen (Fig. 1). These results

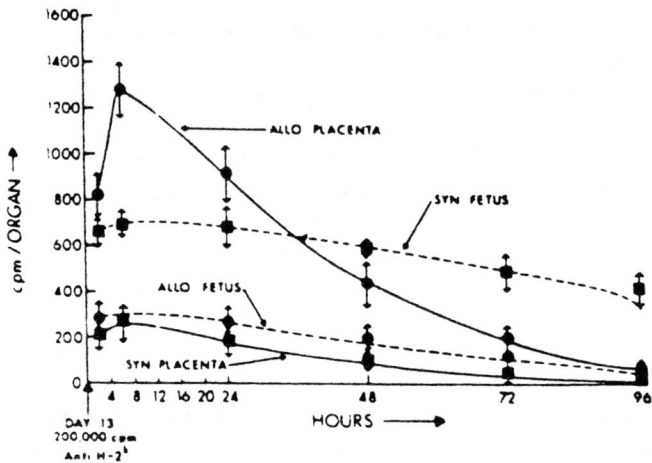

Figure 1 Evidence for the placental immunoadsorbent model. The relationship between the amounts of ^{125}I present at various time periods in control and target placentas and fetuses after a single pulse of [^{125}I]anti-H-2 Kk antibody on day 13 of pregnancy. Each point represents the mean (±SD) radioactivity cpm/organ. ●——● = Target dxk placenta; ■——■ = control dxd placenta; ●---● = target fetus; ■---■ = control fetus. Reproduced from reference 9, with permission

indicate that not only is the placenta removing antifetal MHC antibodies from the maternal bloodstream, but that it is preventing their entry into the fetus.

The results with the control animals, as well as with F (ab)'$_2$ preparations, rule out Fc binding as an explanation for these studies and indicate that the placenta in fact does bear the fetal MHC antigens of the paternal type, in a functionally exposed position. From Figure 1 it may be observed that anti-MHC antibody binding to the placenta reaches a peak 8 hours after injection and then declines. One can conclude that there is a rapid turnover of these antibodies in the placenta, and this has been verified by other experiments in which the placental binding has been blocked by cold antibodies. These experiments indicate that the capacity to bind the antibody is rapidly restored thereafter[8]. Other experiments indicate that the antibody that binds to cells in the placenta is digested intracellularly, and then released as fragments back into the circulation of the pregnant female[9]. An interesting observation is that the placenta is not an immunoadsorbent for monoclonal antibodies directed against Class 2 MHC antigens, although not all specificities have been tested. Autoradiography studies, performed on females injected with radiolabelled antibodies and then perfused *in vivo* indicate that there are two major sites of localization of the Class I antigens. One is in the lateral aspect of the placenta, where the yolk sac inserts into the fetal side of the placenta. A much weaker but definitely positive binding (when compared with non-antigen bearing controls) is seen in the region of the spongiotrophoblast[10]. This localization confirms previous observations localizing antipaternal antibodies in the placenta by immunofluorescence studies[11]. These studies indicate that the placenta can serve as an immunoadsorbent, and also indicate that paternally derived Class I MHC antigens are in direct contact with the maternal circulation. The conclusions presented here are basically in agreement with work reported by others using a variety of techniques[12–15].

THE PLACENTA AS A BARRIER TO MATERNAL CELLS

There are a number of reports of cellular immune traffic from the mother to the fetus during murine pregnancy, although in some of the cases these observations could not be repeated. Perhaps the most recent report of this sort was that of Collins *et al.*, who claimed that as high as 30% of the cells dividing in the liver of newborn animals were of maternal origin, using MHC antigens as markers[16]. Recent unpublished observations of Hunzinger, Gambel, and Wegmann failed to confirm these claims, using the glucose phosphate isomerase isozyme marker, which can distinguish as few as 1% maternal cells mixed with 99% fetal cells, in an objective assay employing gel

Table 1 Occurrence of transplacental passage of cells as revealed by electrophoretic analysis of glucose phosphate isomerase isozymes, of fetal liver, blood, and/or spleen lysates*

	Days' gestation					
Strain combinations	15	16	17	18	19	+1[†]
(Balb/c × C3H)F$_1$♀ × Balb/c♂	5(5)[‡]	10(10)	10(10)	25(26)	15(15)	30(30)
(A/J × B6)F$_1$♀ × A/J♂	ND	10(10)	5(5)	ND	4(5)	ND

ND = Not done.

* From Hunzinger, Gambel and Wegmann (unpublished observations).

† 1 day postpartum.

‡ No evidence of trafficking (less than 1.0%); numbers in parentheses indicate the number of samples analysed.

§ In one embryo, assayed in each of these groups, the electrophoresis lysate shows that 30% of the cells obtained from fetal liver are maternal GPI in phenotype. Thus, significant trafficking is a rare but real event and is being analysed further.

scanning (Table 1). This indication of the existence of a cell barrier formed by the placenta was confirmed by failure to find fluorescinated lymphocytes in the fetus after injection of large numbers of them into the maternal bloodstream at various times during pregnancy, using a fluorescence-activated cell sorter, an assay that can detect one cell in a thousand. There are some well-documented clinical examples of apparent GVH in newborn males caused by maternal lymphocytes bearing XX chromosomes markers, associated with exfoliative dermatitis and other signs of GVH disease, frequently terminating in death[17]. These are very rare exceptions that prove the rule that the placenta must be a fairly effective barrier to the entry of maternal lymphocytes. The mechanism by which it excludes maternal lymphocytes awaits clarification.

VACCINATION AGAINST ABORTION IN MOUSE AND MAN

Having presented evidence that the placenta is a barrier to the entry of cells from the mother to the fetus, the question arises as to how this cell barrier works. It could provide an anatomical barrier, or could work by local active suppression[1,2]. In order to discover how it works, an experimental model must be found in which immunological manipulations influence fetal survival. Such a model is now available[2] (Chaouat, Kiger and Wegmann, unpublished observations), as described below.

A number of investigators have reported that human females suffering from repeated spontaneous abortions can have successful term pregnancies if they are vaccinated with white blood cells from either their husband or from a donor pool[18-20]. These observations are of importance, not only because of their potential contribution to the families involved, but also because they may provide insight into the mechanisms of fetal protection from maternal immune rejection. In order to realize that goal rapidly, as well as to define the genetic and cellular requirements for the vaccination effect, an animal model showing a similar pattern would be of great utility. The model arises from observations of D. A. Clark and associates[21]. They described that when CBA/J female mice are mated with DBA/2 J male mice, there is a high resorption rate for the fetuses. They found in addition that a non-specific suppressor factor was absent from the lymph nodes draining the uterus in the pregnancies with complete abortion,

Table 2 Effect of vaccination upon the rate of spontaneous resorption in CBA/J female mice*

Experiment	Source of spleen cells used for vaccination			
	None (sham vaccination)	CBA/J♂	DBA/2 J♂	Balb/c♂
Villejuif				
1	3R, 12F (20%)	–	6R, 14F (30%)	0R, 7F (0%)
II	12R, 40F (23%)	8R, 32F (20%)	7R,31F(18%)	1R, 18F (5%)
III†		–	4R, 13F(23%)	1R, 14F(7%)
IV	4R, 13F(23%)	7R, 16F(30%)	–	1R, 16F(6%)
Total	19R,68F(22%)	15R, 48F (24%)	17R, 58F (23%)	3R, 55F (5%) (p = 0.001)
V (Nice)	11R, 58F(16%)	10R, 68F(13%)	13R, 71F(15%)	4R, 74F (5%) (p = 0.001)

* CBA/J female mice were vaccinated with 1/10th of a spleen (about 10^7 white cells) from CBA/J, DBA/2 J or Balb/c males, usually 1 week prior to mating with DBA/2 males. Animals were killed at day 12 of gestation, and the number of resorbing fetuses (R) and viable conceptuses (F) recorded. Percentage resorbtion = R/(R+F). Statistical evaluation was carried out by paired t test analysis (Chaouat, Kiger and Wegmann, unpublished observations).
† Mice were alloimmunized 1 month prior to mating with DBA/2 males.

211

but present in the non-aborting pregnancies. This suggested the possibility that vaccination of CBA/J female mice with allogeneic spleen cells prior to mating with DBA/2 males could prevent the abortion, perhaps by increasing the suppressive effect in the vicinity of the placenta.

Evidence for the effect of vaccination in preventing abortion is shown in Table 2. In order to make sure that this phenomenon was not confined to one source of mice in a single experimental centre, the experiment was carried out separately in two different laboratories, in Villejuif and Nice, using mice derived from different sources. CBA/J females and males were derived from the Jackson Laboratory, and inbred at Villejuif. These CBA/J females were mated with DBA/2 J males, also locally inbred in Villejuif. They showed 23% resorption. This was reduced to 5% by vaccinating with 1/10 of a Balb/c spleen cell suspension i.p. 1 week prior to mating. Vaccinating by CBA/J or DBA/2 J spleen cells had no effect. The vaccination effect was highly significant ($p < 0.001$ by paired t test analysis). All the mice used in Nice were obtained from Böm Molgard (Copenhagen). These CBA/J female mice showed 12–15% spontaneous abortions when mated with DBA/2 males. This was reduced to 5% upon vaccination with Balb/c spleen cells ($p < 0.001$).

The availability of this animal model for vaccination against spontaneous recurrent abortion should allow a more rational protocol to be developed for humans. In addition, the basic mechanisms underlying fetal protection from maternal immune rejection can be approached using this model, or similar ones, without the ethical constraints attendant on the human situation. For example, adoptive transfer of serum and/or cells can be done to find out which immune component mediated the effect. One can also examine local suppressor phenomena in the placenta and draining nodes with and without vaccination. Such experiments are now in progress.

In conclusion, there is no doubt that the placenta serves as an immunological barrier to the maternal immune response. Currently available experimental models in mice should soon provide a fairly complete picture of how that barrier functions *in situ*.

Acknowledgements

This work was supported by grants from the Canadian MRC, Alberta Heritage Trust Fund for Medical Research, and INSERM. I thank my colleagues Drs W. H. Fridman, C. Neauport-Sautes and G. Chaouat for their hospitality and help in completing the latter aspects of this work.

References

1. Wegmann, T. G. and Gill, T. J. (eds.) (1983). *Immunology of Reproduction*. (New York: Oxford University Press)
2. Chaouat, G., Kolb, J. P. and Wegmann, T. G. (1983). The murine placenta as a immunological barrier between the mother and the fetus. *Immunol. Rev.* (In press.)
3. Croy, A., Rossant, J. and Clark, D. A. (1981). Is there maternal immune rejection of the fetus in failed murine interspecies pregnancy? *J. Reprod. Immunol.*, S1
4. Rossant, J., Mauro, V. M. and Croy, B. A. (1982). Importance of trophoblast genotype for survival of interspecific murine chimeras. *J. Embryol. Exp. Morphol.*, **69**, 141
5. Swinburne, L. M. (1970). Leucocyte antigens and placental sponge. *Lancet*, **1**, 592
6. Wegmann, T. G., Mosmann, T. R., Carlson, G., Olignik, O. and Singh, B. (1979). The ability of the murine placenta to absorb monoclonal anti-fetal H-2K antibody from the maternal circulation. *J. Immunol.*, **122**, 270
7. Wegmann, T. G., Barrington-Leigh, J., Carlson, G., Mosmann, T. R., Raghupathy, R. and Singh, G. (1980). Quantitation of the capacity of the placenta to absorb monoclonal anti-fetal H-2K antibody. *J. Reprod. Immunol.*, **2**, 53
8. Raghupathy, R., Singh, B., Barrington-Leigh, J. and Wegmann, T. G. (1981). The ontogeny and turnover kinetics of paternal H-2K antigenic determinants on the allogeneic murine placenta. *J. Immunol.*, **127**, 2074
9. Raghupathy, R. (1982). Expression and relevance of paternal MHC antigens on the murine placenta. *Ph.D. Thesis*, University of Alberta, Edmonton, Alberta, Canada
10. Anderson, D. J., Sandow, B. A., Raghupathy, R., Singh, B. and Wegmann, T. G. (1983). Localization of cells constituting an immunological barrier in the placenta. *J. Reprod. Immunol.* (In press.)
11. Voisin, G. A. and Chaouat, G. (1974). Demonstration, nature and properties of maternal antibodies fixed on placenta, and directed against paternal antigens. *J. Reprod. Fertil.*, **21** (Suppl.), 89
12. Jenkinson, E. J. and Owen, O. V. (1980). Ontogeny and distribution of Major Histocompatibility Complex (MHC) on mouse placental trophoblast. *J. Reprod. Immunol.*, **2**, 173
13. Sellens, M. H., Jenkinson, E. J. and Billington, W. D. (1978). Major Histocompatibility Complex and non-Major Histocompatibility Complex antigens on mouse ectoplacental cone and placental trophoblast cells. *Transplantation*, **25**, 173
14. Chatterjee-Hasrouni, S. and Lala, P. K. (1979). Localization of H-2 antigens on mouse trophoblast cells. *J. Exp. Med.*, **149**, 1238
15. Chatterjee-Hasrouni, S. and Lala, P. K. (1982). Localization of paternal H-2 antigens on murine trophoblast cells *in vivo*. *J. Exp. Med.*, **155**, 1679
16. Collins, G. D., Chrest, F. J. and Adler, W. H. (1981). Maternal cell traffics in allogeneic embryos. *J. Reprod. Immunol.*, **2**, 163
17. Seemayer, T. A. (1979). The graft versus host reaction: a pathogenic mechanism of experimental and human disease. *Perspect. Pediatr. Biol.*, **5**, 93
18. Beer, A. E., Quebberman, J. F., Clyers, J. W. T. and Haines, R. F. (1981). Major Histocompatibility Complex antigens, maternal and paternal immune response, and chronic abortion in humans. *Am. J. Obstet. Gynecol.*, **141**, 982

19. Taylor, C. and Faulk, W. P. (1981). Prevention of recurrent abortions with leucocyte transfusions. *Lancet*, **2**, 68
20. Gill, T. J. (1983). Immunogenetics of spontaneous abortions in humans. *Transplantation*, **35**, 1
21. Clark, D. A., McDermott, M. and Sczewzuk, M. R. (1980). Impairment of host *vs.* graft reaction in pregnant mice: II. Selective suppression of cytotoxic cell generation correlates with soluble suppressor activity and with successful allogeneic pregnancy. *Cell. Immunol.*, **52**, 106

20
Detection of immunoreactive materials in body fluids

K. BROGAARD HANSEN and T. HJORT

During the past 25 years there has been an increasing activity in the search for immune reactions with anticonceptional effects. The interest has been stimulated by the need to explain infertility in couples with otherwise unexplained infertility and by a demand for new methods of fertility regulation.

Immune responses to many different antigens in the reproductive tract have been considered, but the only responses so far found to be clinically relevant in relation to infertility seem to be those directed against antigens located on the surface of the spermatoza. Thus, such antibodies – systemically and locally produced – have been detected in increased frequencies in men and women from infertile couples, and experimental studies have clearly revealed effects of the antibodies which could reduce fertility, chiefly impairment of sperm penetration into cervical mucus.

METHODS

For detection of circulating antibodies against spermatozoal surface antigens the agglutination techniques are still the most widely used. They are rather easy to perform and by investigation of the same sera in different laboratories a remarkable agreement was found[1]. These remarks refer particularly to the gelatine agglutination test (GAT) and the tray agglutination test (TAT). Both can be used for testing of serum, seminal plasma, and cervical mucus, in the last case after liquefaction of the mucus by treatment with bromelin[2]. The TAT has two advantages over GAT; it requires only small volumes of sperm and it visualizes the mode of agglutination, i.e. head-to-head, tail-to-tail or mixed agglutination. Moreover, the TAT is more sensitive in detecting head-to-head agglutination than GAT, and this seems to explain why TAT is more convenient for testing of sera from women where this mode of agglutination dominates. Generally GAT and TAT reveal the same antibodies. The complement-dependent sperm immobilization test is also a reliable and reproducible technique for testing of sera, although with a lower sensitivity than the agglutination tests. However, it is not suitable for testing of seminal plasma and cervical mucus, since a significant proportion of the antibodies in these fluids is often of the IgA class, which do not activate complement and which will therefore not be detected in this test. Some laboratories have always found immobilizing sera also to cause agglutination, whereas others have described immobilizing, non-agglutinating sera[3].

Modern immunological techniques, such as RIA and ELISA, have also been applied for detection of antibodies to sperm membrane antigens, but the clinical relevance of these tests has not yet been firmly established. In our hands the ELISA technique has revealed results which turned out to be of little clinical interest.

Recently, detection of antibodies, bound *in vivo* to the spermatozoa, has become a popular way of diagnosing autoimmunity to sperm. Most commonly the mixed antiglobulin reaction (direct MAR test) developed by Jager *et al.*[4] is used. In this very simple technique, which can be carried out in a few minutes, a drop of fresh semen is mixed with a drop of a suspension of indicator cells (for instance erythrocytes sensitized with an IgG anti-Rh antibody or coated with purified IgG) and anti-IgG is added. If the spermatozoa are covered with IgG-antibodies, erythrocytes will stick to them, and the percentage of the living spermatozoa carrying antibody on their surface can thus be determined. In the same way the spermatozoa can be examined for IgA antibodies.The recording of the immunoglobulin classes of the antibodies seems of importance for the evaluation of the fertility status of the patient, since antibodies of the IgA class may impair sperm penetration into cervical mucus more effectively than IgG antibodies[5].

The MAR test can also be applied as a so-called indirect test, in

216

which donor spermatozoa are first incubated with serum or genital secretion for binding of antibody and then tested as described.

In a recent investigation in our laboratory GAT was carried out on serum and seminal plasma from 227 men, referred for infertility problems, and independently direct MAR test for IgG and IgA was performed on the fresh ejaculates (Jensen and Hjort, unpublished observations). The purpose was to evaluate which of these methods was the most useful for routine screening of men for autoimmunity

Table 1 Comparison of direct MAR-test and GAT

	GAT in serum		GAT in seminal plasma	
	Positive	Negative	Positive	Negative
MAR +	14	2	11	5
MAR −	16	173	0	189
Total	30	175	11	194

No. of patients = 227 (MAR testing not possible in 22).
MAR-testing performed: 205
GAT = Gelatine agglutination test; MAR = mixed antiglobulin reaction.

to sperm (Table 1). Due to azoospermia or poor motility the MAR test could not be performed in 22 cases. Among the remaining 205 men, 30 had sperm agglutinins in serum. In 11 of these cases agglutinins were found also in seminal plasma and the MAR test was positive, at least for IgG. The MAR test was positive in another five cases; in three men with sperm agglutinins in serum and in two men where no antibody activity had been detected neither in serum nor in seminal plasma. However, in both of the last cases the MAR reactions were weak with less than 30% of the spermatozoa carrying antibody on their surface (mainly IgA antibody). On the other hand, 16 men with sperm agglutinins merely in serum had negative MAR tests, but in most of these cases the titre was low (≤16). The conclusion was therefore that all cases of stronger immunization – and probably of clinical significance – could be revealed by both techniques.

The main antifertility effect of the antibodies in both men and women is most likely impairment of penetration of the spermatozoa into cervical mucus, but also other mechanisms such as interference in the sperm–ovum interaction may play a role. The reduced penetration of antibody-covered spermatozoa can be observed *in vivo* in the post-coital test and *in vitro* in the sperm penetration test performed in capillary tubes and in the sperm–cervical mucus-contact test (SCMC test)[2]. There is a connection between occurrence of antibodies and reduced migration of spermatozoa in the sperm penetration test and the SCMC test, but the advantage of these methods is that they include a combined evaluation of the sperm quality, the cervical mucus quality, and the antibody effect. However, a regular semen analysis and a sperm/cervical mucus crossed hostility test[6] can help in distinguishing between bad quality of the semen and impaired penetration caused by antibodies to spermatozoa.

INTERPRETATION OF RESULTS

Large investigations from several countries with testing of sera from men, mainly by means of GAT, have shown that the frequency of positive reactions, particularly strongly positive reactions (titre $\geqslant 64$), is significantly higher in men from infertile couples than in fertile men. In men from couples with otherwise unexplained infertility the percentage of strongly positive sera increases to about ten[7]. Less information is available on the significance of antibody levels in seminal plasma, but the presumption has been made that pregnancy is rarely achieved when the titre of sperm agglutinins exceeds 16[8].

In 1974 Rümke *et al.*[9] studied the fertility of men with sperm agglutinins in serum and revealed a highly significant inverse relation between antibody levels and fertility, but even some men with antibodies in relatively high titres had induced pregnancies. By follow-up examination of vasovasostomized men Linnet *et al.*[10] observed significantly more pregnancies induced by men without than by men with sperm agglutinins in seminal plasma.

We have studied the fertility of a group of men who had previously been examined for fertility problems and in whom the GAT had revealed sperm agglutinins in serum and in some cases also in seminal plasma[11]. The observation period ranged from 4 years to 8 months. Among 43 couples with otherwise unexplained infertility, as evaluated by the clinical routine procedures, pregnancy had been achieved by 16 couples (37%). To our surprise the pregnancy rate was the same in the group of 19 couples with agglutinins in low titre ($\leqslant 16$) in the husbands' serum as in the group of 24 with agglutinins in high titre ($\geqslant 64$). However, looking at the antibody concentrations in seminal plasma there was a difference in fertility between men with (23 cases) and without (20 cases) antibodies in seminal plasma, the pregnancy rates in the two groups being 22% and 55%, respectively. It has to be stressed that the rather good fertility prognosis in these patients must be compared with the fact that the husbands' spermatozoa had shown a good motility in all cases. Thus, a good sperm motility may to some extent compensate the impairing influence of the antibodies and maintain a good sperm penetration in cervical mucus. On the other hand, the effect of the antibodies will also vary, depending not only upon the number of antibody molecules bound to each sperm cell (antibodies to one or more than one antigen) and the immunoglobulin class of the antibodies, but also upon the affinity of the antibodies, which has not yet been studied.

Recently, these considerations gained some support from a follow-up study of the men who had induced pregnancies in spite of the previous presence of sperm agglutinins.The purpose was to reinvestigate these men with immunological tests (GAT and MAR test) as well as with tests for sperm migration in cervical mucus to find an explanation for their fertility. The results are summarized in Table 2, where the men are divided into two groups; one without and one with sperm agglutinins in seminal plasma. In some cases, originally with low serum titres, the agglutinins had disappeared. The reactivity ranges in the different tests were wide, but only half of the motile spermatozoa showed presence of IgA antibodies on their surface in the MAR test, and the majority of the men had a fair sperm penetration, i.e. over $20\,\text{mm}\,(2\,\text{h})^{-1}$. A poor penetration was in two of three cases combined with many immotile spermatozoa or a relatively poor motility.

Thus, in the evaluation of the significance of the antisperm antibodies in the individual patient the best guidance may still be achieved by investigation of the ability of the spermatozoa to penetrate into normal cervical mucus. A fair penetration indicates that the fertility prognosis might be rather good.

Investigations on immunological infertility in women, caused by antisperm antibodies, have revealed rather divergent results in different countries[3]. This relates both to the frequency and apparent significance of the antibodies. By follow-up studies of women, tested for agglutinating or immobilizing antibodies in serum, significant differences in occurrence of pregnancy between women with and without circulating antibodies have not been demonstrated. Therefore, it seems that little is obtained by routine screening of infertile

Table 2 Findings in men previously found to have antisperm antibodies and who have induced pregnancy

| No. of patients | GAT titre | | MAR test (% positive) | | SCMC (% shaking) | Penetration (mm (2h)$^{-1}$) | Semen | |
	Serum	Seminal plasma	IgG	IgA			% immotile sperms	Degree of motility
7	0–256	0	2–90	0–49	8–54	<20, 1 man >20, 6 men	25–60	2–4
7	4–1024	4–256	36–93	18–51	36–88	<20, 2 men >20, 5 men	20–80	2–4

GAT = Gelatine agglutination test.
MAR = Mixed antiglobulin reaction: percentage of motile spermatozoa reacting.
SCMC = Sperm cervical mucus contact test: percentage of motile spermatozoa showing 'shaking phenomenon'.
Penetration = sperm penetration into cervical mucus in capillary tubes.
Degree of motility: 1 = poor; 2 = fair; 3 = good; 4 = excellent.

women for antisperm antibodies in serum. On the other hand, local sperm antibodies in the cervix, mostly of the IgA class, are obviously capable of reducing the chance of conception by inhibiting sperm penetration in cervical mucus. Cases of immunologically caused infertility in women are therefore also revealed by the techniques recording the sperm–cervical mucus interaction, for instance the SCMC test where 'shaking' of normal spermatozoa can be observed. If other causes for a bad result in these tests can be excluded, such as scanty, non-optimal, cell-invaded, or acid mucus, testing for agglutinating and immobilizing antibodies should be performed on bromelin-liquefied cervical mucus. At least in Denmark the occurrence of female infertility due to antisperm antibodies seems to be rather rare with an incidence of about 0.5–1%.

References

1. Boettcher, B., Hjort, T., Rümke, Ph., Shulman, S. and Vyazov, O. E. (1977). Auto- and iso-antibodies to antigens of the human reproductive system. I. Results of an international comparative study. *Clin. Exp. Immunol.*, **30**, 173
2. Kremer, J., Jager, S. and Kuiken, J. (1977). The clinical significance of antibodies to spermatozoa. In Boettcher, B. (ed.). *Immunological Influence on Human Fertility*, p. 47. (Sydney: Academic Press)
3. Ingerslev, J. (1981). Antibodies against spermatozoal surface-membrane antigens in female infertility. *Acta Obstet. Gynecol. Scand.*, **100** (Suppl.)
4. Jager, S., Kremer, J., Kuiken, J. and van Slochteren-Draaisma, T. (1980). Immuno-globulin class of antispermatozoal antibodies from infertile men and inhibition of *in vitro* sperm penetration into cervical mucus. *Int. J. Androl.*, **3**, 1
5. Hendry, W. F., Stedronska, J. and Lake, R. A. (1982). Mixed erythrocyte-spermatozoa antiglobulin reaction (MAR-test) for IgA antisperm antibodies in subfertile males. *Fertil. Steril.*, **37**, 108
6. Morgan, H., Stedronska, J., Hendry, W. F., Chamberlain, G. V. P. and Dewhurst, C. J. (1977). Sperm/cervical mucus crossed hostility testing and antisperm antibodies in the husband. *Lancet*, **1**, 1228
7. Husted, S. (1975). Sperm antibodies in men from infertile couples. *Int. J. Fertil.*, **20**, 97
8. Rümke, Ph. (1982). Auto- and isoimmune reactions to antigens of the gonads and genital tract. In Fougereau, M. and Dausset, J. (eds.). *Progress in Immunology IV*, pp. 1065–1092. (London: Academic Press)
9. Rümke, Ph., van Amstel, N., Messer, E. N. and Bezemer, P. D. (1974). Prognosis of fertility of men with spermagglutinins in the serum. *Fertil. Steril.*, **25**, 393
10. Linnet, L., Hjort, T. and Fogh-Andersen, P. (1981). Association between failure to impregnate after vasovasostomy and sperm agglutinins in semen. *Lancet*, **1**, 117
11. Hjort, T. and Brogaard Hansen, K. (1983). Seminal antigens in man with particular regard to possible immunological contraception. In Shulman, S. and Dondero, F. (eds.). *Immunological Factors in Human Contraception*, pp. 47–56. (Field Educational Italia – Acta Medica)

21
Immunological methods of birth control

V. C. STEVENS

INTRODUCTION

Despite the widespread availability of many highly effective methods of contraception, most scientists in the field of family planning agree that new methods of birth control are needed to meet the increasing demand for global population regulation. The development of immunological means of preventing or disrupting human fertility is one of several approaches to the acquisition of new antifertility methods.

There are three basic strategies that might be used to develop an immunological antifertility procedure: (1) active immunization against a component of the reproductive system; (2) passive immunization with antisera against a reproductive component; or (3) manipulation of the maternal immune mechanisms to abrogate the acceptance of the early conceptus and thus prevent the establishment of a successful pregnancy. This last approach is still highly theoretical and is far removed from any practical application but may be a viable procedure in the future as our ability to regulate the immune system becomes more sophisticated. Passive immunization, the administration of exogenously produced antibodies raised against a reproductive substance, has until recently been limited to the use of sera derived from non-human species. In the case of such application to birth control in humans, the repetitive use of animal sera has been considered hazardous because of possible reactions to foreign proteins. However, the recent development of new technology for producing human immunoglobulins *in vitro* from hybridomas opens the door for reconsideration of passive immunization as a safe method of immunological birth control.

While passive immunization procedures have the advantage of allowing control over the nature of antibodies employed and duration of use of the method, they have certain practical disadvantages. The major disadvantage is that the duration of effectiveness from a single application is usually only a few days. On the other hand, active immunization against a reproductive component could offer prolonged protection from pregnancy by a single immunization. This advantage, together with a number of practical considerations, has stimulated most of the research in this area toward the development of antifertility vaccines. To date, few opportunities have arisen to devise an antifertility vaccine for men and most effort has been expended for the development of vaccines for use by women.

POTENTIAL ANTIGENS FOR VACCINE DEVELOPMENT

The possibilities for antifertility vaccine development, as well as the numerous problems and limitations likely to be encountered, have been eloquently reviewed by Jones[1]. It is readily apparent from our current knowledge that the most promise for a vaccine in the immediate future is the use of an antigen considered foreign to the maternal immune system such as sperm or placental components. Excepting for research on ovum antigens, the bulk of research and development work has concentrated on developing a vaccine from these sources. In this report, discussion will be limited to the areas of research most advanced in the development of antifertility vaccines.

Ovum antigens

Most research on ovum antigens is directed toward the zona pellucida. This acellular, gelatinous layer surrounding the ovum offers perhaps the most promise as a source of antigens for specific immunological inhibition of ovum viability. While no specific components have been isolated from this structure, antibodies specific to it have been prepared. Such antibodies block fertility in several rodent species, sometimes for long periods. The mechanism of fertility inhibition could be either the prevention of sperm penetration, or if fertilization occurred the blocking of implantation by interfering with zona shedding.

Antifertility effects have been observed from immunizing female animals with antigens from porcine zona pellucida. Pig zona contain antigens immunologically similar to zona from many species, including monkeys, baboons, chimpanzees and man. Using such antigens, an effective vaccine could be developed and tested in non-human primates before human application. The availability of abundant supplies of pig zona, obtained from pig ovaries, would provide a practical source of antigen for large-scale vaccine use.

Data available from recent studies involving immunizations of female marmosets and baboons with crude pig zona pellucida preparations have revealed that these antigens are very immunogenic and no pregnancies have occurred in immunized females. Thus it appears that a vaccine against the zona pellucida would be very effective in preventing pregnancy in women. The question of possible autoimmune damage to ovarian cells and/or alteration in ovarian function must be carefully assessed in non-human primates, however, before it can be concluded that zona antigens could be used in a vaccine for the regulation of human fertility. More details of research in this area can be obtained from reviews of the subject[2,3].

Sperm antigens

The idea that human fertility could be inhibited by immunological means probably originated from observations of effects of injecting women with sperm or semen components[4,5]. Despite these early promising leads, the lack of defined sperm-specific antigens and the inadequacies of methodology for evaluating effects of immunization resulted in few studies pursuing the development of an anti-sperm vaccine for three decades. Some progress has been made in the isolation of sperm components and development of analytical techniques for assessing immune responses to sperm, experiments on the effects of immunization with a few of these purified sperm antigens on fertility have been conducted.

Most promise for immediate vaccine development exists using an isoenzyme of lactate dehydrogenase (LDH-C_4) isolated from sperm cells of several species. While this enzyme is an intracellular component, antibodies to it react with the surface of intact sperm. This isoenzyme is found only in sperm cells but sperm LDH-C_4 from several species have common immunological determinants. Female baboons have been immunized with mouse LDH-C$_4$ and significant antibody levels attained. Mating of the animals revealed a significant reduction in fertility and pregnancies were correlated with low antibody levels[6]. Since these data were most encouraging, work has proceeded to determine whether synthetic peptides, representing a surface component of mouse LDH-C$_4$ will elicit antibodies to the intact molecule. These studies have produced positive results. Studies are now proceeding to evaluate a potential vaccine utilizing synthetic peptides of the sperm specific enzyme. Use of these materials would eliminate the necessity of isolating vaccine components from natural sources and greatly facilitate the production of suitable quantities of antigen for large-scale use. A major advantage of a sperm vaccine would be that if it destroyed the viability of sperm prior to fertilization it would be a truly contraceptive vaccine. This mechanism would probably make it more acceptable to many populations.

Placental antigens

From the point of view of antifertility vaccine development, the placenta is a rich source of antigens that meet the general criteria of being 'non-self' components and that are present within the woman for a brief period. Extensive experimental evidence has shown that immunizations of laboratory animals with crude placental extracts can inhibit fertility. However, severe non-specific reactions, including nephritis, have resulted from such treatment, and efforts have been made in the past decade to evaluate the effects of immunizations with highly purified antigens from placentas.

The most extensive studies conducted for developing an antifertility vaccine have been those using hCG antigens. Model studies have demonstrated that hCG can be rendered immunogenic in humans[7]. One of the major problems with the use of hCG as an immunogen is the well-known cross-reactivity of anti-hCG antibodies with the pituitary hormone LH. Fearing disturbances of the menstrual cycle and even worse, autoimmune damage to the pituitary, no attempts were made to develop a vaccine with the intact hCG molecule. However, when data became available that antibodies raised to the β subunit of hCG (hCG-β) could discriminate between hCG and hLH, studies were initiated to test the feasibility of using hCG-β for vaccine development.

Female baboons were immunized with hCG-β and antibodies generated reacted with both hCG and baboon CG (bCG). Despite antibody reaction with hLH, these females exhibited normal menstrual cycles since antisera showed no detectable cross-reaction with baboon LH. When the animals were mated with males of proved fertility, no sustained pregnancies were observed, suggesting a highly efficacious antifertility effect from the treatment. Immunizations of marmosets with hCG-β also resulted in a complete fertility inhibition[8]. The duration of effective immunity in these animal experiments has lasted from 1 to 3 years from their last injection.

Women have also been immunized with β-hCG. The subunit, conjugated to tetanus toxoid, has been administered to approximately 60 individuals previously sterilized by tubal ligations. Antibodies reactive to hCG were reported as: 17 subjects attained 'fairly good' titres, 30 moderate responses, and 13 poor responses[9]. Most women continued to menstruate regularly despite a low level of cross-reactivity of antibodies to hLH. Plasma progesterone levels in the luteal phase of the cycle indicated that the women remained ovulatory. Some of these subjects were monitored for more than 4 years and showed no abnormal parameter of kidney, liver, thyroid, adrenal, pituitary or haematopoietic functions. These data offer encouraging evidence that despite the relative non-specificity of hCG-β antibodies, there may be no serious side-effects from immunization of women with the hormone subunit. However, it must be realized that the immune responses in these women were very low and immunizations of fertile women with the same vaccine formulation was ineffective at preventing fertility[10].

Cross-reactions of antisera to β-hCG with hLH encouraged the author and his colleagues to seek more specific hCG antigens for vaccine development. Identification of the primary structure of the β subunits of hCG and hLH revealed that most of the amino acid sequences of the two subunits were identical except at the COOH-terminal portion. With this information efforts were begun in 1974 to evaluate peptides from the COOH terminal portion of hCG-β as potential antigens for antifertility vaccine development.

Antisera generated to a large number of peptides have been assessed for reactivity to both peptide and intact hCG. The results can be summarized by stating that antibodies to peptides representing the 35–37 C-terminal amino acids of hCG-β react to hCG on a molar basis nearly equivalent to the peptides used for immunization. None

227

of the antisera to COOH-β-hCG peptides have shown significant reactivity with hLH or any other purified pituitary hormones[11]. Extensive testing for cross-reactivity of antisera with non-placental organs and tissues has not yet been completed.

Antisera raised to these peptides have significant actions when administered to pregnant baboons. The intravenous instillation of 100 ml of an antiserum from a baboon immunized with peptide β-hCG 111–145 to a non-immunized pregnant baboon promptly disrupted gestation as evidenced by menstrual bleeding and a rapid

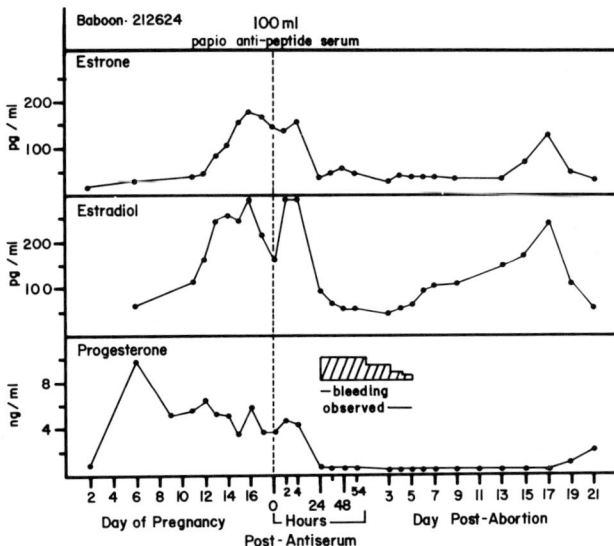

Figure 1 Disruption of pregnancy in a baboon by the intravenous administration of baboon anti-hCG peptide serum on day 18 of gestation. Hormone levels, within the normal range prior to the passive immunization, dropped markedly within 24 hours and menstrual bleeding was initiated. The animal began a new menstrual cycle, with normal hormonal patterns and sex skin changes, a few days after the induced abortion

decline in serum hormone levels (Fig. 1). Despite the limited cross-reactivity of anti-β-hCG peptide antibodies with baboon CG, disruption of placental function at an early stage of pregnancy can be induced. These observations strongly suggest the feasibility of using a synthetic β-hCG peptide as an immunogen for an antifertility vaccine. Antibodies to hCG peptides are not species specific. Fortu-

228

nately, antisera raised to COOH-peptides will react with CG from baboons and chimpanzees, albeit at a lower level than to hCG. Without this cross-reactivity it would not be possible to evaluate the efficacy and safety of a vaccine based on hCG peptides in animals.

Several adult fertile female baboons have been immunized with numerous conjugates of the β-hCG peptides. Significant antibody levels were generated to both hCG and baboon CG. Results of one breeding experiment of carrier immunized females and females

Table 1 Comparison of fertility rates for female baboons immunized with tetanus toxoid to those immunized with tetanus toxoid conjugated with β-hCG (109–145) synthetic peptide. Matings commenced during the course of the third menstrual cycle following primary immunization

Baboons immunized with:	Mating cycle			Totals
	1	2	3	
Tetanus toxoid:				
No. mated	15*	5	1	21
No. pregnant	10	4	1	15
Fertility rate (%)	66.7	80.0	100.0	71.4
Tetanus toxoid: β-hCG (109–145):				
No. mated	15*	14	13	42
No. pregnant	1	1	2	4
Fertility rate (%)	6.7	7.1	15.4	9.5

* Includes one anovulatory menstrual cycle.

immunized with peptide–carrier conjugates are shown in Table 1. Some immunized females were mated only once and others as many as three times if no pregnancy resulted. The antifertility effects of immunizations were related to the antibody level at the time of mating. Sera from animals that remained pregnant despite relatively high antibody levels to hCG showed a lower cross-reactivity of the antisera with baboon CG than those antisera from animals not conceiving. While the pregnancy rate in these immunized baboons may not be acceptable for human application, a clear reduction in fertility from control animals is apparent. It must be remembered that the immunogen used here was related to the human antigen and relatively low cross-reactivity with the baboon hormone was present in all antisera. Should these antibody levels represent total reactivity to the homologous CG, a much lower fertility rate would probably have been observed.

PROBLEMS AND PROSPECTS FOR VACCINE DEVELOPMENT

While an hCG antifertility vaccine may be available within the next few years, its final evaluation and the development of other vaccines will encounter numerous obstacles. A major obstacle to the assessment of vaccines is the lack of good animal models for the meaningful evaluation of safety and efficacy. As with any antifertility method, few health risks are tolerable and strong assurance that serious side-effects are not likely to be observed must be provided before clinical assessment can proceed. The design of animal studies to provide such assurances is difficult. Also, many new features, not currently used in conventional vaccines, must be developed and tested for antifertility methods. Employment of synthetic antigens, carrier–antigen conjugates and potent adjuvant compounds have not been clinically tested in any existing vaccine. These 'multivalent' vaccines must be carefully evaluated for safety despite the lack of any previous experience with such products in the medical field.

However, the importance of new approaches to the development of better birth control methods justifies the continued research towards obtaining an immunological antifertility method. The potential impact of such a method on the problem of increasing world population is obvious.

References

1. Jones, W. R. (1982). *Immunological Fertility Regulation*, p. 273. (Melbourne: Blackwell Scientific Publications)
2. Aitken, R. J. and Richardson, D. W. (1983). Active immunization against zona pellucida antigens. Presented at the *38th Easter School, University of Nottingham School of Agriculture*, April 18–21, Nottingham
3. Shivers, C. A. (1976). Antigens of the ovum as potential basis for the development of contraceptive vaccine. In *Development of Vaccines for Fertility Regulation*, pp. 81–91. (Copenhagen: Scriptor)
4. Rosenfield, S. S. (1926). Semen injections with serologic studies. *Am. J. Obstet. Gynecol.*, **12**, 385
5. Baskin, M. J. (1932). Temporary sterilization by the injection of human spermatozoa – a preliminary report. *Am. J. Obstet. Gynecol.*, **24**, 892
6. Goldberg, E., Wheat, T. E., Powell, J. E. and Stevens, V. C. (1980). Reduction of fertility in female baboons immunized with lactate dehydrogenase-C_4. *Fertil. Steril.*, **35**, 214
7. Stevens, V. C. and Crystle, C. D. (1973). Effects of immunization with hapten-coupled hCG on the human menstrual cycle. *Obstet. Gynecol.*, **42**, 485

8. Hearn, J. P. (1976). Immunization against pregnancy. *Proc. R. Soc. Lond.*, **195**, 149
9. Talwar, G. P. (1979). Immunology in reproduction. *J. Reprod. Med.*, **22**, 61
10. Hingorani, V. and Kamar, S. (1979). Anti-hCG immunization – phase I clinical trials. In Talwar, G. P. (ed.). *Recent Advances in Reproduction and Regulation of Fertility*, pp. 467–471 (Amsterdam: Elsevier/North Holland)
11. Stevens, V. C. (1976). Actions of antisera to hCG-β: *in vitro* and *in vivo* assessment. In *Proceedings of the V International Congress of Endocrinology*. International Congress Series, 402, p. 379. (Amsterdam: Excerpta Medica)

231

22
The treatment of immunologically conditioned infertility

W. R. JONES

INTRODUCTION

The literature relating to the management of immunological infertility is beset with confusion, insubstantial anecdotes, reports of uncontrolled studies and unfounded claims of therapeutic success. This chapter attempts to survey this difficult field, to draw conclusions and to suggest future directions. Many of the data summarized or alluded to in this presentation are referenced in a more detailed review[1].

The incidence of immunological infertility lies somewhere between 5 and 30% and varies between the female and the male partner and with the nature and extent of the investigation of sperm antibodies. In general terms when criteria for the diagnosis of immunological infertility are restricted to relatively high-titre antibodies in local sites (e.g. semen and cervical mucus) the true incidence of the problem probably lies well towards the lower end of the quoted range.

The biological significance of sperm antibodies is hard to assess – more so in the female than in the male. This in turn creates difficulties in determining specific therapeutic efficacy for manoeuvres designed to overcome a presumed immunological block to fertility. These difficulties are compounded by the decline in the incidence of apparently 'unexplained' infertility as a result of the increased detection of conditions such as minor endometriosis and luteinized unruptured follicle (LUF) syndrome. In the author's clinic, the incidence of 'unexplained' infertility has halved in the past 4 years. Although immunological factors may occur in combination with other causes of infertility, it is in the 'unexplained' group that therapy for sperm antibodies can be most rationally examined and assessed – this opportunity is now somewhat limited and there are obvious difficulties in any one centre mounting an acceptable clinical trial of therapy for immune factors in otherwise 'unexplained' infertility.

TREATMENT IN THE MALE

Attempts to treat immunological infertility in the male partner can be summarized under the following headings: suppression of spermatogenesis, immunosuppression, sperm washing/insemination, artificial insemination by donor (AID) and antibiotic therapy.

Suppression of spermatogenesis

Testosterone suppression has historical interest only in the management of men with sperm antibodies since there is no evidence of a consistent or specific effect in the few published studies of this form of treatment.

Immunosuppression

Although early reports of this approach to treatment (with ACTH or prednisone) described only indifferent results, there has been a major resurgence of interest in a variety of forms of immunosuppression in the treatment of sperm autoimmunity in the male. An early clue to the possible mode of action and potential effectiveness of immunosuppression was seen in a report by Bassili and El Alfi[2] who described the treatment with high but reducing doses of prednisone of 18 men with oligoazoospermia and somewhat tenuous evidence of cell-mediated immunity to sperm. The sperm count improved significantly in nine of these subjects.

One of the more popular modern regimens has been the exhibition of high doses (96 mg daily) of methyl prednisolone in a cyclical manner given to the male for 7 days either at the end or the beginning of his female partner's cycle. The rationale of this regimen is based on an anticipated effect on autoimmune pathology in the male at around the time of ovulation in the female. In six reports of this form of treatment, in a total of 152 men, pregnancy rates ranged from 11 to 57%.

The author has used an incremental regimen of cyclical methyl prednisolone up to a maximum dose of 76 mg daily in the male partners of seven couples where sperm autoimmunity was the only demonstrable problem. Conception occurred in three instances. In another 12 couples where other problems coincided with the immunological factor, only two pregnancies occurred.

Low or medium dose continuous or intermittent corticosteroid therapy with prednisone, betamethasone or dexamethasone has also been utilized in the management of sperm autoimmunity. In five series, including the author's, totalling 93 cases, pregnancy rates ranging from 0% to 45% have been recorded. The latter figure was obtained by Hargreave and Elton[3] using a regimen of betamethasone decreasing from 2 mg daily to 0·5 mg daily over 7 days and taken on alternate weeks.

Dondero et al.[4] used methyl prednisolone in continuous decremental dosage over 60 days preceded by a testosterone suppression regimen but failed to demonstrate any advantage of this method over the use of corticosteroids alone. Higher dose continuous corticosteroid regimens (e.g. prednisone 30–60 mg daily) appear to have no place in the therapy of sperm autoimmunity.

Levamisole, an immunomodulating agent, has also been employed to suppress sperm immunity, but the results have been variable, and the potential gastrointestinal effects are a source of concern. Indeed the occurrence of side-effects with the various corticosteroid regimens is also a worry, particularly when such treatment is exhibited in individuals for a potential benefit unrelated to their general medical health. The incidence of minor and major side-effects in collected series is summarized in Table 1.

Table 1 Incidence (%) of side-effects with corticosteroid regimens

Therapy	Minor	Major
High-dose cyclical	16–27%	2–6%
Incremental cyclical	25%	0
Low–medium-dose continuous	20%	0

Hargreave and Elton[3] reported a total incidence of side-effects of 63% associated with two different regimens and a majority of men receiving high-dose continuous therapy experienced problems.

In the two largest series of high-dose cyclical methyl prednisolone treatment totalling 126 cases[5,6], there were five instances of major side-effects. These included two cases of severe gastrointestinal discomfort requiring treatment, one case of haematemesis and two cases of aseptic hip necrosis. The latter problem, a relatively rare, but well-recognized serious sequel to corticosteroid therapy, was foreshadowed by the occurrence of hip pain during treatment, but in both cases did not become overtly apparent until 12 months after cessation of the drug. This suggests that further cases may yet come to light.

Minor side-effects include: dyspepsia, oedema and weight gain, rashes and acne, muscle weakness, mood changes, insomnia, urinary frequency, transient joint pains, headaches, tinnitus and flashing lights. This catalogue, together with the spectre of aseptic hip necrosis, calls for a re-appraisal of corticosteroid therapy in sperm immunity.

The mode of action of corticosteroids in suppressing antibody responses is confused. There is some evidence that they increase the catabolism and decrease the synthesis of immunoglobulin G, but no clear indication that they can inhibit specific antibody responses. On the other hand, they appear to modulate cell-mediated immune responses and to promote an improvement in semen quality – that is in sperm count, sperm motility and in spontaneous sperm auto-agglutination.

The assessment of the results of treatment with corticosteroids is complicated by a variety of factors. These include the low incidence of immune factors in infertility, the increasing incidence of other occult causes of infertility, the variable effect of corticosteroids on antibody levels, natural fluctuations in immunity, and the occurrence of pregnancies unrelated to treatment. The situation is further complicated by factors relating to the selection of patients and the incidence of combined immunity in both partners. These considerations highlight the need for controlled trials to examine the efficacy of corticosteroid therapy in the management of immune infertility.

Sperm washing/insemination

Somewhat desultory attempts have been made by several workers over the years to treat sperm autoimmunity using sperm washing and/or insemination procedures. The results in several reported series totalling 77 patients showed pregnancy rates varying from 8% to 39%. Overall this approach does not seem to be as efficacious as the use of immunosuppression. Some improvement in results might be anticipated with further technical modifications such as direct ejaculation into a buffered medium prior to washing and insemination.

Artificial insemination by donor (AID)

The use of AID is clearly an option for treatment where male fertility is significantly compromised by sperm autoantibodies, particularly where other forms of treatment have failed. The author has used this approach in 11 couples, including seven where male immunosuppressive therapy had failed. Only three pregnancies resulted, however, which is in marked contrast to the 70% overall success rate for AID in our clinic for couples with non-immunological male infertility. The poor results with this approach suggest that occult female factors may play a role in contributing to the antifertility effect of autoantibodies, particularly where other forms of treatment have failed.

Antibiotic therapy

The role of genital tract infection in the promotion of sperm autoimmunity is much debated but it remains possible that occult inflammation may mediate adjuvant effects which initiate or perpetuate an immune response to sperm. Antibiotic therapy has been instituted in men with apparent immunological infertility but the results to date have been unconvincing. This is an area where controlled studies might yield helpful information.

TREATMENT IN THE FEMALE

As mentioned above the biological significance of sperm immunity in the female is less well defined than in the male. The assessment of the results of treatment correspondingly has been more difficult to determine. Five approaches to therapy will be summarized: occlusion, intrauterine AIH, immunosuppression, pre-ovulatory oestrogen administration, and antibiotic therapy.

Occlusion therapy

The use of occlusion therapy with the male partner using a condom has a long, but not entirely respectable, history in the treatment of sperm immunity in the female. This approach involves the prevention of antigen exposure in the female for variable periods (usually at least 6 months) to allow a diminution in the immune response such that subsequent unprotected coitus at mid-cycle might achieve fertilization. Jones[7] reviewed eight series reported between 1968 and 1973 where pregnancy rates of between 19% and 68% were claimed. In a personal study reported at that time[7] a pregnancy rate of 16% was achieved which was similar to that in comparable but untreated women. Subsequent reports have highlighted the variable pregnancy rates obtained with condom therapy and some groups have recorded a complete lack of success. In many of these series, treatment has been instituted on the basis of sperm antibodies demonstrable in serum either alone or in the absence of adequate information about local immunity in cervical mucus. The results obtained in such poorly defined situations are of only limited significance. In addition reports of condom therapy are plagued by losses to follow-up and the occurrence of pregnancies unrelated to changes in sperm antibody titres. Although further studies in better selected cases may clarify the place of occlusion methods, this approach is cumbersome, poorly accepted by patients and of uncertain efficacy.

Intrauterine insemination

Another treatment principle has involved the intrauterine insemination of suitable preparations of the male partner's sperm. Once again variable results have been reported, and their significance has been modified by doubts about the relative significance of the female immune factors in a particular couple's infertility, and by uncertainties about the presence and role of sperm antibodies at sites above the cervix – that is, in the Fallopian tube and possibly in follicular and peritoneal fluid. Logically, intrauterine insemination should be reserved for cases where locally produced sperm antibodies are present in the cervical mucus in the absence of circulating antibodies. The author obtained four pregnancies in 10 such women, where the local immune factor was the only demonstrable abnormality, but there was no success in nine patients where semen or pelvic abnormalities complicated the picture. It was also somewhat disarming that a further three of the 10 'purely' immune group conceived subsequent to the cessation of treatment. This serves to illustrate two important points. First, the relative nature of the anti-fertility effect of sperm antibodies; and second, the possible influence on fertility outcome of the well-described natural variation in sperm antibodies in iso-immune women.

Immunosuppression

There have been a few reports of immunosuppressive therapy for sperm isoimmunity in the female. Pregnancy rates of the order of 20% have been described. The author has treated 11 immunized women with either cyclical methyl prednisolone or prednisone in medium dosage. One pregnancy was obtained in three women with uncomplicated immunological infertility but there was no success in eight patients with other infertility factors present. There are at least theoretical concerns about the possible teratogenic effects of corticosteroid therapy, even in the first half of a conceptual cycle, and it is unlikely that this approach will be pursued with any degree of enthusiasm. The use of locally administered (intravaginal) cortico-steroids has been proposed, but in view of the effective systemic absorption of steroids from the vagina this method suffers from similar concerns about safety.

Pre-ovulatory oestrogen administration

The administration of short courses of oestrogen in the pre-ovulatory phase is an established practice to improve the quality and quantity of cervical mucus. As a by-product of this effect immunoglobulin concentrations might be expected to diminish by dilution. There is some evidence that this, in turn, leads to an improvement in sperm–cervical mucus interactions in women with sperm antibodies in their mucus. This simple therapy is worth further evaluation.

Antibiotic therapy

As in the male, there is evidence that sperm isoimmunity in the female may be enhanced by possible adjuvant effects of genital infection and that antibodies may have a contributory therapeutic role to play.

EXPERIMENTAL APPROACHES

There are three approaches worthy of mention. The first relates to prophylactic immunosuppression at the time of vasectomy. Post-vasectomy sperm immunity has been shown to be prevented in Cynomolgus monkeys by the exhibition of corticosteroids in the perioperative period[8]. This approach might find ultimate clinical application.

A somewhat more theoretical approach might involve the therapeutic use, by local intravaginal application, of physiological immunosuppressive factor(s) derived from seminal plasma. Equally speculative would be the possible modulation of sperm immunity by the oral administration of sperm membrane antigens. This approach has its basis in the mechanisms whereby intestinal exposure to membrane antigens, whilst provoking a local immune response, results in the generation of suppressor T-cell populations capable of depressing pre-existing systemic antibody levels.

FUTURE DIRECTIONS

In vitro fertilization (IVF) techniques might find application in the management of some categories of immunological infertility. For example, the use of washed sperm may achieve fertilization in the presence of sperm autoimmunity. IVF may also play an increasing role in the management of isoimmunized women, particularly where the immune response is confined to the genital tract.

There is a continuing and now urgent need to establish relatively large-scale prospective and properly controlled trials of immunosuppressive therapy in the male. National Fertility Societies should logically assume the responsibility for promoting such trials which of necessity would need to be conducted on a collaborative multi-centre basis. In view of the concerns that are now becoming more apparent about the long-term safety of high-dose corticosteroid therapy, future trials should probably be restricted to the use of medium-dose intermittent or continuous regimens.

Acknowledgements

I wish to thank my clinical, laboratory and nursing colleagues in the Fertility Clinic, Flinders Medical Centre, for their assistance in the management of patients reported in this paper, and Mrs Janet Weber for typing the manuscript.

References

1. Jones, W. R. (1983). The treatment of immunological infertility. *Clin. Reprod. Fertil.* (In press)
2. Bassili, F. and El-Alfi, O. S. (1970). Immunological aspermatogenesis in man. II. Response to corticosteroids in cases of non-obstructive azoospermia with a positive blastoid transformation test. *J. Reprod. Fertil.*, **21,** 59
3. Hargreave, T. B. and Elton, R. A. (1982). Treatment with intermittent high dose methyl prednisolone or intermittent betamethasone for antisperm antibodies: preliminary communication. *Fertil. Steril.*, **38,** 568
4. Dondero, F., Isidori, A., Lenzi, A., *et al.* (1979). Treatment and follow-up of patients with infertility due to spermagglutinins. *Fertil. Steril.*, **31,** 48
5. Hendry, W. F., Stendronska, J., Parslow, J. and Hughes, L. (1981). The results of intermittent high dose steroid therapy for male infertility due to anti-sperm antibodies. *Fertil. Steril.*, **36,** 351
6. Shulman, J. F. and Shulman, S. (1982). Methyl prednisolone treatment of immunologic infertility in the male. *Fertil. Steril.*, **38,** 591
7. Jones, W. R. (1974). The use of antibodies developed by infertile women to identify relevant antigens. In Diczfalusy, E. (ed.) *Immunological Approaches to Fertility Control.* p. 376. (Stockholm: Karolinska Institut)
8. Curtis, G. L., Ryan, W. L. and Lacy, S. S. (1982). Sperm-agglutinating and immobilizing antibody formation following vasectomy prevented with dexamethasone in cynomolgus monkeys. *Fertil. Steril.*, **38,** 97

Part I

Section 6
Male Fertility

23
Epididymal function

G. F. MENCHINI-FABRIS, P. L. IZZO, M. BARTELLONI,
P. MESCHINI and D. CANALE

INTRODUCTION

The epididymis is a long duct (6–7 m, width 450–500 μm) where
the spermatozoa coming from the seminiferous tubules undergo
maturation.

The specialized microenvironment they encounter during the passage in the epididymal duct determines a series of changes in them.
As a result of these changes, the spermatozoa coming out of the
epididymis have the capacity for motility and to fertilize[1].

The spermatozoa coming from the rete testis are immotile. They
are passively transported in a fluid, whose movement is assured
by contraction of the duct wall and of testis capsule[2]. The control
mechanisms of the contractile response, though, are not fully understood. Castration or absence of androgens causes a loss of contractile
response in the first part of the duct. The distal part, instead, seems
to be under control of the autonomic nervous system[3,4]. These regional
variations are reflected in the organization of epididymal-wall components. The wall smooth muscle is relatively sparse in the proximal
region of the epididymis and becomes more prominent distally. There
are also regional differences in the electrolyte and water transport and
reabsorption. The caput and proximal corpus of epididymis were
found to absorb NaCl and water and secrete K^+ at a lower rate than
the cauda epididymis[5]. During their passage through the epididymal
duct, the spermatozoa show an increased oxidative and glycolytic

metabolism[6]. They are also exposed to varying biochemical milieu with differing concentrations of carnitine, glycerylphosphorylcholine, glutamic acid, sialic acids, steroids, a variety of enzymes and proteins. Most of these substances are synthesized or secreted by the epididymal epithelium under androgen control or stimulation[7,8].

Several studies tried to identify the epididymal constituents correlated to the initiation and maintenance of sperm motility. Sheth *et al.* (1980) have isolated a Progressive Motility Sustaining Factor (PMSF) from the human epididymis[9]. Hoskins *et al.* (1978) demonstrated the presence of a Forward Motility Factor (FMF) in bovine semen. The FMF is a glycoprotein and has an epididymal origin[10].

Data concerning these factors in human physiopathology are still controversial and not well defined. Only two substances have been considered to represent a valuable marker of epididymal function: glycerylphosphorylcholine and carnitine.

Glycerylphosphorylcholine is secreted under androgen control at the proximal caput level. It is involved in the metabolic activities of the spermatozoa with its choline derivatives[11–13]. Further evidence, though, is needed to clarify its role in sperm maturation and epididymal physiopathology.

Carnitine is a 3-hydroxy-4-trimethylamino-butyric acid. It is synthesized in the liver[14,15], secreted into the blood-stream and transported to organs, such as muscle, heart and epididymis. The active secretion into the lumen is higher in the region of distal caput and corpus, where the epididymis actively accumulates radioactive carnitine from the blood and transports it into luminal fluid[15,16]. This uptake is stimulated by choline and glycerylphosphorylcholine and is stereospecific[17]. The spermatozoa increase their carnitine content as they pass from the caput to the cauda and become impermeable to carnitine as they come out of the epididymis[18]. At the epididymal level, carnitine enters the spermatozoa and is acetylated[19]. The acetylcarnitine formed is, probably, a ready energy source for spermatozoa, which use it during their maturation[20]. Therefore, carnitine seems to play a role in sperm maturation, fertilizing capacity and motility.

Seminal plasma contains free L-carnitine[21]. There are still conflicting results regarding its origin[22–26]: Wetterauer and Heite (1978)[22] refer 94% to the epididymis and 6% to the vesicles.

Our study was carried out to understand the origin of free L-carnitine in human semen and its correlation to sperm motility and sperm count.

MATERIALS AND METHODS

We evaluated the semen free L-carnitine content by the enzymatic–spectrophotometric method first described by Marquis and Fritz[19]. Semen was obtained by masturbation after 4 days of sexual abstinence. All the patients underwent physical examination. Karyotypes were carried on all the azoospermic patients. Plasma levels of FSH, LH, prolactin and testosterone (T) were evaluated by RIA methods. The study was carried out on seven patients with secretory azoospermia due to bilateral agenesis of the vas deferens, three who were vasectomized (from 6 months to 2 years earlier), seven who were affected by Klinefelter's syndrome, one XX male and

Table 1 Semen carnitine concentration in patients with secretory azoospermia

Patient	T (ng ml^{-1})	TS (ml)	pH	Volume (ml)	Carnitine (nmol ml^{-1})	
Agenesis of vas deferens						
V.A.	4.0	20–20	6.0	1.0	41.6	
M.V.	4.8	20–18	6.0	0.3	27.0	
T.V.	6.4	18–18	6.0	1.0	69.2	
P.V.	5.8	20–20	6.3	0.5	10.0	Mean (±SD) value
F.L.	7.1	20–20	6.5	0.5	30.0	31.8±18.8
C.V.	5.8	20–20	6.0	0.5	10.0	
R.L.	6.5	20–20	6.0	1.0	35.0	
Vasectomized						
C.M.	6.1	20–20	8.0	6.0	105.0	
R.A.	5.3	20–18	7.9	2.0	95.0	Mean (±SD) value
N.U.	6.4	20–20	7.6	5.0	115.0	105.0±8.1

T = Plasma testosterone levels; TS = testis size, according to Prader's orchidometer.

eight who were affected by hypogonadotrophic hypogonadism. The semen carnitine content was also assessed in 124 patients referred to our Andrology Centre for fertility problems and having varying degrees of sperm motility and sperm count. Semen samples under 2.0 ml or over 5.0 ml were excluded.

RESULTS

Normal values of seminal free L-carnitine have been estimated to be over 600 nmol ml^{-1} by means of examination of semen from 10 fertile controls (mean (±SD) value 817.05±200 nmol ml^{-1}). Findings by other authors[15] and our data suggest that there is no condition of pathological increase in carnitine concentration.

We have evaluated (Table 1) the semen carnitine content in seven patients with secretory azoospermia due to bilateral agenesis of the vas deferens, whose ejaculate consisted of only prostatic fluid, as the low pH, the semen volume and the surgical exploration showed. The androgenic parameters (testis size, plasma T levels, etc.) were normal. We found in these patients very low carnitine levels: mean (±SD) value 31.8 (±18.8) nmol ml^{-1}, with a range from 10 to 69 nmol ml^{-1}. A second group of patients with secretory azoospermia, but due to vasectomy, was analysed: the mean (±SD) carnitine value was 105.6 ±8.1 nmol ml^{-1}, with a range from 95 to 117 nmol ml^{-1}. The higher values found in the second group show that the seminal vesicles, the ampulla and the distal part of vas deferens contribute to the final amount of free L-carnitine in seminal plasma. This contribution accounts for 10–15% of the final amount. The contribution by the prostate gland is even smaller at about 5%.

We extended our investigation to another group of azoospermic patients. Their azoospermia was due to testicular failure, either primary or secondary: Klinefelter's syndrome (KS), XX male syndrome and hypogonadotrophic hypogonadism (HH). Table 2 shows the results in seven cases of KS and in one XX male. The mean value of semen free L-carnitine content is below the normal limit, indicating a defective function of the epididymis, probably due to an impaired

Table 2 Semen carnitine concentrations in patients with secretory azoospermia due to Klinefelter's and XX male syndrome

Patient	T (ng ml^{-1})	TS (mm)	pH	Volume (ml)	Carnitine (nmol ml^{-1})	
Klinefelter's syndrome						
S.R.	2.5	5–5	7.6	2.0	380.0	
T.P.	2.3	3–3	7.7	2.5	113.0	
G.C.	2.4	5–5	7.8	3.0	150.0	Mean (±SD) value
G.F.	5.5	5–5	8.0	2.0	213.0	196.8±83
L.N.	4.3	3–3	8.0	4.0	181.0	
M.G.	3.5	5–5	8.0	2.5	212.0	
P.G.	3.1	5–5	7.8	2.0	129.0	
XX male						
M.N.	2.2	5–5	8.0	2.0	293.0	

T = Plasma testosterone level; TS = testis size.

androgen activity (mean ($\pm$SD) value 196.8 ± 83 nmol ml^{-1}). The results in the patients affected by HH were similar: mean ($\pm$SD) value 146.2 ± 54 nmol ml^{-1} (Table 3). We followed up four of these patients during the treatment with human menopausal gonadotrophin (hMG) plus human chorionic gonadotrophin (hCG). As shown in Table 4, the semen free L-carnitine content rose with the increase in testicular size, plasma T levels and sperm count.

Finally, we tried to find a correlation between seminal parameters and the semen carnitine content. The latter was evaluated in patients

Table 3 Semen carnitine concentration in azoospermic patients affected by hypogonadotrophic hypogonadism

Patient	T (ng ml^{-1})	TS (ml)	pH	Volume (ml)	Carnitine (nmol ml^{-1})	
S.F.	1.5	8–8	7.9	1.5	284.7	
G.F.	0.8	10–10	7.6	2.0	115.0	
C.D.	1.1	4–4	7.0	0.5	68.7	
B.A.	1.9	8–8	8.0	2.5	156.2	Mean ($\pm$SD) value
D.F.	1.0	2–2	8.0	1.0	135.0	146.2 ± 54
P.A.	1.2	2–2	7.8	1.0	108.0	
F.C.	1.8	6–5	7.5	0.5	159.0	
P.M.	1.0	10–10	8.0	3.0	143.0	

T = Plasma testosterone level; TS = testis size.

Table 4 Variations of semen carnitine concentration in patients affected by hypogonadotrophic hypogonadism during treatment with human menopausal and human chorionic gonadotrophins

Patient	Age (years)	T (ng ml^{-1})	TS (ml)	pH	Volume (ml)	SC	PM (%)	Carnitine (nmol ml^{-1})
D.F.	26	1.0	2–2	8.0	1.0	0	0	135
	27	1.6	8–8	8.0	1.2	25	20	282
	27.5	2.4	14–14	7.8	3.0	30	30	600
P.A.	31	1.2	2–2	7.8	1.0	0	0	108
	32.5	2.2	8–8	8.0	2.0	17	15	271
F.C.	23	1.8	6–5	7.5	0.5	0	0	159
	24	2.3	12–10	7.8	2.5	16	15	470
P.M.	22	1.0	10–10	8.0	3.0	0	0	143
	22.5	1.8	12–12	8.0	3.0	0.6	15	160

T = Plasma testosterone level; TS = testis size; SC = sperm count (millions ml^{-1}); PM = progressive motility.

referred to our Andrology Centre for fertility problems and showing different values of sperm count and motility. We excluded conditions of hormonal dysfunction, phlogosis or genetic abnormalities. We divided the 124 cases considered into classes according to sperm count (Table 5) and to sperm motility (Table 6). The carnitine concentrations rise with the increase in sperm number and sperm motility but there is a statistical significance only in two classes of motility. Then we decided to correlate the two variables (as motile sperm count) with the semen carnitine content. The results are shown in

Table 5 Variations of mean ($\pm$SD) semen carnitine concentration (in $nmol\,ml^{-1}$) related to sperm count

No. of cases	Sperm count (millions ml^{-1})	Carnitine
63	0.1–10	196.0±113.4
22	11–30	361.4±127.8
9	31–50	410.8±112.7
30	>50	580.3±154.0

Table 6 Variations of mean ($\pm$SD) semen carnitine concentration (in $nmol\,ml^{-1}$) related to sperm motility

No. of cases	Motility (%)	Carnitine
65	0–10	216.0±126.3*
29	11–30	436.3±156.4**
14	31–50	550.1±170.7
16	>50	703.6±119.3

Significant correlation: $*p < 0.01$; $**p < 0.05$.

Table 7 Variations of mean ($\pm$SD) semen carnitine concentration (in $nmol\,ml^{-1}$) related to motile sperm count

No. of cases	Motile sperm count (million ml^{-1})	Carnitine
62	0–1	235.9± 98.2*
30	1.1–10	415.1± 75.6*
13	10.1–20	485.7± 78.9*
19	>20	639.9±132.3*

*Correlation significant at $p < 0.01$; $r = 0.446$.

Table 7. We found a positive, statistically significant, correlation between free L-carnitine and the number of motile spermatozoa.

DISCUSSION

Our results show that the seminal free L-carnitine originates mainly from the epididymis. When the contribution by the epididymis to the seminal plasma is taken off (e.g. in vasectomized patients), the semen carnitine content falls to very low levels. Our data accord with those by Wetterauer and Heite[22] and Soufir et al.[23].

Our findings concerning conditions of hypoandrogenism confirm the works by others[27,28] that seminal carnitine content is an androgen-dependent function. Even so, the changes in patients affected by HH monitored during therapy with gonadotrophins showed a better correlation with the increase of sperm count than with the normalization of plasma T levels.

Finally, the positive correlation between number of motile spermatozoa and carnitine could lead to the postulation of a role for carnitine as a marker of a 'good quality' semen. A noteworthy work by Carter et al.[20] shows that bulls with low fertility rate have reduced seminal carnitine concentrations.

Our results suggest that carnitine may represent a valuable marker of epididymal function. Its evaluation may play an important role in the andrology practice, in the diagnosis of blockages of seminal pathways, of epididymal dysfunction and in establishing the semen fertility potentials.

Further investigations and collaborative studies are needed to elucidate the epididymal function and the role of all the substances that influence the spermatozoal maturation during their passage through the epididymal duct.

References

1. Hamilton, D. W. (1975). Structure and function of the epithelium lining the ductuli efferentes, ductus epididymis, and ductus deferens in the rat. In Hamilton, D. W. and Greep, R. O. (eds.) *Handbook of Physiology*. Vol. **5**, pp. 259–301. (Baltimore: Williams and Wilkins)
2. Bedford, J. M. (1975). Maturation, transport and fate of spermatozoa in the epididymis. In Hamilton, D. W. and Greep, R. O. (eds.) *Handbook of Physiology*. Vol. **5**, pp. 303–317. (Baltimore: Williams and Wilkins)
3. Risley, P. L. (1959). Hormone effects on the *in vivo* contractile behavior of the ductus epididymis of the rat. *Anat. Rec.*, **133**, 329

4. Risley, P. L. (1963). Physiology of the male accessory organs. In Hartmann, C. C. (ed.) *Mechanisms Concerned with Conception.* pp. 73–133. (New York: Macmillan)

5. Wong, P. Y. D., Au, C. L. and Ngai, H. K. (1978). Electrolyte and water transport in rat epididymis: its possible role in sperm maturation. *Int. J. Androl.*, Suppl. **2**, 608

6. Czyba, J. C. (1982). Structure et fonctions de l'epididyme humain. In Menchini Fabris, G. F. (ed.) *Epididimo e Fertilità. Aspetti endocrinologici in Andrologia.* pp. 5–17. (Palermo: COFESE)

7. Orgebin-Crist, M. C., Danzo, B. J. and Davies, J. (1975). Endocrine control of the development and maintenance of sperm fertilizing ability in the epididymis. In Hamilton, D. W. and Greep, R. O. (eds.) *Handbook of Physiology.* Vol. **5**, pp. 319–338. (Baltimore: Williams and Wilkins)

8. Tezon, J., Vazquez, M., Pineiro, L., DeLarminat, M. A. and Blaquier, J. (1982). The effect of androgens in the human epididymis in organ culture. In Menchini Fabris, G. F., Pasini, W. and Martini, L. (eds.) *Therapy in Andrology.* pp. 53–60. (Amsterdam: Excerpta Medica)

9. Sheth, A. R., Gunjikar, A. N. and Shah, G. V. (1980). The presence of Progressive Motility Sustaining Factor (PMSF) in human epididymis. *Andrologia*, **13**, 142

10. Hoskins, D. D., Brandt, H. and Acott, T. S. (1978). Initiation of sperm motility in the mammalian epididymis. *Fed. Proc.*, **37**, 2534

11. Dawson, R. M. C. and Rowlands, I. W. (1959). Glycerophosphorylcholine in the male reproductive organs of rats and guinea-pigs. *Q. J. Exp. Physiol.*, **44**, 26

12. Scott, T. W. and Dawson, R. M. C. (1968). Metabolism of phospholipids by spermatozoa and seminal plasma. *Biochem. J.*, **108**, 457

13. Calamera, J. C. and Lavieri, J. C. (1974). Glycerylphosphorylcholine in human seminal plasma of normal subjects and sterile patients. *Andrologia*, **6**, 67

14. Haigler, H. T. and Broquist, H. P. (1974). Carnitine synthesis in rat tissue slices. *Biochem. Biophys. Res. Commun.*, **56**, 676

15. Brooks, D. E., Hamilton, D. W. and Mallek, A. H. (1973). The uptake of L-methyl-^{3}H-carnitine by the rat epididymis. *Biochem. Biophys. Res. Commun.*, **52**, 1354

16. Hinton, B. T. and Setchell, B. P. (1980). Concentration and uptake of carnitine in the rat epididymis: a micropuncture study. In McGarry, J. D. and Frenkel, R. A. (eds.) *Carnitine Biosynthesis, Metabolism and Function.* p. 237. (New York: Academic Press)

17. Yeung, C. H., Cooper, T. G. and Waites, G. M. H. (1980). Carnitine transport into the perfused epididymis of the rat: regional differences, stereospecificity, stimulation by choline and the effect of other luminal factor. *Biol. Reprod.*, **23**, 294

18. Casillas, E. R. (1973). Accumulation of carnitine by bovine spermatozoa during maturation in the epididymis. *J. Biol. Chem.*, **248**, 8227

19. Marquis, N. R. and Fritz, I. B. (1965). Effects of testosterone on the distribution of carnitine, acetylcarnitine and carnitine acetyltransferase in tissues of the reproductive system of the male rat. *J. Biol. Chem.*, **240**, 2197

20. Carter, A. L., Stratman, F. W., Hutson, S. M. and Lardy, H. A. (1980). The role of carnitine and its esthers in sperm metabolism. In McGarry, J. D. and Frenkel, R. A. (eds.) *Carnitine Biosynthesis, Metabolism, and Function.* p. 251. (New York: Academic Press)

21. Golan, R., Setchell, B. P., Burrow, P. V. and Lewin, L. M. (1982). A comparative study of carnitine and acylcarnitine concentration in semen and male reproductive tract fluids. *Comp. Biochem. Physiol.*, **72B**, 457

22. Wetterauer, U. and Heite, H. J. (1978). Carnitine in seminal fluid as parameter for the epididymal function. *Andrologia*, **10**, 203

23. Soufir, J. C., Marson, J. and Jouannet, P. (1981). Free L-carnitine in human seminal plasma. *Int. J. Androl.*, **4**, 388

24. Frenkel, G., Peterson, R. N., Davis, J. E. and Freund, M. (1974). Glycerylphosphoryl-choline and carnitine in normal human semen and in postvasectomy semen: differences in concentrations. *Fertil. Steril.*, **25**, 84

25. Lewin, L. M., Beer, R. and Lunenfeld, B. (1976). Epididymis and seminal vesicles as sources of carnitine in human seminal fluid: the clinical significance of the carnitine concentration in human seminal fluid. *Fertil. Steril.*, **27**, 9

26. Fahimi, F., Bieber, L. and Lewin, L. M. (1981). The sources of carnitine in human semen. *J. Androl.*, **2**, 339

27. Bohmer, T. and Hansson, V. (1975). Androgen dependent accumulation of carnitine by rat epididymis after injection of [^{3}H]butyrobetaine *in vivo*. *Mol. Cell. Endocrinol.*, **3**, 103

28. Bohmer, T. (1978). Accumulation of carnitine in rat epididymis after injection of [^{3}H]butyrobetaine *in vivo*: quantitative aspects and the effects of androgens and antiandrogens. *Mol. Cell. Endocrinol.*, **11**, 213

24
Gossypol

M. R. N. PRASAD and E. DICZFALUSY

Since the publication of recent reviews on gossypol[1-4], a number of papers have been published that reiterate the earlier conclusions. Further, treatment with gossypol for fertility regulation in men has continued in the People's Republic of China. The present review updates and highlights some of the recent advances.

CHEMISTRY

Gossypol, a dimeric sesquiterpene extracted from any of the three species of the cotton plant, Gossypium (*G. herbaceum, G. hirsutum* and *G. arboreum*) is obtained largely in the form of optically inactive racemic (±) material. On the other hand, gossypol extracted from *Thespesia populnea* (family Malvaceae) is optically active and is strongly dextrorotatory (+)[5,6]. A preparation of (+)-gossypol (98% pure) did not inhibit fertility in male hamsters, even when administered at a dose of $40 \, mg \, kg^{-1}$ (for 54 days consecutively)[7], which is several times the minimal amount of racemic gossypol reported to cause infertility in male hamsters[8]. Although (+)-gossypol does not affect male fertility, it still appears to possess some of the toxic properties associated with racemic gossypol[7]. This observation is in contrast with that of an earlier study[8] which did not report any toxicity of (+)-gossypol, perhaps because considerably smaller amounts of gossypol were administered. These data suggest that the (−) optical isomer of gossypol may inhibit male fertility in a stereospecific manner, while toxic manifestations may also be due to non-stereospecific interactions[7]. Attempts are being made by a number of investigators to isolate (−)-gossypol from plant sources or to separate

255

it from racemic gossypol, using a variety of physical and chemical methods. It is crucial to isolate or synthesize the (−) optical isomer of gossypol and determine whether this form is more potent and less toxic than the racemic compound. An efficient synthesis of the gossypol backbone[9] which has been reported may be useful in the preparation of (−)-gossypol and/or of its analogues.

Racemic gossypol acetic acid has been used by most investigators in animal studies and in clinical studies in China. Questions have been raised as to the purity and stability of various preparations of this compound. The World Health Organizations's Special Programme in Human Reproduction and the Centre for Population Research of the United States National Institute of Child Health and Human Development (NICHD) are collaborating in a number of studies to develop an internationally available reference standard preparation of pure gossypol acetic acid and to define methods for the analysis of its purity and stability. Gossypol acetic acid prepared by the NICHD was assessed in four centres of the WHO, and found to be 99.9% pure, on the basis of such criteria as melting point, mass spectrum, nuclear magnetic resonance, thin layer chromatography and high performance liquid chromatography. This preparation has been accepted as a standard for further studies on stability, in powder, solution and tablet form[10]. The reference standard preparation will ultimately be made available to scientists through WHO and NIH for studies on animals[11]. Preliminary data indicate that it is stable in powder form when stored in amber coloured bottles or in the dark, or in solution (in the NICHD steroid suspending vehicle for over 100 days). The stability in solution appears to be dependent on concentration and temperature; higher concentrations and lower temperatures favour stability (H. Kim, H. Fong, and S. Matlin, personal communication). The stability of another preparation of gossypol has also been studied in five solvents at different temperatures[12]. Both the type of solvent and the temperature appear to affect the rate of decomposition. Gossypol was found to be highly unstable at 37 °C and at room temperature while its stability increased as storage temperature decreased[12]; at all temperatures, the rate of decomposition decreased in the order acetone < acetonitrile < chloroform < ethanol < methanol[12]. Tablets of gossypol acetic acid used in clinical studies in the People's Republic of China have been shown to be stable at room temperature for up to 14 months (H. Liang, personal communication).

SYNTHESIS OF ANALOGUES

Gossypol represents a new lead in the development of chemical agents interfering with male fertility. Therefore, parallel with the development of a reference standard preparation of gossypol acetic acid, there is need for the synthesis of analogues of gossypol or related compounds to identify a new chemical entity (not necessarily related to gossypol) exhibiting a more favourable therapeutic ratio than gossypol[9]. From previous, published studies[10] and personal communications (Huang Liang, Beijing), it would appear that the aldehyde and hydroxyl groups are essential for the antifertility effect. Likewise, optical activity (levorotation) seems to be a prerequisite, since racemic gossypol is active and the (+)-isomer is inactive[7]. It is not yet clear whether the hemigossypol moiety is active; structural analogues of hemigossypol can be prepared by total synthesis[9]. An assessment of the antifertility effect of a larger number of analogues will perhaps cast some light on structure–activity relationships and lead to the identification of new classes of antifertility agents. However, it should be noted that a large number of derivatives, including amino compounds, esters and metallic complexes, have been prepared, but none of these showed a better effect than gossypol acetic acid[10].

SCREENING

The only accepted method presently available for the assessment of the antifertility action of gossypol is the *in vivo* assay in hamsters or rats, which requires daily administration for 70–80 days to males and mating sequentially during the treatment period, which is not only time consuming but is also very expensive. Hence, it is necessary to develop alternate methods for rapid screening of the newly synthesized analogues. Gossypol has been found to inhibit acrosomal proteinase from sonicated boar spermatozoa[13] and intact human spermatozoa[14]. It also caused a dose-dependent decrease in the ability of human proacrosin (zymogen form that is present in ejaculated human spermatozoa) to convert to acrosin[15]. Gossypol has also been shown to inhibit sperm-specific LDH-X from mouse, human and other rodent species[16]; it exhibited a dose-dependent inhibition of LDH-C$_4$ from human spermatozoa but was weak in its action on rabbit spermatozoa[17]. A detailed analysis of the gossypol sensitivity of various enzymes associated with energy metabolism in spermatozoa shows that LDH-X, NAD-isocitrate dehydrogenase, succinyl COA-synthetase, fumarate and acrosin are most sensitive, while carnitine acetyltransferase and succinic dehydrogenase are not inhibited[18]. The WHO is evaluating the *in vitro* inhibition by gossypol of some of these enzymes in human spermatozoa. If the specificity of inhibition of any of these enzymes can be established and the assay is able to distinguish pharmacologically active from inactive compounds, the assay system can, hopefully, be used as a quick screening procedure for evaluating the antifertility activity of new analogues of gossypol and related compounds.

PHARMACOKINETICS

The animal pharmacokinetic data obtained earlier by Chinese investigators have been reviewed elsewhere[4].

Studies on the mechanism of action of gossypol and its metabolism in humans and in animals depend on the availability of labelled gossypol with high specific activity. Based on the observations on the biosynthesis of gossypol by excised roots of cotton seedlings[19], or at the enzymic level[20] and its formation by cell suspension cultures[21], [^{14}C]gossypol has been produced by incubating cotton seedlings for 96 hours in a culture medium containing [^{14}C]acetate[22]. While [^{14}C]-gossypol may be useful for pharmacokinetic studies in animals[23], similar studies including the elucidation of the fate of gossypol, decomposition and the molecular identity of decomposition products *in vivo* are essential and will require the synthesis of [^{3}H]gossypol with a high specific activity as well as the development of a specific radioimmunoassay procedure.

TOXICOLOGY

After the discovery of gossypol as an agent that interferes with spermatogenesis in man, a number of studies were carried out in the People's Republic of China to assess the toxicological effects in various animals, such as rats, rabbits, dog, mouse, guinea-pig and monkey[4]. However, none of these studies provide sufficient details of the toxicological studies that are required for review by drug regulatory agencies. Some of the results of these studies are indicated in Tables 1–5.

The results of available toxicology show marked species differences which are likely to be due to differences in pharmacokinetic behaviour, for instance absorption, metabolism and excretion of gossypol and its accumulation in the tissues[23]. The dog is the most sensitive and the rabbit the most insensitive to gossypol. Gossypol is absorbed less and excreted more in monkeys than in dogs; this is perhaps one of the reasons for the high toxicity of gossypol in dogs.

Table 1 Gossypol: single dose, LD_{50} (in mg kg body weight^{-1}) in animals*

Species	LD_{50}
Rat	2400–3340
Mouse	500–1000
Rabbit	350–600
Guinea-pig	280–300
Pig	550

* The compounds were administered as an aqueous suspension. The same effect was seen with at least 10% less of gossypol, when administered in oil. The dose of gossypol administered in the clinical studies carried out in the People's Republic of China was usually 20 mg daily for 60–70 days followed by a maintenance dose of 60 mg weekly.

The dog seems to be an unsuitable model for the toxicological evaluation of gossypol or of its analogues. Monkeys are not sensitive to the toxic effects of gossypol but are sensitive to its antifertility effects. One of the new therapeutic properties of gossypol observed in cynomolgus monkeys[34] is its hypolipidaemic effect. For the time being, the mechanism and site of action of this hypolipidaemic effect is incompletely comprehended. Hamsters are highly sensitive to the antifertility action of gossypol[35], but this species has rarely been used for the toxicological evaluation of contraceptive drugs.

From the practical point of view, a strong case could be made for the use of the rat as a toxicological model for gossypol. However, rats show strain differences in their response to the antifertility action of gossypol[36]. This species is sensitive to the antifertility action of gossypol, but toxic effects are manifested only at 10–12 times the minimum effective dose. Hence it would be justified to carry out a toxicological evaluation of gossypol in rats on the basis of the effective doses used in the clinical studies on more than 9000 men in the People's Republic of China[2]. Based on the effective dose in humans

259

Table 2 Effects of long-term administration of gossypol in rats

Daily dose (mg kg^{-1})	Duration of treatment (weeks)	Effects	Reference
7.5	52	SGPT, Blood urea nitrogen, ECG histology of heart, kidney, liver, Bone marrow and blood picture normal. Mating normal but fertility decreased. Germinal epithelium damaged but not gross degeneration. Leydig cells normal	24
10	25	Bone marrow, blood picture, oil red O staining G6Pase, G6PDH, ATPase, alkaline phosphatase (AKPase), acid phosphatase, glycogen, RNA, DNA of liver normal, same in kidney and Δ^5-3β-hydroxy-steroid-dehydrogenase (Δ^5 3BHSD). Adrenal normal. Fertility suppressed	25
20	39	Alkaline phosphatase, PAS and liver histology normal. Increase in succinic dehydrogenase (SDH). Other changes as with 7.5 mg kg^{-1} dose	24
30	16	No effect on body weight, sex accessories, histology of heart, liver, lungs, kidney. Occasional focal inflammation in some organs. Testicular cells damaged. No change in Leydig cells	26
7.5 15 30	12 12 12	Normal growth rate maintained. Growth rate significantly reduced with 15–30 mg dose. Infertility at all doses. Sperm numbers in cauda epididymis decreased at 6 weeks with 30 mg and after 12 weeks with smaller doses. All sperms had deformed tails and were immotile. No change in serum T, LH, FSH at 7–15 mg. Serum T and LH significantly reduced with 30 mg; FSH normal. All animals recovered fertility in 6–12 weeks after stopping treatment	27*

*Sprague-Dawley strain; strain of rats not known in any of the Chinese studies[24-26].

Table 3 Effects of long-term administration of gossypol in rabbits*

Daily dose (mg kg^{-1})	Duration of treatment (days)	Effects	Reference
16	14–140	6/10 rabbits died during the treatment. Blood, SGPT normal. Abnormal ECG, brady-cardia	28,29
80	8–17	Anorexia, dyspnoea, loss of weight, hind limb paralysis: all animals died in 8–17 days. Congestion of liver/lungs. Fertility normal	30
40	23–35	Same results	30
20	25–84	Same results	30
10	77–250	Despite severe side-effects resulting in eventual death, no changes were seen in sperm motility, morphology or numbers in weekly ejacultes. Mating was normal and fertility was *not* impaired. T levels were reduced at 12–20 weeks but mating was normal	30

*Results show that gossypol has no antifertility effect in rabbits.

Table 4 Effects of long-term administration of gossypol in dogs

Daily dose (mg kg⁻¹)	Duration of treatment (days)	No. of dogs	Effects	Reference
1.0–1.5	60–141	6	Anorexia, loss of weight, tachycardia, dogs died suddenly after 60–141 or 120–130 days of treatment. Post mortem findings showed myocarditis, endocarditis, cardiac dilatation, oedema and lysis and atrophy of myocardium. Congestion of liver, lungs	28
3	30–64	4	Same changes in organs and death of all treated animals	28*
30	18–28	4		
2–5	42–86	6	ECG abnormalities 4 weeks after start of treatment. Four dogs died of cardiac arrest on days 42, 63, 77 and 86. Severe myocardial damage in two dogs which survived, toxic cardiac signs and histological changes disappeared 1 year after withdrawal of gossypol	4

*Breed of dogs used and conditions of their maintenance during these studies are not mentioned.

Table 5 Effects of long-term administration of gossypol in monkeys

Daily dose (mg kg⁻¹)	Duration of treatment (months)	Effects	Reference
1–2	14	Serum/urinary K^+, Na^+, Mg^{++}, creatinine, SGOT, LDH normal; myocardium slightly congested	4*
4	24	Hepatic sinusoids slightly distended with partial vacuolation in central zone; cloudy swellings in proximal renal tubules with decreased ATPase and acid phosphatase. Histology of other organs normal. Germinal epithelium damaged	32*
1.5	3	Fed orally with peanut butter. No change in fertility or sperm counts/motility. Blood chemistry, serum K^+ concentration, normal. Serum T and gonadotrophin levels normal	32†
5–10	6	Arrest of spermatogenesis. Breakthrough in azoospermia with higher dose. No change in plasma T. Temporary diarrhoea an anorexia at higher dose. No clinical and pathological effects	33‡
5–10	6	No change in plasma Na^+ or K^+ or blood pressure. Significant decrease in total plasma cholesterol and low density lipoprotein and very low density lipoprotein cholesterol without any decrease in high density lipoprotein cholesterol	34‡

*Possible rhesus monkeys.
†Rhesus monkeys.
‡Cynomolgus monkeys.

263

$(20 \, \text{mg} \, \text{kg}^{-1} \text{day}^{-1}$ for 60–70 days, followed by a maintenance dose of $60 \, \text{mg} \, \text{kg}^{-1}$ weekly) the lowest dose in rats would be around $300 \, \mu\text{g} \, \text{kg}^{-1} \text{day}^{-1}$, and multiples of this dose would then be $3 \, \text{mg} \, \text{kg}^{-1} \text{day}^{-1}$ (10×) and $15 \, \text{mg} \, \text{kg}^{-1} \text{day}^{-1}$ (50×).

However, a more modern and more rational approach to the assessment of the toxicity of gossypol in different species could be based on pharmacokinetic considerations, rather than on the blind use of arbitrary multiples of the human dose.

Indeed, toxicological studies with doses producing comparable plasma levels to those obtained in the human will provide more meaningful results than the administration of, perhaps realistic, perhaps unrealistic, multiples, which may result in uninterpretable findings, especially in the absence of adequate information on the bioavailability of the drug in different species. What is therefore urgently needed is a comparative in-depth assessment of the pharmacokinetic behaviour of gossypol in various species, including the human. Unless this is done, it will be difficult, if not impossible, to establish which species is a suitable toxicological model for gossypol.

The future of gossypol as a male fertility regulating agent depends on the clarification of the concerns on its safety (hypokalaemia and recovery of fertility) and on the availability of internationally acceptable animal toxicological data. The WHO is initiating toxicological evaluation of the gossypol 'standard' preparation as a prelude to the initiation of clinical studies with this preparation.

CLINICAL STUDIES

The results of the extensive clinical studies carried out in China have been reviewed repeatedly[1–3,37]. Recently, a controlled double-blind trial of gossypol has been initiated in China[38,39]. The study involved 150 male volunteers randomized into a treatment (gossypol) and a control (placebo) group of 75 subjects each. At the end of the loading phase (treatment with 20 mg daily for 75 days), the subjects were transferred to a maintenance dose of 60 mg weekly. Preliminary results of the loading phase showed that serum LH, FSH and testosterone levels were normal; however, fatigue and decreased libido were noted in some subjects. The study, which is still in progress, constitutes the first controlled clinical trial in which the measurement of haemoglobin, serum potassium and hormone levels and semen parameters is compared with pretreatment values. A number of other studies are in progress to monitor the recovery of subjects who have recently stopped treatment with gossypol[11]. When the results of these new studies are evaluated, it should be possible to assess more confidently than at present the clinical safety of gossypol. In discussing the future of gossypol as a male antifertility agent[2], four adverse effects highlighted in the clinical trials need to be considered. These have been reviewed in detail[1-3] and relate to the following.

Blood potassium – The incidence of hypokalaemia accompanied by paralysis (in 0.75%) appears to be related to dietary deficiency of potassium, which can be corrected by potassium supplementation[40]. The mechanism of the onset of hypokalaemia is still not clear. Clinical and animal studies have not provided evidence of change in adrenocortical function following gossypol treatment[2,25,37]. An animal model in which hypokalaemia can be induced remains to be found.

Reversibility – The chances of complete recovery of spermatogenesis and normal sperm count appear to be related to the degree of effect on the testis; the recovery is greater in subjects in whom only oligospermia, but not azoospermia is induced, and the chances of recovery are significantly reduced with a longer duration of treatment over 2 years[1,2,37]. Ongoing studies in China could provide useful data on the temporal relationship between the effect of gossypol on the testis and recovery of sperm counts and fertility[11,39].

Sex hormones – Hormone levels have been reported to be normal in the earlier clinical studies in China, and in recent studies carried out in China[37] and Brazil[41]. However, conflicting results on the decrease of plasma testosterone and gonadotrophins have been reported in some animals treated with high doses of gossypol[2,27,30].

Liver function – Gossypol is concentrated maximally in the liver of animals[4,32]. A transient elevation of SGPT levels has been suggested by the Chinese clinical studies[37], but not by those carried out in Brazil[41]. Further studies on the effects of gossypol on liver function are warranted in view of the reported inhibition on enzymes involved in detoxifying mechanisms[2].

The future of gossypol as a male antifertility agent rests on satisfactory answers to the above concerns.

USE OF GOSSYPOL AS A VAGINAL SPERMICIDAL AGENT

In vitro spermicidal effects and inhibition of sperm motility and enzymes by gossypol have been reported[13-18]. At concentrations ranging from 5.5 to 16.5 μg ml^{-1} semen, gossypol had no effect on sperm motility but a dose-dependent inhibition of the penetration of zona-free hamster oocytes[14] was observed. These studies have led to suggestions to use gossypol as a vaginal spermicidal agent. Further studies will be required to assess the potential usefulness of this approach.

ABSTRACT

The discovery of gossypol and the demonstration of its antifertility effect in a large number of men marks a particularly important milestone in the search for new chemical entities interfering with male fertility. Indeed, a critical assessment of the various leads which, for the time being, are pursued by scientists around the world to develop an effective, safe and inexpensive agent for the regulation of male fertility leads to the conclusion that gossypol represents the only approach which has a reasonable chance of reaching the stage of large scale clinical testing before the end of this decade.

Viewed against this background, it seems logical that the World Health Organization's (WHO) Special Programme on Human Reproduction and a variety of national and international agencies and medical research councils are supporting various research efforts on gossypol.

A collaborative project between WHO and the US National Institute of Child Health and Human Development (NICHD) resulted in the preparation of sufficient quantities of a highly purified (99.9%) and stable gossypol acetic acid, which may serve as an internationally available reference standard, and the WHO has initiated the preclinical toxicological assessment of this product.

The joint WHO-NICHD effort also embraces a major programme for the synthesis and screening of new gossypol analogues.

Animal toxicological studies seem to place an increasing emphasis on the use of sub-human primate models in which the effect of gossypol appears to resemble that in the human. However, it is strongly emphasized that in the continued toxicological assessment of gossypol in various species, the use of doses producing plasma levels of gossypol comparable to those in men will produce more meaningful information than the old-fashioned administration of arbitrarily chosen high multiples of the human dose.

The future of gossypol as a male fertility regulating agent hinges on the availability of internationally acceptable animal toxicological data on its safety and on the clarification of present concerns with regard to hypokalemia and the irreversibility of antifertility effect.

References

1. Prasad, M. R. N. and Diczfalusy, E. (1982). Gossypol. *Int. J. Androl. (Suppl.)*, **5**, 53
2. Lei, H. P. (1983). Is there a future for gossypol as a pill for men? In Diczfalusy, E and Diczfalusy, A. (eds.). *Research on the Regulation of Human Fertility*. (Copenhagen: Scriptor) (In press)
3. Bajaj, J. S. and Madan, R. (1983). Regulation of male fertility – perspective and prospective. In Diczfalusy, E. and Diczfalusy, A. (eds.). *Research on the Regulation of Human Fertility*. (Copenhagen: Scriptor) (In press)
4. Xue, S. P. (1981). Studies on the antifertility effect of gossypol: a new contraceptive for males. In Chang, C. F., Griffin, D. and Woolman, A. (eds.). *Recent Advances in Fertility Regulation*, p. 122. (Geneva: Atar)
5. King, T. J. and de Silva, L. B. (1968). Optically active gossypol from *Thespesia populnea*. *Tetrahedron Lett.*, **3**, 261
6. Datta, S. C., Murti, V. V. S. and Seshadri, T. R. (1972). Isolation and study of (+) gossypol from *Thespesia populnea*. *Ind. J. Chem.*, **10**, 263
7. Waller, D. P., Bunyapraphatsara, N., Martin, A.-M., Vournazos, C. J., Ahmed, M. S., Soejarto, D. D., Cordell, G. A. and Fong, H. H. S. (1983). Effect of (+) gossypol on fertility in male hamsters. *J. Androl.*, **4** (In press)
8. Yuee, W., Yingde, L. and Xican, T. (1979). Studies on the antifertility actions of cotton seed meal and gossypol. *Acta Pharm. Sin.*, **14**, 662
9. Venuti, M. C. (1981). Efficient synthesis of the gossypol binaphthyl backbone. *J. Org. Chem.*, **46**, 3124
10. Wang, N. G., Luo, Y. G. and Tang, X. C. (1979). Studies on the antifertility actions of cotton seed meal and gossypol. Document of the First National Conference of Male Antifertility Agents, Wuhan (September 1972). *Acta Pharmacol. Sin.*, **14**, 663
11. World Health Organization (1982). *Eleventh Annual Report of the Special Programme of Research, Development and Research Training in Human Reproduction*. (Geneva: WHO)
12. Nomeir, A. A. and Abou-Donia, M. B. (1982). Gossypol: high performance liquid chromatographic analysis and stability in various solvents. *J. Am. Chem. Soc.*, **59**, 546
13. Tso, W. W. and Lee, C. S. (1982). Gossypol: an effective acrosin blocker. *Arch. Androl.*, **8**, 143
14. Johnsen, O., Mas Diaz, J. and Eliasson, R. (1982). Gossypol: a potent inhibitor of human sperm acrosomal proteinase. *Int. J. Androl.*, **5**, 636
15. Kennedy, W. P., Van der Van, H. H., Waller, D. P., Polakoski, K. L. and Zaneveld, L. J. D. (1982). Gossypol inhibition of oocyte penetration and sperm acrosin. *Biol. Reprod.*, **26** (Suppl.), 118
16. Lee, C. Y. and Malling, H. Y. (1981). Selective inhibition of sperm-specific lactate dehydrogenase-X by an antifertility agent, gossypol. *Fed. Proc.*, **40**, 718
17. Eliasson, R. and Virjie, N. (1983). Effect of gossypol on the activity of LDH-C$_4$ from human and rabbit spermatozoa. *Int. J. Androl.*, **6**, 109

18. Tso, W. W., Lee, C. S. and Tso, Y. W. (1982). Sensitivity of various spermatozoal enzymes to gossypol inhibitor. *Arch. Androl.*, **9**, 31

19. Smith, F. H. (1974). Preparation of gossypol by incorporation of acetate (1-^{14}C) and acetate (2-^{14}C) by biosynthesis. *J. Am. Chem. Soc.*, **51**, 40

20. Heinstein, F. (1979). Biosynthesis of gossypol. *Rec. Adv. Phytochem.*, **12**, 313

21. Heinstein, F. (1981). Formation of gossypol by *Gossypium hirsutum* in cell suspension cultures. *J. Natl. Prod.*, **44**, 1

22. Wong, S. M., Slaytor, M. B. and Fong, H. H. S. (1983). ^{14}C-gossypol: optimum conditions for synthesis by cotton seedlings. *Acta Pharmacol. Sin.*, **18**, 57

23. Abou-Donia, M. B. (1976). Physiological effects and metabolism of gossypol. *Residue Rev.*, **61**, 124

24. Zhou, L. F., Chen, C. C., Wang, N. G. and Lei, H. P. (1980). Observations on long-term administration of gossypol acetic acid to rats. *Natl. Med. J. China*, **60**, 343

25. Zhou, C. F., Lei, H. P., Gao, Y., Liu, Y., Wang, N. Y. and Guo, Y. (1982). Further observation on the effect of prolonged administration of gossypol acetic acid to rats. *Acta Pharmacol. Sin.*, **17**, 245

26. Xue, S. P., Zhou, Z. H., Liu, Y., Wu, Y. W. and Zhang, S. D. (1979). The pharmacokinetics of ^{14}C gossypol acetic acid in rats: I. whole body and micro autoradiographic studies on the distribution and fate of ^{14}C gossypol in the rat body. *Acta Biol. Exp. Sin.*, **12**, 179

27. Chang, C. C., Gu, Z. and Tsong, Y. Y. (1982). Studies on gossypol: I. toxicity and antifertility and endocrine analysis in male rats. *Int. J. Fertil.*, **27**, 213

28. Jiangsu Coordinating Group on Male Antifertility Agents (1972). Studies on Gossypol. Presented at the *1st National Conference on Male Antifertility Agents*, Wuhan, September

29. Shangdung Coordinating Group (1973). Presented at the *2nd National Conference on Male Antifertility Agents*, Quingdao, August

30. Saxena, S. K., Salmonsen, R., Lau, I. F. and Chang, M. C. (1981). Gossypol: its toxicological and endocrinological effects in male rabbits. *Contraception*, **24**, 203

31. Bardin, C. W., Sundaram, K. S. and Chang, C. C. (1980). Toxicology, endocrine and histopathologic studies in small animals and rhesus monkeys administered gossypol. Presented at the *PARFR Workshop on Gossypol*, Chicago

32. Sang, G. W., Zhang, Y. S., Shi, Q. X., *et al.* (1980). Chronic toxicity of gossypol and the relationship of its metabolic fate in dogs and monkeys. *Acta Pharmacol. Sin.*, **1**, 39

33. Shandilya, L. N., Clarkson, T. B., Adams, M. R. and Lewis, J. C. (1982). Effects of gossypol on reproductive and endocrine functions of male cynomolgus monkeys (*Macaca fascicularis*). *Biol. Reprod.*, **27**, 241

34. Shandilya, L. N. and Clarkson, T. B. (1982). Hypolipidemic effects of gossypol in cynomolgus monkey (*Macaca fascicularis*). *Lipids*, **17**, 285

35. Waller, D. P., Zaneveld, L. J. D. and Fong, H. H. S. (1981). Antifertility effects of gossypol. *Contraception*, **22**, 183

36. Zatuchni, G. I. and Osborn, C. K. (1981). A possible male antifertility agent. Report of a Workshop. *Res. Frontiers Fertil. Regul.*, **1**, 1

37. Liu, Z. Q., Lui, G. Z., Hei, L. S., Zhang, R. A. and Yu, C. Z. (1981). Clinical trial of gossypol as a male antifertility agent. In Chang, C. F., Griffin, D. and Woolman, A. (eds.). *Recent Advances in Fertility Regulation*, p. 160. (Geneva: Atar)

38. Lyde, K. C. (1982). Controlled clinical trial of gossypol: Methodological considerations. *Arch. Androl.*, **9**, 38

39. Liu, G. Z. (1982). Double-blind study of gossypol: the loading phase. *Arch. Androl.*, **9**, 38

40. Quian, K. S. Z., Jeng, G., Wu, X. Y., Li, Y. Q. and Zhou, Z. H. (1980). Gossypol related hypokalemia: Clinico-pharmacological studies. *Chem. Med. J.*, **93**, 477

41. Coutinho, E. M. (1982). Clinical studies with gossypol. *Arch. Androl.*, **9**, 37

Part I

Section 7

New Approaches to Female Fertility Regulation

25
New approaches to female fertility regulation – an overview

S. S. RATNAM AND R. N. V. PRASAD

INTRODUCTION

It has been estimated that in the next 20 years the number of couples in the reproductive age groups in developing countries alone will have grown to nearly 1 billion. The demand for fertility control will necessarily increase and the bulk of current research is aimed at making the currently available methods safer and more acceptable. It is generally believed that no completely new method of fertility regulation will emerge in the next 20 years or so due to restraints placed by drug regulatory agencies and the prohibitive costs of testing a new drug. Given the world-wide recession the trend has been for a declining investment in financial support for research and development of new contraceptive technology[1,2]. Sterilization, steroidal contraceptives and IUCDs are all very effective. The crucial issues in the near future will therefore be aimed at optimizing the use of currently available methods and improving their safety, and, to a lesser extent, efficacy with minor alterations in composition or delivery systems. Nevertheless there is still hope for a novel breakthrough in contraception from the work which is being done at present by independent researchers. Perhaps these may bear fruition in the twenty-first century. This chapter will review briefly these novel investigations but will stress mainly the work presently under way on improving methods of fertility control.

MODIFICATIONS OF CURRENTLY AVAILABLE METHODS

It is accepted that there is no universally acceptable male or female contraceptive. Existing methods are not perfect and can be improved substantially in terms of safety, acceptability and efficacy.

Contraception

Safer oral contraceptives

The combined pill is theoretically very effective but the user-failure rate has proved high in field studies. The safety aspect of the pill has also been foremost in the mind of the public, doctors and research workers. The main areas of research with oral contraceptives (OCs) therefore have been on modifications to enhance safety and health service research aimed at improving patient compliance and acceptability. They can be discussed under the following headings:

  (1)   Reduction in steroid content.
  (2)   Use of natural oestrogens.
  (3)   Slow-release formulations.
  (4)   Tri-phasic preparations.
  (5)   Use of new progestogens.
  (6)   Methods of improving acceptability and compliance.

Reduction in steroid content – The general trend in making OCs safer has been for the dosages of the hormones to be progressively reduced, especially the oestrogenic component because it is this that has been considered[3-7] the major cause of the serious side-effects. Although Goldzieher[8] has thrown some doubts, a recent Finnish study[9] on 2653 women showed a positive link between cardiovascular disease and the pill. All this evidence has resulted in a lowering of the oestrogen content of the pill. Doses of $30\,\mu g$ and $50\,\mu g$ of oestrogen are currently being used but these may be lowered even further to $20\,\mu g$. The problems to be expected with such low doses are breakthrough bleeding and slightly higher failure rates.

Use of natural oestrogens in combined pills – It has been suggested that natural oestrogens (e.g. oestrone, oestradiol) have less tendency to cause cardiovascular and metabolic problems than the synthetic oestrogen pills. However, initial experience with natural oestrogens has been disappointing with nausea and menstrual complaints being the chief problems[10].

Slow-release formulations – Attempts are being made to develop slow-release OCs by using microsphere and other formulations[11,12]. This would enable one to achieve slow, even absorption of steroids and maintain fairly constant blood levels over a 24-hour period and thus allow a lower intake of oestrogens.

Tri-phasic preparations – Here an attempt has been made to decrease the total hormonal content per cycle by varying the doses of hormones through the cycle to mimic natural events. One such commercially available product[11] provides $50\,\mu$g norgestrel and $30\,\mu$g ethinyloestradiol (EE) daily for 6 days; $75\,\mu$g norgestrel and $40\,\mu$g EE daily for 5 days; and $125\,\mu$g norgestrel and $30\,\mu$g EE daily for the remaining 10 days. More widespread clinical use will prove if this pill will stand up to claims that it is a superior standard preparation. Even if it proves similar to the existing pill it is worthwhile pursuing as it contains less total hormone per cycle.

Use of new progestogens – Although oestrogens have been generally blamed for cardiovascular complications it is now realized that the gestogens may be more important in the aetiology of atherosclerosis and myocardial infarction. The ratio of the HDL cholesterol to LDL cholesterol is an important factor and the general tendency is for HDL cholesterol rich fractions to rise with increasing oestrogen dose and decline with increasing progestin dose[13-15]. Larsson[15] and co-workers believe they can maintain the normal HDL:LDL ratio by careful balancing of the norgestrel:ethinyloestradiol content of the OC pill. More recently a new progestogen desogestrel[16] (a norgestrel derivative) has been claimed to have minimal effects on lipoprotein levels whilst being twice as potent as levonorgestrel[17]. The use of desogestrel in the combined pill is undergoing clinical testing in many centres.

Improving pill acceptability and compliance – Whatever the results of laboratory testing and subsequent improvements may be, the final analysis of success depends on results from field testing. User failure, poor compliance and discontinuation rates have plagued many pill programmes. Such rates may differ vastly between two clinics in the same country as WHO trials have shown. No two populations are alike and research into patient characteristics in the form of health service research and controlled clinical trials are needed in assessing the type of pill most suitable for any population. More attractive packaging with easy to follow instructions may improve compliance in some cases. In others, a completely different formulation may be required. The paper pill formulation was shown to enhance compliance in a WHO study[10] on 1400 women over 1000 women years of use when compared with the regular 'pill'.

Improved injectables – The two currently used long-acting inject-ables are depomedroxyprogesterone acetate (DMPA) and norethis-terone enanthate which are active for 3 and 2 months, respectively[18], after single injection. Initial scare reports about DMPA[19] (i.e. the breast lump in beagle dogs and endometrial cancer in Rhesus monk-eys stories) have been hotly rebutted[20] and the WHO Toxicology Review Panel[21] has subsequently opined that it is safe for use in family planning programmes with a reservation that certain long-term studies needed to be conducted in certain aspects. DMPA signifi-cantly decreased serum HDL cholesterol concentrations (Kremer[22]) in women which may be of concern with regard to risk of coronary thrombosis in the long term. The other problems with DMPA are irregular bleeding, amenorrhoea, slow return of fertility and variable increases in plasma glucose and insulin levels. Norethisterone enan-thate has shown to ameliorate some of these problems. Despite all these problems, injectables have been widely accepted over other methods in many countries where the women seem to find injectables very convenient. Since the need is evident, recent research has been aimed at improving the injectable.

The main reason for the attempts to develop newer steroidal injec-tables is due to the fact that the presently available drugs are not released uniformly from the depot site. The drugs are initially re-leased as a burst after injection, reaching high levels which decline slowly after 4 weeks of injection[23]. Many of the side-effects are due to this initial surge and if some drug or formulation could be developed to cause zero-order release, then the total body drug burden could be reduced and the side-effects reduced or eliminated. Some of the approaches currently under investigation with this aim are:

(1) To develop newer steroids with better release profiles.
(2) To increase the number of injections using a smaller dose of existing steroids.
(3) To combine injectables with natural oestrogens.
(4) To pack the steroid in polymers to improve release characteristics.

WHO[24] has sponsored a large-scale programme of synthesis of newer steroids with better release-rate profiles. Four such esters of levonorgestrel have already been synthesized and toxicology studies have been started with the most promising compound, 22Cc.

The second approach to increase the number of injections but with a smaller dose each time has been conducted by Prema (1981)[25] who gave 20 mg of norethisterone enanthate monthly. This has proved successful with low incidence of side-effects. Prasad (1981)[26] showed that ovulation suppression was consistent with this regimen.

Combinations of oestrogens with depot injectables are also being investigated. Cycloprovera (25 mg MPA and 5 mg oestradiol cypionate) and a WHO compound (50 mg norethisterone oenanthate and 5 mg oestradiol valerate) are under test. The WHO compound[21,27] seems superior as far as pharmacokinetic profiles are concerned.

Packaging the steroids in some form of polymer might improve release rate characteristics. Biodegradable polylactide microcapsules, polyglycolides and polydihydropyran are all being investigated. Polylactide microspheres containing norethisterone[28] can be made to last anything from 60 days to 2 years but do not give a truly zero-order release. The release profile is, however, infinitely better than the conventional injectables. Total doses of less than $0.267 \, \text{mg} \, \text{kg}^{-1}$ of norethisterone in a 6-month formulation had no effect on ovarian function or menstrual bleeding but doses greater than $2.3 \, \text{mg} \, \text{kg}^{-1}$ suppressed ovulation and caused long intermenstrual periods.

Whatever improvements are made with injectables it is envisaged that being basically steroids they are likely to have the usual disadvantages, albeit to a lesser extent.

Improved IUCDs

IUCDs have been available for years and their advantages and disadvantages are well known. All attempts to try to reduce their side-effects significantly by altering the configuration and/or by adding active substances have only met with limited success. The major problems with IUCDs have been the menstrual side-effects and high discontinuation rates.

New IUCDs now undergoing clinical trials have been designed to combat these problems. Contraceptive efficacy too has been improved with copper T380A and T220 compared with the standard Cu T200 (pregnancy rates 0.7, 0.8 and 2.6/100 acceptors respectively)[29]. Another improvement with copper devices has been to make them longer lasting. This improvement has been achieved by either increasing the amount of copper, by the use of additional sleeves rather than wire and the use of silver cores to prevent disintegration of the copper wire. The Cu T220 with multiple copper sleeves lasts from 5 to 10 years. The Cu T380A which has 380 mm^2 of Cu surface in the form of arm sleeves and wire stem lasts more than 6 years. The Cu T380 Ag with a silver core has a projected life span of 16 years.

Progesterone-containing IUCDs were made in the hope of combating the heavy bleeding seen in IUCD users. The total blood loss per cycle was reduced but the number of mild irregular bleeding episodes per cycle proved troublesome. More potent gestogen (e.g. levonorgestrel) devices are under development. The Population Council device will release 20–30 μg levonorgestrel daily (enough to inhibit ovulation)[30] whilst the WHO device will release 2 μg daily (and works by a local uterine effect). The optimal daily dose of levonorgestrel has not been resolved but El-Mahgoub[31] has shown that the best cycle control is achieved by a daily release of 10 μg.

Other newer improvizations are also on the horizon. WHO has backed the development of a diamidine device[21] which has reduced blood loss at menses by 25–42%. Other devices fit for postpartum insertion[32] or ones releasing prostaglandin inhibitors, antifibrinolytic agents or protein inhibitors to reduce pain and/or bleeding are under development.

The IUCD which is an excellent reversible method suffers high discontinuation rates due to side-effects. If the new modifications could reduce the complications, compliance will improve and they may prove more promising in future.

Improved barrier methods and spermicides

Barrier methods have several disadvantages, the main ones being low user efficacy, the relation to coitus and the need for messy genital manipulation. Diaphragms and cervical caps presently available seem unlikely to be improved upon in the near future.

Initial experience with the C film (a water-soluble plastic impregnated with a spermicide nonoxynol-9) showed poor efficacy. Studies are also under way for a vaginal collagen sponge[33] but initial results with patient compliance have been disappointing.

Nonoxynol-9 and TS 88 have been the time-honoured spermicides in current use. They are generally safe but may cause vaginal irritation. They are unlikely to be improved on in the near future but in addition to their use presently as foams, aerosols, etc., they may also be impregnated in collagen sponges and vaginal rings[33].

It therefore appears that no novel improvement in barrier contraceptives is going to emerge.

Better methods of natural family planning

Natural family planning methods, unless under strictly controlled circumstances, have been notorious for having high failure rates[34]. However, some women have no choice but to use them because of religious restrictions. Natural family planning methods depend heavily on methods attempting to predict or detect the occurrence of ovulation. This has been discussed in detail by Moghissi[35].

From the practical point of view, the measurements of various hormonal parameters and of temperature seems the best method we have at present. The use of ultrasound is impractical from the patient's point of view and in any case can only show a ruptured follicle (i.e. after the fact) without being able to predict the exact moment of ovulation.

A well-defined rise in luteinizing hormone (LH) level seems to be the best indirect indication[36] of impending ovulation, the median interval between LH rise and ovulation being 32 hours. It has also been shown[37] that there is a clear relationship between mean concentrations of peripheral E_2 and progesterone levels and the mature graafian follicle.

WHO is therefore concentrating on developing a simple kit method for measurement of urinary metabolites (e.g. 3α-glucuronides of oestrone and progesterone) which the patient could use at home. Simple RIA kits for salivary steroid measurements may also be available in the near future. Gould[38] has also described a rapid haemagglutination urine test for detecting mid-cycle LH peak.

Improved basal body temperature measurements may be easily obtained in future with 'intelligent thermometers'[21]. These devices signal the start of the infertile phase of the cycle when the temperature has risen for three consecutive days. A probe to measure back scattering of infrared light in the vagina has also been described. Temperature measurements combined with hormonal kits may provide a safe fairly accurate method of ovulation detection and indirectly improve efficacy of natural family planning methods.

Steroid implants

Steroid implants like injectables are depot contraceptives but unlike depot injectables they have a longer duration of action and have generally better release profiles. Both biodegradable and non-biodegradable implants are under development but Norplant (which releases levonorgestrel from a non-biodegradable sialastic, polydimethylsiloxane) is already undergoing clinical trials in Indonesia and Thailand. These implants (six capsules are placed at one sitting) have a projected life span of 7 years[39] but in the field are recommended for 5-year use till further data are available. As is to be expected, irregular bleeding has been one problem. Implantation of less than six capsules has caused a higher incidence of ectopic pregnancy[40]. Moreover, removal of these implants is also not easy and needs a fair bit of surgical skill[41]. There is still therefore room for improvement.

There is still a 'burst effect' with Norplant with serum levels of hormones reaching high levels before settling down to fairly sustained blood levels. This has been improved by using sialastic capsules containing the drug pellet (norethisterone acetate) surrounded with saline[42]. The release from this is more of zero order.

Research is also under way with newer steroids in implants. Experiments with such a steroid 16-methylene-17α-acetoxy-19-norprogesterone (ST-1435) have proved unsatisfactory so far because rapid release, short life (6 months) and amenorrhoea are problems[43].

Non-sialastic biodegradable implants (e.g. Alzamer, Capronor) have proved clinically unsatisfactory[21,44] although they are good biodegradable compounds with zero-order release. Alzamer caused unacceptable local irritation and Capronor degraded twice as slowly as the rate at which the steroid (levonorgestrel) was released. Nevertheless, Capronor is being developed and phase I studies are under way. It seems therefore that there will soon be one biodegradable (Capronor) and one non-biodegradable (Norplant) implant in routine use.

Vaginal rings

Medicated vaginal rings with either spermicides or steroids are under development. Inadequate funds have led WHO[19] to abandon the development of spermicide-impregnated rings.

Two types of steroid vaginal rings[12] are currently under review. One, sponsored by the Population Council, has a combination of levonorgestrel and oestradiol and inhibits ovulation. The second, called the Varvelo 20, contains levonorgestrel and is designed not to inhibit ovulation consistently, working very like the minipill. The Population Council ring is designed to be worn 3 weeks in and 1 week out whereas the Varvelo 20 is designed to be worn continuously. If initial trials prove successful then these methods may find clinical application in women who do not mind vaginal manipulation.

The use of Collagen bands to deliver steroids (levonorgestrel alone or in combination with oestradiol) was found by Victor[45] to be unsatisfactory in clinical trial.

Postcoital contraception

This form of contraception would be ideal as it is event related and the patient does not have to dose herself daily with hormones. If the method could be combined with accurate prediction or detection of ovulation (see 'Natural Family Planning') then the drug need only be taken if sexual intercourse occurred during the periovulatory period.

So far oestrogens/progestins alone or in combination or the post-coital insertion of the copper IUCD have been used[46] for postcoital contraception. The hormonal methods have in general caused gastro-intestinal upset (especially high-dose oestrogens) or menstrual irregu-larities[47]. Moreover, the high doses required make the use of postcoital oestrogens unsuitable as an ongoing contraceptive method. Postcoital progestins, on the other hand, seem to fit the bill as ongoing contraceptives. A phase I WHO multicentre trial[48] using 0.75 mg levonorgestrel will soon be under way. If it is proved successful and does not cause much undue menstrual upset, it may prove a good method for the couple engaging in infrequent intercourse (say 4–6 times) during one cycle.

Newer compounds are also being investigated for postcoital use. STS-557 (17α-cyanomethyl-17α-hydroxyestra-4-9-(10)-diene-3-one) is a progestin which has shown anti-implantation activity in baboons. The WHO[49] has carried out phase I trials with this drug and results will be ready soon. Anordrin has been investigated extensively in the People's Republic of China for use as a 'vacation pill'. Anordrin acts as an antifertility agent by either its antioestrogenic property[50] or by its action on alteration of tubal motility. It seems fairly promising and derivatives of Anordrin may see clinical use in future. Centchroman[48] similarly is a potent antioestrogen but initial animal studies show that it causes uterine and ovarian enlargement with menstrual derangement. It is as yet unsuitable for use in women.

Progesterone antagonists are also being investigated, but they will be discussed later under the section on new approaches.

Abortion – prostaglandins

Prostaglandin analogues which are potent have been developed for termination of pregnancy (see reference 51 for a review). These drugs are very effective for second-trimester abortion. However, first-trimester abortions (which are medically and socially preferable to mid-trimester abortion) has largely remained a surgical procedure. If self-administrable prostaglandins analogues with minimal side-effects could be developed for termination of first-trimester pregnancy this would indeed revolutionize this field.

For prostaglandins to be competitive, they have to be as safe, effective and cheap as vacuum aspiration. The prostaglandin analogues tried out via the easily self-administrable routes (i.e. orally or vaginally) have so far had unacceptable gastrointestinal side-effects and uterine pain. There may, however, be some promise for the future as Bundy[52] has shown that a new analogue 9-deoxo-16,16-dimethyl-9 methylene PGE_2 has selective action on uterine muscle compared with gut muscle; also Prasad[53] has shown good efficacy with minimal side-effects when using 16,16-dimethyl-trans-Δ^2PGE_1, methylester (ONO 802) for preoperative cervical dilatation prior to vacuum aspiration of first-trimester pregnancy.

One of the reasons that surgical vacuum aspiration has been preferred over prostaglandins for first-trimester abortion in the past was the problem of incomplete abortion and retained products of conception seen with the use of prostaglandins. It is within the realm of possibility for researchers to develop a potent prostaglandin analogue which can consistently procure almost 100% complete abortion in the first trimester. If such is the case, then abortion could become a patient-administered technique.

Sterilization

Surgical female sterilization by minilaparotomy has become so simplified that it is unlikely to be superseded by any surgical innovation in the near future. Carbon dioxide laser techniques may allow for a more circumscribed tubal tissue destruction, which may make the tubes amenable for successful reanastomosis later should it become desirable.

The advances in this field are likely to be in the following areas: (1) reversible female sterilization; and (2) non-surgical methods of sterilization.

Reversible female sterilization

The amenability to recanalization will depend on the primary method of tubal occlusion used. Fimbriectomy, extensive electrocautery and salpingectomy are irreversible. The use of clips, carbon dioxide lasers and ligation procedures causing limited tubal damage will allow for successful recanalization. However, up to the present, recanalization surgery needs special expertise with expensive microsurgical techniques for acceptably high success rates.

At present sterilization is to be regarded as an irreversible method. However, there have been some attempts to develop reversible methods[12]. Fimbriotexy and ovariotexy (i.e. the use of sialastic caps to contain either the fimbrial end or ovary) have been described. Intratubal plugs have also been tried, but they are difficult to place in the tube and difficult to remove, surgery being required both times. These plugs have also caused tissue irritation and prove difficult to anchor. They are therefore unlikely to be of much hope in the future.

Non-surgical methods of sterilization

A variety of chemicals have been examined for their ability to cause tubal occlusion when instilled either blindly or under hysteroscopic control. Richart[54,55] has reviewed the use of silver nitrate, quinacrine, silicone rubber, phenol, ethanol–formaldehyde and methylcyanoacrylate (MCA). Silver nitrate and phenol were toxic and ethanol-formaldehyde was ineffective. Quinacrine, MCA and sialastic are three promising compounds.

Zipper[56] has found a Pearl index of pregnancy of 4.1 when he used quinacrine (as a 4ml suspension of 1g given once or twice) on 638 patients over 14 677 women months. A major drawback of quinacrine is that its application has to be repeated to achieve bilateral occlusion. Quinacrine pellets may overcome this problem[57]. Quinacrine is better than MCA or sialastic in that it does not require any special device for instillation.

MCA is a liquid monomer which polymerizes when in contact with moist living tissue. It then promotes fibrosis by releasing toxic products as it degrades over 6 weeks. Neuwirth[58] produced 72% bilateral tubal occlusion rate in 131 women using MCA. There is a clear need to improve the techniques of instillation and WHO[21] is carrying out multicentre trials with this method. Irreversibility is a disadvantage with this method.

Sialastic has the potential for reversibility. This fast-setting substance has to be delivered hysteroscopically and 86% success has been reported by Houch[59]. This method may therefore become an 'office' procedure in the near future, but is unlikely to become incorporated into family planning programmes in less developed countries because of the surgical expertise required.

NEW APPROACHES FOR THE FUTURE

Researchers in the field of family planning have been looking to several new leads. These are, however, in their infantile stage and may only become reality in the next century. Under this heading the following will be discussed:

(1) LRF analogues for contraception and luteolysis.
(2) Progesterone antagonists and luteal phase agents.
(3) Novel peptides for contraception.
(4) Immunological fertility control.

LRF analogues for contraception and luteolysis

More than 1500 analogues of luteinizing release factor (or hormone) have been made, and according to their activity have been deemed agonists or antagonists. Some agonists which have been used clinically are [D-Tryp[6]]-LRF, [D-Tryp[6], des Gly[10]]-LRF ethylamide and [D-Ser(TBu)[6], des Gly[10]]-LRF (Buserelin). When used in laboratory animals, agonists could be stimulatory or inhibitory depending on the species used.

LRF agonists have been investigated for female contraception from two angles: as ovulation inhibitors and as luteolytic agents. Their action to inhibit ovulation seems more promising then their luteolytic capability.

Nillius[60] (1978) and Bergquist[61] (1979) have investigated the use of Buserelin via the nasal and subcutaneous routes for ovulation inhibition. Results were acceptable with return of ovulation on cessation of LRF agonist. Amenorrhoea was a problem with this treatment and some[62] have raised the possible ill effects of unopposed oestrogenic action on the endometrium resulting from treatment. The use of LRF analogues for luteolysis is not so promising. When given to non-pregnant women, there occurred some shortening of the menstrual cycle[63] but this effect could not be duplicated in pregnant women[64].

LRF antagonists have been less well investigated than agonists because only recently have potent ones been available. Inhibition of ovulation was not consistent when [N-acetyl-D parachloro-Phe[1,2], D-Phe[6], D-Ala[10]]-LRF was given to women[65]. Another compound has recently been synthesized – [acetyl-D-parachloro-Phe[1,2], D-Tryp[3], D-Arg[6], D-Ala[12]]-LRF. Small doses of this compound have been shown to be potent inhibitors of ovulation in rats[66]. We will have to await further testing before any prediction can be made for LRF antagonists.

Progesterone antagonists and luteal phase agents

Interference with the action of progesterone by blocking its receptors in the uterus is one way of early pregnancy termination. Various progesterone antagonists have been experimented with. STS 557 is one such compound which has been discussed under the heading of Postcoital contraception.

More recently, another anti-progestin, RU 38486 [17αpropynyl-11 (4[1]-dimethylaminophenyl)-9,10,-dehydro-19 nortestosterone] described by Hermann[67] (1982) has been used in a dose of 200 mg daily for 4 days in 11 women 6–8 weeks' pregnant and procured abortion in nine of the patients. This compound also has glucocorticoid-receptor

283

blocking action, which is worrying, and the optimum dose to be used has yet to be worked out.

Various steroid oximes, anti-hCG agents, α-difluoromethylornithine and anti-progesterone monoclonal antibodies are under investigation. Prasad[48] (1983) has reviewed these compounds and they have to be further tested before clinical trial.

Plant products too have yielded agents with menses-inducing or abortifacient properties. Some examples are zoapatle (from *Montanoa fomentosa*), trichosanthin (from *Trichosanthis kirilowii*) and yuanhuacine (from *Daphne genkwa*). More work needs to be done on plant products before the active principles can be identified, extracted and used clinically.

Novel peptides for contraception

A detailed analysis of follicular fluid has revealed many constituents that can prevent ovulation. If these peptides could be purified they could provide very potent anti-ovulation agents which act directly on the target organ (the graafian follicle) and which will have none of the complications of steroidal contraceptives.

Other than LRF analogues which have already been discussed, follicular inhibin[68], oocyte maturation inhibitor[69] and FSH binding inhibitor proteins[70] are some of the novel peptides which may show future promise.

Immunological fertility control

Development of contraceptive vaccines which can be given yearly and are reversible have definite attractions for use in family planning programmes. These vaccines have, however, to be proved to be safe, effective and reversible. Three main types of contraceptive vaccine have been investigated:

(1) Anti-HCG vaccine.
(2) Anti-zona pellucida vaccine.
(3) Anti-LDH-C_4 enzyme vaccine.

Anti-HCG vaccine

Two types of anti-HCG vaccine have been tested. The first approach by Talwar[71] saw development of antibodies to the whole B subunit of the HCG molecule. This, however, cross-reacted with LH, FSH and TSH. When given to women they did not show many short-term side-effects but the possible long-term side-effects are worrying. A subsequent efficacy study[72] showed they were also not uniformly effective in preventing pregnancy.

Because whole-molecule anti-β subunit cross-reacted with LH, attempts have been made to develop antibodies to specific peptide chains on the HCG β Subunit in the hope that they may be more specific. These antibodies need further testing and it remains to be seen whether they are active in the human or are too weak for contraceptive purposes.

Anti-zona pellucida vaccine

Antibodies to zona pellucida will disrupt the ovum and procure contraception. Work on this is still preliminary but one advantage of using this method is that it will be readily available as human and pig zona have cross-reacting antigens and porcine zona can provide abundant starting material. Early work[44] in animals showed that it causes cycle disturbance when administered. The antibodies can also act against developing ova in the ovary as well as the matured ova and this action is obviously undesirable as it can cause an irreversible effect.

Anti-LDH-C$_4$ enzyme vaccine

Antibodies to a sperm-specific antigen, the enzyme lactate dehydrogenase C$_4$, were effective in preventing pregnancy when given to female animals. The mode of action is uncertain but may not be via an inhibitory effect on sperm motility or via an effect on ovum development[73]. Very little is known about this vaccine but if they should damage sperms or ova in any way without completely destroying them, there is potential for teratogenesis.

CONCLUSION

It is extremely difficult to predict the future direction of methods of female fertility control. At best only an educated guess can be made from an assessment of the present state of the art. All such pointers from pundits involved in fertility control predict no momentous breakthrough for this century at least. Barring some sudden scientific breakthrough it looks as though we have to be satisfied with current methods for some time yet.

References

1. Atkinson, L. E. (1979). Status of funding and costs of reproductive science research and contraceptive development. In *Contraception: Science, Technology and Application.* pp. 292–305. (Washington, D. C.: National Academy of Sciences)
2. US Congress, Office of Technology Assessment (1982). *World Population and Fertility Planning Technologies: The Next 20 Years,* Vol. 1. (Washington, D.C.: US Government Printing Office)
3. Royal College of General Practitioners (1974). *Oral Contraceptives and Health; an Interim Report for the Oral Contraception Study of the Royal College of General Practitioners.* (New York: Pitman Publishing)
4. Royal College of General Practitioners Oral Contraception Study (1976). The outcome of pregnancy in former oral contraceptive users. *Br. J. Obstet. Gynaecol.,* **83,** 608
5. Royal College of General Practitioners Oral Contraception Study (1977). Effect on hypertension and benign breast disease of progestagen component in combined oral contraceptives. *Lancet,* **1,** 624
6. Royal College of General Practitioners Oral Contraception Study (1977). Mortality among oral-contraceptive users. *Lancet,* **2,** 727
7. Royal College of General Practitioners Oral Contraception Study (1978). Oral contraceptives, venous thrombosis, and varicose veins. *J. R. Coll. Gen. Pract.,* **28,** 393
8. Goldzieher, J. W. (1983). Oral contraceptive hazards – reappraisal. In Chadhuri, S. K. (ed.). *Practice of Fertility Control, A Comprehenisve Textbook,* pp. 108–114. (Calcutta: Current Book Publishers)
9. Salonen, J. T. (1982). Oral contraceptives, smoking and risk of myocardial infarction in young women. *Acta Med. Scand.,* **212,** 141
10. Ratnam, S. S. and Prasad, R. N. V. (1980). Recent developments in steroidal contraception. *Singapore J. Obstet. Gynaecol.,* **11,** 7
11. Ratnam, S. S. and Prasad, R. N. V. (1983). Oral contraceptives. In Chaudhuri, S. K. (ed.). *Practice of Fertility Control, A Comprehensive Textbook,* p. 103. (Calcutta: Current Book Publishers)
12. Harper, M. J. K. (1983). *Birth Control Technologies Prospects by the Year 2000.* (University of Texas Press) (In press)
13. Bradley, D. D., Wingerd, J., Petitti, D. B., Krauss, R. M. and Ramcharan, S. (1978). Serum high-density lipoprotein cholesterol in women using oral contraceptives, estrogens and progestins. *N. Engl. J. Med.,* **299,** 17
14. Larsson-Cohn, U., Wallentin, L. and Zador, G. (1979). Effects of three different combinations of ethinyl estradiol and levonorgestrel on plasma lipid and high density lipoproteins. *Acta Obstet. Gynecol. Scand. Suppl.,* **88,** 57
15. Larsson-Cohn, U., Fahraeus, L., Wallentin, L. and Zador, G. (1981). Lipoprotein changes may be minimized by proper composition of a combined oral contraceptive. *Fertil. Steril.,* **35,** 172
16. de Visser, J., de Jager, E., De Jongh, H. P., Van der Vies, J. and Zeelen, F. (1979). Pharmacological profile of a new orally active progestational steroid: ORG 2969. *Acta Endocrinol. (Kbh) Suppl.,* **199,** 405

17. Viinikka, L., Hirvonen, E., Ylikorkala, O. *et al.* (1977). Ovulation inhibition by a new low-dose progestagen. *Contraception,* **16,** 51

18. Benagiano, G., Diczfalusy, E., Goldzieher, J. W. and Gray, R. (1977). (Coordinators WHO Task Force on long-acting systemic agents for the regulation of fertility). Multinational comparative clinical evaluation of two long-acting injectable contraceptive steroids: Norethisterone enanthate and medroxyprogesterone acetate. 1. Use effectiveness. *Contraception,* **15,** 513

19. World Health Organization (WHO) (1979). *Special Programme of Research, Development and Research Training in Human Reproduction. Eighth Annual Report.* (Geneva: WHO)

20. Benagiano, G. and Fraser, I. (1981). The depo-provera debate. Commentary on the article 'Depo-Provera, A critical analysis'. *Contraception,* **24,** 493

21. World Health Organization (1981). *Special Programme of Research, Development and Research Training in Human Reproduction. Tenth Annual Report.* (Geneva: WHO)

22. Kremer, J. de Bruijn, H. W. A. and Hindriks, F. R. (1980). Serum high density lipoprotein cholesterol levels in women using a contraceptive injection of depot-medroxyprogesterone acetate. *Contraception,* **22,** 359

23. Weiner, E. and Johansson, E. D. B. (1975). Plasma levels of norethindrone after i.m. injection of 200 mg norethindrone enanthate. *Contraception,* **11,** 419

24. Crabbe, P., Arcjer, S., Benagiano, G., *et al.* (1983). Long-acting contraceptive agents: Design of the WHO chemical synthesis programme. *Steroids (Suppl.)* (In press).

25. Prema, K., Gayathiri, T. L., Ramalakshmi, B. A., Madhavapeddi, R. and Philips, F. S. (1981). Low dose injectable contraceptive norethisterone enanthate 20 mg monthly. I. Clinical trials. *Contraception,* **23,** 11

26. Prasad, K. V. S., Nair, K. M., Sivakumar, B., Prema, K. and Rao, B. S. N. (1981). Plasma levels of norethindrone in Indian women receiving norethindrone enanthate (20 mg) injectable. *Contraception,* **23,** 497

27. Oriowo, M-A., Landgren, B-M., Stenstrom, B. and Diczfalusy, E. (1980). A comparison of the pharmacokinetic properties of three estradiol esters. *Contraception,* **21,** 415

28. Beck, L. R., Ramos, R. A., Flowers, C. E., Jr., *et al.* (1981). Clinical evaluation of injectable biodegradable contraceptive system. *Am. J. Obstet. Gynaecol.,* **140,** 799

29. Sivin, I. and Stern, J. (1979). Long acting more effective copper T IUDs: A summary of US experience, 1970–75. *Stud. Family Plan.,* **10,** 263

30. Nilsson, C. G., Lahteenmaki, P. and Luukkainen, T. (1980). Levonorgestrel plasma concentrations and hormone profiles after insertion and after one year of treatment with a levonorgestrel-IUD. *Contraception,* **21,** 225

31. El-Mahgoub, S. (1980). The norgestrel-T IUD. *Contraception,* **22,** 271

32. Laufe, L. E., Wheeler, R. G. and Friel, P. G. (1979). Modification of intrauterine devices for postpartum insertion. *Lancet,* **1,** 853

33. WHO Task Force on Vaginal and Intracervical Devices for Fertility Regulation (1979). Vaginal rings releasing spermicides. In Zatuchni, G., Sobrero, A., Speidel, J. J. and Sciarra, J. J. (eds.). *Vaginal Contraception: New Developments,* pp. 188–93. (Hagerstown, Md.: Harper and Row)

34. WHO Task Force on Methods for the Determination of the Fertile Period (1981). A prospective multicentre trial of the ovulation method of natural family planning. II. The effectiveness phase. *Fertil. Steril.,* **36,** 591

35. Moghissi, K. S. (1980). Prediction and detection of ovulation. *Fertil. Steril.,* **34,** 89

36. WHO Task Force on Methods for the Determination of the Fertile Period (1980). Temporal relationships between ovulation and defined changes in the concentration of plasma estradol-17β, luteinizing hormone, follicle-stimulating hormone and progesterone. 1. Probit analysis. *Am. J. Obstet. Gynaecol.,* **138,** 383

37. WHO Task Force on Methods for the Determination of the Fertile Period (1981). Temporal relationships between ovulation and defined changes in the concentration of plasma estradiol-17β, luteinizing hormone and progesterone. II. Histologic dating. *Am. J. Obstet. Gynaecol.*, **139**, 886

38. Gould, K. G. and Faulkner, J. R. (1981). Development, validation, and application of a rapid method for detection of ovulation in great apes and women. *Fertil. Steril.*, **35**, 676

39. Sivin, I., Robertson, D. N., Stern, J., *et al.* (1980). Norplant: Reversible implant contraception. *Stud. Family Plan.*, **11**, 227

40. Croxatto, H. B., Diaz, S., Quinteros, E., *et al.* (1975). Clinical assessment of subdermal implants of megestrol acetate, D-noregestrel and norethindrone as a long term contraceptive in women. *Contraception*, **12**, 615

41. Population Council (1982). *Norplant Conference – Experiences of its Use in Thailand and Indonesia*, Bangkok, November

42. Kumar, D., Farooq, A. and Laumas, K. R. (1981). Fluid-filled silastic capsules: A new approach to a more constant steroidal drug delivery system. *Contraception*, **23**, 261

43. Coutinho, E. M., da Silva, A. R., Carreira, C. M. V. and Sivin, I. (1981). Long-term contraception with a single implant of the progestin ST-1435. *Fertil. Steril.*, **36**, 737

44. World Health Organization (WHO) (1980). *Special Programme of Research, Development and Research Training in Human Reproduction. Ninth Annual Report.* (Geneva: WHO)

45. Victor, A. and Johansson, E. D. B. (1977). Contraceptive rings: Self administered treatment governed by bleeding. *Contraception*, **16**, 137

46. Prasad, R. N. V. and Ratnam, S. S. (1981). Postcoital contraception. *Singapore J. Obstet. Gynaecol.*, **12**, 18

47. Yuzpe, A. A., Smith, R. P. and Rademaker, A. W. (1982). A multicenter clinical investigation employing ethinyl estradiol combined with dl-norgestrel as a post-coital contraceptive agent. *Fertil. Steril.*, **37**, 508

48. Prasad, M. R. N. (1983). Postcoital agents and menses inducers. Presented at the *Conference on Research on the Regulation of Human Fertility – Needs of Developing Countries and Priorities for the Future*, Stockholm, February 7–9

49. WHO (1982). *Special Programme of Research in Human Reproduction. 11th Annual Report.* (Geneva: World Health Organization)

50. Mehta, R. R., Jenco, J. M. and Chatterton, R. T. (1981). Antiestrogenic and antifertility actions of Anoudrin. *Steroids*, **38**, 679

51. Karim, S. M. M. (ed.). (1979). *Practical Applications of Prostaglandins and their Synthesis Inhibiters.* (Lancaster: MTP Press)

52. Bundy, G. L., Kimball, F. A., Robert, A., *et al.*, (1980). Synthesis and biological activity of 9-deoxo-9-methylene and related prostaglandins. *Adv. Prostaglandin Thromboxane Res.*, **6**, 355

53. Prasad, R. N. V., Lim, C., Wong, Y. C., Karim, S. M. M. and Ratnam, S. S. (1978). Vaginal administration of 16, 16-dimethyl-trans-PGE, methylester (ONO 802) for preoperative cervical dilatation in first trimester nulliparous pregnancy. *Singapore J. Obstet. Gynaecol.*, **9**, 69

54. Richart, R. M. (1980). Female sterilization using pharmacologically active agents. In Zatuchni, G. I., Labbock, M. H. and Sciarra, J. J. (eds.). *Research Frontiers in Fertility Regulation*, pp. 262–69. (Hagerstown, MD: Harper and Row)

55. Richart, R. M. (1981). Female sterilization using chemical agents. *Res. Frontiers Fertil. Reg.*, **1**

56. Zipper, J., Stachetti, A. and Medel, M. (1975). Transvaginal chemical sterilization: Clinical use of quinacrine plus potentiating adjuvants. *Contraception*, **12**, 11

57. Bhatt, R. V., Aparicio, A., Laufe, L. E., Parmley, T. and King, T. M. (1980).

Quinacrine-induced pathologic changes in the Fallopian tube. *Fertil. Steril.*, **33**, 666

58. Neuwirth, R. S., Richart, R. M., Eldering, G., Argueta-Rivas, G. and Nilsen, P. A. (1980). An outpatient approach to female sterilization using methylcyanoacrylate. *Am. J. Obstet. Gynaecol.*, **136**, 951

59. Houck, R. M. and Cooper, J. M. (1983). Hysteroscopic tubal occlusion with formed-in-place silicone plugs: A clinical study. *Obstet. Gynecol.* (In press)

60. Nillius, S. J., Bergquist, C. and Wide, L. (1978). Inhibition of ovulation in women by chronic treatment with a stimulatory LRH analogue – A new approach to birth control? *Contraception*, **17**, 537

61. Bergquist, C., Nillius, S. J. and Wide, L. (1979). Inhibition of ovulation in women by intranasal treatment with a luteinizing hormone-releasing hormone agonist. *Contraception*, **19**, 497

62. Schmidt-Gollwitzer, M., Hardt, W., Schmidt-Gollwitzer, K. von der Ohe, M. and Nevinny-Stickel, J. (1981). Influence of the LH-RH analogue Buserelin on cyclic ovarian function and on endometrium. A new approach to fertility control. *Contraception*, **23**, 187

63. Lemay, A., Labrie, F., Ferland, L. and Raynaud, J. P. (1979). Possible luteolytic effects of luteinizing hormone-releasing hormone in normal women. *Fertil. Steril.*, **31**, 29

64. Casper, R. F., Sheehan, K. L. and Yen, S. S. C. (1980). Chorionic gonadotropin prevents LRF-agonist-induced luteolysis in the human. *Contraception*, **21**, 471

65. Zarate, A., Canales, E. S., Sthory, I. *et al.* (1981). Antiovulatory effect of a LHRH antagonist in women. *Contraception*, **24**, 315

66. Coy, D. H., Horvath, A., Nekola, M. V. *et al.* (1982). Peptide antagonists of LH-RH: Large increases in antiovulatory activities produced by D-amino acids in the six position. *Endocrinology*, **110**, 1445

67. Hermann, W., Wyss, R., Riondel, A. *et al.* (1982). Effet d'un steroide anti-proges-terone chez la femme: Interruption du cycle menstruel et de la grossesse au debut. *C. R. Acad. Sci. Paris*, **294**, 933

68. Chappel, S. C., Holt, J. A. and Spies, H. G. (1980). Inhibin: Differences in bioactivity within human follicular fluid in the follicular and luteal phases of the menstrual cycle. *Proc. Soc. Exp. Biol. Med.*, **163**, 310

69. Tsafriri, A. and Channing, C. P. (1975). An inhibitory influence of granulosa cells and follicular fluid upon porcine oocyte meiosis *in vitro*. *Endocrinology*, **96**, 922

70. Darga, N. C. and Reichert, L. E., Jr. (1979). Evidence for the presence of a low molecular weight follitropin binding inhibitor in bovine follicular fluid. In Channing, C. P., Marsh, J. M. and Sadler, W. A. (eds.). *Ovarian Follicular and Corpus Luteum Function.* (New York: Plenum Press)

71. Ramakrishnan, S., Kumar, S. and Hingorani, V. (1976). Isoimmunization against human chorionic gonadotropin with conjugates of processed beta-subunit of the hormone and tetanus toxoid. *Proc. Natl. Acad. Sci. USA*, **73**, 218

72. Das, O., Talwar, G. P., Ramakrishnan, S., *et al.* (1978). Discriminatory effect of anti-Pr-beta-hCG-TT antibodies on the neutralization of the biological activity of placental and pituitary gonadotropins. *Contraception*, **18**, 35

73. Goldberg, E. (1975). Effects of immunization with LDH-X on fertility. *Acta Endocrinol. (Suppl.)*, **194**, 202

26
Recent progress in the use of copper IUDs

ALAIN J. M. AUDEBERT

INTRODUCTION

An increasing world-wide utilization of IUDs represents one of the main events in the field of contraception during the past decade. This is due to many factors, but some are directly related to improvements in design. A major advance was achieved when medicated IUDs were made readily suitable for clinical use. The initial contribution was made by Zipper et al.[1] and Doyle and Clewe[2], who, simultaneously in 1968, focussed on using the IUD as a carrier for an active antifertility agent: respectively, metallic copper and a synthetic progestin.

Clinical testing and marketing has involved two copper-bearing devices, the TCu and the Cu7; considerable information has been accumulated, confirming the improvement of their clinical perform-ance in comparison with inert IUDs. Recently various newer devices have been tested in order to improve, if possible, simplicity of insertion procedure, efficacy, retention safety, life span and tolerance.

I will review only some IUDs, among the large number of devices created throughout the world, focussing on their main features and some controversial aspects still under debate; I will limit my review to post-menstrual insertions.

EVALUATION OF PERFORMANCES

Clinical performances of an IUD depends upon many factors, such as patient population, experience and motivation of the physician, tolerance to side-effects, clinic attitude and use of supplementary contraceptives[3].

Some variables can be easily included in the analysis for proper evaluation. Clinic attitude and physician experience are more difficult to control, justifying multicentre studies. Fundal positioning and appropriate relationship between the device's size and endometrial cavity geometry greatly influence clinical performance of the IUD; devices easily inserted are more likely to be correctly placed; in this regard the push-in technique of insertion offers some advantages, especially when the person inserting the IUD is less experienced. More accurate assessment of the uterine cavity is required for selecting the proper device; thus measurements with various devices such as the wing sound of Hasson or the Kurtz cavimeter are certainly helpful and need more selective use to evaluate their effect on performance.

The care following insertion plays an important role in preventing some adverse effects. Many studies have proved the beneficial value of ultrasonography in the follow-up and control of IUD bearers; unsuspected lower placement of the device, disclosed by this safe and repeatable investigation, increased the risk of expulsion, unwanted pregnancy and poor tolerance and thus can be properly managed.

All these factors have to be taken into consideration since they influence the use-effectiveness of the IUD. Evaluation should therefore apply to all recommendations in order to reduce the role of variables.

Comparative studies should be conducted on a double-blind, multicentric and multinational basis; criteria for patient inclusion and for termination of IUD use must be standardized; analysis of data must follow proper statistical methods and the percentage of patients lost to follow-up must be as low as possible[4].

On an individual basis selection of patient is a major step to improve performance, taking into consideration the following: past history; clinical parameters obtained by proper examination; sexual activity and social environment; and all risk factors for pelvic inflammatory disease (PID), ectopic pregnancy, perforation, expulsion and bleeding and pain problems.

CONTROVERSIES ON BIOLOGY OF COPPER

Enhancement of the efficacy of copper-bearing IUDs in comparison with inert ones has been proved by various long-term studies, appearing more marked for smaller devices[5].

Scanning and transmission electron microscopy studies indicate that changes of the endometrium are more extensive with copper IUDs, with a direct relationship between the amount of copper incorporated in the device, the degree of ultrastructural changes and the area of endometrium involved[6].

Use of this concept implicates a minimum release of copper ions to assure expected efficacy and leads to the determination of the most suitable load of copper and the acceptance of a limited life span for a particular device.

Load of copper

With the T-shaped plastic skeleton, antifertility effect was related to area of exposed surface of copper, 200 mm² surface area providing optimal results. 300 mm² was thought to be the upper limit above which adverse effects such as expulsion and bleeding might be promoted; despite controversial opinions, it appears more and more likely that increase of the surface area up to 375 or 380 mm² lowers the pregnancy rate, without modifying the rate of expulsion.

Life span

With the TCu 200 and Cu7 duration was limited to 2–3 years. Recent studies indicate that the antifertility effect is produced for a much longer period of time, up to 8 years[7,8]; no decrease of copper concentration in human uterine secretions up to 4 years after insertion of a Cu7 were found[9].

Release of copper depends upon many factors, which are related to the model used and time after insertion. Dissolution of copper leads to corrosion then to breakage; adverse effects due to fragmentation have so far not been demonstrated even if decreased efficacy could be expected.

Release of copper and corrosion might be delayed by calcium carbonate deposit covering the wire; these deposits increase during the first 3 years of use and then seem to remain relatively constant. Breakage may occur after 3 years, but occasionally can be observed after a shorter period of use; the increase of the diameter of the copper wire does not seem to eliminate breakage[10]. Adjunction of a silver core to the copper wire and utilization of a copper multisleeve instead of a wire protects against fragmentation and increases the life span of the device.

NEW IUDS

The TCu380

The classic T-shaped device has been modified by adding collars of copper on the horizontal arms (TCu380) or on both vertical and horizontal arms (TCu220), in order to increase effectiveness and extend duration of protection. The Population Council comparative trials indicated that the TCu380 is the most effective T-shaped device, with no significantly different total termination rate. A randomized clinical study conducted by Diaz et al.[11] in a developing country clearly showed the higher efficacy of the TCu380 when compared with the Lippes loop C as observed in the United States.

A long-term study analysed by Sivin and Tatum[12] gives a cumulative pregnancy rate of 1.9 per 100 women at 4 years; increased load of copper and placement of copper on the horizontal arms close to the fundus region, even in case of downward displacement of the device, seems responsible for this high effectiveness. An effective lifetime of 4 years has been demonstrated. Addition of a silver core to the wire placed on the vertical stem may extend the life span beyond 6 years. If the retention rate is quite satisfactory, the removal rate for bleeding and pain seems increased; this may be due to a decreased flexibility of the horizontal arms bearing the copper sleeves.

The Multiload devices

Designed by Van Os, the Multiload is made of polyethylene and has two flexible side arms which ensure a good retainability. Pre-loaded in its inserter, the Multiload is very simple to insert by a push-in technique, when a sufficient opening of the cervical canal is present, and thus is easily positioned high up against the fundus with a low risk of perforation. The first to be marketed was the MLCu250, loaded with 250 mm^2 of copper wire placed on the vertical stem; it has shown a high effectiveness at 3 years and a low expulsion rate, respectively 1.3 and 3.2. In a comparative study with the TCu220 and the Cu7,

Goh et al.[13] found a lower expulsion rate for the MLCu250, possibly due to the fundal seeking effect of the transverse arms.

Three variations of the Multiload model are now available:

(1) The MLCu short with a shorter vertical stem.
(2) The Mini MLCu250 with a global reduced size.
(3) The MLCu375 with an increased load of copper due to a thicker (0.4 mm diameter) wire.

The mini model has given less satisfactory results; this may be due partially to the reduced flexibility and partially to the high risks recipient with a very small uterus.

The performances of the standard ML and the short model appear very similar[14]. The MLCu375 is the most promising device of the series with a higher effectiveness than the MLCu250 both at 1 year and 2 years, and an equally good retainability[14]; more data are required for evaluating long-term performances.

The Nova-T

The Nova-T is different from the T-shaped IUDs; its main attributes include:

(1) A loop at the end of the vertical stem.
(2) An enlargement at the end of the horizontal arms to prevent penetration in the myometrium.
(3) A silver coil in the copper wire to prevent fragmentation and extend effective life of the device up to 5 years.

The Nova-T has a higher effectiveness despite a copper surface of 200 mm^2 – a comparative study against the TCu200[15,16] demonstrated a lower pregnancy rate of the Nova-T at 2 and 3 years; 1.4 and 1.9, respectively versus 4.0 and 5.0. This lower pregnancy rate was found in every age and parity group; it may be due to a better fundal placement; the other termination rates of these two devices were not significantly different.

One small-scale single clinic study conducted by Fylling and Fagerhol[17] has shown a significantly higher expulsion rate for the Nova-T in comparison with the progestogen system. A similar study[18] against the levonorgestrel IUD shows the same finding: incorrect placement of the device, secondary to insertion procedure not strictly following specific instructions for this device may be partially responsible. Large-scale studies are required to evaluate their respective efficacy and retainability.

The progestasert system

The system is a T-shaped device releasing continuously $65\,\mu g$ daily of pure progesterone for 18 months with a load of 38 mg progesterone, and this period can be extended to $2\frac{1}{2}$ years with a load of 52 mg; the first model is the only one presently available.

Non-touch loading of the device in its supple inserter makes insertion procedure very simple. The progesterone released in the uterine cavity induces specific changes of the endometrium which becomes hypotrophic and shows some decidual reaction; the passage of progesterone in the blood is clinically non-significant.

These endometrial modifications and other specific local effects of the progesterone are responsible for a significant decrease of the menstrual blood loss even in case of hypermenorrhoea and a significant decrease of menstrual cramps, when dysmenorrhoea was present before insertion, as demonstrated by several similar studies from different countries[19]. At 1 year a pregnancy rate of 1.8 and an expulsion rate of 2.7 have been found in a large-scale study. By selecting the more appropriate patients, reinsertion provides significantly better results for accidental pregnancy, expulsion and removal for bleeding and pain[20,21].

However, the risk of ectopic pregnancy with the progestasert is a major matter of concern, and various controversial results have been opposed and do not permit any conclusions; thus one must be aware of such a complication.

The levonorgestrel IUD

The levonorgestrel IUD is made of a plastic vector like the Nova-T bearing a silastic reservoir of levonorgestrel, which is released at a dose of $25\,\mu g$ daily for at least 5 years.

Blood levels of levonorgestrel are fairly constant and induce some hormonal systemic side-effects. However, no significant effect has been demonstrated on ovarian function, or lipids metabolism. The hormonal adverse effects lead to removal of the device in approximately 5% of the patients at 2 years[15].

Menstrual blood loss and menstrual cramps are significantly reduced; however, due to insensitive endometrium, amenorrhoea may be observed in some patients.

This device is highly effective and well retained. Inducing cervical mucus modifications, like oral gestagens, one may expect some decrease in the infection incidence. The main disadvantages of this device are the hormonal side-effects, but the influence on the termination rate is minor; the termination rate is satisfactory and similar to the Nova-T.

FUTURE DEVELOPMENTS

Research on the devices tends to improve tolerance rather than efficacy, which is now quite satisfactory. Technology permits incorporation of any drug in the device. Oestradiol (Van Os, personal communication) or haemostatic agents are being added in an attempt to reduce bleeding problems. Antibiotics may also be incorporated.

If available devices have established a reasonable compromise between retention and tolerance, the search for a better vector is still open. Since all devices require an anchoring system or some rigidity to be retained, which may contribute by mechanical trauma to some side-effects, a very soft polyethylene IUD has been designed. It is a closed device with two vertical lateral arms, and a middle part of the lower junction surrounds the vertical stem which contains the copper; this movement changes the shape of the device, pushing it towards the fundus and resisting expulsion at the isthmic level. Copper IUDs positioned in the abdominal cavity are encapsulated by adhesions so that despite the closed design, the risk of strangulation seems very minimal[8,9].

Insertion procedure is very simple, similar to the push-in technique used for the Multiload.

Preliminary results of this device, called Ombrelle 250, as indicated by number of events at 1 and 2 years' use are quite satisfactory since only two pregnancies and two expulsions have been observed at 1 year in an unselected group of 407 patients (4304 women-months of use); seven devices were removed for bleeding or pain. At 2 years, three pregnancies and four expulsions were observed in a group of 248 women having their insertion at least 2 years before these data were collected.

Indeed more data are needed and proper comparative studies are required to evaluate this device and its expected improvements due to the soft consistency of the polyethylene frame which should enhance endometrial tolerance and facilitate retrieval when needed.

CONCLUSIONS

(1) Newer copper-bearing IUDs offer satisfactory clinical performances; a compromise has been established between effectiveness and tolerance; the duration of use has been increased so that most of the devices can be left in place for at least 4 years. Abnormal bleeding and IUD-related infections still have to be faced. Research is required to minimize them since no major advance has been accomplished for their prevention. All IUDs have shown a good reversibility.

(2) Data obtained from proper comparative studies do not permit us at the moment to claim the superiority of one device in all aspects. The specific advantages of each IUD must be properly judged for individual clinical benefits.

(3) IUDs delivering steroids, by reducing heavy menstrual bleeding and menstrual pain, offer advantages for the patients with these specific complaints; their drawbacks, however, have to be carefully evaluated before clinical use on an individual basis; their possible therapeutic role is still in a research stage.

(4) These relatively optimistic considerations on IUDs should not let us forget that optimal clinical performance depends mainly upon their optimal use; proper selection of patients, insertion procedure, fundal placement, and the last but not least medical care and control after insertion, are mandatory to reach this goal.

References

1. Zipper, J. A., Medel, M. and Prager, R. (1968). Experimental suppression of fertility by intrauterine copper and zinc in rabbits. In *Abstracts of the Sixth World Congress on Fertility and Sterility, Tel Aviv, Israel, May 20–27*, p. 154
2. Doyle, L. L. and Clewe, T. (1968). Preliminary studies on the effect of hormone-releasing intra-uterine devices. *Am. J. Obstet. Gynecol.*, **101**, 564
3. Mishell, D. R. (1975). The clinical factor in evaluating IUDs. In Hefnawi, F. and Segal, S. (eds.), *Analysis of Intra-uterine Contraception*, p. 27. (Amsterdam: North-Holland)
4. Jarvela, S. (1981). Problems in the comparison of clinical performance of IUDs. *Contracept. Deliv. Syst.*, **2**, 87
5. Randic, L. (1980). Comparative evaluation of medicated and non-medicated IUDs of the same size and shape. *Contracept. Deliv. Syst.*, **1**, 87

6. El-Badrawi, M. H., Hafez, E. S. E., Barnhart, M. I., Fayad, M. and Shafeek, A. (1981). Ultrastructural changes in human endometrium with copper and non medicated IUDs *in utero*. *Fertil. Steril.*, **36**, 41

7. Prema, K., Lakshmi, B. A. R. and Babu, S. (1980). Serum copper in long-term users of copper intra-uterine devices. *Fertil. Steril.*, **34**, 32

8. Larsson, B., Astrom, G., Einarsson, S., *et al.* (1981). The possible risks of a copper and an inert intra-uterine device situated in the abdominal cavity: an experimental study in pigs and dogs. *Fertil. Steril.*, **36**, 229

9. Larsson, B., Hagstrom, B., Viberg, L. and Hamberger, L. (1981). Long term clinical experience with the Cu-7-IUD – Evaluation of a prospective study. *Contraception*, **23**, 387

10. Kosonen, A. and Thiery, M. (1983). Corrosion of filamentous intra-uterine copper. The MLCu250 and MLCu375. *Contraception*, **27**, 85

11. Diaz, J., Diaz, M. M., Pastene, L., Araki, R. and Faundes, A. (1982). Randomized clinical study of the T-Cu 380 A and the Lippes Loop C, in Campinas, Brazil. *Contraception*, **26**, 221

12. Sivin, I. and Tatum, H. J. (1981). Four year experience with the TCu380 A intra-uterine contraceptive device. *Fertil. Steril.*, **36**, 159

13. Goh, T. H., Sinnathoray, T. A., Sivanesaratnah, V. and Sen, D. K. (1983). A randomised comparative evaluation of the Copper 7, Multiload Copper 250 and T-Copper-220 C IUDs. *Contraception*, **27**, 75

14. Van der Pas, H., Van Os, W. and Thiery, M. (1983). Performance of multiload IUD models with different copper load. *Contracept. Deliv. Syst.* (In press)

15. Allonen, H., Luukkainen, T., Nielsen, N. C., Nygren, K. G. and Pyorala, T. (1980). Two year rates for NOVA-T and copper T in a comparative study. *Contraception*, **21**, 321

16. Nygren, K. G., Nielsen, N. C., Pyorala, T., Allonen, H. and Luukkainen, T. (1981). Intrauterine contraception with Nova-T and Copper T-200. *Contraception*, **24**, 529

17. Fylling, P. and Fagerhol, M. (1979). Experience with two different medicated intra-uterine devices: a comparative study of the progestasert and Nova-T. *Fertil. Steril.*, **31**, 138

18. Nilsson, C. G., Luukkainen, T., Diaz, J. and Allonen, H. (1982). Clinical perform-ance of a new levonorgestrel-releasing intrauterine device. A randomized compari-son with a Nova-T-Copper device. *Contraception*, **25**, 345

19. Phariss, B. B. (1978). Clinical experience with the intrauterine progesterone contraceptive system. *J. Reprod. Med.*, **20**, 155

20. Gibor, Y. and Mitchell, C. (1980). Selected events following insertion of the Progestasert system. *Contraception*, **21**, 491

21. Wan, L. S. (1981). Clinical experience with Progestasert beyond one year of use. *Contracept. Deliv. Syst.*, **2**, 243

27
Steroid-releasing vaginal rings: a review

P. J. ROWE

INTRODUCTION

The vaginal route of administration of contraceptive steroids offers a number of advantages over oral or injectable preparations. Firstly, the device can be inserted, removed and replaced by the subject herself without the need of medical or paramedical personnel. The fact that it is *in situ* can be easily checked which is not always the case with an IUD. The vaginal rings that have been developed have a constant release rate of drug which results in steady plasma levels which is not the case with oral preparations[1]. The vaginal absorption of the steroid avoids the 'first pass' effect of the liver which means that the drug reaches the target organ without having entered the enterohepatic circulation.

Important in the case of accidental pregnancy, plasma levels of the drug rapidly reach zero following removal of the ring. The removal half-life of levonorgestrel in 26 subjects wearing the WHO 20 μg ring has been reported as 16.1 hours[2]. Obviously this would not be the case in injectable preparations. The intravaginal ring is not coitally related and does not involve the introduction of creams, gels or foaming tablets. Finally, the ring has the potential for 'over the counter' distribution as with condoms, spermicidal agents and diaphragms, which extends the potential acceptor market for the product. This advantage, however, may be confined only to those rings that

301

release only a progestational steroid rather than those rings designed to release both an oestrogen and a progestogen as they may have fewer metabolic side-effects.

It has been recognized since 1918 that the vagina is a suitable site for the administration of drugs that will reach the systemic circulation[3,4] and in 1964 Folkman and Long[5] described the absorption and subsequent release of dyes from silicone polymers. The ability of the polymer Silastic 382 to release steroids over a prolonged period was first observed in 1965 by Dzuik and Cook[7]. These three findings were brought together in the patent issued to Dr Gordon Duncan of Upjohn Ltd. in 1968[7] which describes a vaginal ring composed of a silicone polymer which could release a number of progestational steroids for contraceptive purposes.

The first publication on the use of a vaginal ring releasing a progestational steroid appeared in 1970[8]. In this study women had a vaginal ring releasing medroxyprogesterone acetate placed in the vagina for 28 days. In all subjects ovulation was suppressed, with a rapid return after removal of the ring. In this study, the drug was homogeneously mixed with the polymer which resulted in a pronounced initial release of drug – the burst effect. The rings were moulded around a stiff, flat metal spring similar to that used in diaphragms and the spring was thought to be the cause of erosion and ulceration of the vaginal mucosa in 13 of the 19 volunteers[9].

In 1973, Henzl and co-workers published the first description of vaginal rings that mimicked the minipill approach of low-dose progestogen-only release. In this study, varying thicknesses of the outer membrane of polymer were shown to alter the estimated release rate of chlormadinone acetate. Thirty women were studied over 35 cycles and ovulation was not consistently inhibited.

Three publications on the intravaginal release of medroxyprogesterone acetate have appeared, all of which reported suppression of ovulation[10-12] when the rings were loaded with between 55 and 200 mg of the drug.

From 1972, research on steroid-releasing intravaginal rings has concentrated upon two approaches. The Population Council of New York began the development of a ring that was *in situ* for 3 weeks and then removed for 1 week to induce withdrawal bleeding. This ring is intended to inhibit ovulation and will be described more fully below.

The World Health Organization's Special Programme of Research in Human Reproduction's research has concentrated upon the development of the low-dose progestogen-only approach with a minimum of ovulation inhibition but relying upon local pharmacological effects on the cervical mucus and endometrium.

Initially the WHO research concentrated upon progesterone itself, norethisterone and levonorgestrel[13]. However, as a result of excessive menstrual disturbances and too many involuntary pregnancies, progesterone and norethisterone rings were abandoned[14].

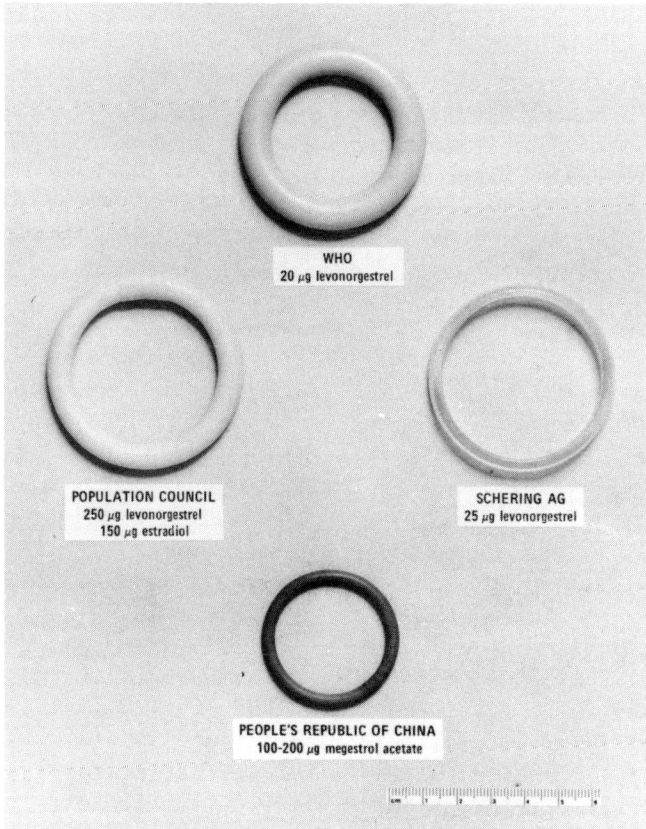

Figure 1 Steroid-releasing vaginal rings

Other progestogens that have been studied in vaginal rings include progesterone itself[15] and the steroid R2323[16,17].

CURRENT CLINICAL RESEARCH

There are four types of vaginal rings under current development that release hormonal steroids and these are shown in Figure 1.

Population Council ring

The Population Council has adopted the approach of developing a ring that releases levonorgestrel and oestradiol in amounts sufficient to inhibit ovulation consistently. Two sizes of rings have been tested – 50 and 58 mm. Each ring has a core of silastic with a layer of drug-loaded polymer containing 100 mg levonorgestrel and 50 mg of oestradiol and this layer is coated with a further layer of silastic. The larger rings release an average of 290 µg levonorgestrel and 180 µg of oestrogen and the 50 mm rings release 250 µg and 50 µg respectively[18].

These rings remain in the vagina for 3 weeks and then are removed by the subjects for 1 week to induce a withdrawal menstrual bleed. After 6 months of use approximately 60% of drug remains in the ring.

Table 1 Clinical results of Population Council vaginal rings. 1-year termination and continuation rates per 100 women*

Result	Rates
Pregnancy	1.0 – 1.8
Medical termination	22.5 – 23.5
Use-related	4.4 – 6.6
Personal reasons	8.8 – 9.7
Continuation	48.8 – 50.4
Expulsions	Not stated
Woman-months (both ring types)	8251

*Adapted from reference 19.

The published clinical results are summarized in Table 1. The two sets of data result from the two rings being studied in the same trial. A control group of subjects were allocated to a conventional low-dose combination oral contraceptive[19]. Pregnancy rates in the three groups were comparable. The continuation rates with the rings were significantly higher than in the pill users. More ring users discontinued for menstrual problems than the pill users as they did for vaginal problems, the commonest of which was vaginal discharge.

More women on the pill discontinued for other medical reasons such as nausea and headaches.

15–21% of ring users experienced one or more expulsions. In all three groups there was an increase in haemoglobin values and little or no changes were seen in blood pressure[20]. There was no evidence of impairment of carbohydrate metabolism or liver function in the ring users but the low-density lipoprotein:high-density lipoprotein ratio was significantly elevated but did not reach the mean value for healthy men[21].

A paper on this ring has been published in which the vaginal bacteriological flora were studied in ring and oral contraceptive users[22]. After 6 months of use there were no statistically significant differences in colony counts between the two age groups and the authors concluded that the use of the ring is not associated with a greater growth of pathogens than with an oral contraceptive.

Progestogen-only vaginal rings

Two types of these rings are currently under development by the World Health Organization and by scientists in the People's Republic of China. The continuous use of these rings, with a near constant zero-order release rate, has the potential of steady plasma levels of the steroid and avoiding the extreme fluctuations found with oral contraceptives and the very high initial plasma levels found with injectable preparations. Both rings have release rates that do not consistently inhibit ovulation.

Table 2 Clinical results of Chinese vaginal rings. 1-year termination and continuation rates per 100 women*

Result	Rate
Pregnancy	8.5
Continuation	43.5
Breakthrough bleeding	23% first cycle
	5% twelfth cycle
Expulsion	131/503 women
	112 women discontinued

*Liu Chi-Ming; personal communication.

The Chinese ring consists of a tube of polymer which is filled with megestrol acetate and then both ends are sealed together to form a diameter of 40 mm. As the walls of the ring are relatively thin the release rate tends to be high initially after insertion. Release rates have been quoted as between 100 and 200 μg per day[23]. A summary of one of the published studies from Shanghai is shown in Table 2. It should be pointed out that other Chinese studies have had much lower pregnancy rates, e.g. 2.15 per 100 women in 16 000 woman-months experience. Intermenstrual bleeding has been reported in between 5 and 8% of treatment cycles. In one study[24] 26% of the woman experienced ring expulsion which happened frequently enough to account for 22% of the reasons for discontinuation. The probable reason for this is that the rings are more likely to be expelled at defaecation especially in those who squat. In view of the relatively high pregnancy rate, consideration is being given to increasing the release rate of megestrol acetate.

Table 3   Clinical results of WHO vaginal rings. 360-day cumulative net life-table rates per 100 women*

Result	Rate	Standard error
Pregnancy	3.6	1.2
Menstrual disturbance	12.7	1.8
Repeated expulsion	3.3	0.8
Non-medical reasons	10.4	1.5
Continuation rate	64.5	2.4
No. of acceptors	689	
Woman-months	4081	

*From 17 centres in 12 countries.

The WHO vaginal ring is constructed differently from the other two types described in this review. A core containing 5 mg levonorgestrel is moulded and then enclosed by two semi-circular rings. The thickness of the outer layer of the silastic determines the release rate, which has been set at 20 μg per day. The ring has an outside diameter of 55.6 mm and a cross-section of 9.5 mm. This device remains in the vagina continuously for 90 days and it is then replaced. The subjects are encouraged not to remove the device for intercourse or menstruation.

The pharmacokinetics and dynamics of this ring have been extensively studied at the WHO centre in Stockholm[2]. Following insertion of the ring, plasma levels of levonorgestrel rose very rapidly reaching a final near steady state of approximately $1 \, \mathrm{nmol \, l^{-1}}$ within 30 minutes. After this, the plasma levels remained stable and diminished very slowly in a linear fashion, corresponding to a daily decrease of 0.2–0.3%. In 69 treatment cycles studied in 20 women, 29% of cycles were judged to be anovulatory, 19% had inadequate luteal function and 52% were considered to be normal. Intermenstrual bleeding occurred most frequently in the anovulatory cycles (37%).

Plasma levels of the drug fell very rapidly after ring removal with a half-life time of 16.1 hours after 90 days use, which emphasizes the need for continuous use of the ring. Table 3 gives details of the ongoing WHO clinical trial which is being undertaken in 17 centres in 12 countries. As can be seen, the commonest reason for discontinuation is menstrual disturbance. In the three Chinese centres, 70% of these complaints related to intermenstrual bleeding or spotting as opposed to 51% in the other centres.

The frequency of menstrual complaints fell from 23% of subjects at 3 months of use to 6% after 1 year of use. The protocol of the study calls for women who have more than three expulsions in any one month to be dropped from the study. This has occurred on 16 occasions.

A total of 130 women (20%) experienced one or more ring expulsions and in 54% of the time this took place at defaecation. With 80% of the subjects who had an expulsion it occurred no more than twice.

Five women discontinued the method because their partners complained of the ring interfering with coitus. There were five discontinuations for excess vaginal discharge and one for vaginal infection. Ten subjects have been lost to follow-up.

Table 4 compares these results with those from WHO randomized multicentre trials[25–27] on a combination oral contraceptive, a levonor-

Table 4 Use-effective life-table rates for involuntary pregnancy at 360 days (WHO studies)

Contraceptive	Rate
Oral contraceptives:	
30 µg LNG only	9.5
150 µg LNG/30 µg EE	3.5
Intravaginal ring (20 µg LNG WHO ring)	3.6
Progesterone-releasing IUD	2.4
(Alza T IPCS 52)	

EE = Ethinyloestradiol; LNG = Levonorgestrel.

307

gestrel-only pill and the Alza progesterone IUD. It can be seen that the 20 μg ring has a 1-year pregnancy rate which is comparable with the low-dose combination pill and the progesterone IUD and very much lower than that found with the levonorgestrel minipill.

Therefore, in summary, the progestogen–oestrogen vaginal ring would appear to be as effective and acceptable as oral contraceptives but with the issue of the changes in the HDL-cholesterol:LDL-chlloresterol ratio unresolved.

The WHO levonorgestrel-only ring – although in the early stages of extensive clinical testing – has the promise of being at least as effective as a low-dose oral contraceptive.

All three types of ring have the potential advantages that were mentioned at the beginning of the chapter: self-administration, ease of insertion and reinsertion, not coitally related, less metabolic side-effects than oral contraceptives and hence the potential for public distribution with minimal or no medical supervision.

References

1. Stanczyk, F. Z., Hiro, M., Goebelsmann, U., Brenner, P. F., Lumkin, M. E. and Mishell, D. R. (1975). Radioimmunoassay of serum D-norgestrel in women following oral and intravaginal administration. *Contraception*, **12**, 279
2. Landgren, B-M., Johannisson, E., Masironi, B. and Diczfalusy, E. (1982). Pharmacokinetic and pharmacodynamic investigations with vaginal devices releasing levonorgestrel at a constant, near zero-order rate. *Contraception*, **26**, 576
3. Macht, D. I. (1918). The absorption of drugs and poisons through the vagina. *J. Pharmacol. Pathol.*, **10**, 509
4. Hartman, C. G. (1959). The permeability of the vaginal mucosa. *Ann. N.Y. Acad. Sci.*, **83**, 857
5. Folkman, J. and Long, D. M. (1964). Drug pacemakers in the treatment of heart block. *Ann. N.Y. Acad. Sci.*, **111**, 857
6. Dzuik, P. J. and Cook, B. (1965). Passage of steroids through silicone rubber. *Endocrinology*, **78**, 208
7. Duncan, G. W. *Medicated Devices and Methods*. U.S. Patent No. 3,545,439
8. Mishell, D. R., Talas, M. and Parlow, A. F. (1970). Contraception by means of Silastic vaginal ring impregnated with medroxyprogesterone acetate. *Am. J. Obstet. Gynecol.*, **107**, 100
9. Mishell, D. R. and Lumkin, M. E. (1970). Contraceptive effect of varying doses of progestogen in Silastic vaginal rings. *Fertil. Steril.*, **21**, 9910
10. Mishell, D. R., Lumkin, M. and Stone, S. (1972). Inhibition of ovulation with cyclic use of progestogen-impregnated intravaginal devices. *Am. J. Obstet. Gynecol.*, **113**, 927
11. Zanartu, J. and Guerrero. R. (1973). Steroid release from polymer vaginal devices. Effect on fertility inhibition. *Steroids*, **21**, 325
12. Thiery, M., Vandekerckhove, D., Dhont, M., Vermeulen, A. and Decoster, J. M. (1976). The medroxyprogesterone acetate intravaginal Silastic ring as a contraceptive device. *Contraception*, **13**, 605

13. World Health Organization's Special Programme of Research, Development and Research Training in Human Reproduction (1979). Intravaginal and intracervical devices for the delivery of fertility regulating agents. *J. Steroid Biochem.*, **11**, 461

14. Gallegos, A. J. (1980). Vaginal steroidal contraception. In Zatuchni, G. *et al.* (eds.). *Research Frontiers in Fertility Regulation.* PARFR series on Fertility Regulation, pp. 230–36. (Hagerstown, Md.: Harper and Row)

15. Victor, A., Jackanicz, T. M. and Johansson, E. D. B. (1978). Vaginal progesterone for contraception. *Fertil. Steril.*, **30**, 631

16. Johansson, E. D. B., Luukkainen, T., Vartiainen, E. and Victor, A. (1975). The effect of progestin R2323 released from vaginal rings on ovarian function. *Contraception*, **12**, 299

17. Akinla, O., Lahteenmaki, P. and Jackaniez, T. M. (1976). Intravaginal contraception with the synthetic progestin R2323. *Contraception*, **14**, 671

18. Jackanicz, T. M. (1981). Levonorgestrel and estradiol release from an improved contraceptive vaginal ring. *Contraception*, **24**, 323

19. Sivin, I., Mishell, D. R., Victor, A. *et al.* (1981). A multicentre study of levonorgestrel–oestradiol contraceptive vaginal rings. I – use effectiveness. *Contraception*, **24**, 341

20. Sivin, I., Mishell, D. R., Victor, A. *et al.* (1981). A multicentre study of levonorgestrel–oestradiol contraceptive vaginal rings. II – subjective and objective measures of effects. *Contraception*, **24**, 359

21. Ahren, T., Lithell, H., Victor, A., Vessby, B. and Johansson, E. D. B. (1981). Comparison of the metabolic effects of two hormonal contraceptive methods: an oral formulation and a vaginal ring. II serum lipoproteins and apoliproteins. *Contraception*, **24**, 451

22. Roy, S., Wilkins, J. and Mishell, D. R. (1981). The effect of a contraceptive vaginal ring and contraceptives on the vaginal flora. *Contraception*, **24**, 481

23. Liu Qui-ming, Zheng Kang-Qi, Xu Xiang-hua, Heseh Chung-ming and Chen Xun (1981). Studies on megestrol acetate intravaginal Silastic ring as a new contraceptive device. *Reprod. Contracept.*, **1**, 29

24. Liu Chi-ming (1983). New long-acting contraceptive delivery system megestrol-acetate silicone rubber vaginal rings. *Presented at the National Symposium on Long-acting Agents for Contraception*, Hangzhou, People's Republic of China, 14–15 January

25. World Health Organization's Task Force on Oral Contraceptives (1982). A randomized double blind study of six combined oral contraceptives. *Contraception*, **25**, 231

26. World Health Organization's Task Force on Oral Contraceptives (1982). A randomized double blind study of two combined and two progestogen-only contraceptives. *Contraception*, **25**, 243

27. World Health Organization's Task Force on Intrauterine Devices (1983). The Alza T IPCS 52 progesterone releasing IUD. Results of WHO-sponsored randomized clinical trials. *Clin. Reprod. Fertil.* (In press)

28
Postcoital contraception: experiences with ethinyloestradiol/norgestrel and levonorgestrel only

K. O. K. HOFFMANN

In May 1976 the Government of the Federal Republic of Germany introduced an important Penal Law Amendment which incorporated a change in the existing abortion law. On the whole it became more liberalized. Furthermore, the new law confirms that 'All methods of birth control used before implantation of the ovum is completed, are not defined as "termination of pregnancy" '. All sorts of implantation-interfering methods can now be used legally during the first 4 weeks following a menstrual period. This law gave the legal basis for an official approach using postcoital methods in Germany.

Now, 7 years after the introduction of this law, the majority of doctors are not aware of the legal position. It is not surprising that the application of morning-after methods is often associated with early abortion and closely linked to the moral and personal conviction of doctors. This timidity to act possibly illegally might be one of the main reasons that the knowledge of postcoital birth control is still not used enough and is even widely opposed.

Many publications about postcoital techniques can be found in scientific literature of the last 10 years. But they have not played a major role in family planning yet. The client-orientated family planning organizations have been challenged to find means and methods

311

for a more generalized application for the benefit of the population of fertile age[1].

These considerations influenced the German Association for Family Planning and Sexual Counselling, Pro Familia, in initiating a Morning-after Service Programme at the end of 1979. It was part of a more comprehensive project concerned with the needs and problems of specific target-groups in the society, especially young couples and the different categories of single people[2]. The disadvantages of continuous and systemic birth control methods – e.g. the pill, injectables and IUDs – are well known, especially in young people. Coitus-related barrier methods, such as condoms, diaphragm or spermicidal preparations, are appropriate for irregular and spontaneous sexual relationships. But in many cases the necessary skill for their application cannot be achieved; and the ruptured condom or the incorrectly placed diaphragm could easily lead to an unwanted pregnancy. Especially for these circumstances, a simple back-up method for the morning after coitus without serious side-effects would be helpful to avoid all the physical and psychological problems associated with therapeutic abortion.

After reviewing scientific literature we found the combined oestrogen/progestogen method as described by Yuzpe et al. in Canada[3] suitable to be used as a good example of reliable postcoital prevention of pregnancy. This method did not have the discouraging side-effects of the concentrated oestrogen application which contributed to the predominantly bad image of 'morning-after vomiting' in the past. The method comprised taking four tablets, each containing 0.05 mg ethinyloestradiol and 0.5 mg norgestrel. The first two tablets were taken not later then 48 hours after coitus and the other two were taken after a further 12 hours.

The original Yuzpe[3] scheme was slightly modified, limiting the use of this method for 48 hours. If we look at the enormous hormone concentration of ethinyloestradiol used in the past (especially in comparison with the amount contained in a normal combined low-dose contraceptive pill) it seems to be quite clear that a more widespread use is definitely not advisable[4]:

(1) Oestrogen/progestogen postcoital treatment (Yuzpe et al.[3]) – ethinyloestradiol, 0.2 mg; norgestrel, 2.0 mg.
(2) Oestrogen-only postcoital treatment (Haspels[4]) – ethinyloestradiol, 25.0 mg.

(3) Progestogen-only postcoital treatment (modified Kesserü *et al.*[5]) – levonorgestrel, 0.6 mg.

(4) Combined low-dose contraceptive pill (21 pills) – ethinyloestradiol, 0.63 mg; levonorgestrel, 3.15 mg.

It seems worthwhile mentioning the recommendation of the combined hormonal method by the Central Council of the IPPF in November 1981[6]. The Medical Committee of Pro Familia is still recommending a progestogen-only postcoital method (one tablet, 600 mg levonorgestrel) within 12 hours after unprotected intercourse.

The idea using progestogens was first described by Kesserü *et al.* in 1973[5]. As long as no suitable single-dose tablet is on the market we are advocating the immediate use of an appropriate levonorgestrel-containing mini-pill.

RESULTS

The evaluation of 737 postcoital applications of two different hormonal methods during the last 3 years in 26 family planning centres of Pro Familia gave the following results.

The age distribution (Figure 1) shows a significant demand for these methods by younger women. 85% of all users were aged under 28 years; almost 30% were teenagers between 14 and 18 years.

The reasons for using a postcoital method were as follows:

(1) Unprotected intercourse (46%).
(2) 'Troubles' with the condom (slipped off, tears, holes) (36%).
(3) 'Troubles' with diaphragm (wrong size, incorrectly placed, etc.) (5%).
(4) Forgetting the 'pill', etc. (5%).
(5) Coitus interruptus (2%).
(6) Spermicide alone used (2%).
(7) Unknown, 'very anxious', calender, basal body temperature, etc. (4%).

What is remarkable is the high percentage of problems associated with using a condom. Even if we expect the majority of the trouble to be due to the users we should consider the advice we are giving with this method becoming popular again, especially in comparison with the time-consuming procedure of instructing how to use the diaphragm.

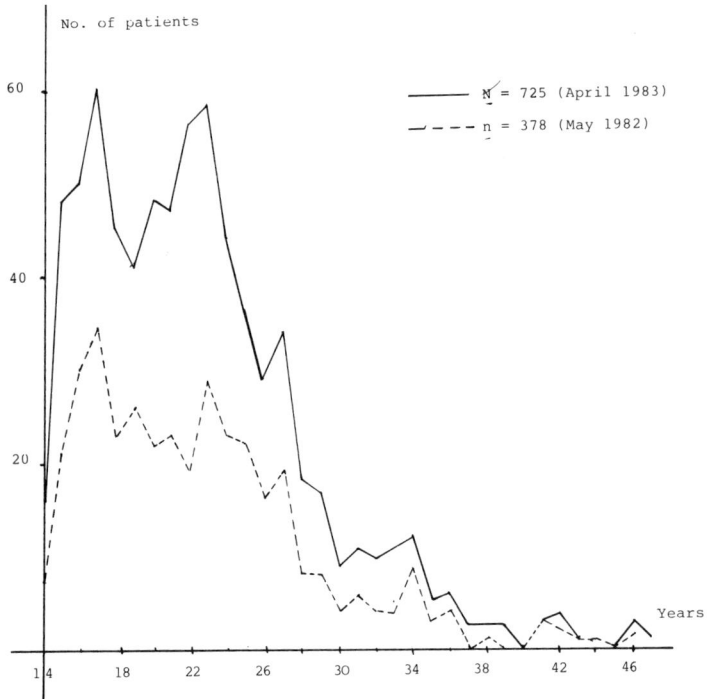

No. of patients

60

40

20

――――― N = 725 (April 1983)

― ― ― ― n = 378 (May 1982)

Years

14   18   22   26   30   34   38   42   46

Figure 1 Age distribution of postcoital-pill users

Approximately 70% of the clients were treated within 24 hours, and 95% were able to contact our advisory centres within 48 hours after unprotected intercourse. 25% began treatment within 12 hours and a further 44% from 13 to 24 hours after intercourse. A further 27% began treatment from 25 to 48 hours; 4% began treatment more than 49 hours after intercourse. In 1% the time after intercourse on starting treatment was not known.

Almost two-thirds of the clients were treated in the middle of the menstrual cycle. In contrast to Yuzpe et al.[7] no special formula correcting different cycle length was used. At mid-cycle there is a 20% risk of pregnancy, according to calculations by Tietze[8] and James[9]. At any other time during the cycle there is an almost 5% chance of pregnancy (Table 1). Therefore, some 102 pregnancies would be expected in this group of 737 women.

314

Table 1 Cycle day of postcoital treatment ($n = 737$)

Day of cycle	No. of patients	Expected no. of pregnancies*	Risk (%)
1–9	54	3	5
10–18	435	87	20
19–27	178	9	5
28 and over	37	2	5
Unknown	22	1	5

* Total = 102.

Among 730 postcoital treatments we found 16 pregnancies *in utero*; no tubal pregnancy was reported. This gave a failure rate of 1.9% for the combined oestrogen/progestogen method, and 2.9% for the progestogen-only postcoital method (Table 2).

Table 2 Pregnancy rate after postcoital treatment ($n = 730$)

Method	No. of patients (%)	Pregnancies (%)
Combined	525 (72)	10 (1.9)
Progestogen-only	205 (28)	6 (2.9)

DISCUSSION AND OUTLOOK

In comparison with previous publications[1,2] we found that there is an increasing demand for postcoital contraception in the young population; infrequent sexual relationship is associated with relatively short experience in appropriate contraceptive methods (e.g. 'troubles' with condom use) or with the widespread 'taking chances'. The use of a highly effective hormonal morning-after method for prevention of unwanted pregnancies is definitely desirable. It seems to be a 'back-up method' in any case of emergency, and does not replace regular and skilfully used means of family planning.

The reported side-effects were nausea, vomiting and irregular cycles that were altogether mild and tolerable. The pregnancy rate of 1.9% for the combined ethinyloestradiol/norgestrel method is in accordance with other results[1,7]. The 2.9% failure rate with a single dose of levonorgestrel needs further investigation and confirmation.

With these results we are quite confident of spreading the knowl-

315

edge about the availability of these less invasive methods for the 'morning-after' to the medical profession as well as to the public. For both, a family planning organization such as Pro Familia is advocated.

Acknowledgements

The author wishes to acknowledge the 26 Pro Familia family planning centres for their great help, and to thank Ms Mia Volling for collecting data.

References

1. Grahame, H. (1983). Postcoital contraception. Methods, services and prospects; presented at a *Symposium in London, Pregnancy Advisory Service*, 15th April 1982
2. Hoffmann, K. O. K. (1982). Erfahrungen mit einem Postkoital-Versorgungsprogramm. *Sexualpädagogik und Familienplanung*, **6**, 13
3. Yupze, A. A., Thurlow, H. J., Ramzy, I. and Leyshon, J. I. (1974). Post-coital contraception – a pilot study. *J. Reprod. Med.*, **13**, 53
4. Haspels, A. A. (1976). Interception: Post-coital estrogens in 3016 women. *Contraception*, **14**, 375
5. Kesserü, E., Larranaga, A. and Parada, J. (1973). Postcoital contraception with D-norgestrel. *Contraception*, **7**, 367
6. IPPF (1981). *Policy Compendium, Appendix D, 2.1.1.0/02 (Nov. 1981)*
7. Yuzpe, A. A., Smith, R. P. and Rademaker, A. W. (1982). A multicenter clinical investigation employing ethinyl estradiol combined with dl-norgestrel as a postcoital contraceptive agent. *Fertil. Steril.*, **37**, 508
8. Tietze, C. (1980). Probability of pregnancy resulting from a single unprotected coitus. *Fertil. Steril.*, **11**, 485
9. James, W. H. (1963). *Pop. Stud.*, **17**, 57

Part I

Section 8

Lactation and Birth Spacing

29
Lactation and birth spacing: an overview

M. A. BELSEY

In many developing countries, the contraceptive effect of breast feeding, more than any other method of control, promotes the larger spacing of births. As shown in the studies reported by McNeilly and his colleagues suckling frequency, i.e. greater than 5 times per day and intensity, i.e. 10 minutes per feed, was associated with failure of follicular growth and ovulation. The decrease in frequency or intensity of ovulation may be brought about by such practices as scheduled rather than on-demand feedings, reduction in night feeds, introduction of bottle feeding, and use of 'pacifiers'.

We thus see a shift in the duration (and probably the intensity and frequency) of breast feeding from the long duration of 15 or more months in more traditional societies, to either a failure to start or only a short duration of breast feeding in more 'modern' urbanized societies (WHO Collaborative Studies).

Lactational anovulation associated with amenorrhoea is highly effective in preventing conception. Thus corresponding to the prolonged duration of breast feeding is a prolonged duration of amenorrhoea.

Once ovulation occurs, it will in most instances be followed by menstruation. Conception, without prior menstruation, however does occur in a small proportion of women. The risk of conception is least during the early post-partum months, but studies have shown that, even after 18 months, no more than 5–10% of women are likely to conceive prior to resumption of menstruation. Even so, in comparison to a discontinuation of breast feeding in the absence of other contraceptive use, breast feeding has an effectiveness comparable to barrier methods and even hormonal contraceptives in some developing country settings.

Prolonged breast feeding is a way of life in many developing countries. Infants often sleep next to their mothers, at times feeding without even waking them, they are with their mothers at all times and thus can be demand-fed without difficulty. Any change in the breast feeding practices in the developing world that reduces the present high incidence and long duration of breast feeding and the high frequency of suckling is likely to increase fertility. The current situation in Kenya is an example: hence the decline in the duration of breast feeding and adherence to post-partum abstinence taboos over the past decades has brought about increased fertility while the adoption of other contraceptive teaching has failed to keep pace. As a result of this rise in fertility and coincident decline in mortality, Kenya today has one of the highest population growth rates in the world, i.e. the population will double in approximately 17 years.

If the duration of breast feeding and the consequent lactational amenorrhoea and anovulation were to decrease in the developing world from their current levels to a mean duration of three months the results would be truly catastrophic. In many instances for these countries to just maintain their already high fertility rates the prevalence of contraceptive use would have to increase to incredible levels in countries where contraceptive practice has increased only slowly. Thus a five fold increase in contraceptive use – from 9% to 52% – would be required in Bangladesh to maintain current fertility rates.

The decrease in birth spacing in turn contributes to the further deterioration of the quality of life for the most disadvantaged groups in our population. The combination of short birth spacing with heavy work demands and poor nutrition contributes significantly to low birth weight which in turn contributes to high perinatal and infant mortality rates. In much of Africa 15% of all infants are less than 2500 g, while in many areas of India the rates are 25–40%. Not unexpectedly the infant and child mortality rates of infants born less than one year after a previous pregnancy are significantly increased.

There are many factors contributing to the decline in breast feeding not the least of which has been the role, status and perceptions of women accompanying what we call social and economic develop-

320

ment. The US, the trend setter for so much of what is perceived of and sought after as 'modern' culture, has been among the trend setters in the decline of breast feeding, to be followed by a decline in other countries.

In most economies women are entering the work force in increasing numbers, such that in many developed countries the majority of women work most often as a consequence of economic necessity but also as an expression and demand for social recognition. Most countries' maternity legislation, even those with the most progressive laws, is geared to the protection of the mother's health or the promotion of fertility. Rarely does such legislation specify the promotion of breast feeding, and with few exceptions rarely exceeds 2 or 3 months, whereas the now recognized duration of full breast feeding without a need for supplementation is 4–6 months. There is rarely any specification or requirement for the provision of creches or allowance for breast feeding breaks in institutions employing large numbers of women. Socioeconomic activity of women in the developing world also affects the patterns of breast feeding and as a consequence infant mortality. Planting or harvesting seasons which require an intense input of additional hands are associated with a decrease in frequency of breast feeding. If, as is often the case, such seasons coincide with the depletion of the last season's food stores, and decreased time availability for the preparation of appropriate weaning foods, the timing or amount of supplemental feeding may be delayed at a time when breast feeding alone is not sufficient to sustain infant growth. Malnutrition may ensue and the early death of the infant result in a further acceleration of the cycle of short birth spacing, low birth-weight, malnutrition and infant death.

Within a community although the more advantaged social classes have often through their role models led the decline in breast feeding, equally so they can and have contributed to the resurgence and return to breast feeding. With the greater understanding of the benefits of breast feeding and the factors contributing to its decline it is hoped that the developing countries will not have to go through the transition of low rates of breast feeding in the mistaken perception that formula-feeding is modern and 'as good as mother's milk'.

One of the major factors in the decline in breast feeding among mothers in the developed world has been the ignorance of health workers as to the multiple health benefits of breast feeding and a lack of understanding of the physiology of breast feeding including ways in which it can be technically supported. As a consequence many of the practices within our own health care systems hinder rather than promote the optimal pattern of breast feeding appropriate to our own society. The wide scope of scientific knowledge on the health benefits of breast feeding has been consolidated only in the last decade or so. Our increasing understanding of the subtle nutrition requirements of newborn infants has caused the infant food industry to continue to invest in the past large sums in research and promotion to find and hopefully to sell the product that is the 'perfect substitute' for mother's milk. The perfect food for infants is breast milk. It is readily available to and economically affordable by all mothers regardless of social class or nutritional status.

The World Health Assembly several years ago discussed and passed, with only one dissenting vote, a resolution on infant and young child feeding in which among other points was recommended an international code of marketing for breast milk substitutes. Among the points recommended was that in their information materials to health professionals and in the labelling of their products the companies should indicate that breast feeding is the best form of nutrition for newborn infants. Virtually all companies producing 'breast milk substitutes' have complied, but all have added a qualifying 'but'. But if for some reason you are unable to breast feed then 'our product is the best substitute'.

The seeds of doubt are widely strewn, when in fact the only real basis, except in very rare instances, for not being able to breast feed, are social circumstance reasons.

Breast feeding promotion and instruction must begin during antenatal care, and not as is the usual case, at the time of the delivery when the physician or nurse, with waiting hormone in hand, asks in a perfunctory way, 'Are you going to breast-feed or not?' Potential problems in breast feeding need to be diagnosed, such as flattened or inverted nipples, and remedial care provided. Explanations as to the why and how of breast feeding are essential. The best providers of supportive information to expectant mothers on breast feeding are women who have already breast-fed, who know the pleasures, the hows and the problems of breast feeding. The information support from such groups of women provides an important psychological boost to mothers wishing to breast feed both before and after delivery. Needless to say the handbooks must be both informed and supportive

322

as well. Such women-to-women education and support is effective in both developed and developing countries.

Maternity practices are frequently counter-productive to the promotion of breast feeding. There is really no scientific nor psychosocial basis for removing the healthy newborn from the mother for a variable number of hours, often 12 or even 18 hours, after delivery. Assuming it is dried and breathing normally, the newborn can be put to breast immediately, even in the delivery room. The effects are multiple. The nipple stimulation results in an almost immediate and potent release of oxytocin contributing to effective uterine contraction and control of post-partum haemorrhage. The mother's body heat serves to assist in limiting temperature loss by the newborn, and, as has been ably shown by Klaus and his colleagues, the immediate and continued contact, or bonding of mother and infant, significantly enhances the development of the infant well beyond the period of breast feeding.

Thus the large 'super-market' newborn nurseries are both outmoded and dangerous. There is no reason for such facilities for healthy newborns in any future maternity hospitals. Those that exist should be re-examined and considered for remodelling to make better and safer use of the space. Rooming-in, even in a bamboo walled, clay packed floored maternity ward is far safer than the supposedly aseptic nursery.

In conclusion it must be re-emphasized that breast feeding associated with lactational amenorrhoea and anovulation is an effective method of birth spacing. It is a birth spacing method available to all mothers, can be practiced by virtually all mothers, and in some again and again even many years after a pregnancy as shown in an instance of relactation in a Zimbabwean grandmother whose daughter died in childbirth.

30
Clinical, hormonal and ultrasonic indicators of returning fertility after childbirth

A. M. FLYNN, S. S. LYNCH, M. DOCKER
and R. MORRIS

INTRODUCTION

It is well known that women enjoy varying periods of infertility after childbirth, depending mainly on whether they breast feed. It is also acknowledged that lactating women are infertile for longer periods than those who do not breast feed[1-3]. To date, what is not so well established is the precise physiological mechanism that regulates this lactational infertility. Several factors seem to be involved, such as:

(1) The high levels of plasma prolactin in lactating women[4].
(2) The influence of the suckling stimulus[5].
(3) The effect of maternal diet and malnutrition in reducing fertility during the lactational period[6].

Longitudinal physiological studies correlating some or all of these factors have already started and are indeed much needed to establish the contribution of lactation to contraception. For persons and programmes involved in providing advice and guidance in natural methods of family planning in the post-partum period there is, however, a more urgent and important question to be answered: can women recognize, by subjective observation of clinical signs and symptoms, the beginning of fertility? If lactation is to play an important role in birth regulation, we must be able to answer this question in the affirmative[7]. This study was designed to provide information in an attempt to answer this question. The study is still ongoing and this chapter presents the results for the first 14 women.

SUBJECTS AND METHODS

Six of the women were 'ecological' breast feeders, four were partial breast feeders and four were non-breast feeders. The title ecological breast feeder is given to those lactating women who fed their babies on demand day and night. The interval between feeds and the time of feeding was regulated by the infant and consequently varies from woman to woman. However, in practice, it is usual for the mother to feed her infant every 3 hours or less and for an average of 10 minutes per feed. When artificial feeding is introduced it is in the form of solid foods so that the infant continues to suckle at the same rate and time as previously. Lactation in this manner is continued for at least 30 weeks and generally for a much longer period.

Those women who breast fed but also introduced liquids and bottle feeding were considered to be partial lactators. The non-lactators never breast fed their infants.

The mean age of the women was 28 years and their ages ranged from 23 to 34. Mean parity was 2, with a range of 1–4. Twelve of the women had a spontaneous vaginal delivery and two underwent caesarean section. All of the infants were healthy. Fourteen of the women had symptothermal charts collected from them, 14 had weekly plasma prolactin estimations, five had estimations for plasma oestrogen, LH, FSH and progesterone values and two of the women had serial ultrasonic measurement of the follicles.

Symptothermal charts

These were charted by the women from the time of delivery until after the first apparent ovulation. Basal body temperature, cervical mucus observations, changes in the uterine cervix and other indicators of fertility such as ovulation pain and breast changes were noted when they occurred. Particular emphasis was placed on detecting changes in the uterine cervix by autopalpation since this appears to

326

be the most distinctive clinical indicator of impending ovulation in the post-partum period.

Infant feeding charts

These indicated the number of feeds and their duration and were kept for the 24-hour period. Anything that upset the infant feeding regimen was also noted.

HORMONAL ASSAYS

Basal prolactin levels

In order to estimate basal plasma prolactin levels, 10 ml of venous blood was collected weekly from each woman from the time of delivery until ovulation was presumed to have occurred. The blood

NON — LACTATORS

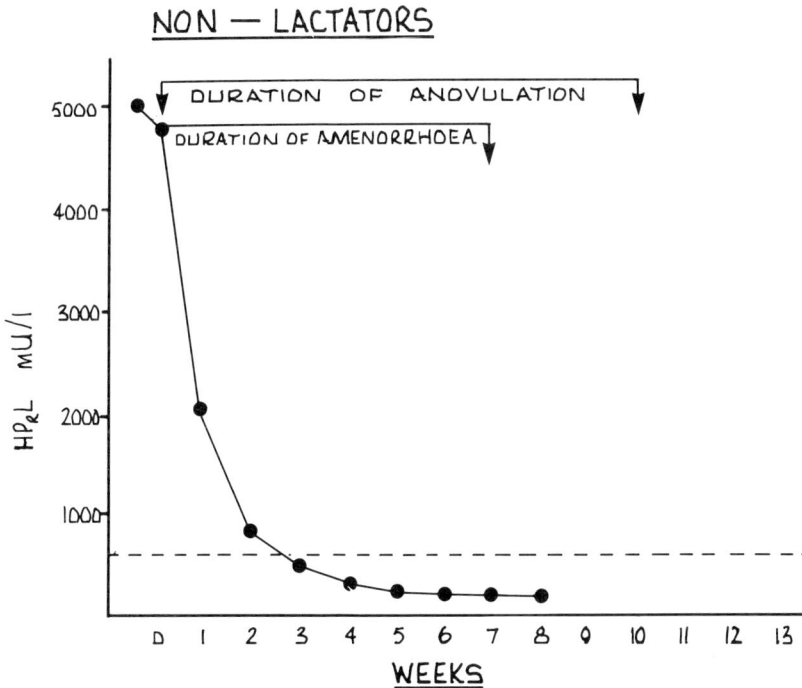

Figure 1   HPrL relative to returning menstruation and ovulation in non-breast feeders

327

was collected at least 2 hours after a feed or at longer intervals if convenient. The number of collections varied between six in some non-lactating women to 80 in one ecological breast feeder.

In addition, five women had daily collections of venous blood taken when they themselves, from their clinical indicators, estimated that fertility was returning. Plasma oestrogen, progesterone, LH and FSH levels were estimated in these samples.

Ultrasonic examinations

Two women had serial ultrasonic measurements of follicular growth when the clinical indicators suggested a return of fertility.

RESULTS

Figure 1 shows the duration of amenorrhoea and anovulation in weeks after delivery in the non-lactators and the basal levels of plasma prolactin over the same period. As other workers have shown, basal prolactin levels reached the non-pregnant state by 3 weeks post-partum.

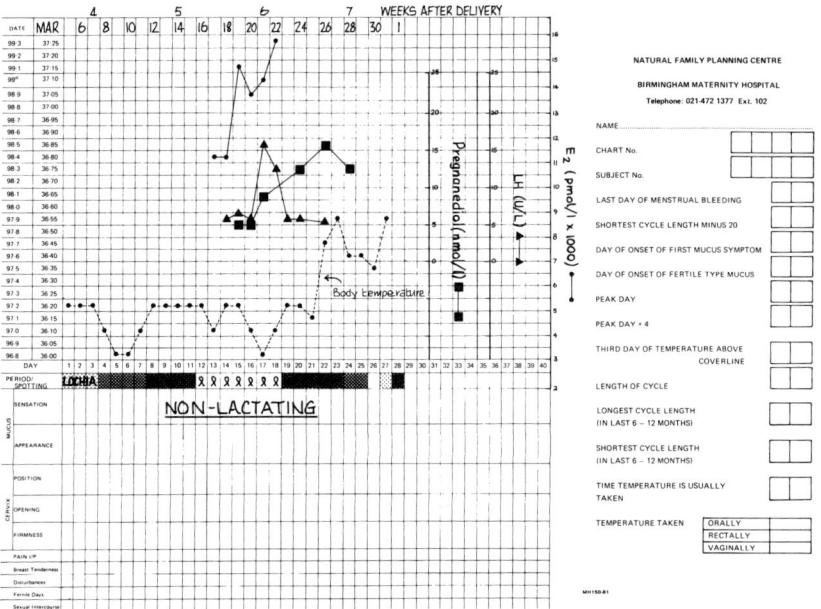

Figure 2   ST chart showing short luteal phase LH peak and high levels of progesterone

Figure 2 shows the symptothermal chart from one of these women. It illustrates the short luteal phase, so characteristic of returning fertility in these subjects. Inset in this figure are the plasma levels of oestrogen, LH and progesterone in this first ovulatory episode. An oestrogen peak of $1721\,pmol\,l^{-1}$, an LH surge from 1.5 to $18\,U\,l^{-1}$ within 24 hours and an increase in plasma progesterone from a pre-ovulatory level of $4\,nmol\,l^{-1}$ to $18\,nmol\,l^{-1}$ 5 days after the LH peak are all consistent with ovulation in our laboratory, and suggest that ovulation did indeed occur.

MIXED FEEDING

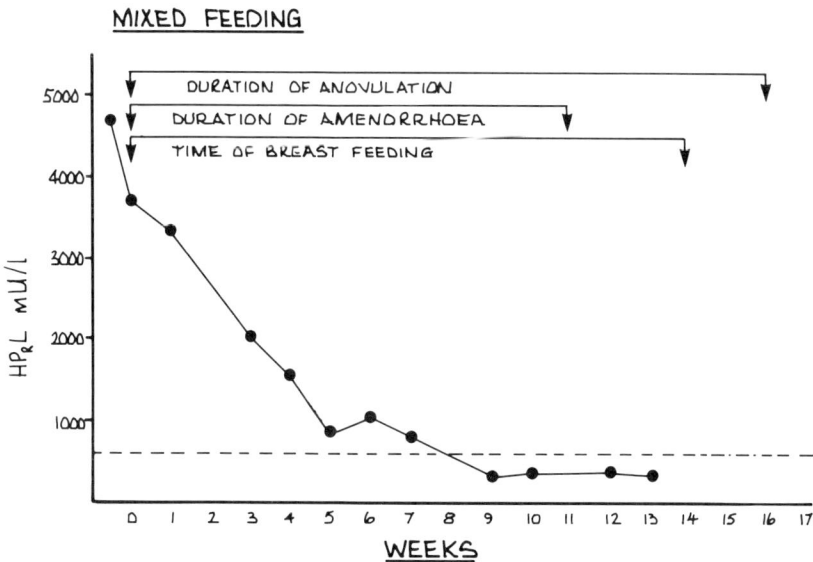

Figure 3 HPrL relative to returning menstruation and ovulation in partial breast feeders

Figure 3 gives the duration of amenorrhoea, anovulation and basal plasma prolactin levels in weeks after delivery for the partial breast feeders. Basal plasma prolactin levels had fallen to pre-pregnant levels at a mean of 8 weeks post-partum, menstruation occurred at a mean of 11 weeks and ovulation at a mean of 16 weeks post delivery. The introduction of bottle feeding caused a rapid return of fertility in these women.

329

Table 1 The duration of breast feeding and time of returning fertility in ecological breast-feeding women

Parameter	Mean (weeks)	Range (weeks)
Duration of breast feeding without supplementation	26	20–33
Total duration of breast feeding	50	42–62
Time from delivery to first significant bleed	44	30–69
Time from delivery to first ovulation (clinical, hormonal or ultrasonic data)	48	32–79

Table 1 gives the mean and range of duration of breast feeding and the mean and range for the period of amenorrhoea and anovulation in the six women who ecologically breast fed.

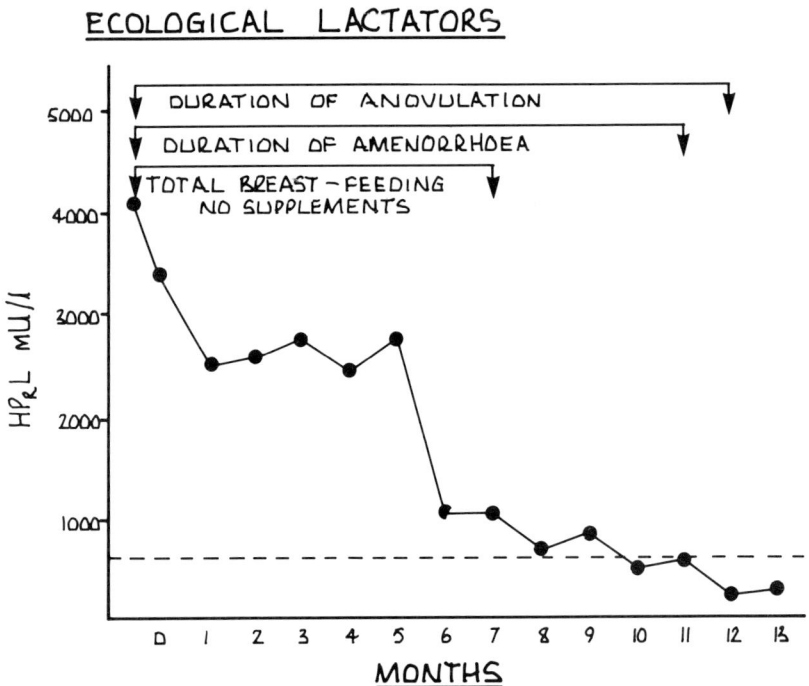

Figure 4 HPrL relative to returning menstruation and ovulation in the ecological breast feeders

Figure 4 shows the mean of the basal plasma prolactin levels for the same women. One can see that although there was a sharp drop in the basal plasma prolactin when artificial feeding was introduced the levels remain higher than the pre-pregnant levels until the 40th week post-partum.

Figure 5 shows the comparative plasma prolactin levels for the three sub-groups – the levels remained consistently elevated in the ecological breast feeders; a fact which may contribute to the prolonged infertility in this group of women.

Figure 6 shows the symptothermal chart of one of these ecological breast feeders at 44 weeks post-partum, a month prior to ovulation. The prolactin measurements are extremely low, well within the pre-pregnant levels. Suckling only occurs once a day yet this single suckling episode seems sufficient to delay the return of ovulation. Finally, when suckling is discontinued completely, fertility quickly returns, indicated by a peak mucus symptom, a clear temperature shift and a luteal phase of normal length followed by the first menstruation 48 weeks after delivery.

It appears, therefore, that in some ecological breast feeders very infrequent suckling can delay the return of fertility. This figure also

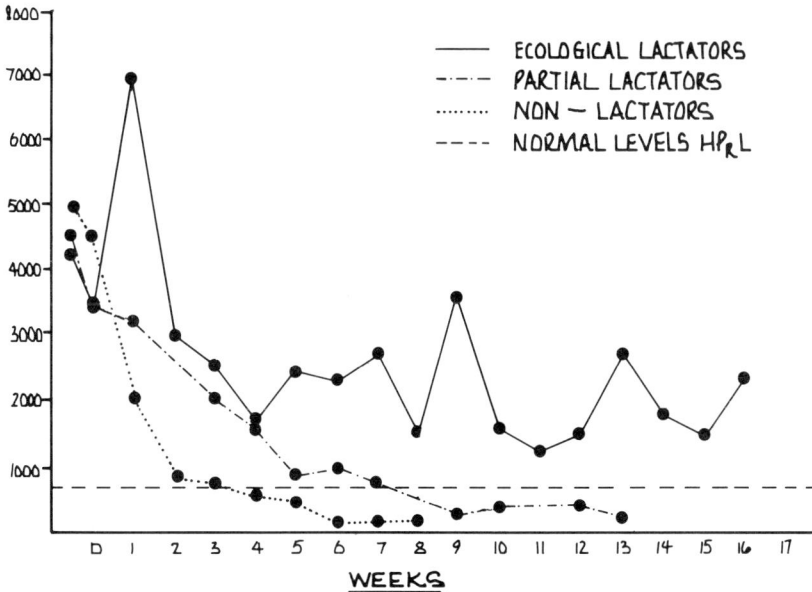

Figure 5 HPrL concentrations in the three groups relative to weeks after delivery

331

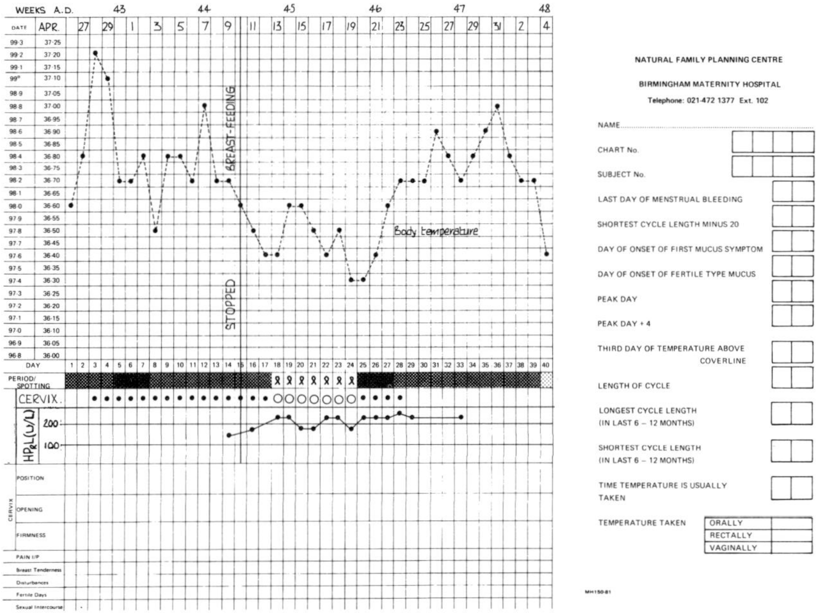

Figure 6 The first ovulation at 45–46 weeks and first menstruation at 48 weeks after delivery (AD). ○ = Fertile mucus; ○ = cervical changes; HPRL = < 300 mU/l

illustrates that although mucus secretions had returned episodically there were no appreciable changes in the cervix until ovulation was imminent.

Figure 7 illustrates the symptothermal chart of an ecological breast feeder who, despite an unchanged suckling regimen, suffered a return of infertile and fertile type mucus when solid food was introduced at 23 weeks post-partum. Ultrasonic examination of the ovaries showed the appearance of myriads of small follicles in both ovaries. Over the following days one or two of these follicles made an attempt at growth. These never proceeded beyond 15–16 mm and then they slowly regressed. A second similar episode occurred. There were no clinical indicators of ovulation such as a temperature shift during either of these episodes. Finally, 10 days after the last episode there were clear clinical indicators of ovulation and a short luteal phase preceded the first menstruation post-partum. Unfortunately, this woman was on holiday during the ovulatory event and ultrasonic measurements were not possible at this time.

332

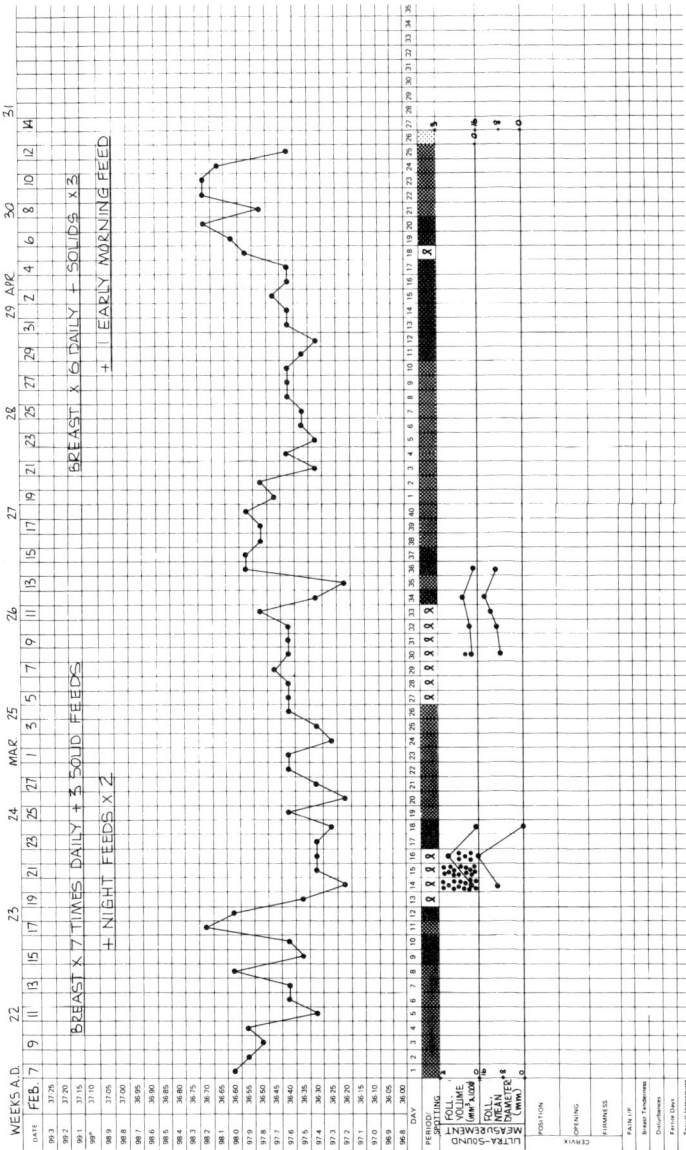

Figure 7 Symptothermal chart of ecological breast feeder. Attempts at follicular growth from 23 weeks after delivery. First ovulation followed by short luteal phase at 30 weeks while still breast feeding

333

Figure 8 illustrates the clinical indices and the ultrasonic measurements of the follicle in a partial breast feeder who was weaning her infant. Her mucus pattern alerted her to a returning fertility, but ultrasonic examination showed follicular growth to be poor and the follicles became atretic without rupture on two occasions. Finally, a further episode of mucus secretion with changes in the uterine cervix characteristic of ovulation occurred. Ultrasonic examination showed a follicle growing to 33 mm diameter, with subsequent rupture. The luteal phase was of normal length and was followed by the first menstruation post-partum.

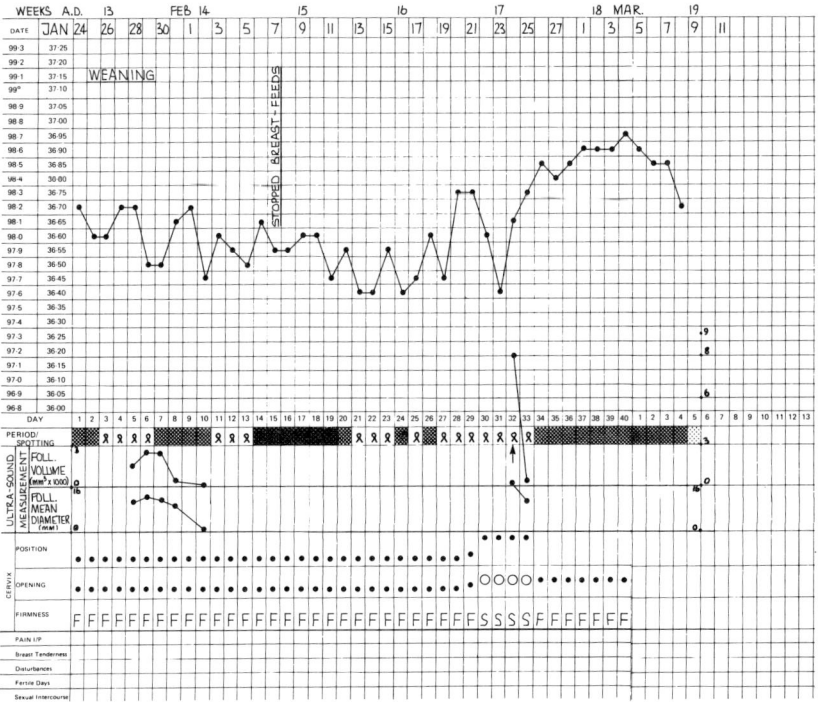

Figure 8 Sympto thermal chart of partial breast feeder. Attempts at follicular growth from 12-13 weeks post-delivery were reflected in the mucus patterns but not in the cervical changes, which only occurred in the ovulatory episode at 17 weeks

CONCLUSION

From these preliminary data, we believe that while high prolactin plasma levels may assist in maintaining post-partum infertility this is not the only mechanism involved. The suckling stimulus, in some instances as little as one suckling episode per day, appears to be an equally important factor in some women. Maternal diet and malnutrition played no part in the prolonged infertility observed in these patients. On the contrary, the behavioural pattern of returning infertility in these well-nourished women shows a great similarity with that of women in developing countries who may be malnourished. It seems, therefore, that it is the pattern of breast feeding in women in developing countries rather than their poor diet that influences the long periods of post-partum infertility seen in these countries. Regarding the most important clinical indicators to detect returning fertility and ovulation in lactating women, changes in the mucus pattern are the first alerting symptom. However, changes in the uterine cervix appear to be the most reliable clinical indicator at present to predict the first ovulatory event after childbirth. Further studies with greater numbers are necessary to confirm these findings.

Acknowledgements

Our gratitude goes to Professor Butt for his advice and encouragement, to the several technicians at the Endocrine Laboratory, Women's Hospital, Showell Green Lane, Birmingham, to those at the NFP Centre who helped recruit the women and finally our most sincere thanks go the the women taking part in the study.

References

1. Bonte, M. and Van Balen, H. (1969). Prolonged lactation and family spacing in Rwanda. *J. Biosoc. Sci*, **1**, 97
2. Hefnawi, F., Ismail, H., Younis, N., El-Sheika, Z. and Badraoui, M. H. (1977). The benefit of lactation amenorrhoea as a contraceptive. *Int. J. Gynecol. Obstet.*, **15**, 60
3. Perez, A., Vela, P., Masnick, G. S. and Potter, R. G. (1972). First ovulation after childbirth – the effect of breast feeding. *Am. J. Obstet. Gynecol.*, **114**, 1041
4. Bonnar, J., Franklin, M., Nott, P. N. and McNeilly, A. S. (1975). Effect of breast feeding on pituitary ovarian function after childbirth. *Br. Med. J.*, **iv**, 82
5. McNeilly, A. S. (1979). Effects of lactation on fertility. *Br. Med. Bull.*, **35**, 151
6. Lunn, P. G., Prentice, A. M., Austin, S. and Whitehead, R. G. (1980). Influence of maternal diet on plasma-prolactin levels during lactation. *Lancet*, **1**, 623
7. Diaz, S., Peralta, O., Juez, G. *et. al.* (1982). Fertility regulation in nursing women: 1. The probability of conception in full nursing women living in an urban setting. *J. Biosoc. Sci.*, **14**, 329

31
Steroidal contraception and lactation

PREMA RHAMACHADRAN

It is estimated that currently about 50 million women use steroidal contraceptives[1]. Over the last few years there has been a trend towards an increase in the use of steroidal contraceptives in developing countries where prolonged lactation is common and a trend towards successful prolonged lactation in developed countries where use of steroidal contraceptives is widespread. Until about 5 years ago most of the users of hormonal contraceptives were from developed countries and information on the consequences of steroidal contraceptive use were derived from data collected in these countries. Since prolon-

Table 1 Prevalence (%) of lactation and oral contraception*

Area	Breast feeding (BF)	BF and using contraception	BF and using HC	Using contraception
Kenya ($n = 77$)	40.1	2.1	0.7	6.0
Bangladesh ($n = 76$)	43.5	4.1	1.9	7.0
Indonesia ($n = 76$)	32.4	10.7	6.6	23.0
Korea ($n = 74$)	22.5	4.7	1.2	32.0
Peru ($n = 77$)	25.7	5.0	0.4	23.0
Costa Rica	6.1	2.9	0.7	58.0

*From reference 1.
HC = Hormonal contraception.

ged lactation was uncommon in these countries during the early 1970s, there is very little information on lactation and steroidal contraceptive interactions. Contraceptive prevalence studies carried

337

out during the last 5 years indicate that in spite of advice to the contrary, hormonal contraceptives are being widely used during lactation[1-3] (Table 1). It is therefore essential that in-depth investigations are undertaken to investigate the consequences of use of steroidal contraceptives during lactation.

Table 2 Effect of lactation on some anthropometric indices*

| Index | Non-lactating | Period of lactation (in months) | | |
		≤6	7–12	>12
Weight (kg)	45.2±8.12[†]	44.1±7.71[†‡]	42.3±7.05[§‡]	42.2±6.26[§]
Arm circumference (cm)	23.1±2.47[‡]	22.8±2.74[‡]	22.1±2.71[§]	22.0±2.31[§]
Skin-fold thickness (mm)	14.0±5.99[†]	12.9±5.72	11.7±4.42	10.4±3.71
No. of women	264	108	170	100

*Values are given as means ±SD.
Values bearing a different superscript are significantly different. From WHO Collaborative Study on Metabolic Side-effects of Oral Contraceptives in Undernourished Women. (Centre: Hyderabad).

Several types of interactions might occur between lactation and use of steroidal contraceptives which might affect the mother, the breast-fed infant or both. The possible interactions include:

(1) Effect of lactation on contraception:
   (a) Alteration in metabolic side-effects on hormonal contraceptives.
   (b) Alteration in maternal nutritional status.
(2) Effect of contraception on lactation:
   (a) Alteration in endocrine milieu.
   (b) Alterations in duration of lactational amenorrhoea.
   (c) Alteration in fertility return during lactation.
(3) Effect of contraception on breast-fed infant:
   (a) Alteration in – (i) duration of lactation, (ii) volume of milk output, (iii) composition of milk.
   (b) Impact of (1–3) on infant growth.
   (c) Consequences of ingestion on steroid excreted in breast milk.

There have been very few studies exploring the possibility of

338

whether metabolic side-effects of hormonal contraceptive use are affected by lactation. The WHO collaborative study on the metabolic side-effects of hormonal contraceptives in undernourished women was one of the first investigations wherein the interaction between lactation and hormonal contraceptives with regard to metabolic side-effects on hormonal contraceptive use were explored[4]. Data from the study indicated that lactation *per se* has some effect on nutritional anthropometric indices, glucose tolerance and serum lipids in the

Table 3 Effect of lactation on some biochemical parameters*

Parameter	Non-lactating	Period of lactation (months)		
		$\leqslant 6$	7–12	>12
Plasma glucose[†]	100.4±32.13	102.0±23.12	96.5±24.86	99.4±45.95
	(260)[‡]	(107)[‡]	(168)[§]	(100)[§]
Triglycerides	85.2±46.09	66.0±26.33	66.3±32.20	58.3±21.35
(mg dl^{-1})	(255)[‡]	(98)[§]	(157)[§]	(97)[§]
Cholesterol	152.6±31.82	157.0±31.12	150.5±32.3	140.7±31.07
(mg dl^{-1})	(258)[‡]	(107)[‡]	(166)[‡]	(100)[§]
Phosphatase	31.0±11.59	39.3±11.24	42.0±13.95	36.4±12.94
(mU ml^{-1})	(261)[§]	(106)[‡‖]	(166)[‖]	(100)[‡]

*Values are given as means ±SD. Figures in parentheses indicate no. of observations. Values bearing different superscripts are significantly different. From WHO Collaborative Study on Metabolic Side-effects of Oral Contraceptives in Undernourished Women. (Centre: Hyderabad).
†2 hours after glucose load of 50 g.

population groups studied (Tables 2 and 3). However, there were no significant differences in the metabolic side-effects of hormonal contraceptives between lactating and non-lactating women (Table 4).

It has been speculated that dual stress of hormonal contraception and lactation might have adverse effects on maternal nutritional status, especially in relation to the energy, mineral and vitamin status. Studies undertaken in the National Institute of Nutrition, Hyderabad, India to explore this possibility indicate that the additional stress on steroid ingestion was not associated with any adverse effect on maternal nutritional status nor did steroid ingestion have any beneficial effect (Table 5) (Prema, unpublished data).

There is very little information on the possible impact of exogenous steroid administration on endocrine milieu during lactation and return of menstruation and fertility in lactating women. The paucity of these data might be attributable to the fact that very few lactating

Table 4 Effect of oral contraceptives (OC) on lactating and non-lactating women*

Parameter	Lactating (n = 38)	Non-lactating (n = 82)
Triglyceride (mg dl^{-1}):		
Initial	61.9±27.11	70.6±26.59
After 12 months of OC use	75.3±28.93	80.3±29.47
Cholesterol (mg dl^{-1}):		
Initial	146.0±30.80	147.1±30.06
After 12 months of OC use	141.3±26.74	147.9±31.11
Alkaline phosphatase (mU ml^{-1}):		
Initial	40.7±9.58	32.6±9.08
After 12 months of OC use	22.5±6.99	22.2±7.77

*Results are given as means ±SD. From WHO Collaborative Study on Metabolic Side-effects of OC in Undernourished Women (Centre: Bombay).

Table 5 Effect of lactation on body-weight, haemoglobin and prevalence of glossitis in oral contraceptive (OC) users*

Parameter	Non-lactating		Lactating	
	Non-OC users	OC users	Non-OC users	OC users
Weight (kg)	44.2±5.72	45.2±6.11	43.2±5.21	43.6±5.51
Haemoglobin (g dl^{-1})	12.1±1.02	12.2±1.06	12.2±1.02	12.4±1.21
Prevalence of glossitis (%)	7.1 (98)	6.3 (64)	8.7 (92)	7.7 (53)

*Results are given as means ±SD.

women were using hormonal contraceptives during early lactation. The effect of four different hormonal contraceptives on the duration of lactation and lactational amenorrhoea (DMPA, 150 mg three monthly; NET, 20 mg monthly; and combination pills containing 150 µg norgestrel with 30 or 50 µg ethinyloestradiol) was investigated. None of the contraceptives had any effect on duration of lactation. Use of any of these hormonal contraceptives resulted in considerable shortening

Table 6 Duration of lactation and lactational amenorrhoea in women using hormonal contraceptives*

Group	No. in group	Previous lactational period		Present lactational period	
		Duration of lactation (months)	Duration of amenorrhoea (months)	Duration of lactation (months)	Duration of amenorrhoea (months)
Control	1917	20± 9.4	11±5.0	20± 9.6	11±5.0
DMPA 150 mg 3 monthly	22	21±10.4	11±5.6	22±11.8	6±3.2***
Neteb 20 mg monthly	51	20±10.5	12±6.0	19±10.9	8±4.1**
Combination pill (150 µg of norge strel and 50 µg ethinyl-oestradiol)	52	19±10.5	11±5.8	21±10.8	9±4.1**
Combination pill (150 µg of norge strel and 30 µg ethinyl-oestradiol)	50	20±11.4	11±5.9	21±11.0	9±4.2
Copper IUD users	68	20±10.8	11±5.8	21±10.8	11±5.6
Tubal ligation	55	21±12.0	11±6.0	22±10.7	12±5.4

Results significantly different (t test): * Values are given as means ±SD. ** $p<0.01$; *** $p<0.001$.

of duration of lactational amenorrhoea (Table 6). These data suggest that though duration of lactation is unaltered, return of 'menstruation' occurs soon after initiation of hormonal contraceptives irrespective of the type, dose, route of administration and time of initiation of contraceptive[7]. Oral contraceptives (OCs) inhibit ovulation by their effect on the pituitary–ovarian axis; DMPA affects the hypothalamic–pituitary axis and inhibits ovulation; low-dosage progestogens do not inhibit ovulation and their contraceptive effect is attributed to changes in the genital tract and its secretions. In spite of the marked difference in mechanism by which contraceptive effect is achieved all these hormonal contraceptives have a similar effect of hastening the return of 'menstruation' without affecting the duration of lactation. Apparently the alterations in hypothalamic–pituitary–ovarian axis produced by contraceptives are sustained and are of sufficient magnitude as to nullify the effect of lactation on the hypothalamo-pituitary axis without having any effect on lactation. Investigations on the hypothalamic–pituitary–ovarian axis in lactating women, including those using hormonal contraceptives, may help to achieve better understanding of hormonal regulation on lactation and lactation-induced changes in hormonal profile.

Table 7 Occurrence of pregnancy in matched pairs of acceptors and non-acceptors of oral contraceptives during lactation

| Pill acceptors | Non-acceptor matches | | |
	Pregnant	Non-pregnant	Total
Pregnant	39	21	60
Non-pregnant	14	19	33
Total	53	40	93

Odds ratio = 1.5.

Attempts to explore the possible fertility implications of the rapid return of menstruation associated with use of hormonal contraceptives during lactational amenorrhoea were few and far between and have not been very successful because regular use of hormonal contraceptives provides contraceptive coverage and renders occurrence of pregnancy unlikely. However, some of the data from Bangladesh[6], where hormonal contraceptives were used during early lactation in women who do not take pills regularly and where discontinuation rates are higher suggest that there are greater numbers of pregnancies occurring in lactating women who were using oral contraceptives irregularly than those who were not using any contraception during lactation (Table 7).

These data suggest that administration of exogenous contraceptive steroids might result in rapid return of menstruation and fertility in lactating women. In many of the developing countries the contacts between health personnel and women are more likely to occur in the immediate post-partum period. Women are thought to be more receptive to contraceptive advice soon after delivery. Therefore many post-partum programmes have been designed for distribution of contraception during early lactation. In poorer segments of the population where motivation of women for continued use of contraception is poor and continuation rates for hormonal contraceptives are low, the fertility implications of distribution of hormonal contraceptives early during lactation need be investigated.

The importance of successful continued lactation in ensuring infant nutrition, health and survival in poorer segments of population in developing countries is well documented. Investigation on the effect of use of hormonal contraceptives on breast milk output, breast milk composition, duration of lactation and infant growth have yielded conflicting results partly because of the complex nature of the problem and partly due to lack of a standardized method for data collection[1]. Most of the studies indicate that use of combination pills containing $50 \mu g$ or more of oestrogen early during lactation is associated with a reduction in milk output and shorter duration of lactation. Data from the WHO sponsored multicentric studies in developed and developing countries suggest that the use of combination pills containing only $30 \mu g$ ethenyloestradiol 6 weeks after delivery is also associated with a reduction in milk output by about 30%. Injectable progesterone and progestational minipills are free from these side-effects[7].

There are, however, some problems inherent in the study design that render the finding rather difficult to interpret. The study design stipulated that milk output was to be calculated from the amount of breast milk expressed from one breast when the infant was suckling in the other breast. The crucial measurement in infant nutrition is not the amount of breast milk output as assessed by manual expression from the breast, but the amount of milk that is ingested by the infant as assessed either by test feeding or by the ducterium oxide

343

dilation method. In recognition of the difficulties in measurement of milk output over 24 hours, the study design stipulated that the amount of breast milk expressed over an 8-hour period be used to compute milk output over a 24-hour period. Infants may suckle more or less in the evening or at night. There is some evidence to suggest that if milk output is low the amount of milk ingested by the infant in the evening or at night might be greater. In OC users more milk intake might occur in the later parts of the day. In view of the importance of breast milk intake in determining the infant growth in poorer segments of the population in developing countries it is imperative that studies are undertaken to obtain actual 24-hour milk intake in infants whose mothers are using combination pills, even though such studies are likely to be difficult, expensive and time consuming.

Studies on the composition of breast milk in hormonal contraceptive users have also yielded conflicting results which might at least in part be attributable to the lack of uniform method of collecting breast milk samples. Most of the available data suggest that there might not be any significant changes in composition of breast milk in OC users[1]. Data from the WHO multicentric study where ample care was exercised in collecting samples under standardized conditions suggest that fat content of milk was higher in OC users and lower in combination pill users (unpublished data). It has been suggested that this might be a compensatory mechanism by which calorie needs of the infants are met even though milk output is recorded in combination pill users. However, there might be a simpler explanation for the observed data. To obtain information on composition of milk the entire volume of milk expressed from the breast was homogenized and fat, protein and lactose estimations were performed in aliquots of the sample. Apparent differences in fat content might, at least to some extent, be attributable to the method of sample collection. Data from this study show that there was a 30% reduction in milk output in combination pill users and a perceptible increase in milk output in DMPA users. It is possible that because of a relatively smaller volume of milk obtained in the OC group vigorous attempts were made to express the breast milk 'completely' and so the sample contained a larger proportion of fat-rich hind milk.

Because of the ease with which an 'adequate quantity' of breast milk was expressed in DMPA users it is possible that less of the hind milk was expressed and this accounted for a reduction in fat content in DMPA users. At the moment there is very little information to verify either of these hypotheses. However, in view of the importance of lipids not only in terms of satisfying the calorie needs of the infant but also in terms of central nervous system development it is essential that further studies on composition of breast milk in hormonal contraceptive users are undertaken.

Data on growth of breast-fed infants from the WHO study suggest that up to 6 months of age growth rate was similar in minipill users, DMPA users and combination pill users and a control group consisting of women not using any hormonal contraceptives, irrespective of the observed differences in milk output between the various groups[7]. The exact reason for the lack of impact of the reduction in milk output on growth of infants in combination pill users is not clear. It is possible that the amount of milk ingested by the infants in each group were not markedly different, though the amount of milk expressed during the limited number of hours was significantly different. More frequent feeds and/or longer duration of suckling might result in infants getting adequate milk intake in spite of apparent lower milk output. There might be differences in the amount of supplementary feeds given to infants in different groups. Hungry infants in the OC group might have consumed more supplements to meet the nutritional needs for adequate growth. It is also possible that the close supervision and adequate health care ensured minimum morbidity in the infants and hence the impact of reduction in milk output on growth was not obvious. Further studies to obtain data on milk intake, the time of introduction of supplement to infants, the amount of supplementary feeds consumed by infants, the morbidity profile and growth need be undertaken to sort out these reported paradoxical findings.

In view of reported data that the use of hormonal contraceptives early during lactation results in reduction in milk output and shortening of duration of lactation, in India it is recommended that a combination pill should not be prescribed to women who are lactating for less than 6 months. Studies undertaken in the National Institute of Nutrition indicate that when OC use was initiated after 6 months of lactation none of the women complained of any significant reduction in milk output in the month after initiation of OCs.

Since the majority of the infants were beyond 6 months of age and had already been receiving supplements before entering into study, information regarding effect of oral contraceptives on the age at which supplements were introduced to infants could not be assessed. There were, however, no significant differences in mean body-weight or mean haemoglobin levels of infants belonging to the control group of non-users of hormonal contraception and study population who were using a combination pill containing 150 μg norgestrel and 30 μg ethinyloestradiol (Table 8). These data suggest that the practice of prescribing the combination pill to carefully chosen lactating women after 6 months of lactation may not have adverse effects on infant growth. However, studies on milk intake and composition of breast milk need to be undertaken to find out whether the relatively late introduction of hormonal contraceptives during lactation has any impact on these parameters.

It has been known that steroidal contraceptives are excreted in breast milk and the amount excreted varies depending upon the dose and type of contraceptives used[1]. There have been a few case reports of breast enlargement in breast-fed infants or children whose mothers were using hormonal contraceptives suggesting that potentially the excreted steroids might exert some biological effect on the infant[8]. The rarity of such case reports suggests that several unknown factors influence the biological activity of steroids ingested. Though there had been speculations regarding the possible biological conse-quences of exposure to steroids in breast milk in relation to type of compounds used, age of infant and duration of exposure, there have been so far very little concrete data. Results of some of the investigations undertaken in the National Institute of Nutrition, Hyderabad, India suggest that there were no alterations in physical growth, nutritional status and morbidity profile of children who were exposed to hormonal contraceptives in breast milk during infancy (Table 9).

However, the sample size investigated is quite small and the children were between 2 and 6 years of age. No information on psychological profile had been collected. An attempt is being made to follow up the cohort at least till sexual maturity and to investigate psychomotor development in these children. Earlier experience with DES exposure *in utero* suggests that some of the sequelae of exposure to steroidal contraceptives might be totally unexpected and appear years after the exposure[9]. It is therefore imperative that studies are undertaken to set up global long-term surveillance programmes

Table 8 Growth of breast-fed infants and children whose mothers were using oral contraceptives (OCs)*

	Age (months)						
Group	7	8	9	10	11	12	13
				Body weight (kg)			
OC users	6.42±0.943 (17)	6.82±0.951 (15)	6.95±0.971 (11)	7.42±0.981 (15)	7.61±0.830 (14)	7.67±0.980 (18)	8.12±1.150 (38)
Control group	6.92±1.413 (36)	7.14±1.040 (30)	7.17±1.013 (22)	7.46±1.102 (30)	7.60±1.030 (28)	7.84±1.150 (36)	8.03±1.160 (76)
Low-income urban group	6.66±0.951 (148)	6.98±0.999 (98)	7.21±1.021 (96)	7.34±1.024 (94)	7.54±1.025 (92)	7.67±1.218 (165)	7.90±1.341 (138)
	7–9			10–12		13–18	
	Haemoglobin (g dl⁻¹)						
OC users	9.5±1.74 (14)			9.2±1.31 (12)		9.3±1.65 (20)	
Control group	9.6±1.59 (46)			9.7±1.56 (48)		9.2±1.63 (62)	
Low-income urban group	9.9±1.86 (199)			9.9±1.86 (199)		8.9±1.80 (93)	

*Values are given as means ±SD. Figures in parentheses indicate number of infants and children.

347

Table 9 Growth of breast-fed infants whose mothers were using oral contraceptives (OCs) during lactation

Group	Weight (kg)	Height (cm)	Head circumference (cm)	Chest circumference (cm)	Arm circumference (cm)	Skin-fold thickness (mm)	Hb (g dl^{-1})
OC:							
Mean	12.4	91.4	46.5	48.1	14.0	7.6	10.2
SD	4.86	20.58	3.18	4.90	1.44	1.71	1.76
No. of subjects	76	78	78	76	73	71	67
Control:							
Mean	12.3	92.2	46.5	48.9	14.1	7.7	9.4
SD	4.65	19.45	3.15	4.52	1.46	2.2	1.94
No. of subjects	76	78	78	76	73	71	67

to monitor breast-fed infants whose mothers are using hormonal contraceptives during lactation.

References

1. Breast feeding fertility and family planning (1981). *Pop. Rep.*, J 527
2. World Health Organization (1981). *Contemporary Breast Feeding Practices. Report of the WHO Collaborative Study on Breast Feeding.* (Geneva: WHO)
3. Strauss, L. T., Speckhard, M., Rochat, R. W. and Senanayake, P. (1981). Oral contraception during lactation – a global survey of physician practice. *Int. J. Gynecol. Obstet.*, **19**, 169
4. Belsey, M. A. (1982). Contraception during postpartum period while lactating. Effect on women's health. Paper presented in the *WHO/NAS Workshop on Breast Feeding and Fertility Regulation: Current Knowledge and Policy Implications*, Geneva, 17–19 February
5. Prema, K. (1982). Duration of lactation and return of menstruation in lactating women using hormonal contraception and IUDs. *Contracept. Deliv. Syst.*, **3**, 39
6. Bhatia, S., Becker, S. and Kim, Y. J. (1982). The effect of pill acceptance on fecundity in the postpartum period in rural Bangladesh. Paper presented in the *WHO/NAS Workshop on Breast Feeding and Fertility Regulation: Current Knowledge and Implications*, Geneva, 17–19 February
7. World Health Organization (1981). *WHO Special Programme of Research Development and Research Training in Human Reproduction, 10th Annual Report.* (Geneva: WHO)
8. Nilson, S. and Nygren, K. G. (1979). Transfer of contraceptive steroids to human milk. *Res. Reprod.*, **11**, 1
9. Herbst, A. L., Scully, F. E., Robbov, S. J. and Welch, W. R. (1978). Complications of prenatal therapy with diethyl stilbestrol. *Paediatrics*, **62**, 1151

349

32
Birth intervals – demographic factors

S. TEPER

At any time the size and structure of a human population reflects the levels of fertility, mortality and migration which have existed in previous periods of time. Often, the level of migration is negligible, or can be assumed to be so, and the population can be treated as a 'closed' system affected only by fertility and mortality. Once mortality has been reduced to approximately the current Western level, then it is fluctuations in fertility which determine the size and structure of the population and dominate any changes in that size and structure. In much of Europe mean family size is now less than two children per woman. In developing societies the *mean* can be as high as 7–8 children per woman, and rapid and uncontrolled fertility remains a major barrier to economic, social and health development.

As a reference point when studying almost any aspect of fertility we can examine the fertility schedules of communities which exhibit 'natural fertility'. Natural fertility means that behaviour which affects fertility is unchanged irrespective of the number of children that have already been born. Controlled fertility is the obverse of this – contraception is used or other behaviour modified depending on the number of children born.

The Hutterites are perhaps the most famous example of a community demonstrating natural fertility. The Hutterites are an anabaptist sect which originated in Europe and then migrated to North America. They now live in a series of interconnected communities in the western United States and Canada. They are healthy and well nourished, and want large families for religious and practical reasons.

351

They do not use contraception, have no postpartum sexual taboos and do not breast-feed for long periods. In a detailed anthropological and demographic study the *mean* number of births was found to be 12.4 per woman. This is the highest natural fertility schedule that is known. There is some evidence that older Hutterite women attempt to limit their families, and it is known that little teenage sexual activity occurs and that teenage marriage is relatively rare. Were the Hutterites to attempt to maximize their fertility, mean fertility could rise by one or two births per woman.

At the other end of the natural fertility scale are the !Dobe Kung, a small group of hunter–gatherers who live in a remote part of the Kalahari desert. Mean age at first birth of the !Kung is 18.8 years (with a median of 19.2 years) and at last birth it is 34.4 years. Each women has, on average, 4.7 births with mean birth intervals (all births) of 4.1 years. Differences between Hutterite and !Kung fertility are explained (in part at least) by factors such as the proportions married and the proportions infertile. For example, the !Kung have a much higher incidence of infertility – and in part this reflects the impact of sexually transmitted diseases introduced by contact with outsiders. The role of diet and critical fatness remains an unresolved element in explaining the extremely low fertility of the !Kung. Menarche is celebrated by a ceremony and has been estimated to occur at a mean age of 16.6 years. It is of interest that menarche has been known to occur at even higher ages in some other hunter–gatherer tribes. In the Bundi, for example, in north New Guinea, it occurs at an average 18.1 years.

Explaining variations in fertility – be it between natural and controlled fertility and be it between or within populations – is obviously a complex task. Many behavioural and biological mechanisms are involved. Once we start to decompose fertility into components – for example, into parity or birth intervals – then the processes of measurement and interpretation become more complex and carry less certainty. An examination of birth intervals demonstrates the complexity of the factors at play.

Birth intervals, as part of demographic structure and change, are themselves affected by a number of demographic, sociodemographic and other factors. For example, migration and female employment patterns affect the timing of conceptions; rural-to-urban migration or male migration for work lead to the temporary separation of husband and wife. Female employment affects the number and tim-

352

ing of births. The effect may operate directly on birth spacing (as with the separation of husband and wife) or indirectly by influencing intermediate variables (that is, by affecting the use of birth control and the duration of breast-feeding, etc.).

The length of a birth interval reflects the circumstances of the individual as well as the impact of natural fertility. A short birth interval can, for example, occur following an optimal period of breast-feeding plus no use of contraception; or after the early death of a previous full-term infant; or after the death of a premature infant, whose risk of death in the neonatal period was high anyway. Maternal nutrition, breast-feeding and weaning also need to be given consideration at this level of analysis. In developed societies short intervals may reflect a late decision to build a family, primary infertility which has been successfully resolved, a decision to minimize the time for which the woman is away from employment, or the inefficient (or non-) use of contraception.

Long birth intervals reflect quite different factors: sub-fertility, for instance, or a new relationship with a baby to consolidate it, or higher maternal age. This last point is of particular importance. Since age is associated with a higher risk of spontaneous abortion and with longer than average intervals between births, the longer birth intervals seen in traditional (non-contracepting) populations may be associated with women who are near the end of the reproductive span. At that point, reproductive 'efficiency' is lower, and the probability of any single pregnancy resulting in a live birth is reduced.

In Western societies, long intervals predominantly reflect the use of contraception. This raises difficulties when studying populations in transition, in which a significant proportion of the population uses contraception and a further significant proportion does not. Mothers who use contraception are likely to be different from those who do not in terms of age, socioeconomic status, health status, health care utilization and infant feeding practices.

In recent years attention has focussed on the implications which birth intervals have for health. Particular interest has been expressed in *short* intervals, and specifically in short intervals occurring in developing countries. However, the health effects of birth intervals remain relatively unknown, despite the fact that we regularly argue for well-spaced pregnancies in order to improve maternal and child health. A number of useful conclusions can be drawn from the current state of knowledge. First, data showing a birth interval effect on health and infant survival should be approached with some scepticism. This is because most studies have not controlled for the many confounding factors which operate on the birth interval/health relationship. Many of the confounding elements have the greatest effect on the shortest birth intervals (those less than 1 year in length), and it is precisely these intervals that have suggested the interval effect of spacing on health. It is particularly important to control for maternal age and parity, socioeconomic status and previous infant death because these factors are themselves associated with differentials in health risks. In addition, an unknown proportion of the excess risk seen in short birth intervals reflects the over-representation of young women of high parity whose children have higher health risks for reasons *other than* the lengths of the birth intervals.

Secondly, we need to know more about the contribution that low birth-weight and/or prematurity make to short birth intervals. Thirdly, we need to know more about the excess risk for siblings in families which have a prior infant death – in particular, can intervention reduce the risk of another death? Fourthly, in societies in which an interval effect on infant mortality has been demonstrated, the majority of births occur with a spacing interval greater than 24 months. In these Third World societies traditional lactation practices result in birth spacing patterns that avoid the worst hazards of short intervals for most children. In these countries it is crucial that traditional patterns of breast-feeding are maintained. Health policy which encourages delaying the first birth and limiting family size once the desired number of children have been born may have as much effect on health as policies aimed at birth spacing *per se*. Fifthly, we do not know as yet how to measure any birth interval effect on *maternal* health. Finally, we do not know whether there are health effects associated with birth spacing in 'low' parity families – for instance, for the woman who has a first birth at age 29 or 30 and then has two more infants at 18-month intervals, a pattern seen increasingly in some parts of the Western world.

The interrelationships between birth intervals, fertility and health are complex. What we can be certain of is that reductions in the prevalence of breast-feeding and in the length of time for which women lactate will undoubtedly – in the absence of contraception – reduce the length of birth intervals and increase fertility. In many parts of the world the pattern of breast-feeding is changing, as is the pattern of contraceptive use. The contraceptive is no longer carried on a woman's hip, but comes from a plastic package of pills. This is likely to disturb traditional patterns of birth spacing, and in doing so has substantial implications for maternal and child health.

Bibliography

1. Eaton, J. W. and Mayer, A. J. (1953). The social biology of very high fertility among the Hutterites. *Hum. Biol.*, **25,** 206
2. Howell, N. (1979). *Demography of the Dobe !Kung.* (London: Academic Press)
3. World Health Organization (1981). *Contemporary Patterns of Breast-feeding. Report on the WHO Collaborative Study on Breast-feeding.* (Geneva: WHO)
4. WHO/UNICEF (1981). *Infant and Young Child Feeding. Current Issues.* (Geneva: WHO)
5. WHO (1983). *Breast-feeding, Fertility Control and Health.* Proceedings of a joint WHO/National Academy of Sciences meeting. (In press)

Part I

Section 9

Psychosocical Aspects of Reproduction

33
The infertile couple and the gynaecologist: psychosocial and emotional aspects

E. V. VAN HALL

INTRODUCTION

The gynaecologist and the infertile couple have the same object in view: to find the cause of infertility and institute a treatment that will lead to pregnancy and eventually to the birth of a healthy child. Unlike other forms of medical care, which are usually directed at the cure of a disease, the management of infertility is aimed primarily at the attainment of a social achievement. It is therefore hardly surprising that during the usually long period of infertility management, emotional and psychosocial factors play an important part in the doctor–patient relationship and even influence the course and results of treatment.

In this chapter, the following aspects will be discussed: the infertility investigation, unexplained infertility, female infertility, male infertility, failure to achieve pregnancy, the achievement of pregnancy, and the interaction between the gynaecologist and the couple.

THE INFERTILITY INVESTIGATION

Although the investigation of an infertile couple includes, in the majority of the cases, very simple procedures (sperm analysis, post-coital test, basal body temperature (BBT), hysterosalpingography

(HSG), laparoscopy), it must be kept in mind that the burden for the patients may be much heavier than the doctor imagines. This holds especially for female investigation. There is a great discrepancy between prescribing and undergoing a procedure. I am afraid that many gynaecologists do not realize what it means for a woman not only to undergo a pelvic examination, but also to keep BBT recordings month after month and have repeated postcoital tests performed – both of which can affect the social and sexual life of the couple. HSG, which usually is, as it should be, performed on an out-patient basis in the cold and technical atmosphere of a radiology department, combines humiliation, pain, and fear, and laparoscopy usually means hospitalization and general anaesthesia while both procedures evoke ambivalent feelings of hope that some treatable cause will be found and fear that a serious untreatable abnormality will be exposed. I have been amazed by the tendency to repeat these procedures without reservation, often without adequate information about the need for and usefulness of such investigations.

Gynaecologists should try to identify with the couple's feelings and use the investigation period to build up a good relationship, their input combining time to listen, sound information, and awareness of unspoken thoughts. At the same time, they should avoid a too paternalistic attitude with the associated risk of increasing the patient's feeling of dependency and thus reducing the couple's own sense of responsibility for the decisions to be taken. An open, knowledgeable, but empathic attitude to the infertile couple during the investigation period will not only safeguard their feelings of well-being and self-esteem but, in my opinion, may well increase the likelihood of the occurrence of spontaneous pregnancy.

In our department the infertility investigation is built up in a systematic way, allowing time to elapse between different steps unless gross abnormalities are found. Under these conditions, we have found that spontaneous pregnancy occurs in approximately 40% of the women within 6 months after HSG and approximately 30% within a year following laparoscopy when these procedures reveal minor or no abnormalities. In my opinion, it is extremely important to exercise patience to allow such spontaneous pregnancies to occur without medical interference for two reasons: (1) medical interference is not necessary and might even be harmful; and (2) a spontaneous pregnancy will be the couple's *own* pregnancy and not the doctor's, which enhances their feeling of self-esteem and independence.

UNEXPLAINED INFERTILITY

When infertility investigation reveals no abnormalities (which is the case in approximately 15% of the investigated couples) a highly frustrating situation arises for both the gynaecologist and the couple. For both sides it is impossible to explain and difficult to accept the failure to conceive in the absence of abnormalities. There is considerable ambivalence in this situation. On the one hand, it is disappointing for the doctor not to be able to say: 'I have found the cause of your problem and will institute treatment'; but on the other hand, there is some relief for the couple that no major obstacle to conception is evident and that pregnancy is physically possible.

Doctors like to solve problems and to *do* something. In dealing with unexplained infertility they should control this drive and accept the situation. Too much unnecessary and sometimes harmful surgery has been performed in the past on women with unexplained infertility, and even now new operations are still being devised, as I heard recently at a meeting on tubal dysfunction where one of the speakers advocated surgical plication of the fimbria ovarica and suspension of the uterus in cases of unexplained infertility. I am personally very much opposed to such technical approaches to a problem I think is more likely to be psychological in nature.

I would like to stress once again here that when no cause for the infertility is found after a complete and thorough investigation, one should refrain from further diagnostic procedures and questionable treatments except as part of a well-controlled scientific study. On the contrary, one should explore the possibility that, especially in long-standing cases of unexplained infertility, there might be no wish at all to have a child. Recently, a woman with primary infertility who for many years had consulted infertility centres all over Europe and undergone many investigations and treatments said to us during a psychotherapeutic session: 'Actually, I never wanted to have a child with *this* man'.

FEMALE INFERTILITY

When the infertility investigation reveals a female cause, a special situation arises. Despite emancipation processes in most Western societies, the majority of couples have a fairly traditional sex-role distribution: the woman is supposed to become pregnant and to have, nurture, and bring up children while the man works and provides the necessary income to maintain his family. When the probable cause of infertility lies in the female partner, her already damaged feeling of self-esteem will be reinforced by feelings of failure and guilt because she is unable to comply with the social expectancy and, moreover, the inability is her fault. When speaking to such couples about the emotional consequences of their infertility I have often heard the husband say: 'I do not care so much; I have my work and the social contact it involves, but it is terrible for my wife because she is so alone'. And the wife would say: 'My husband was unlucky to marry me because I cannot give him what he deserves: a child'. Although I realize that such statements might be influenced by the fact that men have more difficulty in openly expressing their emotions than women, they nevertheless substantially reflect an unfortunate reality, which is further intensified by the general tendency to underestimate the value of housework, thus giving the woman in addition a strong feeling of being useless.

Gynaecologists, who in terms of their specialty might be expected to *help* women, should be aware of these feelings and take a positive attitude toward the emancipation of women at the individual and public levels. In our experience, emancipated and working women with a partner who shares and respects their views have less difficulty in coping with and eventually working through their infertility – which of course does not mean that their grief is less intense.

MALE INFERTILITY

When the infertility investigation reveals a male cause, the resulting situation is in some ways similar – as far as the general and social consequences are concerned – but has very specific aspects at the individual level. Whereas female infertility generally does not affect the woman's sexuality, the opposite is much more likely in male infertility. In our culture, fertility, masculinity and potency are closely related. The traditional linkage of sexuality and reproduction seems to be stronger amongst men than women. Whereas the infertile woman will tend to have feelings of failure and uselessness, infertile men tend to have feelings of not being a man and, even more so, of no longer being a sexual man. It is probably for this reason that there still is a taboo on male infertility, which has historically been kept masked in order to preserve 'masculine pride'. Female partners of infertile men sometimes even say: 'I am so sorry for my husband; I would rather the fault was mine'. The reverse is very seldom heard. The male factor was long excluded from infertility investigation, and fertility research focussed mainly on the female.

Even now, there is still a general tendency among the public to look at the woman when a couple remains childless, although it is well known that the male factor plays a part (either totally or partially) in approximately 50% of the infertile couples. In this respect it is interesting to note how long it has taken the medical profession to overcome its aversion to artificial insemination with donor sperm (AID) compared with the ease and public openness with which *in vitro* fertilization and embryo transfer has been accepted.

Concerning male infertility we have made some interesting observations during group sessions held to prepare and counsel couples for AID. It is important to realize how peculiar the AID situation is: the 'treatment' of male infertility is in practice directed at the female partner, and the real cause of the infertility remains a secret hidden from the outer world.

Most of the couples in our groups have reported a significant decline in sexual activity, and sexual pleasure had often disappeared. The women indicated that they no longer saw the purpose of intercourse, and the men said they could abstain for weeks. Some men said they had completely lost sexual interest after learning about their infertility, and one of them reasoned as follows: 'Since I cannot give proof of my manhood, I even have less sex than I want, as a punishment for myself'. On the other hand, men appeared to be relieved at discovering that other infertile men in the group had a distinctly masculine appearance, being tall and brawny and having a moustache and beard.

All of the couples participating in these group sessions felt relieved that the secrecy surrounding their infertility had been discarded and that they could discuss mutual problems and fantasies with each other. We are of the opinion that greater openness in this respect will promote equality between partners and increase public acceptance of AID as a form of treatment of male infertility. Furthermore, men will be encouraged to accept a more emancipated model of sexuality, one not linked to fertility and masculinity but instead experienced more as pleasure, care, and intimacy. Male infertility will then no longer amount simultaneously to disqualification of men and discrimination of women.

FAILURE TO ACHIEVE PREGNANCY

When pregnancy is not achieved despite long and thorough investigation and intensive treatment, a frustrating situation for both gynaecologist and patient is again created. Often under the pressure from the couple, this situation leads to an endless reiteration of diagnostic tests and often unnecessary additional treatment. Women are operated on over and over again, and couples travel from one doctor to the other unnecessarily prolonging their own torment. Although I know how difficult it is to resist such pressures, it should also be said that it is often the doctor who, unwilling to accept his or her failure to perform, keeps the couple on a string.

There comes a moment at which one should honestly ask the question: 'Who really wants the baby, the doctor or the patient?' It should be realized that the painful working-through of the various phases of the mourning process after infertility is established can only take place adequately if an end has been made to all diagnostic and therapeutic interventions. This decision should be taken with sufficient determination to withstand the couple's natural urge to continue. Gynaecologists should overcome their own frustration, admit their inability, and direct their attention and energy to helping the couple to cope with their grief. Sometimes it is less painful to endure a negative certitude than a positive incertitude.

THE ACHIEVEMENT OF PREGNANCY

As already mentioned, the objective of both the gynaecologist and the infertile couple is the achievement of a successful pregnancy. If this goal is reached, the result is of course highly rewarding for both parties. In our experience, however, the occurrence of conception, especially in cases of long-standing childlessness, is not always received with the joy and enthusiasm that could be expected. Sometimes the news 'You are pregnant' is received with some reservation or even dislike and depressive feelings. These feelings are usually caused by an initial unwillingness to believe the good news out of fear that it might not be true or that something might go wrong with the pregnancy. However, in the course of discussing this reaction with many couples we became aware of another extremely interesting and, in my opinion, understandable mechanism. Although officially these couples pursue pregnancy desperately – partly under the influence of social pressures, the actual knowledge of being pregnant confronts them with the inevitable consequence of this pregnancy: the coming of a child. They suddenly realize that, unconsciously, they have separated their wish to *achieve* a long-desired result (pregnancy) and the real wish to nurture and bring up a child. Quite often they have adapted their social situation and their own relationship to a life without children, and this situation might well be disturbed by a potential intruder, however much the latter has been wanted.

These negative feelings which usually are of transient nature, can be very confusing for both the couple and the gynaecologist, because they are felt as incomprehensible ingratitude and lead to guilt feelings on the one side and irritation on the other. Still, they should be considered as a very natural reaction and not as emotional instability. They represent part of an adaptation process to cope with a completely new situation, and should be met with understanding and empathy. Sometimes this reaction can be extreme, as we recently experienced in our department. A woman of 35 years with a long-standing primary infertility due to tubal pathology underwent a bilateral salpingo-stomy in January 1981. Before that, she had undergone various investigations and treatments in other hospitals, and she desperately wanted a child. In November 1982, she conceived and was deeply confused and disturbed when she heard the 'good' news. The couple could not tolerate the idea of having a child and requested termination of pregnancy. It took us 4 weeks of intensive counselling to reach the difficult decision to comply with their request. At follow-up it appeared that we had made the wrong decision; the couple very much regretted the abortion. Next, despite my advice to use contraception for at least 6 months to have sufficient time to think everything over, the woman conceived again during the first cycle following the termination of pregnancy. Both she and her partner are now very happy with the prospect of having a child. I initially felt frustrated and had guilt feelings about a decision that I had thought was carefully taken but eventually seemed to be wrong. Now I think that the emotionally difficult decision to terminate the first pregnancy (for both parties) helped the couple to accept the consequences of the second pregnancy and to look forward to the birth of a wanted child. The first, more or less unexpected conception was a doctor's pregnancy, whereas the second was perhaps experienced by the couple as an achievement of their own. This case furthermore illustrates that psychological factors can influence the chance of conception. Is it not amazing that this women conceived a second time so quickly although she had to wait nearly two years after tubal surgery for her first pregnancy?

GYNAECOLOGIST–COUPLE INTERACTION

Much of the foregoing concerns the emotional relationship between a gynaecologist and an infertile couple. It should be kept in mind that this relationship has two specific aspects: in the first place, the gynaecologist is (at least in our society) usually a male, and secondly, he usually already has what the couple are seeking: a family. This situation can influence the gynaecologist's attitude toward the problems confronting the couple.

In discussions on the relationship between the male gynaecologist and his female patient, the following point is assumed to hold: the male physician's attitude to his female patient will to a great extent be determined by his attitude to women in general. If the doctor sees a woman as someone whose main function is to serve and reproduce, his feeling of superiority – already present in any doctor–patient relationship – will be intensified.

Under these conditions the patient will be less likely than ever to talk about her real problems, especially if they are concerned with sexuality or are relational in nature. Thus, the position of the male physician relative to his female patient is characterized by a double sense of superiority: the unavoidable superiority of the physician in relation to his patient, reinforced by the traditional superiority of men in relation to women. This combination produces the classic picture of the male physician: paternalistic and sympathetic but stand-offish. He knows what is good for the patient and is not influenced by emotions. These characteristics are not necessarily bad and in some situations can even be valuable. But they are not sufficient to generate adequate communication and can therefore constitute an obstacle to a real understanding of the patient's problems. They lead to what might be called one-way traffic: talking, advising and prescribing predominate, leaving little space for listening, understanding, and empathy.

There is still another aspect of the relationship between gynaecologist and patient that deserves special attention. The woman who is the patient of a male physician will often adopt a passive, accepting, and dependent attitude, and this will not promote communication between them either. In this context one of the important functions

366

of the gynaecologist should be to encourage the female patient to be verbal and independent, and thus greatly increase not only her ability to express her real feelings but also the degree of her involvement in the investigation and the treatment.

Is the foregoing applicable to the relationship between the male gynaecologist and the infertile couple? In my opinion it could be. Acceptance of the proposed model of interaction in relation to an infertile couple has the following advantages:

(1) An equally divided sense of solidarity toward both partners.
(2) A better awareness and understanding of the psychosocial consequences of female infertility.
(3) A better awareness and understanding of the psychosexual consequences of male infertility.
(4) Avoidance of a 'father–daughter'-like relationship with the female patient, especially by enhancement of her sense of responsibility and self-esteem.
(5) Avoidance or at least understanding and handling of the sometimes associated feelings of jealousy in the male partner toward the doctor who is seen as responsible for a pregnancy: 'Doctor, I am so grateful to you; this is in fact your child'.
(6) Last but not least, an easier acceptance of failure of success by putting into proper proportions the social pressures to have a family and by endorsing the emancipation of both men and women in the way described above.

Infertility is not only a personal but also a sociocultural problem, and the virtually inevitable psychological stress is perhaps induced more strongly by current attitudes in our society than by the situation itself.

CONCLUSION

I am well aware that any discussion of the emotional and psychosocial aspects of infertility like the foregoing will encounter some resistance and questioning of the validity of the opinions expressed. We gynaecologists have been trained mainly to deal with the somatic and technical aspects of our profession, and as a result we tend to believe only what has been proved, preferably by statistically significant findings. Without denying the value of such studies, I have gradually come to the conviction – after 15 years' experience in dealing with infertile couples – that sensitivity for and observation of the non-somatic aspects of infertility can improve not only the quality of care but also the actual results of treatment.

Let me close by giving you one example which concerns a highly topical subject: *in vitro* fertilization and embryo transfer. So far, all efforts to improve the results of this new treatment for tubal infertility have been directed at biological factors, such as spontaneous versus induced cycle, the quality of the recovered ovum, and the timing of embryo transfer. We now know that the extracorporeal part of the procedure is usually highly successful but that the intracorporeal part is the bottle-neck, whereas this is not the case if the procedure is performed (for economic reasons) in animals. I wonder whether anyone has ever tried to imagine what it means for a women to undergo such a treatment. She usually has long-standing infertility, has undergone various tubal operations, and has finally been on a waiting list for *in vitro* fertilization for a couple of years. She knows that when her turn comes, she will be given a chance to become pregnant during two or three cycles, and will then go back to the bottom of the waiting list if she does not succeed. I am convinced that the psychological stress during these two or three cycles must be tremendous, and there is no doubt in my mind that psychological stress can affect the delicate mechanism of implantation.

Although I am not yet able to prove the validity of this statement, I dare to predict that more attention to the psychological aspects of embryo transfer and an adequate and professional psychological preparation of these women will improve the pregnancy rates after *in vitro* fertilization.

Bibliography

Horbach, J. G. M., Maathuis, J. B. and Van Hall, E. V. (1973). Factors influencing the pregnancy rate following hysterosalpingography and their prognostic significance. *Fertil. Steril.*, **24,** 15

Van Hall, E. V. and Trimbos-Kemper, G. C. M. (1982). The management of 'unexplained infertility'. *Infertility*, **5,** 105

Van Hall, E. V. (1982). Androgyny: a model for improving gynaecologist–patient interaction. *J. Psychosom. Obstet. Gynaecol.*, **1,** 87

34
Stress in infertile couples

R. F. HARRISON, A. M. O'MOORE, R. R. O'MOORE and
D. ROBB

INTRODUCTION

Involuntary sterility is undeniably a most stressful situation for a couple to find themselves in. However, the role stress itself plays in the aetiology of childlessness and how best this can be treated is unclear. This is hardly surprising for, although stress may be investigated and treated biochemically and psychologically, and while there is a large amount of literature on psychosocial aspects of fertility[1], the optimum approach is yet to be worked out.

We have previously reported on the formation of a psychological stress profile to measure stress levels in infertile couples[2] and of the close relationships that these meaurements have to biochemical stress markers[3,4]. However, our attempts to treat in particular the idiopathic infertile couples who make up 19% of our total clinic population[5] or that sub-group of women who show spikes of hyperprolactinaemia[6-8], especially in the premenstrual phase, have not been over successful. Therapy such as clomiphene citrate[6] and bromocriptine[7] have been disappointing and transcendental meditation has been found unacceptable to the majority of patients[2].

Although a combination of clomiphene citrate plus bromocriptine has been more successful it was obvious that further in-depth biochemical and psychological studies were needed. The results of these further investigations together with the effects of treatment with autogenic training form the basis of this chapter.

MATERIAL AND METHODS

Patients

22 couples with at least 2 years infertility were enrolled into the study. All had a normal fertility profile[5]. The mean age of the women patients was 33.2 years (range 26–41 years), the mean length of infertility 6.6 years (range 4–10 years).

10 control couples were also studied who had had no difficulty in conceiving and who were not on hormonal therapy. The mean age of these was 32 years (range 24–38 years).

Biochemical

Urine-free cortisol and plasma prolactin levels were measured at the same time as psychological assessment. Standard RIA techniques using reagents supplied by the Radio-Chemical Centre, Amersham, and CEA-Sorin, 61y-sun Yvette, France, were used respectively.

Psychological assessment

Four psychological self-report tests were used: (1) the State–Trait Anxiety Inventory (STAI)[8]; (2) the Taylor Manifest Anxiety Scale[9]; (3) the Sixteen Personality Factor (16 PF)[10], in particular emotionality, guilt proneness, tension and motivational distortion; (4) the Eysenck Personality Questionnaire (EPQ)[11] measuring extraversion–introversion, neuroticism–stability, psychoticism and a lie scale.

Study flow sheet

After selection for the study a visit was arranged for the couple between days 25 and 30 of the menstrual cycle. On the day prior to this both partners collected 24-hour urine samples. The psychological profile was measured during the visit and blood taken for prolactin estimation. This process was repeated for the control patients.

13 couples followed the autogenic training programme. This is a series of simple mental exercises designed to diminish responses to stress and enhance the relaxation response. Patients proceed to a gentle exercise in body awareness and physical relaxation, progressively involving the various areas of the body. Hourly group sessions (four couples per group) were given weekly for 8 weeks and couples

urged to practise for a few minutes three times each day. Pregnancy was achieved by one couple during the course and one couple dropped out and were not re-tested. One other couple became pregnant 3 months after finishing the course.

RESULTS

Investigations

Table 1 shows the couples to have higher mean anxiety scores of all the initial emotionality factors. This is particularly true of the infertile women except for the STAI state and the 16 PF tests. Further break-

Table 1 Comparison of emotionality in patients and controls. Combination of comparison of emotionality in the females, males, and couples

Factors	Females		Males		Couples	
	Control (n = 10)	Patients (n = 22)	Control (n = 10)	Patients (n = 22)	Control (n = 10)	Patients (n = 22)
STAI-trait	33.4	40.2*	33.2	36.0	33.3	38.0
STAI-state	33.1	33.8	37.4	35.2	34.2	38.5
Taylor Manifest	6.9	10.2*	5.2	7.4	6.0	8.8
Cattell (Emotionally stable)	4.9	5.0	6.6	5.7	6.3	5.3
EPQ (Extraversion)	13.5	9.5	15.1	13.0	14.3	11.3

*Difference between control and experimental groups significant ($p < 0.05$).

Table 2 Other relevant factors in the 16 PF personality factor tests

	Female		Male	
	Control (n = 10)	Patients (n = 22)	Control (n = 10)	Patients (n = 22)
Apprehension	4.8	6.7	5.6	5.2
Tense, frustrated driven	5.2	6.4	6.5	5.2

down of the 16 PF tests (Table 2) showed the female patients to have higher mean scores than had their controls in respect of tension (6.4 and 5.2, respectively), correlating perhaps with the significantly

Table 3 EPQ Neuroticism

	Female		Male	
	Control (n = 10)	Patients (n = 22)	Control (n = 10)	Patients (n = 22)
	8.9	13*	7.7	8

*Difference between control and experimental groups ($p < 0.001$).

different ($p < 0.001$) neuroticism score (Table 3) in suggesting that infertile women have greater psychological lability than their fertile counterparts. The male patients again had lower mean scores on these factors than had the controls (Tables 2 and 3), which although not significant are a trend that suggests that male patients were more relaxed, tranquil and unfrustrated than their controls.

Table 4 Comparison of 'faking good' patients and controls

	Female		Male	
Factor	Controls (n = 10)	Patients (n = 22)	Controls (n = 10)	Patients (n = 22)
EPQ (Lie)	4.8	8.3	3.6	9.3*
Cattell (Motivational distortion)	3.5	5.4**	4.1	5.8

Difference between control and experimental groups *$p < 0.001$; **$p < 0.05$.

However Table 4 shows that examination of the lie scale (EPQ) and motivational distortion (MD) factor of the 16 PF reveals male patients to have higher mean scores on both tests than their controls with significance reached in the EPQ lie test ($p < 0.001$). The female patients also had higher mean scores than their controls with significance reached in the 16 PF (MD test) ($p < 0.05$).

Therapy

Table 5 shows that after autogenic training there was for the most part a reduction in the mean anxiety scores both in husbands and in

Table 5 Comparison of 'anxiety' of patients before and after autogenic training. Results are given as mean scores

Emotionality factors	Female		Male	
	Before treatment	After treatment	Before treatment	After treatment
STAI A-State	42.9	33.6*	36.0	30.3*
STAI A-Trait	41.1	38.1	33.0	31.0
Taylor Manifest	10.9	8.8	6.63	6.72
16 PF	5.54	5.45	6.2	5.5
EPQ	11.1	10.2	8.0	7.7

*Difference between control and experimental groups ($p < 0.05$).

wives. Statistical significance was, however, only reached with the STAI state test ($p < 0.05$) suggesting that both infertile women and husbands are better able to cope with an anxiety-provoking task after relaxation therapy. The women were also found to be significantly less self-reproaching after autogenic therapy (6.7 v 5; $p < 0.05$) but husbands were found to be more self-reproaching (4.7 v 5.1), although

Table 6 Comparison of 'tension' among infertile couples before and after autogenic training. Results are expressed as mean scores

Patients	Before treatment	After treatment
Females	6.3	6.0
Males	5.3	6.6

this difference was not significant. Table 6 shows a similar pattern for tension, the female patients reporting less tension after treatment and the husband mean scores higher after treatment. None of these differences, however, were statistically significant.

But in conjunction with the pre-treatment scores with the EPQ lie

Table 7 Comparison of 'faking good' among the male patients before and after autogenic training. Results are expressed as mean scores

	Before treatment	After treatment
EPQ (L)	10.9	9.9
16 PF (MD)	5.8	5.45

scale and the 16 PF MD factor, Table 7 shows that the male tendency to fake good had diminished at the post-treatment interview.

Table 8 Biochemical variables in idiopathic infertility

	Females			Males		
Variable	Controls	Patients	Post-treatment patients	Controls	Patients	Post-treatment patients
Prolactin	194	350*	251*	130	205	–
$(mU l^{-1})$	(n = 9)	(n = 14)	(n = 10)	(n = 8)	(n = 12)	
Urine free	291	220	268	302	271	–
cortisol (nmol	(n = 9)	(n = 12)	(n = 9)	(n = 8)	(n = 11)	
$(24 h)^{-1})$						

*Difference between control and experimental groups ($p < 0.05$).

Predictably Table 8 shows that plasma prolactin levels were higher in patients than controls with a significant difference reached in females ($p < 0.05$). This level fell significantly following autogenic therapy ($p < 0.05$) but no significant differences were observed between patients and controls either before or after autogenic therapy in 24-hour urine free cortisol values.

Pregnancies

One patient conceived and delivered a female child.

DISCUSSION

The results of the psychological tests confirm our previous studies in showing idiopathic infertile patients to be biochemically and psychologically more stressed than their fertile counterparts[2-4]. This appears particularly true of the infertile female patients who are more prone to anxiety, are more introverted, guilt prone and tense than their control counterparts. If the high motivational distortion scores are considered it might be argued that the results underestimate the strength of feelings both in the females and in the males. This requires further investigation for it is recognized[12] that distortion in the direction of greater social desirability leads to lower anxiety and slightly elevated extraversion scores. However it also points to the necessity for developing more sensitive test parameters.

Only one pregnancy was achieved during autogenic training[4] but unlike the previous study using transcendental meditation[2] where only three patients stayed the course only one dropped out of this study. The more Westernized approach of autogenic therapy appears therefore to suit the Irish mentality. However, although the results showed a trend towards improved psychological health following therapy, in keeping with other research studies[13,14], significant improvements were only found amongst female patients in anxiety and guilt proneness. However, a significant reduction of mean prolactin levels ($p < 0.05$) in parallel with decreased anxiety scores following treatment is encouraging as is the significant reduction in the anxiety state in the patients ($p < 0.05$) and a decreased tendency to 'fake good' suggesting increased openness after autogenic therapy.

It must be noted that patients were not re-tested until at least 2 months after completion of the autogenic therapy programme by which time the disappointment of two or three further infertile cycles may have been psychologically detrimental. Indeed, bearing in mind the results of a previous study on patients undergoing artificial insemination[15], which showed that perhaps the clinic itself bears a high responsibility for the stress engendered, greater success in investigation and treatment might well be achieved by embarking on such programmes from the initial visit rather than waiting until investigations are complete. Further studies now in progress will show whether this is indeed correct.

References

1. Christie, G. L. (1980). The psychological and social management of the infertile couple. In Pepperell, R. J., Hudson, B. and Wood, C. (eds.). *The Infertile Couple*, pp. 229–247. (Edinburgh: Churchill Livingstone)
2. Harrison, R. F., O'Moore, A. M., O'Moore, R. R. and McSweeney, J. R. (1981). Stress profiles in normal infertile couples. Pharmacological and psychological approaches to therapy. In Insler, V., Bettendorf, G. and Geissler, K. H. (eds.). *Advances in Diagnosis and Treatment of Infertility*, pp. 143–157. (New York: Elsevier, North-Holland)
3. Harrison, R. F., O'Moore, R., O'Moore, A., McSweeney, J. and Carruthers, M. (1980). Correlations between psychological and endocrinological stress profiles in infertile couples. In *Serono Symposia Endocrinology of Human Reproduction*. (Oxford: New Aspects)
4. O'Moore, A. M., O'Moore, R. R., Harrison, R. F., Murphy, G. and Carruthers, M. (1983). Psychosomatic aspects in idiopathic infertility. Effects of treatment with autogenic training. *J. Psychosom. Res.*, **27**, 145
5. Harrison, R. F., Walzman, M., McGuinness, E., Gill, B. and Kidd, M. (1981).

Investigation and treatment of the infertile couple in Ireland. *Clin. Exp. Obstet. Gynaecol.*, **7**, 145

6. Harrison, R. F. and O'Moore, R. R. (1983). The use of clomiphene citrate with and without human chorionic gonadotrophin. *Irish Med. J.*, **76**, 273

7. Harrison, R. F., O'Moore, R. R. and McSweeney, J. (1979). Idiopathic infertility. The trial of bromocriptine versus placebo. *Irish Med. J.*, **72**, 79

8. Spielberger, C. D., Gorsudi, R. L. and Lushane, R. E. (1970). *STAI Manual for the State Trait Anxiety Inventory.* (Palo Alto, Cal.: Consulting Psychologist Press)

9. Taylor, J. A. (1953). A personality scale of manifest anxiety. *J. Abnorm. Soc. Psychol.*, **48**, 285

10. Cattell, R. B. and Eleer, H. W. (1970). *Sixteen Personality Factor Questionnaire.* (Slough: National Foundation for Education and Research)

11. Eysenck, H. J. and Eysenck, S. B. G. (1975). *Manual of the Eysenck Personality Questionnaire.* (London: Hodder and Staughton)

12. Krug, S. E. and Cattell, R. B. (1971). A test of the trait-view theory of distortion in measurement of personality by questionnaire. *Educ. Psychol. Meas.*, **31**, 721

13. Luthe, W. and Schultz, J. H. (eds.). (1969). *Autogenic Therapy*, Vol. **3**, *Applications in Psychotherapy.* (New York: Grune and Stratton)

14. Brown, B. (1977). *Stress and the Art of Bio-Feedback.* (London: Harper and Rowe)

15. Harrison, R. F., O'Moore, A. and O'Moore, R. (1981). Stress and artificial insemination. *Infertility*, **4**, 303

35
Psychosexual problems in infertility

A. D. G. BROWN

Infertility causes considerable physical and psychological strains on a couple and it is well known that a wide range of emotions may be displayed by both partners. The psychological stress may be manifested as a behavioural problem so that sexual activity is affected. The relationship between sexuality and infertility is complex and Elstein[1] observed that infertility may cause sexual problems, sexual dysfunction may masquerade as infertility or there may be coincidental sexual disturbance in the infertile couple.

Steele[2] studied 500 infertile couples and found that 37% had sexual or marital problems. Amelar et al.[3] considered that male sexual dysfunction was the primary or a major contributory factor in about 10% of infertile marriages. In 1981 Bell[4] interviewed 20 primary infertile couples to assess their psychological adjustment to investigation and treatment. Concerning sexual adjustment, four females and one male had diminished sexual satisfaction secondary to their infertility and two females and one male claimed they had never enjoyed coitus. From the Sexual Experience Scales questionnaire it was found that 30% of both sexes had an aversion to sexual experience. The marital adjustment was analysed and seven couples reported a deterioration in their relationship with 25 and 15% of the women and men, respectively, having a low attraction to their marriage. A good correlation ($r = 0.7$) was observed between sexual satisfaction and marital attraction.

The incidence of sexual problems in infertility depends on many factors, including the attitude of the clinician to sexuality, the degree of reluctance by the patient or clinician to discuss the problem and on a detailed sexual history. However the data show that sexual problems are an important factor in the management of infertility.

CLASSIFICATION OF SEXUAL DISORDERS

This has been simplified by Kaplan's[5] concept of the biphasic nature of sexual response. Thus in men, *erectile dysfunction*, which can be primary or secondary, is due to a disordered vasocongestive phase which is under parasympathetic control of the autonomic nervous system; *ejaculatory disorder*, either primary or retarded, results from dysfunction of the sympathetically innervated orgasmic phase. Likewise in women, *general sexual dysfunction* relates to a vasocongestive problem which is separate from *orgasmic dysfunction*. Vaginismus is a psychosomatic condition involving involuntary spasm of the vaginal muscles which prevents penile penetration; it is not related to the biphasic sexual response as both phases are usually normal. General sexual dysfunction involves a variable degree of sexual inhibition characterized by a lack of erotic feelings and reduced vasocongestion so that such vaginal changes as lubrication and expansion do not occur. These women may or may not have orgasmic dysfunction.

The term impotence is widely used to describe impaired erection but its strict meaning is the inability to copulate or reach orgasm. Erectile dysfunction is a more accurate term and is, therefore, recommended[5,6].

EFFECT OF INFERTILITY INVESTIGATION ON SEXUAL FUNCTION

It has been suggested that infertility investigations may cause psychological problems[7] and several workers have implicated particularly the mid-cycle postcoital test (PCT). The effect of this test on 51 infertile couples has been studied by Drake and Grunert[8]. Infertility was present for 1 year at least and the initial interviews excluded sexual dysfunction. Six men had two negative PCTs (no sperm in the vaginal pool or motile sperm in the cervical mucus); of these men one admitted to a 7-year history of impotence while the remaining five had acute dysfunction as their sexual performance between the tests was normal. Two experienced erectile dysfunction which prevented intravaginal ejaculation and the three others had erections but were unable to reach a complete ejaculation.

Drake and Grunert noted some predisposing factors to this mid-cycle problem. The 'This is the night' syndrome is seen commonly in infertile couples and results from the knowledge that mid-cycle coitus may lead to conception; this demand for performance can be threatening to some men.

The change in purpose of intercourse from sex for pleasure to sex on demand affects the spontaneity of love-making and, possibly, the couple's relationship when its primary purpose changes from being an expression of a loving relationship to the need for conception. In the study most affected husbands observed that their wives' interest in sex was concentrated on mid-cycle which provoked hostility and further stress. The use of the helpful basal body temperature chart may also complicate the problem by demonstrating the need for planned intercourse.

These charts and the postcoital test result, usually for the first time, in the couple sharing their sexual behaviour and performance with a third party, the clinician. Some men are unable to perform on demand particularly when a third party is assessing the outcome[7]. Drake and Grunert found that the five dysfunctional couples experienced increased anxiety at intercourse for the postcoital test.

When a male has a sexual problem, for example erectile dysfunction, he becomes worried about his ability to perform well in the future. This anxiety may lead to further failure and thus a vicious cycle is established. The phenomenon has been observed by Masters and Johnson[9].

The treatment recommended for this acute mid-cycle male problem includes the discontinuation of investigation for 6 months, reassurance to the couple that the problem is common and temporary, and a reminder to them that the main purpose of intercourse should be their mutual gratification and a demonstration of affection for each other.

EFFECT OF DIAGNOSING AN ORGANIC CAUSE OF INFERTILITY

The diagnosis of an organic cause for infertility is known to have psychological sequelae. This is well demonstrated by Berger[10], who interviewed 16 couples in whom a diagnosis of azoospermia was made. They had been infertile from 8 months to 4 years and the female and male age ranges were 21–34 and 21–38 years respectively.

Exclusions from the study were couples in whom the male's infertility was known before marriage, when the female was found to have a physical abnormality or when either partner demonstrated severe psychopathology. Berger's interviews focussed on each partner's reaction to the diagnosis and on their dream reports.

Following discovery of azoospermia 10 of the 16 (63%) men experienced impotence which involved failing to institute or maintain an erection to orgasm; the impotence lasted for 1–3 months. Prior to the diagnosis all the men had normal sexual function. Only five of them reported dreams which were of no particular relevance. Of the women, 14 of the 16 (87%) had adverse reactions to the azoospermia diagnosis. Six had feelings of anger towards their husband and 10 had similar dreams of (1) concern for the husband; (2) a wish to be rid of him; and (3) guilt over the wish. When the wife had no symptoms or dreams the husband did not suffer impotence; this suggests an interactional cause for the disorder.

Berger suggested that management of this condition should involve a consultation with the couple, reassurance that the phenomenon is a common and expected reaction to the diagnosis and that it should resolve within 3 months. Discussion should then be directed to the couple's reaction to the diagnosis, namely the husband's depression and feeling of inadequacy and the wife's rage. The couple should be encouraged to continue discussions at home about their feelings and to postpone the decision of what to do about the infertility.

SEXUAL PROBLEMS IN RELATION TO INFERTILITY

A wide range of sexual disorders may be related to infertility, as Elstein[1] has shown. Previously satisfactory sexual activity may be adversely affected by infertility investigation.

Loss of libido may occur when the main purpose of sexual activity changes from the expression of mutual desire and affection to the need for reproduction. This phenomenon affects women more commonly and, as has been shown, the woman may agree to intercourse only in mid-cycle when there is the possibility of pregnancy.

Inhibition of orgasm – The effect of the postcoital test on ejaculation has been demonstrated[8], and the husband may suffer from the impression that his role is to provide semen for his wife's genital tract. In women anorgasmia may result from a preoccupation with conception at the expense of the previously satisfactory response to stimulation.

Erectile disorders (impotence) – Erectile difficulty during postcoital tests or following the discovery of azoospermia has been shown and reassurance that the problem is common and temporary is necessary. Also, masturbation to produce semen for analysis may provoke disorder as many men find the procedure disturbing. Endogenous depression can be aggravated by infertility and cause dysfunction; as with all psychiatric problems the depression must be treated before any success with sexual counselling can be achieved.

Sexual problems masquerading as infertility

Vaginismus results from a phobic anxiety to vaginal penetration. Rarely is a physical factor present thus the classic gynaecological procedures of vaginal dilatation under general anaesthesia, hymenectomy or perineotomy are not indicated or justified. Elstein stresses the well-recognized clinical observation that often a dominant female who finds it hard to submit has a gentle male who will not force her to submit and both have a strong need to maintain the sexual stalemate of non-consummation. Also the male frequently has sexual difficulties such as erectile dysfunction or premature ejaculation. Vaginismus responds well, but often slowly, to the correct treatment of psychotherapy and the use of vaginal stretching techniques by the female and, sometimes, her partner[11].

Erectile disorders – The aetiology of erectile dysfunction includes physical factors, for example fatigue, debility and endocrine or neurological problems such as diabetes or multiple sclerosis. Psychological factors are common and the anxiety following one episode of erectile failure resulting in a vicious cycle of further dysfunction has been cited; also endogenous depression and marital discord may cause a problem but in both cases it is necessary to establish which are the primary and secondary difficulties.

Ejaculatory incompetence – This is also called retarded ejaculation and is present when ejaculation does not occur in spite of a satisfactory erection. Drug therapy with hypotensives or anti-depressants may be the cause but more commonly psychological or relationship problems are involved.

Fears and anxieties result in stress which may cause infertility; however, the mechanism by which this occurs is not fully understood. Nevertheless worries concerning, for example, what is normal sexual activity, fear of pregnancy, etc. can be alleviated by the understanding clinician.

Incidental sexual abnormalities

Incidental sexual abnormalities may be discovered during infertility investigations.

Anorgasmia – Primary anorgasmia has been estimated to occur in about 10% of women. Treatment for the primary or secondary condition may or may not be requested; if so advice on sexual physiology and technique is required.

Premature ejaculation – This is a common problem but its definition varies; Kaplan[5] described its essential features as the absence of voluntary control of the ejaculatory reflex so that arousal is quickly followed by orgasm. Sometimes premature ejaculation may present as a secondary erectile dysfunction due to anxiety caused by inability to control ejaculation. Correct treatment using the squeeze technique[9] gives excellent results.

TREATMENT

It has been shown that there is a relationship between sexuality and infertility, therefore the clinician must be able to recognize a sexual difficulty as the earlier it is diagnosed the easier is treatment. A detailed sexual history is essential and it should be taken in an empathic and non-judgemental way; information should be obtained from each partner about their interest, pattern of activity, arousal, penile penetration and ejaculation.

Sufficient time must be set aside with the couple so that there is full discussion of the many aspects of the problem. Their feelings, anxieties and fantasies can be explained and misunderstandings, for example, about the fertile time of the cycle and coital frequency, can be corrected. Infertility investigations are often complicated, stressful and disruptive so that full explanations are essential if co-operation is to be achieved. The interference and monitoring of the couple's sexual activity should be strictly limited if the problems that have been highlighted are to be avoided.

When the final diagnosis is made an accurate assessment should be given so that the couple have realistic expectations for the future.

Also love-making will be allowed to return to its important role of providing pleasure and an expression of affection for each other.

In treating an established sexual problem the principles involved[6] are similar to those in infertility. There is a mutual responsibility as all problems should be considered shared disorders. For example the man may contribute to his partner's anorgasmia by his lack of appreciation of her needs; when this is understood he may feel inadequate. The emphasis should be on shared responsibility rather than blame.

Ignorance of human biology and effective sexual technique are widespread, particularly among dysfunctional couples. Simple information on basic anatomy and physiology is often necessary and while it may not relieve symptoms it is a prerequisite to successful treatment[12]. A negative attitude to sexual expression may result from the parental or religious or cultural background and is commoner in women, possibly due to Western culture's double-standard morality[13]. The male may have to reassure his partner that respect will grow rather than lessen if she becomes more sexual, but this may be accompanied by anxiety about his ability to cope with her increased demands. Probably most important of all is an encouragement to increase discussion between the couple as undoubtedly communication failure perpetuates and escalates the problem.

The best treatment for sexual disorders uses the behavioural approach and the Sensate Focus technique of Masters and Johnson[9]. They recognized that touch is a basic part of human communication and many feelings are conveyed through it. The basis of this method is a gradual re-learning of sexual, or courting, behaviour which initially involves kissing, then touching, first fully clothed then unclothed and, finally, intercourse. Sensate Focus forms the basis for treatment of most sexual dysfunction.

CONCLUSION

Sexual problems are associated with infertility in a variety of ways thus a detailed sexual history taken in an understanding way is important. Full discussion of all aspects of the problem may be time consuming but will certainly be worth while. Treatments for acute and chronic sexual disorders are available and, in general, give good results.

References

1. Elstein, M. (1975). Effect of infertility on psychosexual function. *Br. Med. J.*, **iii,** 296
2. Steele, S. J. (1976). Sexual problems related to contraception and family planning. In Crown, S. (ed.). *Psychosexual Problems: Psychotherapy Counselling and Behaviour Modification*, pp. 383–401. (London: Academic Press)
3. Amelar, R., Dubin, L. and Walsh, P. (eds.). (1977). *Male Infertility*, p. 202. (Philadelphia: W. B. Saunders)
4. Bell, J. S. (1981). Psychological problems among patients attending an infertility clinic. *J. Psychosom. Res.*, **25,** 1
5. Kaplan, H. S. (1974). *The New Sex Therapy*. (London: Bailliere Tindall)
6. Brown, A. D. G. (1982). Sexual dysfunction in gynaecological and obstetrical practice. In Bonnar, J. (ed.). *Recent Advances in Obstetrics and Gynaecology*, pp. 283–306. (Edinburgh: Churchill Livingstone)
7. Walker, H. E. (1978). Sexual problems and infertility. *Psychosomatics*, **19,** 477
8. Drake, T. S. and Grunert, G. M. (1979). A cyclic pattern of sexual dysfunction in the infertility investigation. *Fertil. Steril.*, **32,** 542
9. Masters, W. H. and Johnson, V. E. (1970). *Human Sexual Inadequacy*. (Edinburgh: Churchill Livingstone)
10. Berger, D. M. (1980). Impotence following the discovery of azoospermia. *Fertil. Steril*, **34,** 154
11. Duddle, M. and Brown, A. D. G. (1980). The clinical management of sexual dysfunction. In Elstein, M. (ed.). *Clinics in Obstetrics and Gynaecology*, Vol. **7,** pp. 293–323. (London: W. B. Saunders)
12. LoPiccolo, J. and LoPiccolo, L. (1978). *Handbook of Sex Therapy*. (New York: Plenum Press)
13. Christensen, H. T. and Gregg, C. F. (1970). Changing norms in America and Scandinavia. *J. Marr. Fam.*, **32,** 616

36
Problems of adoption

L. LEFROY

The title 'Problems of Adoption' is very wide and I must deal with it somewhat superficially and selectively. I will first outline the establishment and structure of adoption services in Ireland. I will then go on to describe the changing needs of the children who need adoptive families and some of the problems these raise. I will discuss adoptive parents and particularly those who are infertile or childless and the problems they raise. I will not use the word 'problem' much since although I will be raising matters for consideration and drawing attention to specific possible difficulties, I would not like adoption and all that surrounds it to be seen too negatively.

Adoption is a permanent arrangement by which adoptive parents assume full legal parental responsibility for the child and it involves the severing of the child's legal relationship with his natural parents and establishes a new legal parent–child relationship between the child and his adoptive parents. In this it is different from fostering in which, no matter how long term or emotionally secure the relationship is between the child and his foster parents, the relationship is not legally binding. It is the legal transfer of parental rights and responsibilities that makes adoption different from fostering. It is often also assumed that as the legal rights and responsibilities are transferred to the adoptive parents, the natural parents cease to have any interest or contact with the child but this need not be so in all cases. I will refer to such a situation later.

Legal adoption was first introduced in Ireland in 1952 after much debate and controversy. It would seem that it was then seen as a way of alleviating problems for unmarried mothers and enabling childless couples to have a child which they could call their own. The child himself was important but his needs were not the primary focus of adoption. It was not until 1974 that the statement was made in adoption legislation that a decision on the making of an adoption order 'shall regard the welfare of the child as the first and paramount consideration'. Social workers are trying to move the focus of adoption more clearly to the needs of the children, although the needs of adoptive and natural parents are important and cannot be dismissed – nor should they be.

The first legislation in 1952 only allowed for the adoption of illegitimate or orphan children under 7 years of age – the age restriction was raised to 21 years in 1964. The 1952 Adoption Act specified the religious denomination of those who were eligible to adopt a child and laid down that children should be adopted by people of the same religion as the child and his parents. This restriction was relaxed in 1974 to allow the natural parents to consent to the adoption of their child by people of a different religion, if any. This made it possible for couples of different denominations or with no religion to adopt legally.

In 1952 the parents' consent to adoption could not be given until the child was at least 6 months old but in 1974 this was altered to at least 6 weeks old. In 1952 the law only allowed for parental consent to be dispensed with if the mother or guardian could not be found or was incapable by reason of mental infirmity of giving consent. In 1974 the Adoption Act gave prospective adoptive parents the right to appeal to the high court in cases where the parent or guardian refused to give consent or withdrew a consent already given.

Children can be placed for adoption by their parents, a registered adoption society, a health board or another person if the child is being placed with a relative. 'Third' party placements are otherwise prohibited. Before legal adoption in Ireland it was common practice for children to be placed with new parents on a long-term basis by a 'third party', usually doctors, priests or nursing home staff.

At present in Ireland there are 19 registered adoption societies and eight health boards but not all health boards place children for adoption and the numbers placed by societies vary greatly. Some registered adoption societies are run by or in conjunction with health boards. All the presently registered adoption societies were registered before the religious restrictions were relaxed and were set

386

up for a specific religious denomination (18 Roman Catholic, one Protestant). The health boards are supposedly non-denominational. That there is no society or health board that readily accepts people of no religion or who are non-Christian is a matter of considerable anger to such people and it is often said that there is an unnecessary emphasis on religion in respect of applicants for adoption. I would suggest that there is such emphasis, but not more so than in other aspects of life in Ireland. Considerable discussion and press coverage was given recently to a situation where a Jewish couple resident and domiciled in Ireland adopted a child in South America, partly because they were unable to find an adoption society or health board in Ireland able to place a child with them. The law still states that the parent in giving consent for adoption must agree to the religion of the prospective parents and most parents appear to choose that the child be brought up in their own religion rather than with a couple of different denominations, non-Christians or of no religion.

In the 30 years since adoption has become legal in Ireland the majority of adopted children have been the children of unmarried mothers and were placed as small babies. They were also usually healthy 'normal' children without great handicaps or possible congenital illness or instability in their background. Handicapped children or those with difficulties in their background were usually reared in institutions or foster homes. It is likely that there were three reasons for this.

(1) That it was assumed it was too great a risk to transfer a responsibility for them to new parents and for there to be no special control/support once an adoption order was made.

(2) It was also felt (often correctly) that adoptive parents wanted 'perfect' children, such as they supposed would have been born to them.

(3) There were as many small 'normal' babies available for adoption as there were prospective adoptive parents.

Recently, attitudes have changed and as the adoption service is, superficially at least, becoming more child focussed attempts are being made by some organizations to place children with handicaps or other difficulties with adoptive parents. The needs of these children are not always understood by people who might consider being adoptive parents and I do not think that we (those involved in childcare) have been successful in making it known to them. The people who might adopt a normal small child are often those who are wanting a child that might have been born to them and may be different from those considering adopting a child with a handicap, a difficult background or an older child.

We still sometimes hear a child referred to as being 'unsuitable for adoption'. What child is there that would be unsuitable for adoption? Probably only the child who has a functioning family already. It might be that the natural parents, while not parenting themselves, would not allow adoption or that adoptive parents could not be found but if we say that the child who is without a functioning family is unsuitable for adoption we are saying that he is unsuitable for family life. That surely can only apply to those with or without a functioning family who are so severely handicapped as to need constant nursing care.

As in other countries, but less so here, the number of unmarried parents who seek adoption for their child is decreasing in proportion to the increase in illegitimate births. This means that, although there are still small healthy babies in need of adoptive homes there are an increasing number of older or handicapped children becoming available. In some instances the children will be older because their parents have tried to keep them and have found themselves unable to do so or, in the case of some handicapped children, their parents have not felt able to care for them and authorities did not consider adoption for them.

It is likely that in the future, but how far away I cannot tell, legitimate children will also be available for adoption in this country and this too will increase the number of children in need of adoptive families. In some cases the legitimate children would be very young and their parents' marriage will have broken down but more common will be those whose parents initially intended to keep them but for some reason parted temporarily at a time of crisis and the contact was not maintained or they feel totally unable to cope. At present these children have to remain in institutional care, children's home, hospital or in a foster home. This also means that they will not be babies; they may even be teenagers.

To some people the idea of a teenager being adopted is very strange; after all, could a teenager accept a new family? Most want to have a family of their own even if they fear the adjustments, emotional and physical, that this would entail. It is our job to help them with this and to help them build up their confidence. This also means we must have confidence both in them and in their prospective adoptive parents. We need to be able to help them to make the commitment, to understand what it is and to do it in their time, not hold them back when they are ready or push them on too hard before they are ready. I think this is sometimes difficult; those in the services tend to have rules to regulate when this decision is to be made. Sometimes these rules are not openly acknowledged. As an example many agencies would automatically place a child as a foster child 'with a view to adoption' or directly for adoption knowing that the adoption order will not be made for over a year. These rules do not take account of the different pace we all have for making decisions, nor to put the confidence in the people most affected by the decision, i.e. the adoptive family and the child, to make the decision. Such rules do not acknowledge the insecurity that can be built into extended 'trial periods' unless all want, understand and can tolerate the trial. Of course ensuring a long trial may be reassuring to those with the responsibility for placing the child; they can wait until the child is fully grafted into the family and the relationship relatively trouble free before releasing them for adoption. However the relationship is already forming and the worker's responsibility should be to help those most closely involved to have the confidence to make the decision and the commitment. Sometimes the commitment is necessary before they can start to feel secure.

I will not spell out all the needs of adopted children as most of their needs are the same as children who live with their natural parents, i.e. love, physical care, stimulation, respect, security, companionship. However, adopted children have some extra needs due to their past experiences and their two sets of parents, the natural and their adoptive parents (whether they knew their natural parents they still have them). Even small babies placed for adoption have had changes in their care before placement. It is possible, though rare, for children to go to their adoptive parents straight from the hospital. It is also rare though not impossible for a baby to be breast fed by the adoptive mother. Many babies go from hospital to a nursery or a foster home while the agency selects and prepares the prospective adoptive parents and the natural parents confirm their decision.

Those who are not small babies have inevitably lacked continuity of care – to the child changes and rejections are similar and the child will need more reassurance and a greater sense of security often while they are testing out their new parents and are confused by the different handling and responses.

This is often particularly difficult for inexperienced parents who themselves need to acquire confidence in their handling of the child. They may be learning and building up their confidence together.

With increasing awareness of children's relationships and childrens' need for understanding of their origins we need to ensure that we can fulfil those needs. Social workers arranging adoption must ensure that they acquire the necessary information and are prepared to hand it on and to help adoptive parents to handle this as confidently and completely as possible. It is also important that natural parents of children placed for adoption should understand the child's needs and be helped to provide the necessary information. Adopted children need to know what their natural parents, father and mother were like, what they looked like, what they felt about the child, what type of occupation they had, their age and family experience. This information builds the picture which helps the child to form a confident self-identity.

Older children may have had other parent–child relationships and have known their natural families. It is increasing practice for social workers to help children to build up life story books to fill in any gaps they may have in their knowledge of their own life experiences. Children who remain in the family in which they were born have all this fairly automatically, their families discuss their early experiences and the family's photograph album is important. The child who has had disruptions in family and parent–child relationships needs these also.

At present in Ireland adopted people do not have access to the birth records officially, but in the UK and many other countries adopted people can obtain a copy of the entry of their birth when they are adult. This would give the name of their natural parent and the name that their natural parent gave them when they were born. Whether this should be allowed in Ireland is controversial and the subject of considerable discussion. Many fear that if this was available the natural parents' lives could be damaged irreparably by the sudden appearance of the child they had parted with, possibly without telling their immediate friends and relations. Some adoptive parents fear that this could jeopardize the security of their relationship with the child they had raised and possibly confuse him by allowing him to compare his natural and adoptive parents. There is considerable evidence that adopted people have wanted to be able to obtain their birth record but there is very little evidence to indicate that where it has been available it has been significantly damaging. There is always a danger and difficulty when two people's needs and wishes affect each other and yet may be in conflict and there are some occasions when we have to decide which is the more necessary or important. Many social workers find that even where a natural parent has wanted complete secrecy or help to forget at the time of parting the same person wants later reassurance about the child and is prepared to help the child provided that contact is sensitively handled. The adoptive parents who have felt able to discuss and inform the child confidently as he grows up and wants information and who have had a satisfying relationship with the child are usually the least threatened by a sudden and desperate need on the adopted person's part to know about his origins.

This brings me back to the adoptive parents and the qualities needed in adoptive parents. Most people who want to adopt a child, want to do so because they have no children or would like more children than they can have naturally. Those who adopt an older or handicapped child often have other reasons such as a particular interest in that child or type of child. With the gradual decrease in small babies available for adoption there is inevitably an increase in the number of childless couples who will not have a child ever or who will be only able to adopt a child with specific difficulties. This means that increasingly childless couples will not be adopting a child similar to the one that they feel would have been born to them or young enough for them to feel that the child was almost born to them. As I suspect many of you are concerned with childless couples I will concentrate on them as adoptive parents. It has been automatically assumed that once a couple found that they could not have children they would adopt a child. Now each couple are asked to think whether they have the extra qualities needed to adopt a child, the understanding of the extra needs of an adopted child and whether they and their family could accept totally a child born to another couple. Social workers in adoption placement agencies have the often difficult task of assessing their marriage, their future parenting ability and their ability to be adoptive parents. There is a constant demand, rightly, for ever improving and increasing the agencies' ability to make such assessments.

We all know that the journey to the discovery of infertility can be a long and painful one for couples. They can go through real decisions about their wish for parenthood individually and as a couple, the sexual side of their marriage becomes one regulated by charts and temperatures and the emphasis of their relationship moves from a friendly sharing relationship to one that has to prove fertility. Some couples can cope with this difficult process relatively comfortably; for others it is frightening and threatening to their relationship and to each of them individually.

Most childless couples go through periods of great emotional distress, and feelings of depression, guilt, anger and lack of self-esteem are very usual. There may be feelings of blame of infertility or – which is often just as difficult – one spouse may have such protective feelings towards the infertile partner that they are unable to share their separate and joint feelings. Many couples immediately plan adoption as soon as they realize or are told that conception is unlikely. This is very natural; apart from a need to cure their childlessness they have a need to take their thoughts from what they are missing to what they can have.

This is very understandable but does not really meet their long-term needs – nor, if they do decide, on adoption, their needs as adoptive parents. They experience in different ways a deep sense of loss not only of their expected fertility and place in posterity but also their social expectations and, of course, their hope of a child, a child made by both of them. Marital relationships are often badly strained and their envy of their 'fertile' friends is at its highest. These must be alleviated and they need the opportunity to mourn. This is not the time to venture forth to adoption even though they have for some time considered it a possibility. Adoption itself will not ease the pain or bring the couple closer. Many couples need help at this time; many need professional help which is often not readily offered or available.

It is not unusual for adoption workers to find that, in considering a couple as adoptive parents, they first need help in coming to terms with their childlessness. It is difficult and unsatisfactory for adoption workers to do this as the couple are so firmly focussed on presenting themselves as good parents to the adoption worker, who they see as having the baby they want. It is also difficult for them to express their distress and negative feelings in this context.

A real dilemma for couples who recognize their need for time is that they often recognize also that there may not be much time for them. As more couples postpone attempts to start a family, when there is no pregnancy they may be quite old before they have started and completed their fertility tests. Most adoption societies will not place a child with people over 40 – many have a waiting list and therefore the latest safe age for couples who want to adopt a baby to embark on an adoption application is 35.This means that there is not endless time for them to recover from their feelings about infertility before applying for adoption and the timing therefore is very important.

I have said that adoptive parents need to have the extra aspect of parenting ability to love a child not born to them and to accept that he was born to someone else. This is not always as easy as it sounds. Firstly, they may have extreme feelings of envy towards the child's parents, who had a baby by their standards too easily. Secondly, they must be able to accept with understanding and equilibrium the child's testing questions about his conception, birth and, as he may see it, rejection by his natural parents. Most adoptive parents say they feel as if the child was born to them and by this are indicating the bond between them and the child. This bond and feeling is important but it is equally important for the child that they recognize a part of him that they do not and cannot share and they must be able to explain and describe this to him comfortably for them and for him.

It is sad but not unusual for us to see adopted people who want to know about their origin and say they cannot discuss this with their adoptive parents. They usually give the same reasons: they don't want to remind their parents they did not give birth to them or any child, they don't want their parents to feel that their love for each other is questioned or threatened, they sense a feeling of embarrassment (to put it mildly) about their parents' infertility or jealousy towards those who gave birth to them. These people may have picked up through emotional and unspoken contact negative feelings about sexuality and the security of their relationship with their adoptive parents.

I therefore return to what I said about the adopted child's need to understand his origins and to gain this understanding from those with whom he has a close and warm relationship. It is a deeply sensitive subject to all: the adoptive parents' need to be confident parents, confident that they are 'real' parents. Despite the fact that the child was not born to them they have done the parenting and are

393

none the less real for that. They must have the confidence as parents to feel entitled to form a full parenting relationship.

All parents go through periods of stress and difficulty and variations in their degree of confidence in themselves as parents. Natural parents do not have the same vulnerability to lack of confidence in their entitlement to be parents to their children as adoptive parents do.

I do not list all the other qualities needed by parents such as stability and security which of course apply to adoptive parents as much as any parents. I have referred particularly to the extra aspects of relationships and attitudes which are needed by adoptive parents because they do not apply so much to natural parents who start with a confidence about their procreative capacity and entitlement to a family.

In selecting adoptive parents, adoption placement agencies must assess the potential of prospective adoptive parents. This is not easy as it can be very difficult for prospective adoptive parents to understand what the agencies are looking for. It puts a great onus on the agencies to make it clear and to respect the needs and sensitivities of people applying to them. Adoptive parents formed an adoption parents' association in 1976 to provide support to adoptive parents and to highlight difficulties in the adoptive system. This organization has done much to help in highlighting difficulties found by its members in adopting children and by those who were not happy with the service they had received.

I have inevitably had to deal with the wide area of 'problems' somewhat superficially and selectively. I have tried basically to outline the establishment and structure of the adoption service in Ireland; the children who require adoption and the extension of availability of adoption from only small babies to include any children who need a permanent family. These children could be any age, and of either sex.

The gradual changes that have taken place and the type of children available for adoption have occurred as a result of the focus on adoption being children who need permanent families whatever the children's background, age or physical or mental condition or past experiences. There is now a growing acceptance that no child should be unadoptable. The child may only be unadoptable in so far as it has not been possible to find suitable adoptive parents for him. I have referred to, superficially I realize, the needs of adopted children which are extra to the needs of children reared in their natural families and relate particularly to their origins; also the needs and qualities of adoptive parents which are extra to those of natural parents. Adoption should essentially be a service for the children taking into account the needs of the parents both adoptive and natural and these should be complementary. Adoption is an alternative for childless couples but not always the right option for them, nor always available.

References

1. Adoption Act, 1952, Dail Eireann, Government Press, Dublin, Government Publications, Dublin, Ireland
2. Adoption Act, 1974, Dail Eireann, Government Press, Dublin, Government Publications, Dublin, Ireland

37
Psychosocial aspects of fertility control

T. STANDLEY

The control of human fertility is probably the most widespread example of conscious regulation of a normal physiological process. The psychosocial factors that affect these decisions are very numerous and are frequently interrelated. They include variables that are reasonably easy to define such as age, parity, marital status, education, occupation, and urban/rural residence. They also comprise personal factors, such as husband–wife communication, influence of other members of the family and perceptions of bodily factors and of sex, that are much more difficult to define. Cultural factors also intervene, for instance the value of children, preference for male children, the dependence of social status on continued procreation, and religious prescriptions.

Rather than attempt the practically impossible task of discussing the relative importance and interrelation of these factors, I will try to show how an understanding of at least some of them can help clarify issues relating to the three main components of family planning, and how psychosocial data may in fact be of practical use to the physician, the policy maker and to the scientist working on methods of birth control. One might describe the three main components of family planning as being:

(1) Motivation for family planning, that is decisions on whether or not to practise birth control.

(2)   Choice and use of specific family planning methods.
(3)   Provision of family planning services.

Rather than embark on a theoretical discussion I will briefly describe some studies and their findings under these three headings.

MOTIVATION FOR FAMILY PLANNING

Most psychosocial research on motivation for family planning is
at present carried out in developing countries, where, with a few
exceptions, levels of contraceptive practice are much lower than in
the industrialized world. I will cite two examples of research on this
issue, one from a large quantitative study, the World Fertility Survey,
the other from a small qualitative project in Kenya, a country with a
very high fertility rate.

The World Fertility Survey, conducted in 70 developing countries
during the past decade, has yielded a vast amount of psychosocial
information which has been and is being subjected to sophisticated
statistical analysis. One of its recent publications[1] discusses, *inter
alia*, the relationship between fertility and education, based on data
from 22 developing countries.

Until recently, it had been generally accepted that education was
negatively related to fertility, or, in other words, that higher educational attainment led to greater motivation for and practice of family
planning. The World Fertility Survey data have shown that the
relationship does not prevail universally and is not a straightforward
one. There appears to be an 'educational threshold' prior to which
fertility either is not affected or in fact increases as level of education
rises.

The strength and form of the relationship also appear to be associated with general socioeconomic development. In countries at the
highest level of development, the effect of education on fertility is
most manifest. A corollary of this is that countries at the lowest end
of the development spectrum should expect no change, or perhaps
even an added impetus to marital fertility as an initial result of raising
the educational level of the population.

The extent to which such generalizations, based on the processing
of large quantities of data from different countries, help in understanding the factors at work in specific communities is always a matter of
debate. Certainly the mechanisms of decision-making in the Kenyan
communities studied in a WHO project could not have been elucid-

ated except by an observational study. The study was designed to involve the community in defining its family planning needs and the type of services it desired, as well as to secure its participation in providing such care. The results of the study showed clearly the conflict in these communities between, on the one hand, the high esteem in which fertility was held and, on the other, the realization of the economic constraints of large families and of the health hazards of grand multiparity. Family planning to space pregnancies and to avoid the dangers of grand multiparity was acceptable, whereas slogans such as 'two (or for that matter four) children is enough' met with general laughter and incomprehension.

It was apparent from the study that these communities had been left in a state of confusion by the introduction of the concept of planning their families without any attention being given to planning other components of their lives. This had confirmed their opinion that family limitation was in the interest of 'other people' with ulterior motives, not in their own interest. The men in the community asked why 'strangers are so concerned with stopping us from having children when they don't bother about our leaking roofs'.

Another factor that emerged was the ready acceptance in the family circle of extramarital children and of the children of other relatives who brought them to 'fill out' the smaller families. These practices weakened the economic rationale for limiting family size since the family that had adopted birth control simply spent more of its resources on other people's children that were brought to them. The need for group acceptance and group practice of family planning emerged very clearly from the study, and also the fact that the community, rather than the individual or family, was the appropriate target for information and education.

CHOICE AND USE OF FAMILY PLANNING METHODS

Unlike other areas of therapeutics, where the physician prescribes, in family planning the choice basically lies with the user: the woman, man or couple. A whole range of personal factors enter into the choice of method, such as preferences for certain routes or frequency of administration or perceptions of effectiveness and side-effects. An understanding of these factors helps with counselling individuals on choice of method, with successful practice of the method by the user, and with research and development to improve existing and develop new methods of fertility regulation.

A number of methods of birth control such as the pill, IUDs or injectables affect menstrual bleeding either by decreasing or eliminating it entirely, or by increasing its amount or duration, or cause intermenstrual spotting. To what extent do these side-effects influence the choice by women of these methods or lead to discontinuation of use? In developing new methods, which of these side-effects is it particularly important to avoid? Are women sufficiently aware of when their next menses are due for it to be worth while trying to develop a menses inducer? Most people have opinions on these matters but there has been relatively little scientifically collected data on menstruation. This led the WHO Special Programme of Research in Human Reproduction to organize a cross-cultural study of patterns and perception of menstrual bleeding[2]. Over 5000 women of reproductive age were included in the study from Egypt, India, Indonesia, Jamaica, Korea, Mexico, Pakistan, Philippines, the United Kingdom and Yugoslavia; they belonged to 14 different cultural groups.

The majority of women in 12 of the cultural groups believed that menstruation was an essential characteristic of femininity; the only exceptions were the United Kingdom and Pakistan (Sind), but even there 42% and 33% respectively held this belief. For many women menarche was the time when one 'became a woman'. In spite of this, a substantial proportion of women (41–93%, excluding the United Kingdom) also believed that menstruation was 'dirty'. This paradox may be partly explained by the notions of pollution and impurity that surround menstrual blood in many cultures and that exist alongside the positive connotations of continuing youth and fertility.

The women were aware of the duration of their blood loss, the nature of menstrual blood, the physical discomforts and, to a lesser extent, mood changes associated with menstruation. The majority in all cultural groups did not wish either an increase or a decrease in the amount of blood loss. Furthermore, when a hypothetical contraceptive method that induced amenorrhoea was discussed, most said they would not use it.

Women often confused the concepts of 'duration' and 'amount' of menstrual bleeding. In all cases, light bleeding was equated with 1–3 days' duration and heavy bleeding with 6 or more days' duration. The confusion between duration and amount has important consequences for those concerned with assessing the effect of contraceptive technology on the menstrual cycle. For example, a contraceptive may reduce the actual volume of menstrual blood, but if the frequency or number of bleeding days is increased the user is likely to perceive the volume of blood loss to have increased. If potential users of contraceptives see amount of blood loss in terms of duration, they are likely to misunderstand, and perhaps resent, claims that it reduces the amount of blood loss.

Only a third of women in the sample were able to predict accurately when their next menses were due. They could, however, predict how long it would last. This may be due to the fact that the majority of women experienced little variation, as recorded on their menstrual diary cards, in the length of their bleeding episode but almost one-third experienced a variation of one week or more in the length of the bleeding-free interval. This suggests that fertility regulating methods, such as a menses inducer, may not be used effectively if they require the woman to predict the onset of menstrual bleeding with reasonable accuracy.

A paradox discovered in the study was that the beliefs expressed about menstruation were often inconsistent with behaviour. Those holding the belief that menstruation was like an illness did not necessarily behave as if they were unwell. Conversely, those not holding the sickness belief were among those demonstrating the greatest behavioural changes during menstruation. Therefore, it is understandable that although most respondents said they would not use contraceptives causing increased or decreased bleeding or amenorrhoea, large numbers of women do in fact use such contraceptives in many parts of the world. The effect on menstrual bleeding is only one factor among many affecting the acceptability of a contraceptive method. Other characteristics of the method, such as effectiveness in preventing pregnancy, may be seen as so advantageous as to outweigh the changes in the menstrual cycle it might cause.

USE OF FAMILY PLANNING SERVICES

For family planning practice, as well as motivation and acceptability of methods of fertility control, the acceptability of the services, including the service providers, is an equally important component. Factors that have been identified as being important psychosocially are sex of the provider; in India, caste of the provider; attitudes of the providers to family planning, to specific methods and to the user;

privacy during consultations; whether the service outlet is specifically for family planning; and so on.

One may illustrate the force of these factors by reference to studies carried out in the UK by the Office of Population Censuses and Surveys[3]. Despite availability of services from general practitioners and NHS and other clinics, in 1975 the proportion of unwanted pregnancies remained substantial. Frequent reasons cited for non-use of services were embarrassment at having to deal with a male doctor and dislike of an internal gynaecological examination. Lack of privacy militated against use of clinics, although it was also complained about with respect to GPs. It was felt at times of reception, in the waiting room, and in the lack of seclusion during or after undressing. Most of these shortcomings can be remedied at little or no cost. The author of the report felt that it might also be worth reconsidering the routine use of the gynaecological examination, except when required by the method to be provided. The survey also suggested that the needs of one group at great risk, the teenager, would in part be met by special clinics for the unmarried, possibly held in the evenings.

In most developing countries, the problem may be thought to lie maybe more with availability than with fine shades of acceptability of services. This has led to seeking unconventional approaches to service delivery, such as home-visiting by various types of personnel, or use of commercial outlets or of community organizations for provision of family planning services. In each of these, however, the psychosocial factors that affect their acceptability are just as important and do require research.

CONCLUSION

I have artificially isolated three components of fertility regulation: motivation, use of methods, and use of family planning services. Clearly, all three are interrelated in real life. For example, improving the acceptability of services will affect motivation, and thus use of methods. I have also dealt separately with psychosocial factors such as education, or perceptions of body functions affected by contraceptive technology, that are themselves interrelated and also affected by other psychosocial factors such as age, socioeconomic status or culture. Regression analysis can help in showing which, among these factors, are the most important, but the methodological difficulties, particularly of accurate data collection, must not be underestimated. In the present state of development of the art the best studies may still be those with clearly stated hypotheses and a fairly simple study design.

References

1. United Nations (1983). *Relationships Between Fertility and Education: A Comparative analysis of World Fertility Survey Data for twenty-two Developing Countries.* (New York: UN)
2. Snowden, R. and Christian, B. (1983). *Patterns and Perceptions of Menstrual Bleeding.* (London: Croom Helm)
3. Bone, M. (1978). *The Family Planning Services: Changes and Effects.* (London: HMSO)

Part I

Section 10

Social and Demographic Problems of Fertility*

* Sponsored by the Draper Fund

38
Social and political factors in fertility control

E. M. MARTIN

It is too often overlooked that family planning means just what it says: 'planning', i.e. a conscious choice of goals for the future and of the best means of achieving them. Good planning for the family, or as some like to put it, 'responsible parenthood', must be based on both 'macro' and 'micro' considerations. 'Macro' ones involve the impact of decisions as to family size made by each family in a society on the achievement of the goals of that society. 'Micro' factors concern the impact of such family decisions on the goals of that family.

Essential in each case is a real concern about the future, a willingness to sacrifice present well-being to some extent to protect or promote the future happiness of those now only children or even the children of one's children.

Turning to specific obstacles to more effective family planning, a basic point that cannot be overemphasized is the variation in situations from country to country and even within the same country between rural and urban communities, between ethnic and tribal units and between families at different income levels.

I shall comment on 'macro' considerations of a political and of an economic nature, previous speakers having dealt with religious and moral aspects. I shall then turn to 'micro' factors within the family.

At the national political level one can still find leaders whose policies on family planning are dictated by the simple belief that more is always better. Even in the supposedly sophisticated USA, one can hear otherwise intelligent people refer to country X as strategically important because it has a population of over 100 million. A comparable position is that of the political or military leaders of a few countries who believe that they need a rapidly growing population to man their armed forces against a neighbouring enemy, overlooking the fact that military power is today even more capital intensive than modern industry.

Occasionally, a political leader will adopt the position taken with me once by the top economic adviser to the president of a middle-income LDC* – a Harvard PhD in economics I regret to say – that their farmers had to have big families to ensure expanding markets for their urban industries so that they could benefit from the lower costs of large-scale industrial production. Where the money to buy more industrial products would come from after the additional children had been fed and educated and kept healthy he could not say.

A more frequent economic argument for large rural families has been the need for the extra labour, often starting at a very early age. In some circumstances it is a good point, but population growth has rapidly reduced the size of each farmer's holding making labour a surplus commodity in the rural areas of most countries and causing excessive migration to already overcrowded cities.

Despite these factors plus the religious ones already described, the net result has been that 95% of the LDC population now lives in countries that have adopted national policies designed to reduce population growth. So why has not more been achieved? At the national Government level, there have been four main reasons:

(1) Most important has been the absence of an efficient bureaucracy able to provide to all families the information needed to plan family size wisely and the means to carry out family decisions by safe, modern methods. This is especially difficult in rural areas and 75% of the LDC population is still rural. Private initiatives can help but not on a nationwide basis – Government resources are needed.

(2) Some political leaders have been weak supporters of their own policies because they have not been willing to stand up against the opposition of well-organized and vocal opponents, even though they may represent a small minority of the popula-

*LDC = Less Developed Country

tion. This has reflected in part the not unnatural tendency of politicians to take a short view of the world, focussing more on the next election than the next decade or so when current rates of population growth would become disastrous.

(3) As an example of minority pressure, some Governments have had ineffective programmes because of the policies of the organized medical profession. It has opposed the use of para-medics for relatively simple procedures, even in rural areas when there are no MDs. It has elsewhere required acceptance of developed country standards for medical practices even though the morbidity rates of pregnancies in their countries, and even more from abortions, is far higher, as is the infant mortality rate. There has also been a preference to use their skills for curative medicine rather than preventive measures such as family planning.

(4) Partly because of these pressures some otherwise intelligent leaders have fallen back on the theory that if they concentrate on economic and social development and achieve a better educated and wealthier population, families will act to reduce family size without any help or guidance from the Government – the traditional population transition of the developed countries. The evidence so far is that the financial and personnel resources in most developing countries are not available to achieve such progress for all their people, largely because progress on it cannot keep ahead of their current population growth rates.

The Communist parties often use a similar argument to join right-wing religious groups in opposition to family planning, saying that equalization of incomes by a communist revolution will solve the problem in the same way. There is no evidence it will; rather, as in Cuba, population growth is reduced by massive attempts to emigrate.

At the 'micro' level of the family the principal problem is men, the male parent. His opposition has several causes of varying importance in different societies:

(1) More children flatter his public image of virility; and
(2) it is essential to perpetuate the male name by having plenty of sons, thus making his wife
(3) feel that her standing in the family and the community is determined by the number of children she bears.

409

(4) He fears that if his wife is protected against pregnancy she can cheat without being caught.

(5) Sexual matters like birth control are not considered to be proper subjects for her to talk about with anyone, sometimes not even with him.

(6) He does not always pay much attention to the effect of pregnancies on the health of his wife, another aspect of the common maldistribution of food in the family with females much more subject to malnutrition than males.

Finally, I may be expected to criticize the branch of the medical profession concerned with fertility and sterility for helping more babies to be born. If so, I shall be disappointing, for their activity is in my judgment entirely useful. 'Responsible parenthood' cannot take place without parents having children. It's how many that matters. In addition, in some parts of the world, especially in West Africa, infertility is comparatively frequent. In such communities it is natural that being able to conceive has first priority. How many children to have takes second place, as it should. If family planning programmes are to be accepted there at all they must tackle both problems, but as infertility is cured family planning becomes even more important.

Moreover, I am sure that your great research efforts on the human reproductive system have made and will continue to make important contributions to family planning means, especially by helping to find simpler techniques to reverse sterilizations. Making it easier to do this would give a substantial boost to the use of this procedure, almost 100% effective and increasingly popular in nearly all countries. Most important is the fact that being a 'one-time' procedure, it requires less bureaucratic efficiency to deliver and fewer debates between parents. Achieving this would earn the thanks of all those who are concerned with achieving more quickly and by more humane means population growth rates in all countries which will bring within reach of all their people the enjoyment of full and useful lives.

39
Population trends and prospects

L. R. KEGAN

I propose to deal with world population trends and prospects as a background for pointing out the importance of work on contraceptive development and clinical research.

Recent trends have been favourable. At the end of World War II, there was a sudden sustained decline in death rates starting from 50 per thousand. This, combined with little change in birth rates of around 50 per thousand, produced an unprecedented growth rate of 2% in 1965. But since then, the rate of population growth has declined to 1.75% per year. As a result, the news media for the last few years have been making a grand fanfare about 'the end of the population crisis'.

Nevertheless, there is simply no precedent in world history for the absolute numbers still being added to the world's population. It took hundreds of thousands of years to reach the first billion (1000 million) early in the last century. The fourth billion took place in only 15 years, from 1960 to 1975, but it took only 12 years to reach the fifth billion. As a consequence, about 80 million people are added every year, the equivalent of an additional Mexico or Nigeria.

The basic reason for this population momentum is the continued high, even though declining, birth rates and rapidly falling infant mortality rates in recent decades. As a result, taking account of births that have already occurred and of current life expectancies and barring any nuclear catastrophe, more than one billion people will reach their peak productive years – the ages of 15–29 – during the next two decades.

Before appraising the prospects for world population, it is useful to consider the reasons for the fertility decline. One set of reasons relates to the motivation of families, and particularly women in the developing world, to have smaller families than the six or eight children they had previously. These motivations are associated with the substantial declines in infant mortality, the increased education and status of women (with more entering the job market), fewer choices to breast feed, or breast feeding for shorter lengths of time, and some increased availability of family planning services and contraceptives. Another element in some parts of the developing world, and particularly in the rapidly urbanizing sections, is the increasing limits of housing and in obtaining adequate food at prices that are affordable.

Another set of reasons has to do with the perception by Governments and leading citizens that the recent trends in population growth distribution and structure are out of balance with social, economic and environmental factors. They create difficulties for the achievement of sustained development, including limited resources, food distribution problems, high rates of debilitating disease and infant mortality, lack of proper sanitation, scarcity of investment capital and shortages of educational facilities and work opportunities. The need to increase food and fuel production for rapidly increased numbers of people has led to denuding of forests, transformation of productive land into desert, and waterlogging and salinization of irrigated land. The balance-of-payments deficits and increased debts of most oil-importing developing countries in recent years have further depressed their rates of economic development. Rapid population growth definitely diverts resources from potentially productive investments to support the expanding dependent population. As a result, social services such as education and health cannot keep pace with the burgeoning need and production of materials for export markets is seriously hindered. Finally, the urban crowding and unemployment greatly increase the instability of governments and generates conditions of unrest and intensified immigration and refugee issues.

It is this perception of obstacles to national development that has led the governments in the developing world to announce population policies and to undertake serious efforts to control their population growth. Strong commitment by government leaders is essential to the success of any national programme of family planning services

412

and public education on population issues. Wherever major changes in fertility have occurred, strong national commitment by leaders and in budgets to reduce population growth combined with widely available family planning services have existed.

Governments that once deemed rapid population growth as incidental to their well-being now realize that development itself is not a contraceptive, but can only influence contraceptive usage. As a result, they have been seeking help with their population problems from the more developed countries and the United Nations Fund for Population Activities, who have been providing population planning assistance as part of general development aid to countries who need and want help in reducing their birth rates. 118 Governments now officially support the provision of family planning information and services. There is now an international consensus that access to contraceptive services is a basic human right.

The turning point in this recognition and commitment took place at the World Population Conference that was held in 1974, where all 137 governments adopted, by consensus, a World Population Plan of Action which states:

> Population and development are interrelated: population variables influence development variables and are also influenced by them; thus the formulation of a World Population Plan of Action reflects the international community's awareness of the importance of population trends for socioeconomic development, and the socioeconomic nature of the recommendations contained in this Plan of Action reflects its awareness of the crucial role that development plays in affecting population trends.'

They also agreed with the basic principle of responsible family planning which takes account of needs of the individual, the family and the community:

> 'All couples and individuals have the basic right to decide freely and responsibly the number and spacing of their children and to have the information, education and means to do so; the responsibility of couples and individuals in the exercise of this right takes into account the needs of their living and future children, and their responsibilities towards the community.'

413

There will be another World Populations Conference in 1984, which is expected to affirm the World Population Plan of Action and recommend further implementation.

On the basis of all this experience, it is clear that contraception and development are both necessary to produce a better contraceptive record. Successful family planning programmes occur when there is strong commitment by the host Government to tackle its population problems, an infrastructure with capacity to deal with these services and social and cultural acceptance of the concept of family planning. Since there is no ideal method of family planning, and there is no ideal contraceptive, a combination of methods suitable to different conditions and stages in life comprises the best family planning programme. Surveys show that the number using contraception falls very short of the number who have a knowledge of available family planning methods. There are limitations to current contraception technologies. This fact and their unavailability cause many women in all parts of the world to seek induced abortion.

The prospects, therefore, for future population growth depend on Government commitment, increased contraceptive availability and improved methods of contraception.

If the current rate of increase of 1.75% per year is maintained, the world's population would double in 40 years. This would mean that by the year 2020, the current population of 4.6 billion would grow to 9.2 billion. However, it is expected that Governments will undertake to implement more effective programmes in family planning. In many places such as Bangladesh, India, Nepal, Pakistan, Egypt, and parts of Sub-Saharan Africa and Latin America, the pressures of population against limited resources continue to mount, but the family planning programmes have not yet been very effective. Furthermore, some observers believe that the fertility reductions achieved during the 1970s represent the easy phase because they covered city dwellers and better educated people. Bringing fertility down further will involve more extensive and expensive efforts in education, motivation and extension of family planning services throughout the rural areas.

When all this is taken into account, the world's population is expected to grow to about 6 billion by the year 2000. More than 90% of this growth will occur in the developing countries. This increase alone is almost as much as the entire population of the world as recently as 1930, and will add more people in the year 2000 than were added last year.

But what about the longer run and the possibility of achieving stabilization which is associated with fertility rates of about 2.2 births per couple, or one daughter per woman? The process of development involves a process of demographic transition from a balance of 50 deaths against 50 births per thousand to a full-life equilibrium in which people can have adequate food, be in good health, be literate and live to their four-score years on a sustainable basis. This ultimately involves a balance closer to 10 deaths against 10 births per thousand.

The concern of many of us today is the time it is taking to move through this demographic transition. The longer it takes, the greater the global population will be when we get there. The United Nations estimate is 11–12 billion some time in the twenty-first century. Others believe that there is a serious question whether our planet can support much more than 6 billion at anything near current standards of living. The question therefore is: under what conditions of human life will the eventual stabilization take place? The number will depend on the decisions of hundreds of millions of families, and on the policies and programmes of Governments. But the longer the delay in taking action, the greater the total number will be because of the effect of the population momentum.

For these reasons, it is important that effective population policies and programmes should have an overriding priority on the world's agenda. Greater resources should be marshalled and co-ordinated for research and development of contraceptives that have less serious drawbacks from the standpoints of safety, effectiveness and acceptability than existing family planning methods. Efforts to produce safe, effective and cheap contraceptives, and to design clinical and distribution systems that make them more desirable to couples within their economic, cultural, national and religious settings therefore make an important contribution to world human welfare.

415

40
Fertility, population and development

A. McCORMACK

These congress proceedings have naturally been technical. I would like to put their content, and indeed the work of gynaecologists and obstetricians in the field of fertility, in a wider perspective: that of population growth, development and social welfare, especially in the developing countries. Population growth, and in some cases lack of it, is a grave preoccupation of the international community. Two factors determine such growth (apart from migration, which is not significant for the global picture): fertility and mortality. For all practical purposes, annual population growth is equal to crude birth rates minus death rates.

This century has witnessed a veritable population explosion, however some may dislike the term. It is true that the term is not a strictly accurate one because this 'explosion' is a silent one. But it is apt enough when we consider the explosive rate of population increase in the second half of this century which is steadily continuing in developing countries.

The population of the world was 1.6 billion (a billion is regarded as 1000 million) at the beginning of the century. It was 2.5 billion in 1950. It was 4.6 billion in 1982 and projections call for 6.1–6.4 billion by the year 2000. To appreciate these figures truly it should be realized that it took from the beginning of human history until 1830 for the number of people on earth to reach 1 billion people.

The reason for this unprecedented growth is that a considerable reduction in mortality has been achieved while, especially in many developing countries, birth rates have remained high.

The demographic situation is often regarded as a world population problem, which indeed it is. But it would be more accurate to regard the present position as composed of a number of different problems. In the developed countries, for example, population growth has declined so that in some cases it has reached replacement level. There is no country which has a population rate of increase in the industrialized world of more than 1% annually. On the other hand, there are only a handful of countries in the developing world which have population rates of growth *below* 1.5% per annum. Very many are over 2% annual increase: quite a number are above 2.5% and there are over 30 countries with a rate of increase of 3% or more (several are above 3.5%).

The significance of these rates of increase can be appreciated by recalling that annual rates of increase are compounded. This means that a country with a population rate of increase of 1% will double its present population in just under 70 years; with an increase of 2.5% the doubling will take place in 27 years: a rate of increase of 3% will produce a doubling in just over 20 years.

The importance of these cold statistics is that many of the countries that are already desperately poor and that can least afford or sustain a rapid population increase are the ones which, within the next 20–27 years, are going to be subject to it.

The population of the world in mid-1982 of 4.6 billion people included 3500 million in the developing countries. These formed nearly two-thirds of the world's population. It is projected that by the year 2000, 17 years from now, three quarters of the total population of the world of between 6.1 and 6.4 billion will be in the developing countries. These figures are taken from the best United Nations and other international sources. It is interesting that the monumental World Fertility Survey which was organized and supervised and recently completed by Sir Maurice Kendall, who died a month or so ago, substantially confirmed the figures that have been quoted.

In the past, large birth rates were regarded as a good thing and were endorsed by most religions as such. In fact, the love of life stimulated by the birth of a child is a good and wholesome value which must never be lost. However, we have to realize that we are in a completely new era. As Sir Julian Huxley first warned in 1950; that high birth rates can hinder the economic and social development

418

of the developing countries. An example of this could be taken from the 1960s which produced a remarkable average annual rate of economic growth in the developing countries of 5% per capita. However, the real net increase was 2.5% per capita because the average growth of population in the developing countries at that time was 2.5%.

Another example is taken from the latest world population figures. The bad news was that economic growth had not kept up with population increase in the developing world. In other words, instead of there being growth which could enable poorer countries to give a better standard of living to their people there was a decline in growth. The net result was that there was not economic growth but economic loss as the annual per capita income growth was offset by the annual population growth. These figures indicate on a macro-level the problem that demographic increase causes.

Perhaps I may be permitted here to go right down to the micro-level which illustrates also social consequences. I was in a slum in Haiti in the Caribbean some time ago. I was charmed by the fact that even in the midst of the poverty there were lovely children playing about: obviously the parents were loving and caring. In spite of the fact that Haiti is a desperately poor country and its rate of growth will mean a doubling of its already poor population in 25 years, I felt that it seemed a shame to contemplate any programme which would lessen the numbers of these attractive little children. But then I looked round and I did not see many children over the age of 10; I saw no teenagers. When I asked the reason for this I was told that because of large families and the poverty-stricken nature of the houses, there were only so many of their children that the parents could keep. The rest, when they reached their teens, were turned out of their homes, not out of any lack of love, but merely to make room for other children and to enable these to be fed and cared for. The boys went on the streets and became members, sometimes, of gangs, or otherwise lapsed into a state of unemployment and semi-starvation. The girls became prostitutes. It is clear that a real love for children which was effective would suggest having a lower number because in the forseeable future a very great improvement in living conditions is not to be expected.

One could summarize the whole demographic situation and its consequences by saying that over-rapid population increase, especially when combined with the already considerable numbers, is one of the causes and indeed one of the principle complicating factors of that terrible poverty that one sees in the slums of the overcrowded cities of the third world and the less obvious poverty of the rural areas which drives people to the already densely populated urban areas. Rapid population increase makes it more difficult to feed and nourish children; to give them a decent education; to provide health care for the whole family; to make effective strides towards eliminating grinding poverty, the like of which we can hardly conceive of in the West; to give decent housing instead of the hovels which a vast number of the world's people live in; to give useful employment and dignity to children when they emerge from childhood and are ready for work.

It is ironic that the Population Council of New York did a study of Kenya's population in 1965. It warned that unless stringent measures were taken to reduce population increase, the problems now facing Kenya would occur. They also forecast the exact rate of increase, 3.9% by 1980, if their Report was disregarded. It was. One might well ask in considering attitudes to population and development 'Why look into a crystal ball when you can read the book?'

At country level, Charles Njonjo, Kenya's Minister of Community Affairs, recently told Parliament that a family should have no more than three children. An editorial in Kenya's largest newspaper, *The Daily Nation of Nairobi*, said that 'stringent population measures are absolutely vital, if we are to have a future in which there will be enough food for all, enough jobs to go round and enough room in which to live.' (It is projected that Kenya's population will be 34 million by the turn of the century.)

Population growth is, of course, only one factor in the poverty situation. I once worked out, with regard to one large third world country, that there were about 24 different causes of poverty, of which population increase was only one. To deal with the other 23, however, and neglect the population factor would have been just as much a recipe for disaster as to deal with population and neglect all the other elements of the problem.

One of the reasons why the population explosion has become such a problem is that there is so much reluctance to face it. There are a number of reasons for this: religious, ideological, social and cultural. For example, although Mao Tse Tung was warned in 1954 by Ma Yin Chiu, the Chancellor of the University of Peking, that China's increasing population would rapidly cause very serious problems,

Mao kept to the ideological tenet that the population explosion was a capitalist myth and that a Communist country would always be able to produce enough food to feed and cope with the population increase.

Now we see the results of this failure to face the facts and reasonable projections from them. The present birth control campaign in China has aroused the horror of those familiar with it because of the ruthless way it is carried out. The excuse given is that even with such drastic measures, the population of China will be over a billion and a quarter people by the year 2000 and this will be a very great strain on resources. Ma Yin Chui was rehabilitated after 28 years of exile recently. But the damage had been done.

Developing countries were not keen to admit their population problems because it looked as if, somehow or another, they were to blame for their poverty and that Western nations were using their population increase as an excuse for increasing programmes of population reduction and neglecting programmes for development. In most cases this was not true but it was widely believed.

Not only that but family planning and its methods were regarded by many developing countries as foreign interference with their way of life based on a foreign ideology which should be resisted. The Vice President of Kenya, a Minister for Home Affairs, Mr Mwai Kibaki has now warned Kenyans against dismissing family planning as a foreign interference and he said, 'family planning has already been proven in numerous other societies in the world so we accept it and are ready to apply it in Kenya and apply it effectively.' It is a pity it took so long for this prejudice to be overcome.

But above all, perhaps, was the difficulty that people found in accommodating to the idea that while in the past a large family had been regarded as a blessing and even a necessity because disease carried off so many children and adults and great epidemics served the purpose of birth control, this idea was no longer valid where a considerable reduction in mortality had been achieved in the Third World in a relatively short time. For example, between 1944 and 1955 malaria was almost completely eradicated from Ceylon. The result was an increase of 1% in the natural growth rate because birth rates remained more or less at the same level of 3% and death rates declined by 1%. In fact, it would not be too sweeping a generalization to say that the population explosion of this century, especially in the developing countries, was the result of fertility remaining high and

421

mortality being substantially reduced. There are some who divide those concerned with population and development into population-ists and anti-populationists. But these terms are virtually meaning-less except on a primitive time scale. It is surely axiomatic that in a finite world high birth rates cannot co-exist for long with low death rates.

An example comes from Brazil, the fifth largest country in the world. If the population of Brazil in 1974 of nearly 100 million were allowed to continue at its rate of increase of over 3% its population would be 19 times as great in 100 years' time. Brazil has already reduced its rate of growth by a family planning campaign which has brought the rate down to 2.4% per year. And just as population growth is a spiral upwards when births are increasing, it is a spiral downwards when they are decreasing. Radical political parties main-tain that birth control is being imposed on the people of Brazil by multinational companies, but actually it is the logic of facts that is imposing these programmes. The alternative to birth rates being lowered is that high death rates will take their toll long before saturation point is reached.

The urgency of the need to reduce population increase, at the same time working as hard as possible to improve the living conditions of people in the poorer countries of the world, is great. As I have already pointed out, it was not really recognized until the mid-1960s when the United Nations World Population Conference of population experts alerted people to the fact that there really was a veritable population explosion going on. This had not been realized until the censuses of 1960 and 1961 even by the experts themselves. It took a very consider-able time for countries, for reasons I have indicated, to realize it and to act.

In 1969 a dramatic event took place when the United Nations Fund for Population Activities started with a budget of well below 10 million pounds. Already a trend had been started by the New Delhi Conference of 1965 to reduce rates of growth. The efforts of the United Nations Fund, together with numerous other organizations in the world, some governmental, some voluntary, have resulted in a con-siderable change in the population picture. Whereas in 1965, when the rate of population increase was 2%, it was projected (not proph-esied) that at that rate of growth the 3.5 billion people in the world at that time would increase to 7 billion by the year 2000, the present rate of 1.7% means that there will probably be 900 million less than anticipated by AD 2000.

One final reflection: sometimes population regulation is regarded as anti-life, a refusal to accept life, a kind of selfishness. But this is not so. The stress nowadays must be on *quality* not on *quantity* if we wish to overcome grinding poverty. To have many children may not mean, in present circumstances, a great and really genuine love of life. Personal problems and the problems of rapid population growth indicate nowadays that a love of life may show itself by a smaller number of children which can be better looked after and given the prospect of a more human life in keeping with human dignity.

Part II

Workshop Reports

41
Workshop on the standardized investigation of the infertile couple

MODERATOR: P. ROWE*
CO-ORDINATOR: M. DARLING

Since 1974 the World Health Organization has been concerned with research on infertility. Initially this was confined to epidemiological studies which were undertaken at the request of member governments and took place mainly in sub-Saharan Africa, where infertility was considered to be a major problem in certain communities. In the late 1970s there was increasing scientific interest in the WHO Special Programme of Research in Human Reproduction assuming an active role in research on the aetiology of unexplained infertility, the simplification of diagnostic procedures, evaluation of certain controversial treatments in large-scale multinational trials and continuing research on the prevalence of infertility.

In 1977, the Task Force on the Diagnosis and Treatment of Infertility was established. It was immediately apparent that the lack of standardization of investigative procedures and definitions was the first problem the Task Force had to face. After much discussion between the clinicians involved in the Task Force planning, a manual for the investigation of the infertile couple was developed. This has now been tested in 33 centres in 25 countries and the four presentations in the Workshop discussed the rationale behind the standardized investigation and some preliminary analyses of the data. It was

*Presented by the World Health Organization's Special Programme of Research in Human Reproduction's Task Force on the Diagnosis and Treatment of Infertility.

stressed that since the study was not yet complete not all information is available in some subjects and the results presented at the Workshop were based on the numbers of subjects for whom that particular data item was available.

The first paper was presented on behalf of the Task Force by Professor Bruno Lunenfeld in which the need for a standardized approach to the investigation of the infertile couple was emphasized.

THE NEED FOR A STANDARDIZED APPROACH TO THE INVESTIGATION OF THE INFERTILE COUPLE

The possibilities for classifying infertile patients are virtually unlimited, depending on the clinical and laboratory facilities available. For any classification to be valuable it must be well defined and ethically acceptable, and requires a reasonable compromise to be achieved between the accuracy, clinical usefulness, the effort and cost required.

However, the extent of the investigation of both partners varies in different clinical situations. Since the criteria used to reach certain diagnoses are only vaguely defined, and the patient's history, clinical findings and laboratory results are often interpreted differently, data collected on infertility vary in their reliability and in their uniformity. Often the information collected is excessive and irrelevant for the diagnosis and appropriate therapy and in other instances insufficient, and furthermore may differ from patient to patient even within the same centre.

The lack of uniformity, the extent of the investigation of the couple, the selection of the infertile patient for treatment, the choice of therapy, the treatment scheme, the monitoring, and the follow-up seldom allows a meaningful comparison of data reported from different centres. There are a large number of variables involved, all associated with the problem or problems causing infertility and thus related directly with the success or failure of subsequent therapy. They must be considered when attempting to arrive at the correct diagnosis and in designing studies for the assessment of diagnostic procedures, and the appropriate drug therapy used in the treatment of infertility. Co-ordinated multicentre research using standardized procedures helps to clarify many issues, as well as to improve diagnostic precision and the results of subsequent management in terms of effectiveness, risk, and cost. Furthermore, such research provides the basis for an unbiased assessment of procedures and therapies for which no consensus has yet been reached.

The principal objective of the Task Force approach was to devise a standardized approach to the investigation of the infertile couple, using, in a logical sequence, a minimum of procedures that will result in a rational diagnosis being made. Within the framework of this objective, a manual has been developed for use with forms and flow charts which hinge on three main components for a rational diagnosis – history taking of the couple, physical examination of each partner, laboratory and diagnostic procedures.

While the basic framework of the methodology remains constant, the definitions of factors affecting infertility and diagnostic procedures are under continuous review by the Task Force Steering Committee.

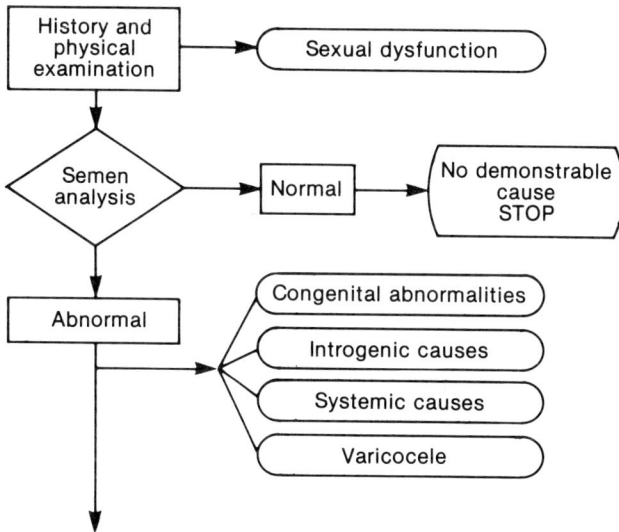

Figure 1 Part of the flowchart for the diagnosis of male accessory gland infection

Multicentre collaboration in 25 countries throughout the world involving to date more than 6000 couples complaining of infertility has permitted the feasibility of this approach to be assessed and the definitions and algorithmic schemes to be revised in the light of the knowledge gained.

For example, certain male diagnoses can be arrived at after history taking and clinical examination and the analysis of semen. These include the diagnoses of sexual dysfunction, congenital abnormalities, iatrogenic causes, systemic causes and varicocele. Due to shortage of time Professor Lunenfeld concentrated on two specific examples – one for the female which is not controversial (hyperprolactinaemia) and one for the male (male accessory gland infection) which is controversial.

The part of the flowchart for the diagnosis of male accessory gland infection is shown in Figure 1. The relevant components from the history and physical examination concern a history suggestive of infection such as any reported urinary symptoms, painful ejaculation, epididymo-orchitis, a history of sexually transmitted disease or physical signs such as abnormal epididymides, or vas deferentia, evidence of past infection, inguinal scars or lymphadenopathy, an abnormal prostate or seminal vesicles. The laboratory indications of infection are positive prostatic secretion culture or cytology or leukocytes or significant bacteria in the urine. Semen analysis signs include abnormal seminal fluid biochemistry, increased viscosity, or repeatedly elevated WBCs (more than 1 million per millilitre) in the semen sample, and positive seminal fluid culture. The conditions required for the diagnosis of male accessory gland infection requires that at least two signs of infection are found from the three groups (Table

Table 1   Male accessory gland infection

The diagnosis requires:

(1)   Either a history or physical sign with a urinary or prostatic sign;
(2)   Or a history or physical sign with an ejaculate sign;
(3)   Or a urinary or prostatic sign with an ejaculate sign;
(4)   Or at least two ejaculate signs.

1). This is a working definition used by the Task Force, but it is under continuous review. The treatment of this condition is another area of controversy and the Task Force is addressing this problem by evaluating antibiotic therapy in a randomized study.

The diagnosis of hyperprolactinaemia in the female partner is more straightforward. Whereas much essential information can be gained from the history and clinical examination to suspect hyperprolactinaemia such as amenorrhoea, short menstrual cycles, or galactorrhoea, the diagnosis rests on one factor alone – repeatedly elevated prolactin levels. The assessment of prolactin values is an essential step in the evaluation of the female partner. The WHO Special Programme's Matched Reagents for the Standardization of Gonadotrophins and Hormone Assays ensures external quality control of all laboratories participating in this and other multicentre studies which permits comparisons between laboratories. However, whether the prolactin values are considered to be elevated or not depends upon each centre's 'normal ranges'. The aetiology of hyperprolactinaemia requires that a pituitary lesion be excluded as well as the rare possibility of hypothyroidism since each of these conditions requires different treatments. Prior to initiating treatment for the patient's infertility, any mechanical problems such as tubal blockage must be excluded.

In the time available it was not possible to go into all the diagnostic categories and many of the diagnostic procedures are available in textbooks. This standardized approach is expected to make a major contribution to the diagnosis and management of the infertile couple and will result in a low cost, highly effective and time saving method of evaluating this emotional and unfortunate condition. It was emphasized that the investigation of infertility involves the couple rather than the individual. This approach requires close collaboration and co-ordination between those responsible for the investigation of both the male and the female partner.

The second presentation was given by Professor Oscar Mateo de Acosta on a general description of the study population and the major diagnostic categories.

STANDARDIZED INVESTIGATION OF THE INFERTILE COUPLE: DESCRIPTION OF STUDY POPULATION AND MAJOR CATEGORIES

Age distribution

The age range for the males was 17–66 years with 90% of men between the ages 24 and 40 and a mean age of 31 years. Similarly, the females' ages ranged from 15 to 47 years with 90% of the subjects within the range 21–35 years and a mean age 27.4 years.

Parity and type of infertility

80% were nulliparous and the highest parity was 7. 68.4% of women had primary infertility.

Type of centre, recruitment pattern, duration of infertility

All centres admitted couples to the study provided they had at least 1 year's duration of infertility and both partners agreed to be fully investigated according to the standardized protocol. Certain centres are primary referral centres seeing a wide range of infertile couples. Other centres are secondary or even tertiary referral centres specializing in particular aspects of treatment of male or female infertility and again the same criteria for admission to the study have been applied. A third group of centres see a mixture of primary or secondary referrals for infertility and it is clear that the patterns of infertility and the characteristics of the infertile couples seen by those different types of centre will be substantially different. There is no basis for extrapolating the results of this study or the prevalence of certain conditions to the general population.

Diagnoses

Each partner was fully investigated and all factors considered to be related to infertility were identified; however, not all couples had completed all investigations and almost half the male and female partners had no demonstrable cause for infertility – these were the subjects in whom all the necessary investigations had been completed and no cause for infertility could be found. For 46.4% of the couples there is insufficient information for a final diagnosis to be made and to exclude the diagnosis of no demonstrable cause – these are couples in whom the investigations are still continuing. However, of these, there are 430 couples (7.2%) who have not given their full co-operation for all the diagnostic procedures to be carried out and have been discontinued from the study. In the remaining 3193 couples there were 489 pregnancies (15.3%) during the course of the investigation and in many of those couples there was again incomplete data on all aspects of the infertility investigation – however, those couples have *ipso facto* demonstrated that whatever causes of infertility could have been identified, they can no longer be classified as infertile.

Table 2 shows the distribution of female diagnoses. Just under half the subjects have no demonstrable cause for infertility, while bilateral tubal occlusion and other acquired tubal or ovarian abnormalities including adhesion is the most common diagnosis seen in 13.1% of subjects. Note that subjects may fall into more than one diagnostic group so that the percentages in the table add up to more than 100%. Inadequate ovarian function other than congenital abnormalities, but including hyperprolactinaemia and hypothyroidism, accounted for 24.4% of subjects.

Table 2 Female diagnostic groups

Diagnostic group	No. of diagnoses	Percentage of subjects (n = 3306)
No demonstrable cause	1583	47.9
Tubal occlusion and other acquired tubal or ovarian abnormalities, including adhesions	755	22.8
Anovulation without amenorrhoea	600	18.1
Hyperprolactinaemia	190	5.7
Endometriosis	168	5.1
Ovulatory oligomenorrhoea	139	4.2
Amenorrhoea with either normal or low FSH, elevated FSH or normal endogenous oestrogen	114	3.4
Acquired uterine or cervical abnormalities or pituitary lesion	69	2.1
Congenital abnormalities, including abnormal karyotype	38	1.1
Systemic causes, including hypothyroidism	21	0.6
Sexual dysfunction	30	0.9
Iatrogenic causes	13	0.4
Endometrial tuberculosis	13	0.4

Table 3 shows the male diagnoses and again just under half have no demonstrable cause for infertility. The most common factor is varicocele which is seen in 17.2% of cases. The diagnosis is made on the basis of abnormal semen quality and varicocele found (either visible, palpable or valsalva positive) at physical examination. Three idiopathic conditions describing semen quality – abnormal sperm morphology, idiopathic low sperm motility and primary idiopathic testicular failure – are the next most common conditions seen in 16.8%, and 16.1% of males, respectively. It is interesting to note that

81.2% of males have either no demonstrable cause of infertility or an idiopathic, rather than a congenital or acquired condition.

The preliminary data presented on the diagnostic groups show that tubal lesions including bilateral obstruction to be the commonest female factor and varicocele the commonest male factor. There were more couples in which only one partner had one or more factors identified than couples in which both had one or more factors. Further analyses are necessary to identify any associations between male and female causes that may occur more frequently together.

Table 3 Male diagnostic group

Diagnostic group	No. of diagnoses	Percentage of subjects (n = 3438)
No demonstrable cause	1662	48.3
Varicocele	593	17.2
Abnormal sperm morphology, idiopathic low sperm motility or immotile cilia syndrome	578	16.8
Primary idiopathic testicular failure	553	16.1
Male accessory gland infection	138	4.0
Congenital abnormalities including abnormal karyotype	72	2.1
Obstructive azoospermia or partial obstruction	62	1.8
Suspected immunological factors	56	1.6
Systemic causes, iatrogenic causes or retrograde ejaculation	44	1.3
Sexual dysfunction or ejaculatory disturbance	35	1.0
Pituitary lesion or gonadotrophin deficiency	19	0.6

The next paper, presented by Professor David de Kretser, described the characteristics of the semen analyses.

CHARACTERISTICS OF SEMEN ANALYSIS

Criteria for a normal semen analysis

Table 4 shows the eight criteria that have been adopted to characterize a 'normal semen analysis'. Each semen sample was classified separately (Table 5) as normal or abnormal according to whether or not all its characteristics fell within the defined normal limits, and a male was considered to have normal semen if at least one sample was normal. This is the working definition adopted by the Task Force for this study. Using this classification 51.8% of the 3591 men on whom semen data were available were considered normal and 41.3% abnormal; the remainder had either azoospermia or aspermia.

Table 4 Criteria for a normal semen analysis

Appearance	Normal or yellow
Viscosity	Normal
Agglutination	No
Density	$\geq 20 \times 10^6\,ml^{-1}$
Morphology	$\geq 50\%$ normal forms
Motility	$\geq 40\%$ progressively motile
Viability	$\geq 60\%$ live
WBCs	$\leq 1.0 \times 10^6\,ml^{-1}$

Table 5 Classification of semen samples

Semen classification	No. (%)
Normal	1859 (51.8)
Abnormal	1483 (41.3)
Azoospermia	240 (6.7)
Aspermia	9 (0.3)
Total	3591

Difference between samples

All male partners were requested to supply two semen samples with at least a 2-week interval. There was very little difference between the sperm densities or the morphology in the first and second samples, but the motility was significantly higher in the second sample – however, the importance of this is not great since the mean difference is only 1% motile sperm. The standard deviations for the square-root transformed sperm density (which results in a more normal distribution), motility and morphology are considerably greater between subjects than within subject from the first sample to the next. Thus, most of the differences observed are due to the differences in semen quality between the men rather than to the variability within the same person.

It appears that if one of the three characteristics is normal in the first sample then it has a chance of between 90 and 95% of being normal in the second sample, but if it is abnormal in the first then it only has a 15–25% chance of being normal in the second.

Pregnancies

Of the 5952 couples enrolled in the study there were 489 female partners who became pregnant during the investigation. For almost 30% there is no semen data available since there was no longer any need to continue investigating the couple's infertility once pregnancy was achieved. There were two men (0.4%) with azoospermia in both samples. Of the 228 men in the study who were azoospermic in the first semen sample, 12 (5.2%) had sperm present in the second and in two cases the second sample was well within the range of normality, indicating that azoospermia in one sample does not necessarily preclude adequate semen quality in the next.

Semen quality with reference to diagnostic categories

Table 6 shows the semen characteristics for those men in whom no demonstrable cause for infertility was found, compared with those

Table 6 Semen characteristics by diagnosis group

Semen category	No demonstrable cause No. (%)	One or more male factors identified No. (%)
Aspermia	0 (0)	8 (0.5)
Azoospermia	0 (0)	229 (13.0)
Sperm present	1647 (100)	1530 (86.7)
Total	1647	1767

Mean semen characteristics	No demonstrable cause	One or more male factors identified	Statistics	
			t test	p value
Density ($\times 10^6\,\mathrm{ml}^{-1}$)	85.8	43.0		
Back transformed square-root density	77.6	30.3	28.9	< 0.001
Motility*	61.6	35.4	37.8	< 0.001
Morphology†	71.7	46.6	34.0	< 0.001

*Results are expressed as percentages progressively motile.
†Results are expressed as percentages of normal forms.

in whom one or more factors were identified. One of the conditions for no demonstrable cause for infertility was that at least one semen sample was judged normal by the criteria adopted by the Task Force. The semen quality in this group is uniformly better than the group with one or more factors identified.

In discussing semen quality in relation to the most common diagnostic groups it was noted that in the group with 'male accessory gland infection' there is a very marked reduction in sperm motility and morphology, with a comparatively smaller reduction in density, whereas those men with varicocele also had an appreciably lower sperm density.

Semen quality in relation to clinical findings

The diagnostic group 'varicocele' consists only of those men in whom a varicocele was detected during clinical examination and who provided two abnormal semen samples. In order to see the effect of varicocele on semen quality the semen characteristics of men were divided according to grade of varicocele (Table 7). The most severe

Table 7 Semen characteristics in relation to varicocele

		Varicocele grade		
Characteristic	None	Valsalva positive	Palpable	Visible
	No. (%)	No. (%)	No. (%)	No. (%)
Semen category:				
Azoospermia	206 (7.1)	11 (4.3)	19 (6.3)	4 (4.3)
Sperm present	2692 (92.9)	242 (95.7)	281 (93.7)	134 (95.7)
Total	2898	253	300	140
Mean semen values:				
Density ($\times 10^6\,\mathrm{ml}^{-1}$)	7.0	51.5	48.6	45.2
Back transformed				
square-root density	56.9	40.8	36.8	32.6*†
Motility§	50.6	41.1	44.0	39.5*‡
Morphology‖	61.4	52.1	54.4	52.0*‡

*Differences between control and experimental groups significant ($p < 0.1$).
†Decreasing trend significant ($p < 0.1$).
‡Difference between varicocele and no varicocele groups significant ($p < 0.1$), but no difference between grades of varicocele.
§Percentages progressively motile.
‖Percentages of normal forms.

437

of the two grades is taken if a varicocele was visible on examination. The percentage of cases with azoospermia did not change significantly with grade of varicocele, but semen quality (for those men with sperm present) deteriorates as the severity of varicocele increases. There is a very strong trend ($p < 0.001$) of reduced density, while for the motility and morphology there is a marked drop ($p < 0.001$) when there is a varicocele, but the differences in motility and morphology are not significantly different according to the severity of the varicocele. It appears that grades of varicocele should be considered as a factor potentially influencing fertility since they all clearly affect semen quality.

Another factor related to semen quality is the testicular volume. The percentage of men with aspermia or azoospermia decreases from 66% in the group with total testicular volume less than 12 ml to 4.1% in the group with total volume greater than 44 ml. Similarly, the semen density increases uniformly with increasing testicular volume as does the motility and morphology. It is only for volumes greater than 22 ml that the mean semen characteristics on all three measurements fall within the 'normal ranges' defined earlier.

There is no association between high fever in the past 6 months and azoospermia but semen quality is reduced considerably – mean density from 53.1 to 34.6×10^6 ml^{-1}, motility by 9.8% and morphology by 9.7%. All these differences are significant at $p < 0.5$, and the mean motility and morphology drop to the border-line of normal semen defined earlier. Unfortunately, information is not available on the time since the episode of high fever and therefore the rate of return to normal semen values in those men cannot be evaluated.

The final paper was presented by Professor Ian Cooke.

PRELIMINARY OBSERVATIONS ON OVULATORY DISORDERS DERIVED FROM THE INFERTILITY TASK FORCE DATA

Menstrual category

A regular pattern of menstruation from 25 to 35 days was described in 83.2% of women, oligomenorrhoea in 13.4% and amenorrhoea in 3.4% (total 5731 patients). Of 3055 couples who had their ovulatory status recorded, 69.8% were described as ovulatory as their plasma progesterone value was greater than $18 \, \text{nmol} \, l^{-1}$, or urinary pregnanediol greater than $8 \, \text{nmol} \, l^{-1}$ or having secretory phase endometrium; 27.1% were classified as anovulatory whereas 3.1% were uncertain. This sub-group of patients included some who were oligomenorrhoeic and 'uncertain' frequently may have applied to patients who were at one time ovulatory and another anovulatory, although mostly the allocation was made according to the first cycle which was adequately investigated.

There were 3038 for whom coding was complete. Almost 20% of regular cycles are anovulatory whereas 60% of oligomenorrhoeic patients were anovulatory, at the time that the blood sample was taken.

Secondary amenorrhoea

There were 225 of 5628 patients (4.0%) who were categorized as having secondary amenorrhoea. There was considerable variation in the number of patients with this characteristic in different centres. Of 196 patients who had the duration of secondary amenorrhoea listed, 78 had from 6 to 11 months, 38 from 12 to 23 months and 80 more than 24 months; 5.1% had more than 98 months' amenorrhoea.

Ponderal index

From the basic data of weight and height, it was possible to calculate the Ponderal Index; this is weight $(\text{kg})/\text{height}^2(\text{m})$. According to the Garrow scale, a British Standard, the normal Ponderal Index is from 19 to 24. Less than 19 is regarded as thin and more than 24 as obese. In the overall study, from 5729 completed data sets, 55.5% were considered to have a normal female Ponderal Index, 12.8% to be low and 31.7% to be high.

Cycle irregularity or amenorrhoea are more likely to be associated with a high Ponderal Index. When oligomenorrhoea and amenorrhoea are combined and compared with the group with regular cycles, there is no significant difference between those with a low and those with a normal Ponderal Index ($\chi^2 = 0.08$). On the other hand, when comparing those with a high Ponderal Index against those with a normal index, there is a highly significant difference ($\chi^2 = 39.1$; df = 1; $p < 0.001$). This suggests that obese women are more likely to have cycle irregularity, whereas underweight women do not have such a clear-cut association.

Patients can be divided according to weight change. Comparing those who have lost more than 10% of their body-weight in the past year with those in whom there has been no change, showed a highly significant difference (χ^2 = 10.3; df = 1; $p < 0.001$) in the percentage with regular cycles. Similarly, there is a highly significant difference between those who have gained more than 10% of their body-weight in the past year compared with those whose weight has not changed. Thus there is a greater chance of a patient having an irregular cycle if her weight has fluctuated by more than 10% in the past year. It is well documented in the literature that acute weight loss results in amenorrhoea, but an association with weight gain has not been so clearly documented.

Other associations

Two other clinical conditions were noted to have an inverse association with ovulatory status and these were *tubal damage* and *endometriosis*. For each of these tabulations, menstrual status and ovulation were categorized as 'ovulatory regular, anovulatory regular, ovulatory oligomenorrhoea, anovulatory oligomenorrhoea and amenorrhoea' and were cross-tabulated according to patency of both tubes, one tube or having both tubes blocked. There was a highly significant inverse correlation (χ^2 = 49.3; df = 10; $p < 0.001$) indicating that tubal damage was less likely in women with anovulation or cycle irregularity. This was further demonstrated with respect to peritubal adhesions in the presence of patency which again was less likely to be present in amenorrhoeic patients (6.9%) than in those with regular ovulation (19.5%) (χ^2 = 37.4; df = 10; $p < 0.001$). A similar association was noted with the absence of endometriosis in amenorrhoeic women in comparison with a 7.9% frequency in regularly cycling women. This inverse association with ovulation was also highly significant (χ^2 = 39.9; df = 10; $p < 0.001$).

Male pattern of hair distribution

The observation of a male pattern of hair distribution is a common clinical observation and was found in 9.1% of patients who did not have a regular cycle in comparison with 3.4% of those who did

($\chi^2 = 61.2$; df $= 1$; $p < 0.001$). This was equally found in oligomenorrhoeic patients (9.2%) and amenorrhoeic women (9.7%). The male pattern of hair distribution was found overall in 4.4% of 5725 patients, the principal final diagnoses of these patients being anovular regular cycles (14.4%), anovulatory oligomenorrhoea (21.2%) and no demonstrable cause (39%).

Galactorrhoea

There were 382 patients (6.7% of 5736) who had a history of discharge from the nipple. In six of these it was said to have been blood stained. Galactorrhoea was not confirmed in 97 cases whereas in 295 it was found in one or both nipples on physical examination when it had not been suspected from the history. Thus, those in whom nipple discharge was volunteered represented only 49% of those with galactorrhoea. Of those with a past history of breast discharge but who denied it was currently present, 66% still had demonstrable galactorrhoea.

It is notable that only 25.6% had bilateral galactorrhoea associated with repeated prolactin estimations above the upper limit of normal. Seventeen abnormal skull X-rays have been found, 12 in those who had two elevated prolactin levels but five in those who had both prolactin values recorded as normal. Only about half of the data have been coded with respect to skull X-rays and it is too early to analyse this further.

Family history of diabetes mellitus

It was noted that a family history of diabetes mellitus was associated with hyperprolactinaemia ($\chi^2 = 4.06$; df $= 1$; $p < 0.05$). The severity of the diabetes has not been recorded, but this is an unexpected association that will require further investigation.

DISCUSSION

In the discussion periods that followed each presentation the following points were raised.

It was stressed again that this study was not a study on the incidence or prevalence of infertility in particular communities – such a study requires a different approach and there were WHO-sponsored epidemiological studies underway to measure this. It was pointed out by one member of the audience that between-centre comparisons of prolactin values may be problematic in view of the known difficulties and variability in the assay. In reply, Professor Lunenfeld said that the majority of centres in the study participated in the external quality control scheme of the WHO Matched Reagents Programme and that each centre provided WHO with their individual range of normal values. In addition, the protocol called for each centre to state whether the prolactin value was considered to be elevated or normal according to the individual laboratory's values.

The practice of combining the results of semen analysis from different centres was questioned in the light of the fact of large variability between one sample and another. Members of the panel pointed out that the semen samples had to be collected at not less than a 2-week interval and no more than 3 months apart and in each case preceded by 3 days abstinence. In fact, the results obtained which were described in Professor de Kretser's paper showed good reproducibility from one sample to the next.

A member of the audience stressed the importance of investigating infertility thoroughly both in the male and in the female and that infertility is a problem for the couple rather than the individual. In addition, infertility had considerable psychosocial ramifications both within the family and the community.

WORKSHOP

42
Monoclonal antibodies in human reproduction

MODERATORS: L. METTLER and P. M. JOHNSON
CO-ORDINATOR: K. HANNON

This workshop centred on the effect which monoclonal antibodies (mAbs) are now beginning to make in various fields of research in human reproduction. An introduction by the chairperson, L. Mettler (Kiel, W. Germany), outlined the background to much of the technology involved in the production of mAbs based from the original work of Köhler and Milstein in 1975[1]. The relative advantages now recognized for mAbs over conventional polyclonal antibodies were listed – notably their monospecificity, lack of background effects, and potentially immortal production. The laboratory usage of mAbs is now widespread and, of particular relevance to fertility regulation, the fast-moving areas of interest have focussed on the identification, localization and assay of antigens present on sperm, zona pellucida, reproductive hormones, the early embryo and trophoblast. This has involved the application of mAbs in a variety of roles including as assay reference material, as means for biochemical approaches to antigen purification, for immunohistological localization procedures, for passive contraception models, for laboratory diagnosis of infertility, for the study of maternofetal interactions, for the identification of reproductive tumours and delivery of cytotoxic agents. Many of these applications were illustrated in the subsequent presentations in the workshop.

443

F. Kohan (Rehovet, Israel) described extensive studies on the use of various mAbs reactive with sites on steroids and steroid metabolites in very sensitive radioimmunoassays, enzyme-linked immunoassays (ELISA) and chemiluminescence immunoassays[2,3]. The minimization of cross-reactivity between α-testosterone and 5 α-dihydrotestosterone, as well as oestriol and oestradiol, was described – the former situation using a mAb with only 2% cross-reactivity. An anti-oestrone mAb with titres of up to $1:10^6$ was mentioned. This presentation highlighted the new-found specificity and, particularly, the rigorous standardization and quality control that may now be achieved with mAbs.

S. Isojima (Hyogo, Japan) briefly mentioned earlier work with an mAb to a human seminal plasma antigen which had been used successfully in affinity chromatography to isolate the antigen at up to 200-times purification from seminal plasma. He went on to describe his experience with five mAbs raised to porcine zona pellucida antigens, and assessment of their cross-reactivity with human, hamster, rat and mouse zona pellucida[4]. It is clear that different zona pellucida antigens, defined by mouse mAbs, are distributed differently between the species and may or may not also localize on the oocyte membrane. The ability of these mAbs to block sperm binding was also compared. It was concluded that most anti-porcine zona pellucida mAbs do not block human sperm penetration of zona pellucida, but do if a second antibody (anti-mouse Ig) is used to make a precipitate with the mAb on the zona pellucida surface. As was raised in subsequent discussion, this would suggest a steric hindrance of sperm penetration rather than the mAb being reactive with (and hence directly blocking) the receptor site. In line with this are observations showing that Fab fragments of mAbs do not block sperm penetration.

P. M. Johnson (Liverpool, UK) discussed the application of mAbs to dissect individual components of the complex surface of human fetal trophoblast that may be relevant in maternofetal interactions[5,6]. Studies of the degree of specificity and selectivity required for cell surface antigens had not previously been practical with polyclonal antibodies. One mAb (H315) was described in detail. This mAb is unreactive with oocytes, sperm or components of male reproductive tract, whereas it does react with a 36 000 molecular weight protein (the p36 trophoblast membrane protein) on human placental villous trophoblast, cytotrophoblast of the surrounding chorion and extravil-

444

lous cytotrophoblast populations within the maternal endometrium. This had included study of pregnancy tissues as early as 12 days' gestation. Since this antigen is represented at all maternofetal interfaces and not on any other adult or fetal cell type, and also since maternal blood levels are low (<200 ng ml^{-1} at term), it was considered that it might be a suitable target for immunological approaches to contraception. However, very recent work has shown this and other trophoblast antigens to also be expressed by columnar epithelium of glands within the maternal endometrium. The full significance is not yet clear, but this would indicate some local regulatory control influencing the expression of these antigens within the uteroplacental bed and extraembryonic membranes. Nevertheless, these antigens are also expressed by some tumours, particularly of the female reproductive system, and there is preliminary indication that mAbs such as H315 will prove useful for the detection, histological localization and radioimaging of these tumours, and perhaps even eventual cytotoxic targeting. Furthermore, there is obvious scope for the use of mAbs selective for fetal trophoblast in a fluorescence-activated cell sorter to separate trace trophoblastic elements from maternal blood – which would greatly facilitate means for the identification of fetal genetic abnormalities.

T. G. Wegmann (Paris, France and Edmonton, Canada) described the *in vivo* use of mAbs to histocompatibility antigen (H-2) specificities in murine models to identify how the placenta may serve as an immunological barrier[7]. Using intrinsically labelled ascitic cells (tritiated amino acids or [^{35}S]methionine) to obtain high-activity radiolabelled mAbs, it was possible to inject pregnant mice with anti-H-2 mAbs to demonstrate the localization and ontogeny of various histocompatibility antigens on different trophoblast populations. A separate application of mAbs reactive with histocompatibility antigens was also described, based on the approach of R. Hunziker and P. Gambel in Edmonton. Mouse chimaeras had been established following a bolus injection of anti-histocompatibility antigen mAb to F1 animals, followed by reconstitution with parental stem cells. Analysis of uterine decidual cells in these mice, when subsequently pregnant, had demonstrated no significant numbers of cells of bone marrow origin. This is in contrast to the studies of P. Lala on deciduoma in pseudopregnancy of bone marrow chimaeric mice established following lethal irradiation. There was then a vigorous but unresolved discussion on the paradoxical contrast of these results, debating whether these cells were in granulomatous or decidual reactions in pseudopregnancy and also commenting on the contrasting results between lack of detection of decidual cells of bone marrow origin in mice using enzyme markers (referred to by T. G. Wegmann) and detection of such cells in man using mAbs to cell surface antigen markers (referred to by P. M. Johnson). The resolution of this question is fundamental to understanding any maternal immunocompetent cellular response to fetal cells within the placental bed.

A. Hinrichsen (Munich, W. Germany) described a large series of mAbs raised against human spermatozoal pellets, which had been screened in ELISA using spermatozoa immobilized on solid-phase with poly-L-lysine[8]. Most of these mAbs recognized acrosomal antigens, but some bound also to the equatorial segment. Nine mAbs had been particularly studied, of which five reacted with isolated acrosin and none apparently reacted with any component in seminal plasma. This group is now using these mAbs to elucidate the biochemistry and physiology of sperm maturation and fertilization.

S. Paul, L. Mettler and V. Baukloh (Kiel, W. Germany) also described a large series of mAbs raised against human spermatozoa but, in contrast, the large majority were reactive with both spermatozoa and seminal plasma[9,10]. Fifteen mAbs were sperm immobilizing and seven reacted with antigens represented only on sperm or in seminal plasma. Like the study by Hinrichsen, cross-reactivity had been assessed by immunohistology on various human tissues. One mAb (III-3) had been studied in particular detail. The relevant antigen (molecular weight 45 000) was not restricted only to the acrosomal region of sperm, and had been isolated by affinity chromatography. That this antigen might be relevant to human anti-sperm antibody responses was shown by the fact that 70% of such sera showed at least some inhibition by the purified III-3 antigen. Evidence was also presented that the III-3 antigen exists in serum at 13–$18\,\mu g\,ml^{-1}$ and may bind to peripheral blood T cells, suggesting some fundamental immunobiological role pertinent to fertility. The concentration of this antigen in seminal plasma was given as over $280\,\mu g\,ml^{-1}$.

There followed broad discussion around the technical aspects of maintaining hybridoma cell lines in culture or as ascitic tumours, as well as the relative merits of different methods for using mAbs to identify or quantitate their respective antigens. It was clear that most groups used ELISA for their primary screening procedures, and immunohistology to assess cross-reactivity, prior to adapting the most optimal mAbs into the laboratory research for which that mAb had been obtained. The following eight potential applications of monoclonal antibodies to reproduction research were discussed.

(1) As well-defined, cheap reference material in immunoassay for reproductive hormones, sperm antibody, zona antibody, etc.

(2) For the relatively facile isolation of reproductive tract antigens by immunoaffinity methods, elucidation of their importance in immunological infertility and their potential as immunological contraceptives.

(3) Mapping of antigens on cell surfaces and along the reproductive tract; determination of cross-reactivity with other tissues.

(4) Achievement of passive contraceptive effects with for example the local application of sperm cytotoxic antibodies, block of fertilization with anti-sperm/zona antibody, interference with the hormonal milieu with anti-HCG antibody, etc.

(5) Diagnosis of antibody specificity in immunological infertility using analogous monoclonal antibody based immunoassay systems; therapy utilizing the relevant antigen to neutralize the antibodies.

(6) Study of maternofetal immunological interactions during pregnancy, for example in definition of the mechanism and specificity of antibody transport by the trophoblast, in elucidation of enhancement/rejection reactions.

(7) Localization of reproductive tract tumours and their metases with antibody coupled to a suitable dye.

(8) Specific delivery of cytotoxic drugs to the target tissue with antibody–drug conjugates.

References

1. Köhler, G. and Milstein, C. (1975). Continuous cultures of fused cells secreting antibody of predefined specificity. *Nature (Lond.)*, **256,** 495

2. Kohan, F., Lichter, S., Eshhar, Z. and Lidner, H. R. (1982). Preparation of monoclonal antibodies able to discriminate between testosterone and 5α-dihydrotestosterone. *Steroids*, **39,** 453

3. Lidner, H. R., Kohan, F., Eshhar, Z., Kim, J. B., Barnard, G. and Collins, W. P. (1981). Novel assay procedure for assessing ovarian function in women. *J. Steroid Biochem.*, **15,** 131

4. Isojima, S., Koyama, K. and Hasegawa, A. (1981). Production of monoclonal antibody to zona pellucida from porcine oocytes. *Acta Obstet. Gynecol. Jpn.*, **33,** 1995

5. Johnson, P. M., Brown, P. J., Molloy, C. M., Bulmer, J. N. and Czuppon, A. B. (1983). Identification of a human trophoblast-specific membrane associated antigen by

a monoclonal antibody. In Shulman, S. and Dondero, F. (eds.), *Immunological Factors in Human Contraception*, pp. 95–102. (Rome: Field Educational Italia Acta Medica)

6. Johnson, P. M. (1983). Immunobiology of human trophoblast. In Crighton, D. B. (ed.). *Immunological Aspects of Reproduction in Mammals*. (London: Butterworths) (In press)

7. Chaouat, G., Kolb, J.-P. and Wegmann, T. G. (1983). The placenta as an immunological barrier. *Immunol. Rev.*, **75** (In press)

8. Hinrichsen, A. C., Hinrichsen, M. J. and Schill, W. B. (1983). Topographical Analysis of the Spermatozoal Surface by means of mAbs – VIII Human – vekerinär med. Gemeinschaftsgung, Verhandlungsberichte, München (In press)

9. Paul, S., Baukloh, V., Baillie, M. and Mettler, L. (1982). Generation of monoclonal antibodies against human spermatozoa and seminal plasma constituents. *Clin. Reprod. Fertil.*, **1**, 235

10. Mettler, L., Paul, S., Baukloh, V. and Feller, A. (1983). Monoclonal sperm antibodies: their potential for investigation of sperms as target of immunological contraception. *Am. J. Reprod. Immunol.* (In press)

43
Therapeutic approaches to male infertility

MODERATOR: J. P. PRYOR
CO-ORDINATOR: P. O'DONOVAN

The first aspect of treatment is to reassure the patient who has been given false information about their prospects of fertility – such information has usually been based on results of a single seminal analysis and a mistaken belief that the normal range of sperm concentration is synonymous with fertility. It is important to identify the specific causes for infertility in both partners as only then is it possible to offer treatment with a high prospect of success. The couple should be informed of the overall prognosis and be advised of the possibility of artificial donor insemination and adoption.

The assessment of any treatment for infertility not only requires the cause to be identified, but also that other factors in both partners should be excluded. It is important that the treatment is given for a sufficient period of time (4–6 months) and that any improvement is based upon statistical analysis of results in each patient. The detection of improvement in semen quality is a different matter from the conception rates and these should be related to a given period of time. The psychological benefit of any new form of treatment on semen quality should be appreciated and in view of this it is essential that any trials should be carried out on a controlled double-blind basis.

Professor W. Schill (Munich, West Germany) spoke of the specific indications for hormonal therapy. The treatment of hypogonadotrophic hypogonadism with a combination of human chorionic gonadotrophin (hCG) and human menopausal gonadotrophin (hMG) is particularly successful, but unfortunately it is only applicable in a small number of patients. Those patients with a hypothalamic hypogonadic defect leading to hypogonadotrophic hypogonadism may be treated with LH releasing hormone. Patients with hyperprolactinaemia respond to treatment with bromocriptine, but such patients are rarely encountered in the infertility clinic.

The identification of men with androgen insensitivity (high luteinizing hormone level and high testosterone level) and occasionally men with a form of andrenogenital syndrome (high testosterone levels, but with a low level of gonadotrophic hormone) will present a small group of patients who may occasionally respond to treatment.

Mr W. F. Hendry (London) spoke of the role of antisperm antibodies in the treatment of the infertile male and emphasized the risks associated with high-dose steroid therapy. Not only must the diagnosis of antisperm antibodies be made with precision – MAR test to detect antibodies in seminal plasma, elevated levels of circulating antibodies by gel or tray agglutinating test – but there must also be an abnormal post-coital test and abnormal crossed sperm mucus penetration test. Furthermore there should be no contraindications to steroid therapy in the man and his wife should have been fully investigated to ensure that she is ovulating and has no problem with the Fallopian tubes. The current practice is to prescribe prednisolone 20 mg twice daily for the first 10 days of three consective cycles in the wife. The role of antibodies as a cause of oligozoospermia was mentioned in discussion. All members agreed that a clinical trial for the treatment of antisperm antibody problems was long overdue.

The question of genital tract infection in male infertility was briefly discussed and should always be eliminated – particularly when there are problems of poor concentration, poor motility, or both.

Dr J. Paulsen (Virginia, USA) discussed the use of glass filtration in an attempt to improve fertility rates. The treatment would appear to be particularly useful in men with increased semen viscosity when it was possible to recover the spermatozoa without loss of semen volume. He emphasized that in one third of infertile couples there were multiple factors causing the problem.

Dr M. Glazerman (Beir Shiva, Israel) briefly discussed the role of varicocele in infertility and there was general accord that whilst there is still a role in treatment of the varicocele, it is important to detect and treat the causes of infertility that may be present.

Dr W. Schill in his presentation has emphasized the empirical nature of most forms of medical treatment and Mr W. Hendry reminded the audience that in order to treat anaemia it was first necessary to diagnose the cause. The treatment of male infertility is improving as we are able to diagnose more specific disorders causing the problem. Unfortunately many causes are irreversible and these couples so afflicted should be offered the possibility of artificial donor insemination.

44
Artificial insemination

MODERATOR: C. D. MATTHEWS
CO-ORDINATOR: A. I. TRAUB

Dr Robertson (Sydney, Australia) discussed the changing pattern of couples requesting AID. Highlighted was the dramatic change in circumstances surrounding the requests for help over the last 20 years. 20 years ago, artificial insemination was hardly drawing-room conversation and practitioners of it were themselves considered quasi-ethical by their colleagues. The adoption of healthy babies was facile so there existed an outlet for the frustrations of infertility. The requests in 1960 for AID originated from clearly defined self-motivated couples who were generally 'strong, stable, law abiding people of the community'. With the changes in the law relating to abortion, the cult of the single mother and the increasing scarcity of babies for adoption, the scene changed. Fears have existed that frustrated, impatient couples demanding AID might not allow the best long-term decisions. Dr Robertson allayed such fears by showing that the skills of parenting were still strong. He admitted that the guidelines for AID used by his own clinic were conservative by comparison with some regions of the world but perhaps liberal by others. They included the requirement for two parents of different sex having entered into a marriage contract or who had a long-term stable *de facto* relationship. Requests for surrogate motherhood were not currently acceptable. Dr Robertson indicated other concerns, including the mixing of natural and donor children and the increasing but still small percentage of couples referred for genetic reasons. Dr Robertson believed that the length of treatment should be decided

453

by mutual decision between the doctor and the couple and that the presence of minor infertility factors in the female played an important role in the success or otherwise of the programmes.

Dr Marik, of the Tyler Medical Clinic, Los Angeles, California, spoke on the selection of donors, reporting on a new study of donors from California and relating, in particular, their very interesting attitudes to their sperm donation. Donors were recruited from the university campus population. The results of the survey contained several unexpected attitudes, including a long-term responsibility for the semen donation which included expressions of concern for the children generated from their semen donations. In parallel with this was a liberal attitude towards the use of their semen, with some donors not being averse to their semen being used for couples outside of marriage and even in homosexual relationships.

Dr Sherman (Arkansas, USA) reviewed the history and development of AID, and in particular the history of preservation techniques. He drew together data derived from an international study, which demonstrated the wide acceptance of preserved semen for artificial insemination and its considerable advantages for practice and scientific advancement.

Dr Kobayashi of Japan presented a factual follow-up of 40 children derived from AID in Japan. This represented about 10% of the parents and children approached to provide information about their present-day situation, having been derived by donor insemination up to 15 years previously. The clinic at Keio University was the principal centre in Japan for AID and commenced the procedure in 1948 and has used frozen semen since 1958. So far, more than 6000 patients had become pregnant by AID since 1949. The insemination technique used employed 0.5 ml of semen inseminated into the uterine cavity used a specially made silver flexible needle. The follow-up of the children indicated clearly that as far as their mental, physical, emotional and behavioural characteristics were concerned AID children were above average compared with age-matched control children. The mental development of the children was estimated using a Developmental Quotient for infants under $2\frac{1}{2}$ years, and an Intelligence Quotient for the older group. School records were analysed for behavioural and academic achievement. The explanation of the improved performance of the AID children included genetic reasons, the semen having been almost wholly derived from the medical student population, together with the possibility that these children

454

were very much desired, and generally were from smaller families with parental devotion, commitment and expenditure.

Dr Snowden (England) considered a very wide ranging number of issues relating to what he termed 'artifical reproduction'. He saw the possibilities of considerable interaction between the mother, the child, the AI practitioner, the donor and the husband. Many questions were raised but in particular the question of whether the child has a right to a knowledge about his/her origins. Other dangers were inherent in revealing to a child his/her AID status. There was a need for legal changes to allow the AID child to become legitimate in law. From the societal point of view, Dr Snowden questioned whether commercial sperm banks should be permitted and whether the secrecy and deception surrounding AID might undermine the values of society. Furthermore, he questioned whether it was proved that AID did not constitute a danger for the institution of marriage and the family and how AID could be effectively regulated; he questioned the adoption model as the right one to judge AID. Dr Snowden believed that a formal structure should be established in which artificial reproduction could be practised in a way that was acceptable to society and in his view this included the need for married persons being involved with artificial reproduction and that at least one partner should be the genetic parent, the carrying mother or the nurturing parent. He believed that counselling should include alternative ways of coping with childlessness and to include close relatives in the decision-making process. In addition donors of gametes should also be independently counselled and assessed.

The role of AIH was discussed briefly. Dr Kobayashi (Japan) showed that sperm washing and sperm concentration using Ficol was a simple and useful method of using oligospermic semen and reported seven pregnancies.

The discussion period centred around the secrecy issue for children derived from AID and it was evident from the many countries represented and contributing to the discussion that nationalistic and cultural attitudes were very different on this issue. In many countries the male ego was such that infertility was still firmly linked with the lack of virility and for these cultures a secrecy of AID was paramount.

Further discussion took place on the spectre of sex election using AIH and it was indeed recognized that when reliable methods become available for this area, the potential demand was hard to comprehend.

455

WORKSHOP

45
Luteal-phase insufficiency

MODERATOR: I. D. COOKE
CO-ORDINATOR: N. HEASLEY

Dr F. Zegers produced data for the plasma progesterone profile in a normal cycle. He obtained data in 22 patients who were stopping barrier contraception and, using these patients (who subsequently proved to be highly fertile), he was able to show no difference between the non-conception cycles and the progesterone profile in the subsequent conception cycles (at least in the first half before corpus luteum rescue).

By serial daily ultrasonic scanning, he was able to describe antecedent follicle characteristics which were associated with a normal progesterone profile in the luteal phase. The mean maximal follicle diameter in those who conceived was 19.6 mm. Rupture occurred within 24 hours of the LH surge and the follicle diameter was stable in the 24 hours prior to rupture, varying by no more than 5% from that of the preceding day. This provided a difference from follicle characteristics in non-conception cycles which were not stable for the last 24 hours although they did ultimately reach the same size at the time of the LH surge. If the normal characteristics of ovulation occurred as described above, luteal dysfunction was not seen.

Dr E. Lenton reviewed long-term follow-up data and described a 63% cumulative conception rate at 12 years in 125 infertile patients with unexplained infertility. A significant number of these patients had suboptimal plasma progesterone concentrations during a luteal phase of normal length. She found that the best way to describe this was with a progesterone index which was the mean concentration of plasma progesterone over the 4 days from +5 to +8 of the luteal phase with respect to the LH surge. She presented the ranges of progesterone indices in conception cycles ($n=27$); the range was 31–73 nmol l^{-1}, median 47 nmol l^{-1}. In control cycles in women not attempting conception ($n=62$), the range was 16–62 nmol l^{-1} with a median of 40 nmol l^{-1}. In infertile women ($n=127$) the range was 16–49 nmol l^{-1}, median 33 nmol l^{-1}, approximately 50% having a progesterone index below two standard deviations. If patients were grouped according to the time taken to conceive and whether any form of treatment was given, it was noted that early spontaneous conceptions without treatment were characterized by a higher progesterone index than those who conceived spontaneously but over a longer time. Similarly, those that conceived with any form of therapy had lower progesterone indices but those that conceived early in any such regimen had a higher progesterone index than the lowest group which took a long time to conceive on any form of treatment. This suggests that fertility is related to the progesterone index. She hypothesized that follicle growth anomalies were frequently associated with abnormalities of timing of growth and of the LH surge and with luteal-phase abnormalities. Follicular volume was correlated with peripheral plasma oestradiol concentration ($r = 0.89$), and she described comparisons of follicular volume and follicle growth rates in different abnormalities. Follicular oestradiol excretion was calculated in pmol l^{-1} of peripheral plasma ml^{-1} of follicle volume. Thus the characteristics of ovarian function could be defined by follicular volume estimation and the progesterone index which defined the abnormalities of luteal phase, premature follicular rupture, delayed follicular rupture and late pre-ovulatory follicle growth. This provided a basis for a classification of abnormalities of follicular function.

Dr Acosta described ovarian manipulations in women enrolled in an *in vitro* fertilization programme. He emphasized that he was treating 'normally' ovulating women with sequential hMG/hCG. These were not abnormal cycles such as anovulatory ones. He related the response to hMG to subsequent pregnancy rates using *in vitro* fertilization dividing plasma oestradiol concentrations at the time of the ovarian follicular peak into three groups, low (reaching 300 pg ml^{-1}), intermediate (reaching 500 pg ml^{-1} – comparable with normal) and high responders (reaching 800 pg ml^{-1}). These variations were seen despite the fact that plasma progesterone concentrations were not significantly different. The pregnancy rates associated with these three groups were 23% for the high responders, 19% for the normal or intermediate and 16% for low responders. He described five separate patterns of follicular oestradiol concentration, the optimal being associated with a 27% pregnancy rate. Among these was a pattern characterized by a fall in oestradiol concentration on stopping daily hMG, resulting in a 16% pregnancy rate. Another was characterized by an early fall of oestradiol before stopping the daily hMG, which resulted in a 12% pregnancy rate. Sometimes there was a secondary rise of oestradiol values, indicating recruitment and functioning of a second crop of follicles; but despite these variations, luteal-phase oestradiol and progesterone patterns were not significantly different. Therefore, differences must be related to the oocyte and follicle function.

Luteal-phase insufficiency was associated with traumatic aspiration of granulosa cells from the follicles at laparoscopy and attempts had been made to remedy this problem by providing progesterone pessary supplementation. This improved luteal function but a normal luteal-phase profile was obtained only when follicle stimulation preceded aspiration and was followed by pessary supplementation. If an early rise in progesterone is noted there may be an early fall and it may not be possible to rescue the corpus luteum and this he described as 'delayed' luteal-phase defect. Hyperstimulation within the cycle usually gave rise to an early rise and early fall.

Professor E. del Pozo calculated a progesterone index over the whole of the luteal phase and defined normal values as over $107 \, \text{ng ml}^{-1}$, an integrated value. He selected patients by their basal temperature record and described 10 patients who presented with galactorrhoea who had a normal progesterone index re-established on treatment with bromocriptine. He had demonstrated a similar phenomenon on treatment of patients with demonstrable pituitary microadenomas and their abnormal progesterone index had returned to the pre-treatment value on stopping bromocriptine. He hypothesized that prolactin had a central regulatory role related to LH pulsatility and probably did not only have a local influence on luteal function. In his experience, hyperprolactinaemia rarely caused luteal dysfunction. Short luteal phases occurred in 6% of patients and about 10% of these were caused by hyperprolactinaemia. Moderate hyperprolactinaemia needed to be present before treatment of the hyperprolactinaemia with bromocriptine could be expected to normalize the luteal phase. He had found that estimation of plasma progesterone on days 3, 6 and 9 after elevation of the basal temperature record provided a value that bore a good relation to his total luteal-phase progesterone index.

46
Secondary sterility

MODERATOR: S. ROBERTSON
CO-ORDINATOR: R. F. HARRISON

The Moderator opened the session by defining the scope and the relative position of secondary sterility in New South Wales, Australia. It then became evident that this problem presents in very different ways in different parts of the world, being 50% in the Australian figures and falling as low as 10% in some of the Belgian figures; the World Health Organization figure is 30%.

It was indicated in the Australian figures that 66% of the patients had previously delivered a viable child and 33% had not and the prognosis for each group differed to a significant degree on that account alone, and the most frequent group of all secondary sterility was that of 'one child only' problem. It was indicated that the most frequent pathological cause was occult pelvic infection which had now reached epidemic proportions in Sydney and certainly is ensuring a steady future for the tubal surgeon and for the IVF programme.

MALE FACTOR

The first of the principal speakers was Dr Comhaire, whose topic was the male factor in secondary sterility. Though many more couples consult for primary than for secondary infertility, the latter may be as disturbing to the couple as the former. In the specialized male infertility referral centre run by Dr Comhaire, 10% of cases consult for secondary infertility.

This is remarkably less than the frequency for all secondary infertility problems found in a systematic multicentre survey performed by

WHO and including both male and female. In the latter, nearly 30% of cases consulted for secondary infertility. This difference could indicate the male factor to be rather uncommon in secondary infertility.

Dr Comhaire's group studied the test sample of patients with primary or secondary infertility and compared the frequency of aetiological diagnosis as well as semen characteristics in both groups.

RESULTS

It appears that only two remarkable differences were present in the two populations.

(1) A higher incidence of varicocele amongst men with secondary infertility.

(2) Absence of cases with azoospermia in the secondary infertile group. Other diseases occur with almost the same frequency in both groups, though we did not find any patient with male adnexitis in our group with secondary infertility as against 7% in primary infertility cases. This, however, could be due to the rather small sample-size.

Our observation of an increased incidence of varicocele amongst men with secondary infertility confirms data reported earlier by Schoysman, but is not corroborated by the results of the WHO study.

Varicocele causes progressive deterioration of testicular function, the severity of which has been documented to be age related. Therefore, varicocele patients with a relatively minor problem of infertility could have had no, or little problems in obtaining the first conception, but as the seminal quality continues to deteriorate with time, they could well experience problems in obtaining a second or third conception.

CONCLUSION

The male factor in secondary infertility should not be neglected, and particular attention should be focussed on the detection of varicocele. Investigation and treatment of men with secondary infertility should be performed with the same care and strategy as in men with primary infertility.

Table 1 Causes of primary and secondary infertility in men

Cause	Primary (90% of cases)	Secondary (10% of cases)
Varicocele	31	58
Idiopathic	24	18
Immunological	8	8
Normal	11	8
Cryptorchidism	4	8
Adnexitis	7	–
Azoospermia	15	–

The second speaker was Dr Cohen, who spoke on the tubal factor from two different points of view. Firstly, in relation to repeat tubal surgery; and secondly, related to the updated view on ectopic pregnancy.

REPEAT TUBAL SURGERY

Many patients who have undergone an unsuccessful tuboplasty have difficulty in accepting their infertility and therefore request a new tuboplasty. A reasonable counselling of these couples is difficult because the results of repeated tuboplasties are contradictory, and because *in vitro* fertilization may be a better treatment.

An analysis of recent publications shows a fertilization rate of 18–40% in repeat tubal surgery with an intra-uterine rate of 8–22% and ectopic rate of 2–13%.

The failure of a previous tubal surgery should not be considered as a contraindication for repeated surgery in some cases selected by previous hysterography and laparoscopy. The best results seem to occur in pure terminal salpingostomies and in proximal anastomosis and reimplantations. The operation must prepare the ovaries for a possible IVF (careful ovariolysis and often temporary suspension). The operation as a rule must preserve the ovaries to have the best possibilities for IVF.

SURGERY OF ECTOPIC PREGNANCY

Today, conservative procedures are being recommended even if the contralateral tube appears normal, and total salpingectomy for an

unruptured tubal pregnancy is being seriously questioned as a procedure for a woman who wishes to bear children.

From the analysis of recent publications, it is reasonable to conclude that salpingotomy and evacuation of the tubal contents is a
safe procedure unlikely to impair tubal function further and likely
to maintain fertility.

Results of conservative surgery for ectopic pregnancy in sole patent
oviduct suggest an average rate of 57% intra-uterine pregnancy and
20% ectopic. Unruptured ampullary pregnancies have been successfully removed laparoscopically. Manual expression is associated with
the highest incidence of recurrent ectopic pregnancies. Segmental
resection and repair (primary or secondary) have been successfully
accomplished, with contradictory results. The options must always
be discussed with the couple before operation.

HABITUAL ABORTION

The final speaker was Professor R. Harrison, who discussed habitual
abortion, its investigation and the related hormones in early pregnancy. He then discussed a double-blind placebo-controlled trial
which was being carried out with hCG as a form of therapy. The final
results of this will not be known until the code is broken and more
cases are required, so only an outline is presently available. However,
he was able to state that in a previous open trial, using a regime of
an initial loading dose of 10000 IU i.m., as early in pregnancy as
possible, followed by 5000 IU i.m. twice weekly up to week 12, and
once weekly up to week 16, treatment of threatened abortion resulted
in an abortion rate of only 6% and in habitual abortions (three plus
consecutive) a rate of 7%.

DISCUSSION

Lengthy discussion followed these papers relating to immunology,
follow-up laparoscopy, post-operative therapy and other post-operative investigations as to their nature and the timing of them. The
conservation of right ovaries where possible for the future IVF
Programme was stressed.

Lengthy discussion took place on cervical suture for incompetent
cervix and particular emphasis was placed on the internal cervical
suture in cases where difficulty has previously occurred.

47
Sexually transmitted diseases and infertility

MODERATOR: W. CATES, Jr.
CO-ORDINATOR: P. McKENNA

The major preventable cause of infertility today, for both men and women, is sexually transmitted disease (STD). Infection-related infertility constitutes not only an individual problem for the infertile couple, but also a public health challenge. Pelvic inflammatory disease, due to sexually transmitted infection, probably accounts for half of all female infertility in many regions of the world. Low sperm count, often the result of infection, is the most important preventable male factor.

The workshop addressed a spectrum of female and male infections leading to subfecundity. The papers discussed epidemiological aspects of infertility, clinical approaches to the diagnosis of salpingitis, microbiological content of semen, therapeutic regimens for salpingitis and the role of prostititis in male infertility.

W. Cates (Atlanta, Georgia) presented an overview of infertility in the USA and other countries. A relatively large number of married American couples of reproductive age are infertile. In 1976, over 1 in 10 couples had failed to conceive after at least 1 year of marriage during which no contraceptives were used. In the USA, the estimated number of visits to private physicians' offices for infertility-related consultation increased from approximately 600 000 in 1972 to over 900 000 in 1978; it remained near that level through 1980.

The epidemiology of infertility in the developing world differs from that in the developed countries. While infertility is probably most common in tropical Africa, it also occurs frequently in some Asian countries and the Caribbean region. In Sudan, Indonesia, and Jamaica, for example, more than 6% of married women reach the age of 40–49 without having any children. Higher percentages of couples in the developing countries become infertile after they have had one or more children, apparently related to infections developed during pregnancy and delivery. Regardless of the level of infertility, however, wherever preventable diseases such as STD or postpartum infection are major causes of infertility, public health programmes can play an important role in helping couples avoid this tragic problem.

J. Henry-Suchet of Paris, France, reported on her experience with the use of immunology, laparoscopy and histopathology to diagnose chronic chlamydia salpingitis. Her group used the microimmunofluorescence test to measure IgM and IgG antibodies against *C. trachomatis* among infertile women. She compared those with laparoscopic evidence of chronic tubal inflammation but with no clinical or historical evidence of salpingitis to those with clinical evidence of salpingitis. IgM antibodies were not found in any of the patients undergoing an infertility work-up. IgG antibodies, however, were more common in women who were previously asymptomatic. She concluded that silent chlamydial infection was an important cause of tubal factor sterility; moreover much of the chlamydial infection had probably occurred in the distant past. Even after treatment with tetracyclines, she noted most of the antichlamydial titres did not change.

Her position was supported by histological evidence of persistent chronic inflammation in women with tubal obstruction. Morphologically, she found a predominant lymphocytic invasion, fibrinoid exudate and areas of necrotic tissue surrounded by inflammatory cells. Women with this chronic inflammation were more likely to have positive culture for any bacteria, positive abdominal cultures for chlamydia, and an elevated IgG antibody level to chlamydia. She inferred a strong connection between histological chronic inflammation and previous chlamydial infection.

H. Riedel (Kiel, W. Germany) reported on his results of infertility and semen bacteriology. He discussed the bacterial contamination of human semen, collected through his *in vitro* fertilization (IVF) programme. Nearly 60% of cultures of male ejaculates were negative or had bacterial counts of less than $10^4 ml^{-1}$. However, over 40% had bacterial concentrations of $10^5 ml^{-1}$. While *Ureaplasma urealyticum* was the main agent isolated, a wide range of organisms was found among the group with positive cultures. No correlation was found between ejaculates with positive cultures and leukocyte count or sperm quality. No direct effect of micro-organism contamination of human semen could be demonstrated in reduced fertilization rates or on other outcomes of the IVF programme. Thus, he questioned the appropriateness of bacterial screening of semen in IVF programmes.

A. Ingelman-Sundberg (Stockholm, Sweden) discussed the role of therapy for acute PID. PID refers to the clinical syndrome attributed to the ascending spread of micro-organisms from the vagina and endocervix to the Fallopian tubes and contiguous structures. Therefore, it includes the clinical entities of endometritis, salpingitis, parametritis, and/or peritonitis. Clinical diagnosis usually involves a history of lower abdominal pain, lower abdominal tenderness, cervical tenderness on movement and adnexal tenderness.

Advances in microbiology, combined with the use of culdocentesis or laparoscopy to evaluate patients with acute PID, have broadened traditional concepts of the microbiological aetiology of the disease. Although we formerly felt *N. gonorrhoeae* was the key agent involved in PID, we now realize that many organisms play a role in the pathogenesis of this syndrome. *C. trachomatis, M. hominis* and other anaerobic bacteria contribute to PID. Therefore, treatment regimens should be initiated which are active against the broadest range of these pathogens.

The treatment of choice is not established. No single agent is active against the entire spectrum of pathogens. Several antimicrobial combinations provide broad-spectrum activity against the major pathogens *in vitro*, but most have not been adequately evaluated for clinical efficacy in PID. Many current recommendations include a cephalosporin regimen combined with a tetracycline agent.

E. Johannson and R. Eliasson (Stockholm, Sweden) reported preliminary results from their study of the cytology of fluid obtained by prostatic massage. Using as their baseline a threshold of 10 leukocytes per high-power field, they found over one-third of infertile men demonstrated abnormally high leukocyte counts in prostatic fluid. These abnormal findings could not be correlated with clinical history or physical examination. They postulated that low-grade, clinically inapparent prostatitis may be an important contributor to infertility.

467

Dr Eliasson also emphasized the use of seminal plasma as an indicator of male infertility. Unfortunately, few laboratories have considered a function other than sperm motility as contributing to male infertility. The recent investigations in Stockholm have examined such factors as chromatine stability, the uptake by DNA of specific stains, the stability of the spermatozoa membranes against lipid peroxidation and other biochemical properties of the seminal plasma. Normal values for seminal plasma have not yet been determined, and thus there is a need to identify and quantify them. To date, the Stockholm investigators have not found any association between the concentration of fructose, zinc or citric acid in seminal plasma and male factor infertility.

In discussion at the workshop, the audience underscored the important role of infection as the main preventable cause of infertility. Because treatment of infertility is expensive, and its success uncertain, increased attention should address prevention. Infection-related infertility can be reduced by attention to the major reasons for infection: STD, poor obstetric care and illegal abortion. However, participants felt public health programmes aimed at these three major causes of infertility are not easy to implement. They require a level of political support that is difficult to achieve in the developing world. For example, STD programmes have usually been unpopular among policy makers. STD initiatives compete for funding with other programmes affecting the entire population, such as malaria, schistosomiasis and tuberculosis. Moreover, information about STD is not always available in those regions where infertility is the greatest.

Further discussion also emphasized both the role of a team approach in reducing preventable STDs, and also the need for outreach programmes to interrupt chains of transmission within communities. The absence of much behavioural research from the Congress was noted, and participants expressed interest in more involvement of behavioural scientists at the next World Congress on Fertility and Sterility in Singapore in 1986.

48
Genetics in reproduction

MODERATOR: N. C. NEVIN
CO-ORDINATOR: N. O'HANRAHAN

Genetic factors are involved in many aspects of reproduction. The workshop considered the problems in reproduction of patients with genetic disease, genetic aspects of fetal wastage, the role of H-Y antigen in sex differentiation, and factors affecting the sex ratio. The large burden of undesirable mutations in man, reproduction in patients with genetic disease, and the genetic aspects of fetal wastage was presented by Dr A. Kuliev. Some 38.0–46.0 per 1000 newborn infants have a genetic disorder, of which 6.9 per 1000 are chromosomal anomalies; 11.7–14.0 per 1000 have a gene defect; and 26.0–32.0 per 1000 have a congenital malformation or complex disorder. This relative increase in genetic disorders presents a major challenge in the field of prevention. With improving care, an increasing number of patients with genetic disease survive until reproductive age. Many genetic disorders compatible with reduced or normal levels of female reproduction are modified in their expression by gestation. In some disorders, gestation may be altered by direct or indirect effects of the disease on the mother or fetus. Patients with genetic diseases may thus pose particularly complicated problems when reproduction is contemplated. For example, the survival of patients with Down's syndrome (mongolism) has improved dramatically in the last three decades. In Down's syndrome, there has been no report of a male with trisomy 21 having offspring. Females with trisomy 21 are capable of reproduction; 24 patients have produced 15 chromosomally normal and 10 trisomy 21 offspring. Twelve mosaic fathers and 24 mothers have produced 38 chromosomally abnormal and 12 normal offspring in 50 progeny. In phenylketonuria (PKU), affected females have an extremely high risk of having children with mental retardation, microcephaly, and congenital abnormalities. In all, a total of 524 pregnancies in 155 mothers with PKU or some degree of hyperphenyl-alaninaemia have been documented. In addition, women with PKU also have an increased frequency of spontaneous abortion. With preconceptional counselling and dietary management, it may be possible for phenylketonuric females to produce normal offspring. Male infertility is a feature of cystic fibrosis, the commonest autosomal recessive gene disorder in European communities. High rates of spontaneous abortion and neonatal death occur in dystrophia myotonica. The survival of patients who have sickle-cell anaemia and thalassaemia will become a major problem in developing countries.

Genetic factors play a major role in fetal wastage. Although it is difficult to estimate accurately human reproductive loss, the extent of fetal death in man is likely to be about 25% among those that reach the third week of gestation. From earlier studies of the fate of human eggs in contact with sperm, it has been calculated that the rate of sterility may be as high as 42%, and that of infertility as high as 16%. If the combined infertility and sterility rate of 58% is added to the 25% of fetal loss, the reproductive loss or failure in man is an astonishing 83%. Some of the causes of this loss have been recognized. The role of chromosome abnormalities has been well documented. The prevalence of chromosomal abnormalities in the early abortions is about 61.5% and in later ones about 5%. The overall prevalence of chromosomal abnormalities in spontaneous abortions is very close to 50%, and that one in 13 conceptuses has a chromosomal abnormality of some kind. Recently, with developments in *in vitro* fertilization, some light has been shed on early loss of embryos. A recent paper described the chromosomal examination of 11 embryos fertilized *in vitro*. Of the three oocytes in which chromosomal analysis was possible, two were chromosomally abnormal, and in a further eight oocytes examined by flow cytometry approximately 20% were haploid. Other possible factors resulting in fetal loss were considered; consanguinity, temperature-induced mutations, rhesus blood groups, chromosomal polymorphisms, and so-called multifactorial factors.

Recurrent abortion is not an infrequent problem.Chromosomal

abnormalities in couples with a history of three or more spontaneous abortions are probably 12 times higher than in the general population. This figure is even higher if the couple also have had a child with a birth defect. Some 3.5% of couples with habitual abortion have a balanced chromosomal translocation which can be implicated in the repeated fetal loss. It is of interest that females are more likely than males to have the balanced chromosomal translocation carrier reflecting the fact that structural chromosomal rearrangements that are compatible with fertility in the female may be associated with sterility in the male. Some of the recent advances in prenatal diagnosis of genetic disorders and congenital abnormalities were considered, particularly the use of trophoblastic villi biopsy in early gestation which would make tissue available for cytogenetic, biochemical, and DNA analysis.

The role of H-Y antigen and abnormal sex differentiation was considered by Professor Haseltine. The process of sex determination has become, at least, partially clarified in the last 10 years. By 1970, it was clear that a Y-chromosome was necessary to mediate testicular development. However, it was uncertain how the Y-chromosome carried out this function, and the search for a factor(s) controlled by the Y-linked gene intensified. A possible candidate was the H-Y antigen. Professor Haseltine reported on experiments in mapping the H-Y antigen. It is now clear that more than the structural gene on the Y-chromosone is involved; X-linked or autosomal loci may play a part. The association of gonadal tumours and the presence of a Y-chromosome in the female was considered. It was concluded that if the child with a Y-chromosome has an abdominal gonad, it is reasonable to remove the gonad so that he does not develop a tumour. No patient with normal Y and who was H-Y antigen negative developed a tumour. Of 47 individuals with Y-chromosome and H-Y antigen positive, 15 developed gonadal tumours but of 23 with Y-chromosomes and H-Y antigen negative only two developed gonadal tumours. Some patients with an abnormal X-chromosome may be H-Y antigen positive; in these patients the gonad should not be removed.

It is of interest to know whether the sex ratio at very early stages of pregnancy is different from the ratio at birth. In early induced abortions it has been demonstrated, with banding and fluorescence techniques, that the sex ratio is not as high as has been believed. Some of the numerous factors relating to variation in the sex ratio were discussed by Mr M. Hull. Several factors influence the sex ratio, including frequency of intercourse, time of fertilization, and nutritional status of the individual. At birth, the sex ratio may or may not truly reflect the ratios at fertilization. The association of coital timing and sex ratio is well established, a male being more likely to be conceived 1 or 2 days before ovulation. Some have speculated as to the role of hormonal factors. The proportion of males is said to be reduced in women who have received clomiphene and hCG. This reduced sex ratio has been attributed to an increased circulating hormonal level at the time of conception. Mr Hull presented data of his own studies of the relationship of hormone treatment and sex ratio. In bromocriptine-treated patients there was a relatively high sex ratio of 49.8%, whereas in those treated with gonadotrophin and clomophene the ratio was reduced. In artificial insemination, some have found a reduced sex ratio with donor insemination, especially with frozen rather than with fresh seminal fluid. However, the biggest factor in determining the sex ratio will still be chance.

The workshop also considered the role of parental age and reproduction. There is little doubt that congenital malformations, particularly chromosomal abnormalities, occur more frequently in older mothers. The underlying defect is chromosomal non-disjunction.

Recently, by using a variety of staining techniques for the cytogenetic analysis, it has been shown that non-disjunction also may occur in the father. From several studies, it has been estimated that some 10–15% of cases of Down's syndrome are due to non-disjunction in the father. Increasing age of the father is also an important factor in gene mutations. It has been estimated that the likelihood of mutation leading to sporadic cases of achondroplasia, fibrodysplasia ossificans progressiva, Apert's syndrome and haemophilia increases by ten-fold from the third to the sixth decade of paternal age.

It was concluded that a greater understanding of the genetic factors in reproduction greatly facilitates the management of patients with sterility and infertility problems, and would help in preventing the numerous birth defects that afflict man.

49
Occupational hazards in reproductive health

MODERATOR: M. J. ROSENBERG
CO-ORDINATOR: M. MOLONEY

The recent realization that the working environment can lead to decreased fertility, increased fetal loss, and a variety of other reproductive impairments has been reflected by mounting scientific interest in this field. This session reviews preliminary work in three important areas: genetic surveillance to monitor reproductive hazards, to agents suspected of causing spermatogenic impairment, and the relationship of energy requirements to favourable pregnancy.

Kuliev discussed routine surveillance of genetic changes among workers which presents the possibility of determining the degree of risk that may be present on a more timely basis than by other methods such as monitoring of fertility and fetal loss. Genetic techniques involve determination of sister chromatid exchange and base-pair alterations which might alter the shape of chromosomes. However, such techniques require a good deal of additional work before the normal frequency of genetic abnormalities and their relationship to clinical events such as fetal loss can be defined. Since these are sophisticated techniques, their potential use is probably limited to certain high-risk groups as defined by animal or epidemiological studies. These techniques are discussed in the World Health Organization monograph on occupational hazards to reproduction. This document, now in final preparation, reviews the literature and discusses the epidemiological evaluation of such problems.

Comhaire stated that carbon disulphide (CS_2) has been identified as inhibiting spermatogenesis in animals, but results of studies in humans have been conflicting. A preliminary study of 28 CS_2 workers and 38 age-matched controls indicated that, as compared with control subjects, exposed men had lower sperm concentration (75.6 million ml^{-1} vs 107.3 million ml^{-1}, respectively), increased proportion of abnormally shaped sperm (75.7% vs 34.6%), and decreased sperm motility. There was, however, no suggestion of increasingly abnormal sperm parameters with increased length of work, and exposure levels were not recorded.

Aribarg described how lead has also been implicated as impairing spermatogenesis in man. In a Thai battery plant, 39 men were tested from different areas of the plant by comparing blood and semen lead levels. Both levels were related to ambient levels, and higher levels were found among men who had worked longer. Thirteen of the 39 men had greater than 'normal' blood lead levels.

Prema stated that for women in developing countries, food intake and manual labour are important considerations in ensuring a healthy outcome of pregnancy. Although precise measurement of both these factors is difficult, an increasing body of literature indicates that favourable outcome requires a progressive increase in energy intake as compared with the non-gravid state in pregnant women. When increased work or steady or decreased caloric intake precludes extra energy to support a pregnancy, the general outcome is decreased fertility, increased rates of fetal loss, or children born prematurely and/or with low birth-weight.

WORKSHOP

50
Principles of training in human reproduction

MODERATOR: M. ELSTEIN
CO-ORDINATOR: G. OYAKHIRE

The purpose of this workshop was to produce a working document to be presented to IFFS for approved use as a working basis for the promotion of education of physicians in the field of human reproduction. The document which is reproduced below was adopted unanimously by the IFFS General Assembly during IFFS Dublin '83. Other members of the working party were A. Mendiz Abal, C. Ng, U. Arai and K. Semm.

UNDERGRADUATE (see Figure 1)

1. Not all aspiring medical students, like any other member of society, will ideally have had some teaching during their school years in human reproduction in preparation for adulthood.

2. The introduction of Human Reproduction teaching early in the curriculum is desirable, since it meets the individual medical student's personal needs at a formative time in his development and his relationship with his peers.

3. In newly established schools or where curricula are being reviewed, integrated system teaching with physiologists, anatomists, biochemists, geneticists, behavioural scientists and their clinical counterparts should be encouraged. The co-ordination

should be the responsibility of the clinician who is involved in this practice. In most cases this would be a gynaecologist, and perhaps an andrologist or endocrinologist especially if they are part of an integrated service team in fertility regulation. Where orthodox division between basic sciences and clinical subjects exists, involvement of clinicians, by invitation, to the basic courses would provide a bridge and relevance. This interest has an important fringe benefit in encouraging recruitment into the speciality of obstetrics and gynaecology.

Primary and Secondary Schools

Medical Schools	–	Early in curriculum
	–	Human reproduction integrated system courses
	–	Involvement of clinicians in basic sciences
Clinical teaching	–	Family planning
	–	Human sexuality
	–	Sexually transmitted diseases
	–	Interpersonal relationships

Figure 1 Undergraduate education in human reproduction

4. In clinical programmes the emphasis should be on normality. Human reproduction must be taught within broad concepts to include human and family relationships, sexuality, contraception, infertility, sexually transmitted infections and genetic counselling. The related disciplines of psychiatry, andrology, endocrinology should be involved, bringing in the background of the continued contribution of the basic sciences.

POSTGRADUATE (Figure 2)

Postgraduate training must be related to the needs of the population served. While in some communities the need is for fertility control, in others, this is for fertility enhancement. The provision of services depends on available resources such as trained personnel, dispersion of the population, and clinical and research facilities. Cognizance needs to be taken of the influence of political and religious factors and the ethical ethos.

1. Primary medical care

The value of providing services related to the human reproduction needs of a population, by the primary medical care team is

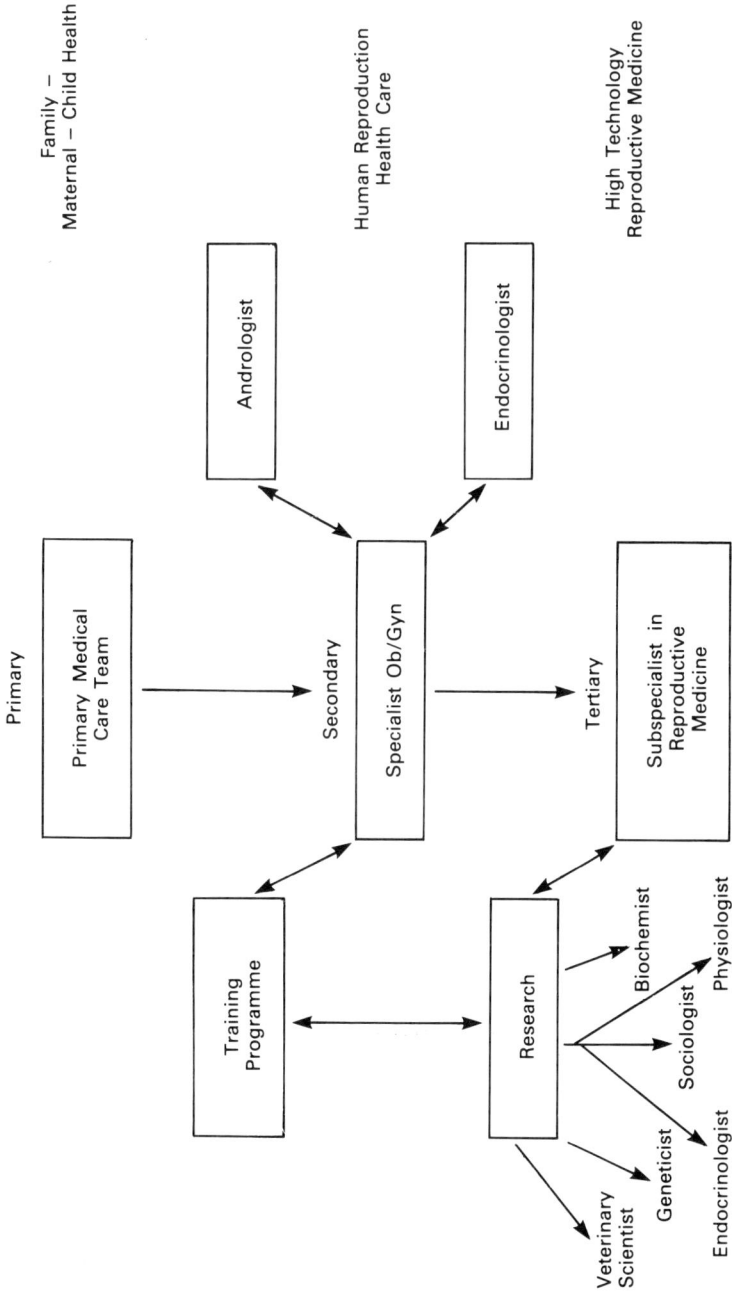

Figure 2 Provisions of human reproduction

now well recognized. Resources of manpower will dictate this provision. Irrespective of their background, it is essential that the caring professionals providing primary care have been trained in the broad aspects of human reproduction and its regulation and where appropriate in the prevention of sexually transmitted disease and their aftermath. They can make a valuable contribution to the education of the public in these matters.

2. Specialist obstetrician/gynaecologist

While the consensus was that obstetrician/gynaecologists were in a prime position to provide health care in human reproduction and teaching in the subject, in many instances a team of specialists including andrologists and endocrinologists provide valuable service. Interrelations with genetic and psychosexual counsellors enhance this contribution and stimulate research.

3. Training programmes

In the training of the specialist obstetrician/gynaecologist the importance of broad aspects of human reproduction needs to be stressed. There is value in an exposure to research during this training in order to instil its disciplines particularly of data collection and involvement in the field. There would be some who will pursue such a training programme at depth in order to follow a career in the subspeciality of reproductive medicine, devoting their major energies to this. The training would enter the high technology frontiers of the speciality in which exciting developments are occurring.

In this training, exposure to related disciplines such as genetics, biochemistry, reproductive physiology and endocrinology will occur. Collaboration with colleagues in veterinary medicine with an interest in reproductive medicine should facilitate the development of animal models to answer research problems.

The economic and sociological implications will require airing.

4. Subspecialist in reproductive medicine

Subspecialists in reproductive medicine will play an important role in training in human reproduction. High technology developments in reproductive medicine should occur in those countries where there is need. This must of course be related to resources available. Where these are limited, research and technological endeavour should be centralized.

5. Training requirements and proficiency examinations

There appear to be considerable differences in the way in which specialists providing human reproductive services were recognised in different parts of the world. Because of these variations it was felt that each country should define its own criteria. However, each should move to the establishment of appropriate standards, relevant to their needs.

Part III

Special
Symposia

Part III

Section 1

Prolactinomas and Pregnancy*

* This special symposium was sponsored by Sandoz

51
Introduction: prolactinomas and pregnancy

H. S. JACOBS

The last decade has seen a revolution in the treatment of anovulatory infertility and nowhere has this been more obvious than in the diagnosis and management of patients with hyperprolactinaemia. Notwithstanding the remarkable increase in our understanding of the neuropharmacological control of prolactin secretion (detailed by Dr Crosignani in the opening chapter of this section), the single most reliable diagnostic guide to a disturbance of prolactin secretion remains the basal serum prolactin concentration. While much confusion and uncertainty exists in the exact interpretation of the normal range, the simple point to remember is that with prolactin concentrations, as with all clinical investigations, correct evaluation demands that one takes into account the clinical context in which the measurement is made. Thus because it is known that oestrogen stimulates prolactin release and that women with amenorrhoea due to hyperprolactinaemia suffer from oestrogen deficiency, a minor elevation of the serum prolactin concentration in an oestrogen deficient patient with amenorrhoea is of much greater clinical significance than a considerable elevation in a well oestrogenized patient with an intact menstrual cycle.

At least half the women presenting with hyperprolactinaemic amenorrhoea have a prolactin-secreting pituitary tumour (prolactinoma). The exact proportion diagnosed depends upon the imaging procedure used and Dr Hall outlines with great clarity the information that can be obtained from the various procedures presently in use (Chapter 53). The advantages of CT scanning, in which the pituitary itself rather than its bony carapace is imaged, are clearly described. In addition Dr Hall describes the advantages of the direct coronal scan compared with multiple axial scans with computer reconstructions in the coronal and sagittal planes. This is a fascinating article in which the limits of current radiological techniques are also drawn.

Several modalities of treatment exist, but undoubtedly surgical extirpation and medical treatment with bromocriptine are the two most frequently used. Professor Teasdale and colleagues (Chapter 54) address the type of clinical information endocrinologists and gynaecologists find particularly helpful. Thus in contrast to the majority of articles by surgeons, this chapter describes the outcome both in terms of rates of normalization of prolactin concentrations and in terms of pregnancy rates. He shows that in experienced hands surgical removal of prolactinomas confined to the pituitary fossa continues to provide a reliable method of treatment, with a remarkably low rate of endocrine (and indeed surgical) complications.

Drs Franks and Jacobs describe some aspects of the use of dopaminergic agonists (Chapter 55). In addition to describing the familiar story of the success of bromocriptine in normalizing prolactin secretion and reconstituting fertility, they provide long-term follow-up data on patients originally treated with bromocriptine 6–8 years ago. Naturally such data are only now becoming available and for some patients the picture is looking quite optimistic, even for long-term remission of symptoms in patients who have discontinued their medical therapy.

Drs Bergh and Nillius deal directly with the problem of the prolactinoma that expands during pregnancy (Chapter 57). In fact, it turns out that this is a rare problem. At first it seems remarkable that a complication we all worried about so much should not eventuate, or only so as a rarity. In my opinion the reason is the remarkable shrinkage of prolactin-secreting pituitary tumours that occurs on treatment with bromocriptine. As described by Franks and Jacobs, the tumour quite rapidly shrinks away from the walls of the expanded fossa and so any tendency for it to enlarge during pregnancy can be readily accommodated. Of course, in the past, when ovulation was induced with drugs that were not dopaminergic agonists, such shrinkage did not occur and therefore room had not been made for pituitary

486

expansion during pregnancy, a phenomenon that of course occurs normally. Should clinical symptoms of pituitary expansion occur in a patient with a prolactinoma (whether or not she was originally treated with bromocriptine) it does seem, however, that using bromocriptine during pregnancy is safe to both mother and fetus, based upon the excellent report of the extensive post-marketing surveillance of the use of bromocriptine in pregnancy reported by Drs Krupp and Turkalj (Chapter 56).

In conclusion the following chapters describe most aspects of the management of patients with prolactinomas in relation to their infertility and their progress through pregnancy. I commend them to you as up-to-date accounts by experienced authors of problems faced by all clinicians treating this common condition.

52
Medical investigation of abnormal prolactin states

P. G. CROSIGNANI, C. FERRARI, P. RAMPINI,
P. ADELASCO, C. ZAVAGLIA, G. BRAMBILLA,
M. BOGHEN and A. PARACCHI

In hyperprolactinaemic patients, despite the large amount of clinical data, radiological studies and biochemical testing, the most useful diagnostic criteria remain the basal serum prolactin (PRL) levels and the results of radiological investigation of the sella and suprasellar region. High-resolution CT scans are especially helpful. These statements are supported by our experience with several diagnostic tests of prolactin secretion, which have been carried out in a large population of hyperprolactinaemic subjects over the last 7 years.

PATIENTS AND METHODS

Patients with hyperprolactinaemia of different origin have been studied for basal serum PRL determination, radiological studies of the sella and in most cases for different functional tests of PRL secretion. On the basis of clinical and radiological findings, patients' conditions have been classified as follows:

(1) Idiopathic hyperprolactinaemia, when conventional tomography and CT scans of the sella and suprasellar region were normal.

(2) Microprolactinoma, by the presence of typical radiological

findings; surgical confirmation has been subsequently obtained in the 30 patients undergoing operation.

(3) Macroprolactinoma, on the basis of CT-scan findings.

(4) Acromegaly, as shown by concomitant GH and PRL hypersecretion; all these patients had evidence of pituitary macroadenoma.

(5) Empty sella syndrome, as diagnosed by CT scans.

(6) Hypothalamic lesions, as suggested by CT scan and confirmed by surgery.

(7) Uraemia; these patients were studied during chronic haemodialysis.

The following functional tests were used:

(1) TRH test (200 µg i.v.). Individual responses were classified as normal when the maximum increase over baseline was in the range of normal subjects, as absent when this increase was less than 50%, and as impaired when the increase was greater than 50% but below the normal range.

(2) Sulpiride (100 mg i.m.) or domperidone (2 or 8 mg i.v.) test. The criteria for judging the individual responses were also derived from parallel studies in control subjects, with definition of normal, absent or impaired responses as for the TRH test.

(3) Directly acting dopamine agonists or dopamine precursors:
   (a) dopamine ($5 \mu g\,kg^{-1}min^{-1}$ infused i.v. during 120 min),
   (b) L-dopa (500 mg by mouth),
   (c) bromocriptine (2.5 mg by mouth),
   (d) dihydroergocristine (6 mg by mouth).
   The criterion for a normal response was a lowering of PRL value to below 50% of the baseline concentration after either dopamine, L-dopa or bromocriptine. Dihydroergocristine was observed not to lower PRL levels significantly in normal subjects at this dose when given by mouth[1].

(4) Central nervous system acting dopaminergic drugs:
   (a) L-dopa (100 mg by mouth) plus carbidopa (35 mg by mouth) after pretreatment with carbidopa 50 mg by mouth six hourly for four doses,
   (b) nomifensine (200 mg by mouth).
   The criteria for a normal response were PRL lowering to below

50% of baseline after carbidopa plus L-dopa, or to below 65% of baseline after nomifensine.

RESULTS AND DISCUSSION

Basal PRL levels in the various categories of hyperprolactinaemic patients examined are reported in Figure 1, showing that values

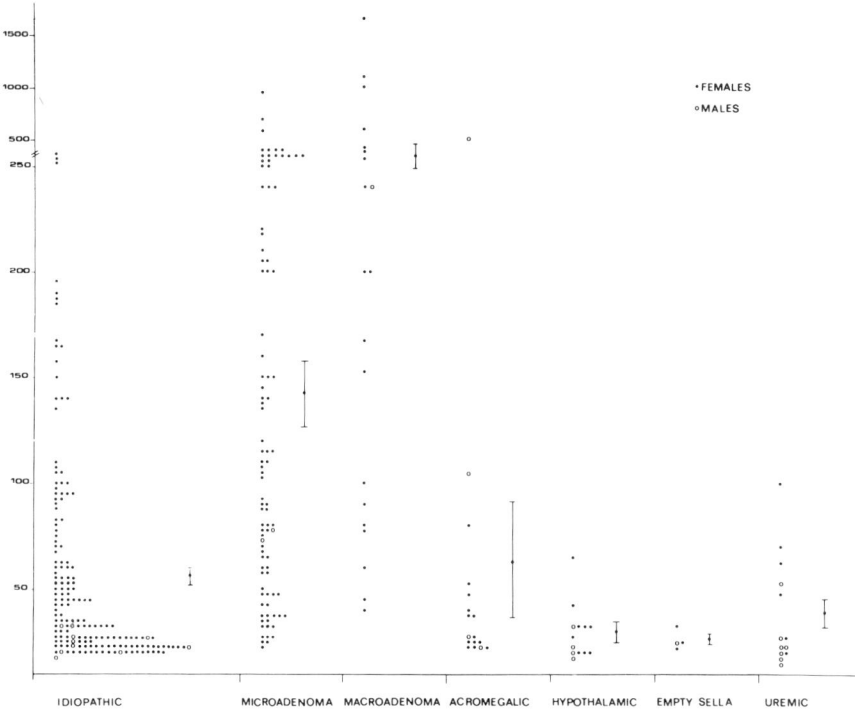

Figure 1 Basal serum prolactin concentrations in individual subjects with hyperprolactinaemia of different aetiology. Mean ±SE values are also shown

above $200 \, \text{ng} \, \text{ml}^{-1}$ are almost solely found in patients with prolactinoma. This is in agreement with many previous studies, but much overlap exists between the different aetiologies.

TRH test

The mean PRL response observed in the various groups of patients was always significantly lower, on a percent basis, than that of

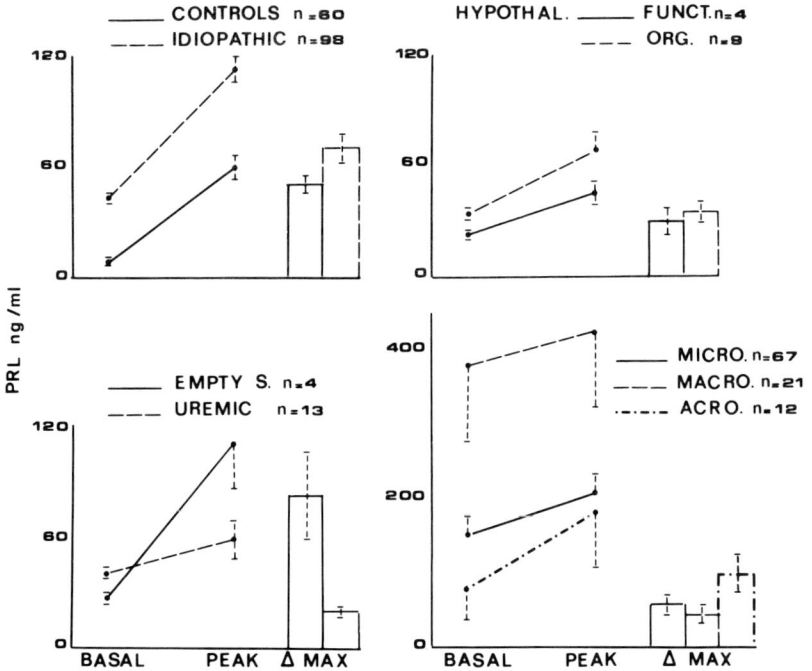

Figure 2 Serum prolactin (PRL) response to TRH in healthy controls and in patients with hyperprolactinaemia of different aetiologies. Micro = microadenoma; Macro = macroadenoma; Acro = acromegaly

healthy controls (Figure 2). Within the hyperprolactinaemic patients, the highest responses were found in the idiopathic group. The patterns of PRL response to TRH in 228 hyperprolactinaemic subjects indicate that most but not all patients with prolactinoma or with uraemia do not adequately respond to the stimulus; a large overlap between groups is, however, evident.

Sulpiride and domperidone tests

Both these antidopaminergic drugs elicited normal PRL responses in many patients with idiopathic hyperprolactinaemia but only in a few with prolactinoma. It is noteworthy that none of the 19 subjects

492

with hypothalamic disease or acromegaly responded adequately to dopamine receptor blockade[2]. An important finding was the normal PRL response obtained in five patients with radiological evidence of microprolactinoma, in two of whom the diagnosis was confirmed at surgery.

Since exogenous dopamine infusion restores the normal PRL response to sulpiride in unresponsive subjects with either idiopathic, adenomatous or hypothalamic hyperprolactinaemia[3] a defective concentration of dopamine at the lactotrophs seems to be the cause of the failure of dopamine antagonists to stimulate PRL secretion in these patients.

Some interesting information may be derived by comparing the responses to TRH and sulpiride tests in the same hyperprolactinaemic subjects. In fact a higher PRL increase is elicited by sulpiride than TRH in patients with idiopathic hyperprolactinaemia as well as in the controls, while prolactinoma patients appear unresponsive to both stimuli, and those with hypothalamic disease show a positive response to TRH associated with an absent response to sulpiride. These data suggest that the combination of the two tests may be of some practical value in subjects with mild to moderate hyperprolactinaemia and no radiological evidence of pituitary adenoma[4].

Direct dopamine agonists or precursors

All of the three substances used (dopamine, L-dopa and bromocriptine) induced a substantial lowering of PRL value in most patients irrespective of the underlying aetiology, as previously reported[5]. However, a certain proportion of subjects showed partial or total resistance to the drugs; this is reminiscent of the findings obtained with chronic bromocriptine treatment[5].

This resistance to dopamine action may be caused either by defective dopamine receptors at the lactotrophs or by a postreceptor defect[6]. Nevertheless, compared with the relatively uncommon dopamine resistance, the large majority of hyperprolactinaemic patients are responsive, or even hyper-responsive, to the action of dopamine. This is suggested by the recent finding that an oral dose of the relatively weak dopamine agonist dihydroergocristine can suppress PRL levels significantly in hyperprolactinaemic states of different aetiology but not in healthy controls[1]. These data are reminiscent of previous findings obtained with subemetic doses of apomorphine[7].

Central nervous system acting dopaminergic drugs

Most patients in the various groups had an impaired or absent suppression of PRL in both the carbidopa plus L-dopa and the nomifensine tests, as previously reported[8].

The failure of nomifensine administration to lower PRL levels in most hyperprolactinaemic patients was initially attributed to defective activation of brain dopaminergic pathways in these subjects[8,9]. However, the recent finding that nomifensine elevates serum growth hormone (GH) levels in hyperprolactinaemic as well as in healthy subjects[10,11] makes this hypothesis unlikely and suggests that the impairment lies in the dopamine transport to the lactotrophs, prob-

Table 1 Prevalence (expressed as percentages) of: (A) Pituitary dopamine resistance*, (B) Pituitary dopamine concentration defect[†], and (C) CNS dopamine inhibition defect[‡]. Number of subjects tested is given in parenthesies

Group	Idiopathic hyperpro- lactinaemia	Micro- prolactinoma	Macro- prolactinoma	Acromegaly	Hypo- thalamic hyperpro- lactinaemia
A	17 (54)	15 (59)	33 (18)	0 (7)	0 (7)
B	38 (50)	92 (58)	100 (19)	100 (8)	100 (11)
C	70 (34)	82 (24)	80 (20)	50 (4)	75 (4)

*As assessed by impaired PRL inhibition by dopamine, L-dopa or bromocriptine.
[†]As assessed by impaired PRL stimulation by sulpiride or domperidone.
[‡]As assessed by impaired PRL inhibition by carbidopa plus L-dopa or nomifensine.

ably due to alterations in the microcirculation. Table 1 summarizes the prevalence of the three dopaminergic defects discussed above in the different groups of hyperprolactinaemic patients we have studied. These data show that dopamine resistance is relatively uncommon in hyperprolactinaemia, while evidence of pituitary dopamine deficiency is quite common and almost uniformly found in patients with prolactinoma. These conclusions are in contrast with reports suggesting that dopaminergic tone is increased in hyperprolactinaemia on the basis of thyrotrophin (TSH) hyper-responsiveness to dopamine antagonists[12] and that hyperprolactinaemic subjects may be more resistant to the PRL-lowering effect of dopamine infusion than healthy controls[13]. The results of TSH testing, however, cannot simply be extrapolated to the PRL secretion system, and different results have been obtained with dopamine infusion by other groups with both *in vivo* and *in vitro* experiments[6,14]. These discrepancies probably result from the small number of patients studied and from the variable prevalence of subjects truly resistant to the action of dopamine in the different investigations. This is a particularly important bias in studies like that of Bansal *et al.*[13], which were performed in a small number of subjects.

Acknowledgements

This work was supported in part by C.N.R. Special Program 'Control of Neoplastic Growth'.

References

1. Ferrari, C., Romussi, M., Benco, R., Rampini, P. and Mailland, F. (1983). Effect of dihydroergocristine administration on serum prolactin and growth hormone levels in normal, hyperprolactinemic, and acromegalic subjects: further evidence for pituitary dopamine deficiency in these conditions. *Acta Endocrinol.*, **103**, 1
2. Ferrari, C., Scarduelli, C., Rampini, P. *et al.* (1983). Prolactin response to the dopamine antagonists sulpiride and domperidone: further evidence for pituitary dopamine deficiency in hyperprolactinemic disorders of different etiology. *Gynecol. Obstet. Invest.* (In press)
3. Crosignani, P. G., Reschini, E., Peracchi, M., Lombroso, G. C., Mattei, A. and Caccamo, A. (1977). Failure of dopamine infusion to suppress the plasma prolactin response to sulpiride in normal and hyperprolactinemic subjects. *J. Clin. Endocrinol. Metab.*, **45**, 841
4. Ferrari, C., Rampini, P., Benco, R., Caldara, R., Scarduelli, C. and Crosignani, P. G. (1982). Functional characterization of hypothalamic hyperprolactinemia. *J. Clin. Endocrinol. Metab.*, **55**, 897
5. Crosignani, P. G., Ferrari, C., Liuzzi, A., *et al.* (1982). Treatment of hyperprolactinemic states with different drugs: a study with bromocriptine, metergoline, and lisuride. *Fertil. Steril.*, **37**, 61
6. Bethea, C. L., Ramsdell, J. S., Jaffe, R. B., Wilson, C. B. and Weiner, R. I. (1982). Characterization of the dopaminergic regulation of human prolactin-secreting cells cultured on extracellular matrix. *J. Clin. Endocrinol. Metab.*, **54**, 893
7. Martin, J. B., Lal, S., Tolis, G. and Friesen, H. G. (1974). Inhibition by apomorphine of prolactin secretion in patients with elevated serum prolactin. *J. Clin. Endocrinol. Metab.*, **39**, 180
8. Crosignani, P. G., Ferrari, C., Malinverni, A., Barbieri, C., Mattei, A., Caldara, R. and Rocchetti, M. (1980). Effect of central nervous system dopaminergic activation on prolactin secretion in man: evidence for a common central defect in hyperprolactinemic patients with and without radiological signs of pituitary tumors. *J. Clin. Endocrinol. Metab.*, **51**, 1068
9. Müller, E. E., Genazzani, A. R. and Murru, S. (1978). Nomifensine diagnostic test in hyperprolactinemic states. *J. Clin. Endocrinol. Metab.*, **47**, 1352
10. Dallabonzana, D., Spelta, B., Botalla, L. *et al.* (1982). Effects of nomifensine on growth hormone and prolactin secretion in normal subjects and in pathological hyperprolactinemia. *J. Clin. Endocrinol. Metab.*, **54**, 1125
11. Ferrari, C., Caldara, R., Barbieri, C. *et al.* (1981). Central nervous system and

pituitary mechanisms in dopaminergic stimulation of growth hormone release in women. *Neuroendocrinology*, **32**, 213

12. Scanlon, M. F., Rodriguez-Arnao, M. D., McGregor, A. M. *et al.* (1981). Altered dopaminergic regulation of thyrotrophin release in patients with prolactinomas: comparison with other tests of hypothalamic-pituitary function. *Clin. Endocrinol.*, **14**, 133

13. Bansal, S., Lee, L. A. and Woolf, P. D. (1981). Abnormal prolactin responsivity to dopaminergic suppression in hyperprolactinemic patients. *Am. J. Med.*, **71**, 961

14. Reschini, E., Ferrari, C., Peracchi, M., Fadini, R., Meschia, M. and Crosignani, P. G. (1980). Effect of dopamine infusion on serum prolactin concentration in normal and hyperprolactinemic subjects. *Clin. Endocrinol.*, **13**, 519

53
Neuroradiology of prolactinomas

K. HALL

The neuroradiological methods that can be used in the detection and delineation of known or suspected prolactinomas are numerous. They include relatively non-invasive techniques such as skull radiography, sellar tomography and CT scanning. Sometimes more invasive procedures are deemed to be necessary, such as cerebral angiography, basal cisternography and cavernous sinus venography.

FACTORS INFLUENCING THE CHOICE OF NEURORADIOLOGICAL TECHNIQUES

The decision as to which of these methods should be used in any individual case will depend on several factors. The first is the skill and expertise of the radiologists, allied to the sophistication of the apparatus that they have available. One important point is that all of the invasive methods mentioned above are potentially dangerous and may, in some circumstances, be avoided if a third- or fourth-generation CT scanner is in use.

The second factor influencing the choice of radiological investigations is what sort of treatment will be used. Thus if medical treatment alone is to be used very little radiological investigation will be necessary. In our experience, all that is required prior to the initiation of bromocriptine therapy for prolactinomas is a plain radiograph of the skull to exclude a large tumour. If, however, the surgical removal of a prolactinoma is contemplated, either as the primary form of therapy or because bromocriptine has failed or has not been tolerated by the patient, then the surgeon may demand more information from the radiologist. He will probably wish to confirm the presence of a tumour in the gland and may want to know where it lies. In addition, if it is large he may wish to have some advance information about the precise relationships of the lesion to adjacent structures such as the optic nerves and chiasm and the carotid arteries and their branches. Some surgeons may wish to know about the anatomy of the cavernous sinuses, and their interconnections, prior to surgical exploration via the transsphenoidal route. The demand for such information will, obviously, depend on past experience during surgical exploration of the pituitary fossa.

The neuroradiological techniques that are thought necessary will also depend on the size of the prolactinoma. Pituitary adenomas are fairly arbitrarily divided into either microadenomas (diameter $\leqslant 10$ mm) or macroadenomas (diameter > 10 mm), the importance of this distinction being that microadenomas probably tend to become macroadenomas and that the smaller tumours are easier to remove, with less risk of recurrence. The one basic radiological difference between these two subdivisions of pituitary adenomas, and this applies to prolactinomas in particular, is that macroadenomas tend to enlarge the sella whereas the microadenomas do not. The large tumours tend to exert effects on adjacent structures, such as arteries and nerves, and to demonstrate these changes the invasive techniques may be necessary.

THE DETECTION AND DELINEATION OF MACROPROLACTINOMAS

Sellar radiography

As already mentioned, macroprolactinomas tend to enlarge the pituitary fossa and this can be readily assessed if it is fairly gross. However, if there is any doubt about sellar expansion an arbitrary method can be used to calculate the 'sellar volume'[1]. In this the length and height of the pituitary fossa are measured on the lateral film, and its width is determined from the posteroanterior (PA) film. These figures are multiplied together and then divided by two to arrive at this so-called volume, a figure of 1500 mm^3 usually being taken as the upper limit of normal.

A pituitary adenoma is not the only cause of an enlarged sella. It can be enlarged by pressure from a dilated third ventricle in chronic hydrocephalus, by a craniopharyngioma or by a large intrasellar aneurysm. However, the commonest cause of an expanded sella turcica, after a pituitary adenoma, is an empty sella. This is the term used for an intrasellar arachnoid herniation in which a CSF-filled sac bulges downwards through a defect in the diaphragma sellae, into the fossa, causing compression of the pituitary gland as well as symmetrical, globular sellar enlargement.

A macroadenoma in the pituitary fossa is often not central in position and any enlargement will produce asymmetry and depression of the sellar floor. The floor will often become thinned and eroded and the tumour may bulge down into the sphenoidal sinus.

If a large adenoma grows upwards out of the pituitary fossa it will tend to distort the anterior clinoid processes and push the dorsum sellae backwards. Thus an erect dorsum sellae may indicate a fairly large suprasellar extension of the tumour. When the tumour becomes extremely large the dorsum sellae and the top of the clivus can be destroyed completely.

When the sella is definitely abnormal sellar tomography is rarely indicated. We only perform tomography in such circumstances if the surgeon wishes to see the sellar floor and the anatomy of the sphenoidal sinuses, prior to transsphenoidal surgery, if these have not been shown by the CT scan.

CT scanning

When CT scanning was first introduced it rapidly became established as the next radiological investigation to carry out, after the initial skull radiograph, in the detection and delineation of pituitary adenomas. The older generations of scanners, by means of scans in the axial and coronal planes, could demonstrate very adequately large intrasellar tumours and those with extensions into the sphenoidal sinus and the suprasellar regions.

With these scanners pituitary tumours of all types tend to be slightly denser than surrounding brain and show fairly homogeneous enhancement, i.e. following the administration of intravenous contrast medium they appear whiter on the scans. Some tumours, however, show a more cystic or necrotic appearance, having a central darker area surrounded by an enhancing white ring.

A CT scan can also demonstrate, and sometimes distinguish from a pituitary adenoma, other lesions in or near the sella, such as a craniopharyngioma, a meningioma or a large aneurysm. An empty sella can often be suggested by the low CSF density in the sella, though sometimes a cystic or necrotic tumour produces a similar appearance and can be misdiagnosed as an empty sella.

CT scanning is of value in the follow-up of pituitary adenomas, whether they have been treated or not. Thus, a decrease in tumour size can be readily appreciated on repeat scans when a patient with a large prolactinoma is treated with bromocriptine, or other medical treatment.

Only fairly large tumours, and quite marked changes in tumour size, can be detected with these older CT scanners. A small macroadenoma, or other small lesion in the sellar region, can be missed, making other radiological methods such as basal cisternography necessary. The newer third- and fourth-generation scanners can, however, demonstrate these lesions much more reliably, as described later in the section on the CT scanning of microprolactinomas.

Cerebral angiography

Bilateral carotid angiography may be demanded by the surgeon before surgical removal of a macroprolactinoma, by the transsphenoidal or the intracranial approach. This angiogram should show the relationship of the tumour to the adjacent arteries, which may be quite markedly distorted and displaced by a large tumour. Sometimes the adjacent artery may be encased by a prolactinoma, making removal impossible.

When a transsphenoidal approach is to be used the surgeon may want to know that the carotid arteries in the cavernous sinuses are not too tortuous and are not bulging into the pituitary gland. Also, he may wish to be certain that there are no small aneurysms arising from these arteries and bulging into the gland. These precautions should prevent disastrous arterial haemorrhage during the operation because, if an arterial anomaly is found, a different approach can be chosen.

Rarely, the angiogram may show that rare cause of an enlarged sella, a huge intrasellar aneurysm, another potentially dangerous lesion for the pituitary surgeon.

Basal cisternography, with CT

In the basal cisternogram, a positive contrast medium, such as metrizamide or iopamidol, is introduced into the basal subarachnoid cisterns, especially those adjacent to the sella. These cisterns and their contents, normal or abnormal, are then visualized by lateral radiography or tomography and also by axial and coronal plane CT scanning. This technique was developed to supplement conventional CT scanning on the older generation scanners in an attempt to demonstrate smaller tumours, etc.[2].

The cisternogram should show quite small macroprolactinomas with small suprasellar extensions. It will also demonstrate the relationship of small or medium-sized tumours to the optic nerves and chiasm, which the surgeon may find of value at operation. An empty sella, be it large or small, can be readily demonstrated by this technique and small changes in prolactinoma size are easily seen[3]. If more sophisticated CT scanners are available basal cisternography is of more limited value.

Cavernous sinus venography

In some centres cavernous sinus venography is used instead of carotid angiography to demonstrate arterial anomalies in the sellar region[4]. The carotid arteries show as filling defects in the opacified cavernous sinuses and anomalies such as tortuosity and aneurysms can be detected. Sometimes, however, an angiogram may still be required to confirm the abnormality shown on the venogram. The advantage of the venogram over the angiogram is that it is less invasive, it is simpler to perform and can be performed on out-patients.

THE DETECTION OF MICROPROLACTINOMAS
Sellar radiography

Microprolactinomas do not enlarge the pituitary fossa and in reality plain skull radiographs are only of importance in such cases to exclude a large tumour.

The 'classic' feature on the plain skull radiograph that is said to suggest a microadenoma is the 'double floor' to the pituitary fossa. This is said to be due to a small bulge produced by the tumour growing close to the floor, or even at some distance from it. However, this is a very unreliable sign and appears to be as common in patients who are having their skulls radiographed because of head trauma as in those with a clinical suggestion of a prolactinoma.

The causes of this 'double floor' include:

(1) *Poor radiography*; if the film is not a true lateral one, with the anterior clinoid processes superimposed, even a perfectly flat floor will look double because of the angle of the X-ray beam relative to it.

(2) *A normal central or off-central depression in the sellar floor*, usually associated with the insertion of one or more sphenoidal sinus septa into the floor of the sella.

(3) *A normal slope to the sellar floor* (see below).

(4) *A carotid sulcus.* This is the impression on the side of the upper part of the body of the sphenoid that is fairly common and is caused by the carotid artery; it may even show an anterior curve, easily confused with the sellar floor, corresponding to the anterior curve of the artery to pass medially to the anterior clinoid process.

(5) *Accessory spenoidal sinuses* below and anterior to the sellar floor.

Sellar tomography

The principle behind the use of sellar tomography in the detection of microprolactinomas is that this technique can show minor changes in the bone of the sellar floor that are supposed to indicate the presence of a small tumour nearby. These changes include focal bulges and erosions, which have to be distinguished from normal variations in this region.

These tomograms are usually obtained by using fairly sophisticated equipment that produces a complex movement of X-ray tube and film to blur out adjacent structures and produce a thin section of bone in focus. The movement is usually hypocycloidal but can be circular or spiral and quite a long X-ray exposure is necessary. The tomographic slice thickness is usually 1 or 2 mm and to cover the whole sella up to 10 or 12 slices may be required in both the axial and the coronal planes. As a result of all this, the radiation dose received by the patient, especially to the radiation-sensitive lenses of the eyes during coronal plane tomography, can be appreciable.

Several authors have claimed, over the years, a very close correlation between the positive findings at sellar tomography and their results of transsphenoidal surgery for microprolactinomas[5–7]. However, recently more papers have appeared casting a great deal of doubt on the true value of sellar tomography in the management of patients with suspected microprolactinomas.

The *facts suggesting that sellar tomography is of limited value in detecting microprolactinomas* are:

(1) Quite *marked variations in the configuration of the sellar floor are common*[8,9], on plaiñ radiography or tomography; thus there can be a prominent slope to the floor, a fairly marked central depression and even bone thinning is common normally[10]; these changes can be very difficult to distinguish from pathological features.

(2) *Interpretation of these abnormal findings can be extremely difficult*, even by the most experienced radiologist; in one study[11] two neuroradiologists, with much experience in this field, evaluated the tomograms of a group of patients with suspected microprolactinomas independently and on two separate occasions; they found an inter-observer agreement of only 63–75%, and even the intra-observer agreement was quite poor at 76–85%.

(3) *Post-mortem examination of the pituitary gland, by tomography and microscopy*, has revealed a very poor correlation between the two[12,13]; in one study[12] 32 out of 120 pituitaries were found to contain microadenomas. 41% were prolactinomas but tomography suggested this in only six; a false-negative result in 83%. There was also a false-positive figure of 24%.

(4) *Many normal persons harbour microadenomas in their pituitary glands*, as first described by Costello[14] and confirmed in many other studies since, and as mentioned above in which the prevalence was 27%. These persons, if they were to be tomographed, would be expected to show similar sellar-floor abnormalities making the distinction from those with clinically significant tumours even more difficult.

As a result of all this work, there must be a great deal of doubt about the validity of sellar tomography in the detection of microprolactinomas. We have tried tomography in a large number of cases and found it very disappointing indeed. We found very few definite abnormalities and sometimes when one was identified the surgical exploration revealed no tumour. As a result, we abandoned sellar tomography several years ago and now feel fully vindicated.

CT scanning

High-definition CT scanning of the sella is becoming the investigation of choice in the detection of microprolactinomas. The technique requires a very sophisticated scanner of the third or fourth generation so that really fine detail of the sella turcica, its contents and the adjacent structures can be seen. The big difference between this type of CT scanning and sellar tomography is that the gland itself is seen, as well as small tumours within it, in addition to indirect features suggesting a mass lesion. Sellar tomography only shows one indirect sign suggesting an intrasellar lesion, namely the rather dubious bony changes in the sellar floor disscused above, that may be at some distance from the tumour itself.

It is generally agreed that the most valuable plane in which to perform these high-definition scans of the sella is the coronal[15]. The sagittal plane is also of value but axial plane scans on their own are of little value as adjacent bone and CSF produce spurious areas of high and low density in the pituitary gland. Coronal-plane scans show the bony sellar floor, as well as the top of the gland, outlined by CSF.

It is possible to carry out the scans in the axial plane and then produce, from these slices, reformatted images in the coronal or sagittal plane, However, the reformatting process tends to degrade the images and the numerous axial plane slices that may be necessary may pass through the eyes. This gives a large radiation dose to the sensitive lenses. We, however, prefer to scan in the direct coronal plane whenever possible, though it is a little more awkward for the patient as the head has to be tilted back into the head-rest to obtain a suitable position. Also, the scanner gantry has to be angled to avoid teeth fillings which produce marked streak artefacts if included in the scan slice, making the scans of little diagnostic value. Sagittal plane scans can be reformatted from these coronal plane scans, if necessary.

Using our pituitary scan protocol we have recently calculated the absorbed radiation dose to the eyes, skin and gonads during pituitary scanning. These measurements were carried out during both axial plane scanning, with the slices passing through the eyes, and direct coronal plane scanning in which the slices are well away from the eyes. The radiation dose to the eyes during axial plane scanning was 45 mGy (4.5 rads or 4500 mrads) but during coronal plane scanning it was only 0.32 mGy (32 mrads), i.e. the dose was 140 times greater for the axial plane scans than for the coronal ones. The dose to the gonads was less than $10 \mu Gy$; almost unmeasurable.

The scans are obtained with intravenous contrast medium which is infused before and during the scanning procedure. This contrast medium shows the carotid arteries, the arteries in the circle of Willis and the cavernous sinuses due to the circulating opacified blood. It is also taken up by the pituitary gland and the infundibular stalk to a similar degree as the cavernous sinuses. Thus the lateral extent of the gland is difficult to determine, though its top and bottom are well shown. The optic nerves and chiasm do not take up the contrast

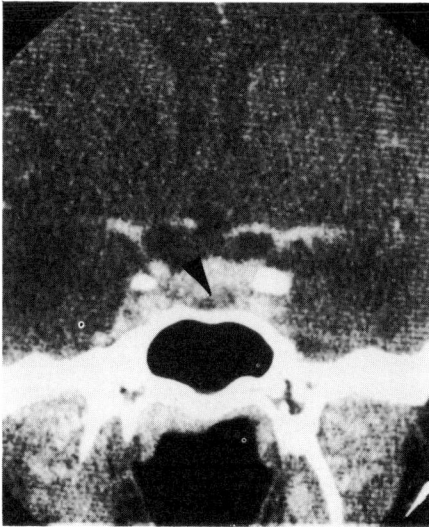

Figure 1 Direct coronal plane high-definition CT scan of the pituitary gland, showing a microadenoma near the sellar floor (arrowhead); this is seen as a low-density area in the enhanced gland

medium and are quite difficult to see in the suprasellar region. However, the cranial nerves III to VI can usually be seen as negative filling defects in the walls of the cavernous sinuses (Figure 1).

The CT features suggesting a microprolactinoma[15,16] are:

(1) *Enlargement of the pituitary gland,* the normal height being up to 7 mm in the female and a little less in the male.
(2) *Upward convexity* to the upper surface of the gland.
(3) An *area of low density,* the microprolactinoma itself, in the enhanced gland; some microprolactinomas may be the same density as the gland, or even denser, but most appear to be of lower density[17]. Sometimes there is more than one tumour.
(4) *Displacement of the infundibular stalk* away from the low-density prolactinoma; normally the stalk is fairly central.
(5) *Sloping sellar floor* under the tumour.
(6) *Erosion of the floor* in the same region; however, these last two features have to be treated with the same caution as the sellar tomography changes described previously.

Probably, when all or most of these features are present, with the appropriate biochemistry, a microprolactinoma can be fairly confidently diagnosed.

There is some recent evidence suggesting caution in the interpretation of microadenomas in the pituitary gland:

(1) *Normal women may show similar changes.* In a recent study[18] 50 normal women volunteers were scanned in the direct coronal manner and 44% showed an upward convexity to the gland; in addition, 36% showed low densities in the gland that could have been interpreted as a microadenoma and the height of the gland was up to 9.7 mm, with a mean value of 7.1 mm.
(2) *Low-density areas in the enhanced pituitary gland* can be produced by lesions other than microadenomas[19], such as pars intermedia cysts (present in 20% of one postmortem series), infarcts, metastases and even a partial empty sella.

In addition the images produced by the scanner may be 'noisy', with alterations in the gland density which, if they are large, may be easily confused with a small adenoma. Hence some caution has to be used in interpreting these high-definition CT scans, especially until more work has been done on the subject. However, at the moment this type of radiological investigation is the best available for detecting microprolactinomas.

References

1. Di Chiro, G. and Nelson, K. B. (1962). The volume of the sella turcica. *Am. J. Radiol.*, **87**, 989
2. Hall, K. and McAllister, V. L. (1980). Metrizamide cisternography in pituitary and juxtapituitary lesions. *Radiology*, **134**, 101
3. Hall, K., McGregor, A. M., Scanlon, M. F. and Hall, R. (1980). Metrizamide cisternography in the assessment of pituitary tumour size, with special reference to the demonstration of tumour (prolactinoma) shrinkage on bromocriptine therapy. In Hubinont, P. O. (ed.). *Progress in Reproductive Biology*. Vol. **6**, pp. 232–43. (Basel: Karger)
4. Teasdale, G. and Macpherson, P. (1982). Use of cavernous sinography to detect aneurysms or anomalies of the infraclinoid carotid artery. *J. Neurosurg.*, **57**, 637
5. Richmond, I. L., Newton, T. H. and Wilson, C. B. (1980). Prolactin-secreting pituitary adenomas: correlation of radiographic and surgical findings. *Am. J. Neuroradiol.*, **1**, 13
6. Raji, M. R., Kishore, P. R. S. and Becker, D. P. (1981). Pituitary microadenomas: a radiological–surgical correlative study. *Radiology*, **139**, 95
7. Vezina, J. L. and Sutton, T. J. (1974). Prolactin-secreting pituitary microadenomas. Roentgenologic diagnosis. *Am. J. Radiol.*, **120**, 46
8. Bruneton, J. N., Drouillard, J. P., Sabatier, J. C., Elie, G. P. and Tavernier, J. F. (1979). Normal variants of the sella turcica. Comparison of plain radiographs and tomograms in 200 cases. *Radiology*, **131**, 99
9. Dubois, P. J., Orr, D. P., Hoy, R. J., Herbert, D. L. and Heinz, E. R. (1979). Normal sellar variations in frontal tomograms. *Radiology*, **131**, 105
10. Rhoton, A. L., Harris, F. S. and Renn, W. H. (1977). Microsurgical anatomy of the sellar region and cavernous sinus. *Clin. Neurosurg.*, **24**, 54
11. McLachlan, M. S. and Banna, M. (1979). Observer variations in interpreting radiographs of the pituitary fossa. *Invest. Radiol.*, **14**, 23
12. Burrow, G. N., Wortzman, G., Rewcastle, N. B., Holgate, R. C. and Kovacs, K. (1981). Microadenomas of the pituitary and abnormal sellar tomograms in an unselected autopsy series. *N. Engl. J. Med.*, **304**, 156
13. Turski, P. A., Newton, T. H. and Horten, B. H. (1981). Sellar contour: anatomic–polytomographic correlation. *Am. J. Radiol.*, **137**, 213
14. Costello, R. T. (1936). Subclinical adenoma of the pituitary gland. *Am. J. Pathol.*, **12**, 205
15. Taylor, S. (1982). High resolution computed tomography of the sella. *Radiol. Clin. N. Am.*, **20**, 207
16. Syvertsen, A., Haughton, V. M., Williams, A. L. and Cusick, J. F. (1979). The computed tomographic appearance of the normal pituitary gland and pituitary microadenomas. *Radiology*, **133**, 385
17. Hemminghytt, S., Kalkhoff, R. K., Daniels, D. L., Williams, A. L., Grogan, J. P. and Haughton, V. M. (1983). Computed tomographic study of hormone-secreting microadenomas. *Radiology*, **146**, 65
18. Swartz, J. D., Russell, K. B., Basile, B. A., O'Donnell, P. C. and Popky, G. L. (1983). High resolution computed tomographic appearance of the intrasellar contents in women of childbearing age. *Radiology*, **147**, 115
19. Chambers, E. F., Yurski, P. A., LaMasters, D. and Newton, T. H. (1982). Regions of low density in the contrast-enhanced pituitary gland: normal and pathologic processes. *Radiology*, **144**, 109

54
The outcome of pituitary exploration in patients with hyperprolactinaemic infertility

G. TEASDALE, A. RICHARDS, R. BULLOCK and
J. THOMSON

INTRODUCTION

The achievement of fertility is a major aim in the treatment of patients with hyperprolactinaemia. When this is considered to be due to a prolactin-producing pituitary adenoma, beneficial effects of treatment may also include removal of the risk that the tumour will enlarge and cause compression on adjacent important structures, either during any subsequent pregnancy or in later life. Of the various methods of treatment that are available, only operation offers the prospect of combining a rapid resolution of hyperprolactinaemia in the short term with the likelihood of long-term avoidance of tumour expansion.

In the last decade, operations on the pituitary gland have become much safer and much more effective. This reflects the swing from performing operations intracranially, gaining access by a standard frontal craniotomy, to approaching the pituitary transsphenoidally and employing the operating microscope. The transsphenoidal route avoids the risks of epilepsy, intracranial haematoma and other neurological complications of intracranial operations and also provides a more direct approach to the face of the gland within the fossa. The operating microscope provides a high illumination and magnification and this has made it possible to identify that in many patients with

509

hypersecretion of pituitary hormones the cause is a small (<1 cm) adenoma contained within an otherwise normal gland. Microsurgical techniques allow the selective removal of the offending lesion, while at the same time preserving normal pituitary tissue. Experience in acromegaly and Cushing's disease has made it clear that the best results are obtained when the tumour is still small – before gross radiological abnormalities appear. The latter herald the enlargement of the tumour to a size such that little normal gland remains – so that a selective operation is more difficult – and also expansion of the tumour into structures outside the pituitary capsule so that the prospects of cure are considerably reduced.

A major problem is the difficulty in the diagnosis of a prolactin-secreting pituitary adenoma while it is small. The problem with the radiological methods is that the first signs are merely minor abnormalities of the fossa on conventional tomograms, or within the tissues of the pituitary gland when studied by modern high-definition CT scanning. Unfortunately, each of these can be seen in between a quarter and a third of otherwise apparently normal young women. Endocrinologically, however, although a very high serum prolactin concentration (>4000 mU l^{-1}) is virtually diagnostic of a tumour, when most patients with a microadenoma first present the level is only moderately raised. By itself this does not discriminate a tumour from various 'functional' types of hyperprolactinaemia.

This chapter reports the results in a series of patients who were considered, on the basis of dynamic endocrine tests, to be likely to have a prolactin-secreting pituitary adenoma and who elected to undergo pituitary operation. Most reports of the surgery of prolactinomas have concentrated on the effect on prolactin secretion, often measured only in the immediate post-operative period. The present series is distinctive because patients who desired to conceive have been followed up for long periods and the outcome assessed in respect of pregnancy rate or by their ovulatory status. We also report the course of the 42 pregnancies achieved after operation.

PATIENTS AND METHODS

The diagnosis of a prolactinoma was based on endocrine criteria: a serum prolactin concentration consistently greater than 360 mU l^{-1} and impaired responses to TRH and metoclopramide, agents that normally produce several-fold increments in serum prolactin concentration[1]. Negative radiological studies[2] did not preclude operation, which was performed by a standard sublabial paraseptal transsphenoidal microsurgical technique. The aim was to identify any tumour, and to remove it; because it is known that adenoma may infiltrate the normal gland, a 1 mm rim of the latter was usually also removed. No patient received radiation therapy before or after operation.

Pituitary function was determined before and after operation according to standard methods and serum prolactin concentrations were determined during and after any pregnancy. Patients with hyperprolactinaemia persisting after operation received bromocriptine treatment, but this was discontinued after conception. In patients who did not conceive, a rise in late cycle of the serum progesterone concentration of more than $20 \, mU \, l^{-1}$ was taken as an index of ovulation.

RESULTS

The patients' serum prolactin concentrations before operation ranged from 560 to $70\,000 \, mU \, l^{-1}$ with a median value of $2280 \, mU \, l^{-1}$. Only 16 patients had a distinct radiological abnormality; in 11 this was a minor definite change in conventional tomography but in five patients CT scanning showed a tumour with a suprasellar extension. At

Table 1 Operative findings and postoperative outcome in 40 patients with hyperprolactinaemia and abnormal responses to TRH and metoclopramide

Adenoma at operation	No. of patients	'Normal' post-operative PRL*	Fertility			
			Operation only		Operation + BCr	
			Pregnancy	Ovulation	Pregnancy	Ovulation
Micro[†]	30	23	18	6	4	2
Macro	7	2	1	–	4	–
None[‡]	3	1	2	–	1	–

*Normal serum prolactin $< 360 \, mU \, l^{-1}$. Data about ovulatory state were missing in two patients.
[†]Microadenoma $< 1 \, cm$.
[‡]Includes one patient with a pituitary granuloma.
BCr = Bromocriptine.

exploration of the pituitary a tumour was found in 37 patients. In seven cases this was a macroadenoma ($> 10 \, mm$). Only one patient developed a potentially serious operative complication; 1 week after operation she developed headache and pyrexia, a lumbar puncture showed a leukocytosis and the presence of *Staphylococcus albus*. This patient recovered fully after antibiotic treatment and has since conceived.

Twenty-six of the 40 women (65%) had a normal basal serum prolactin concentration after operation. The most successfully treated group were patients in whom the tumour was found to be microadenoma, of whom 77% had a normal prolactin level and either conceived or were ovulating after operation (Table 1). After additional bromocriptine treatment all of the remaining patients with a microadenoma became fertile – an overall rate of 100% fertility in this group.

A slightly raised serum prolactin concentration after operation did not preclude fertility. One woman, however, received gonadotrophins before conceiving. Otherwise endocrine deficiency after operation was restricted to two patients both with a large tumour, and persisting diabetes insipidus, and one patient, with impaired reserve before operation, who required cortisone.

Forty-two pregnancies have so far been achieved by 29 women. Of these, only four have miscarried and there were no major congenital malformations:

    (1)   Result of pregnancy:
           term delivery, 34; continuing pregnancy, 3; miscarriage, 4; termination, 1.
    (2)   Complications:
           multiple pregnancies, 3; antepartum haemorrhage, 1; premature labour, 1; congenital malformation, 0; tumour expansion, 0.

The serum prolactin concentration was normal throughout pregnancy on all but three occasions. This was despite no patient having received bromocriptine treatment during pregnancy. No patient had symptoms during pregnancy that could have been related to an increase in the size of the tumour. On the other hand, two patients whose serum prolactin concentration was normal after operation had recurrent hyperprolactinaemia after delivery, but both have conceived again without further treatment. Another patient, whose serum prolactin concentration had been $1793 \, \mathrm{mU \, l^{-1}}$ after operation, had a level of only $280 \, \mathrm{mU \, l^{-1}}$ after delivery.

In none of the patients who failed to conceive was the reason related to a complication of the operation. Six patients had a normal serum prolactin concentration and four of these who had been tested showed biochemical evidence of ovulation. Two patients, each with a large tumour, had persisting hyperprolactinaemia, despite bromocriptine treatment.

DISCUSSION

This review shows that an offer of surgery to a patient with biochemical evidence of a prolactinoma results in the majority becoming fertile and also that any subsequent pregnancy is free of complications. The morbidity of the operation is low and no patient has remained infertile as a direct result of a complication of operation.

The relatively favourable results reflect the large proportion of patients who were found to have small tumours, in whom removal of the adenoma was easy to achieve while preserving normal function. Almost all the patients with persisting hyperprolactinaemia had either very large tumours, or a small tumour that had been situated very laterally and had already eroded through the wall of the pituitary and into the cavernous sinus at the time of operation. The large number of small tumours reflects our policy of operating on patients on purely endocrine criteria, but this had the consequence that in three of the 40 patients a tumour was not found. One of the three did have a pituitary granuloma and her prolactin was reduced to normal.

Reports of surgically treated patients include pregnancy rates of 68% in 19 women[3]; 25% in 12 women[4], and 36% in 64 women[5]. Other reports with shorter follow-up bear out the safety and efficacy of the operation in reducing serum prolactin to normal while preserving function in patients with a small adenoma[5,6]. It is clear, therefore, that operation is a more rapid and reliable method than X-ray treatment in the treatment of hyperprolactinaemia due to a prolactin-producing pituitary adenoma. Because operation was followed by freedom of complications in pregnancy, it removes the need for irradiation to guard against this complication occurring in a pregnancy subsequent to bromocriptine therapy, an approach recommended by some authorities.

Reports of medically treated series are difficult to compare with the present series. One reason is that the precise diagnosis in many patients treated medically is uncertain. This is a reflection of the limitations of endocrinological and radiological tests for distinguishing between a tumour and 'functional' hyperprolactinaemia. Moreover, few reports of drug treatment include in their outcome an analysis of the patients who discontinued treatment because of intolerance and who should also be counted as failures of the method.

An operation to explore a normal sized pituitary fossa for a prolactinoma should not be undertaken lightly and is a technically demanding procedure. Nevertheless, these and other reported results suggest that when performed by an experienced surgeon it offers a reasonable alternative to medical treatment. There is clearly a need for further long-term studies of the results of the two approaches.

Acknowledgements

We thank our many colleagues in the departments of Endocrinology, Obstetrics and Gynaecology, Radiology, and Biochemistry, who have been responsible for the diagnosis and management of the patients included in this report.

References

1. Cowden, E. A., Thomson, J. A., Doyle, D., Ratcliffe, J. G., Macpherson, P. and Teasdale, G. M. (1979). Tests of prolactin secretion in diagnosis of prolactinomas. *Lancet*, **1,** 1155
2. Teasdale, E., Macpherson, P. and Teasdale, G. (1981). The reliability of radiology in detecting prolactin-secreting pituitary microadenomas. *Br. J. Radiol.*, **54,** 566
3. Landolt, A. M. (1981). Treatment of pituitary prolactinomas: post-operative prolactin and fertility in seventy patients. *Fertil. Steril.*, **35,** 620
4. Guibout, M., Jaquet, P., Lissitzky, J. C., Grisoli, F. and Vincentelli, F. (1978). Resultats de l'exérése transsphenoidale des adenomas hypophysaires secretonits. *Ann. Endocrinol. (Paris)*, **39,** 95
5. Randall, R. V., Laws, E. R., Abboud, C. F., Ebersold, M. J., Kao, P. C. and Scheithauer, B. W. (1983). Transsphenoidal microsurgical treatment of prolactin producing pituitary adenomas. *Mayo Clin. Proc.*, **50,** 108
6. Hardy, J. (1981). Le Prolactinome. *Neurochirugie*, **47,** (Suppl.), 1

55
Medical treatment of prolactinomas

S. FRANKS and H. S. JACOBS

The place of dopamine-receptor agonist drugs in the management of hyperprolactinaemic states has now been firmly established and in the last few years these drugs have been used increasingly as primary treatment in patients with small and large prolactinomas. The purpose of this chapter is not to argue the relative merits of medical and surgical treatment of prolactinomas, but to review the effects of dopaminergic drug therapy in patients with prolactinomas with respect to (1) their effectiveness in restoring normal fertility in hyperprolactinaemic women; (2) their effect on tumour volume; and (3) their effect on the natural history of hyperprolactinaemia. We shall refer, briefly, to the use of low-dose, pulsatile therapy with the luteinizing hormone-releasing hormone (LH-RH) as an alternative means of induction of ovulation in hyperprolactinaemic patients in whom dopaminergic drug treatment has been unsuccessful.

EFFECTIVENESS OF BROMOCRIPTINE IN HYPERPROLACTINAEMIC AMENORRHOEA

Treatment with bromocriptine rapidly reduces serum prolactin concentrations to normal or near normal and results in ovulatory menses in most women with hyperprolactinaemic anovulation. In our original series of 40 patients (11 with pituitary tumours) on long-term treatment, 36 menstruated and all of these ovulated[1]. Four out of eight patients who had previously received pituitary ablative therapy did not respond – all were gonadotrophin deficient. Seventeen out

515

of 21 infertile patients who received primary treatment with bromocriptine became pregnant; in three of the remaining four there were defined, non-endocrine factors preventing conception. An updated analysis showed that the cumulative conception rate in treated patients was no different from that in the normal population[2]. Recently Bergh and Nillius[3] have reviewed the results of bromocriptine therapy in 120 women with hyperprolactinaemic amenorrhoea (75% of whom had radiological evidence of a prolactinoma). Ovulatory menses occurred in 94% of pre-menopausal women and the pregnancy rate in 54 infertile women was 91%. Thus, in a total of 160 patients (101 with pituitary tumours) from these two series, the overall ovulation rate was 93% and the pregnancy rate 88%.

Treatment with other long-acting dopamine agonists including lisuride, metergoline and pergolide may in the future produce similar results in terms of ovulation rate. Lisuride and metergoline are effective short-acting drugs[4]; pergolide mesylate is a potent, synthetic ergoline derivative with a prolonged action and can therefore be given in a low, once-daily dose[5]. Ovulation occurred in 11 of 14 patients during long-term treatment with pergolide. Side-effects were similar to those of bromocriptine; some patients who had previously had to stop bromocriptine because of side-effects were able to tolerate pergolide but the reverse was also true. Further clinical trials are in progress.

EFFECTS OF DOPAMINE AGONISTS ON PITUITARY TUMOUR SIZE

One of the most important advances in the management of patients with prolactin-secreting pituitary adenomas is the finding that bromocriptine and other dopamine agonists not only lower prolactin levels but may also cause regression of the tumour (see references 3 and 6 for extensive reviews). This has prompted an increasing number of clinicians to consider bromocriptine as primary therapy in patients with pituitary macroadenomas. A number of case reports, dating from that by Corenblaum et al.[7], showed that bromocriptine treatment was associated with an improvement in the visual-field defects. These reports were followed by studies using radiological criteria to monitor tumour size during treatment and confirmed that there was indeed shrinkage of the prolactinoma. Bergh and Nillius[3] have recently collected data from ten series in which a total of 49 cases have been treated with bromocriptine or lisuride. In 44 (90%) there was evidence of tumour regression during treatment and in many cases the response was very rapid. The reduction in tumour volume seems to be due to a decrease in cell size (the major change being in the cytoplasm) rather than in cell number[8]. Dr A. G. Frantz presented data at the American Endocrine Society in San Francisco (1982) showing that of 105 patients treated in eight series the overall rate of tumour shrinkage was 73%. In the non-responders, tumour growth was noted in five patients in whom there was no significant fall in prolactin and in two of these the tumour increased in size despite a fall in prolactin concentrations. Those patients whose tumours did not shrink on treatment with bromocriptine may in fact have had secondary hyperprolactinaemia associated with a large non-functioning tumour rather than a true prolactinoma. There is no general agreement about the dose of bromocriptine that should be used to shrink tumours but in our experience a dose that is sufficient to keep prolactin levels within the normal range (often as little as 5 mg daily) is also effective in reducing tumour volume.

FOLLOW-UP OF PATIENTS ON LONG-TERM DOPAMINE AGONIST THERAPY

Limited data are now available concerning the effects of bromocriptine and other dopamine agonists on the natural history of hyperprolactinaemia in patients with and without pituitary tumours. Bergh and Nillius[3] stopped treatment with bromocriptine in 49 patients (37 with pituitary tumours) who had received treatment for at least 12 months. Within 2 months of stopping the drug, prolactin concentrations had returned to pre-treatment levels in 42 (86%) patients. This is consistent with the report from Thorner et al.[9] on two patients in whom rapid return of prolactin levels to pre-treatment concentrations was associated with re-expansion of the tumour. However, the tumour may not necessarily re-grow after bromocriptine treatment is stopped. In one patient in our series bromocriptine was stopped after 6 months of treatment during which there had been significant reduction in the tumour volume. Six months later there has been no radiological recurrence on high-resolution CT scanning in this patient despite the fact that the prolactin concentrations have risen to pre-treatment levels. Five out of 7 patients who had lower post-treatment values were studied by Bergh and Nillius for 1–2 years after therapy was stopped, and in all five prolactin concentrations steadily rose towards pre-treatment levels. Bergh and Nillius noted that most of the patients with prolonged suppression of prolactin following treatment were those with large tumours. Ferrari[4] in a study of 69 patients (most with either microadenomas or idiopathic hyperprolactinaemia) found that although prolactin levels were significantly lower than pre-treatment values after bromocriptine treatment had been stopped, only five resumed ovulatory menses – i.e. a similar remission rate to that observed in an untreated series of hyperprolactinaemic women[10]. This is in contrast to the results following pregnancy in bromocriptine-treated women (*see* below).

LONG-TERM FOLLOW-UP OF BROMOCRIPTINE-INDUCED PREGNANCIES

A number of groups have shown that prolactin concentrations following bromocriptine-induced pregnancies may be lower than the pre-treatment levels[3,11-13]. Bergh and Nillius reported persistent reduction in prolactin concentrations in 19 out of 28 women (a mixture of tumour and non-tumour patients), and three of these patients resumed spontaneous ovulatory menstruation.

We have recently reviewed our own series of 27 patients with normal pituitary X-rays who had previously been treated with bromocriptine and in whom treatment was discontinued. Sixty per cent of women with amenorrhoea and normal pituitary X-rays whose prolactin concentrations were less than $2000\,mU\,l^{-1}$ were cured, in the sense that basal prolactin levels were normal and ovulatory cycles resumed after stopping bromocriptine[12]. When these patients were tested with TRH before treatment with bromocriptine the response of prolactin was impaired, i.e. showing a similar abnormality in regulation of prolactin secretion as in other hyperprolactinaemic patients (Figure 1). Thus although most patients with hyperprolactinaemia will require further treatment with bromocriptine, a significant proportion of those with normal pituitary X-rays appear to be cured following pregnancy. This may represent persistent shrinkage of a small prolactinoma or perhaps resolution of true 'functional' hyperprolactinaemia.

INDUCTION OF OVULATION WITH LOW-DOSE
PULSATILE LH-RH IN HYPERPROLACTINAEMIC WOMEN

A number of studies have shown that the mechanism of the reproductive disorder in hyperprolactinaemia is related to an abnormality in the hypothalamic regulation of gonadotrophin secretion[14-16] which manifests itself as a grossly abnormal pattern of pulsatile LH secretion[17,18]. The importance of the hypothalamic abnormality is illustrated by the fact that ovulation can be induced in women with

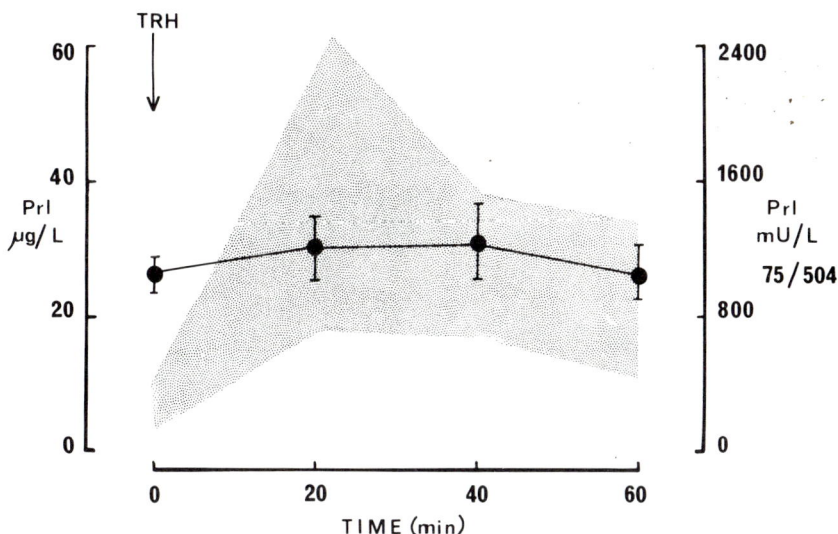

Figure 1 The prolactin response to 200 μg of TRH prior to therapy in those patients who subsequently underwent cure. The shaded area indicates the range of responses in normal women

persistent hyperprolactinaemia by low-dose pulsatile LH-RH[19]. This is also of practical importance since this form of treatment may be used to induce ovulation in women in whom dopamine agonists have failed either because of unacceptable side-effects or (as in a very few patients) because the hyperprolactinaemia appears 'resistant' to bromocriptine.

References

1. Franks, S., Jacobs, H. S., Hull, M. G. R., Steele, S. J. and Nabarro, J. D. N. (1977). Management of hyperprolactinaemic amenorrhoea. *Br. J. Obstet. Gynaecol.*, **84**, 241

2. Hull, M. G. R., Savage, P. A. and Jacobs, H. S. (1979). Investigations and treatment of amenorrhoea resulting in normal fertility. *Br. Med. J.*, **1**, 1257

3. Bergh, T. and Nillius, S. J. (1982). Prolactinomas: follow up of medical treatment. In Molinatti, G. M. (ed.) *A Clinical Problem: Microprolactinoma*. pp. 115–30. (Oxford: Excerpta Medica)

4. Ferrari, C., Mattei, A., Rampini, P., *et al.* (1982). Long-term effects of drug treatment on hyperprolactinaemic disorders: a study after discontinuation of bromocriptine and metergoline. In Molinatti, G. M. (ed.) *A Clinical Problem: Microprolactinoma*. pp. 141–48. (Oxford: Excerpta Medica)

5. Franks, S., Horrocks, P. M., Lynch, S. S., Butt, W. R. and London, D. R. (1983). Effectiveness of pergolide mesylate in long term treatment of hyperprolactinaemia. *Br. Med. J.*, **286**, 1177

6. Nillius, S. J. (1980). Medical therapy of prolactin secreting pituitary tumours. *Progr. Reprod. Biol.*, **6**, 194

7. Corenblum, B., Webster, B. R., Mortimer, C. B. and Ezrin, C. (1975). Possible antitumour effect of 2-bromoergocryptine (CB-154 Sandoz) in two patients with large prolactin-secreting pituitary adenomas. *Clin. Res.*, **23**, 614A

8. Tindall, G. T., Kovacs, K., Horvath, E. and Thorner, M. O. (1982). Human prolactin producing adenomas and bromocriptine: a histological immunocytochemical, ultrastructural and morphometric study. *J. Clin. Endocrinol. Metab.*, **55**, 1178

9. Thorner, M. O., Perryman, R., Rogol, A. D., *et al.* (1981). Rapid changes in prolactinoma volume after withdrawal and reinstitution of bromocriptine. *J. Clin. Endocrinol. Metab.*, **53**, 480

10. March, C. M., Kletzky, O. A., Davajan, V., *et al.*, (1981). Longitudinal evaluation of patients with untreated prolactin-secreting adenomas. *Am. J. Obstet. Gynecol.*, **139**, 835

11. Rjosk, H. K., Fahlbusch, R., Huber, H. and Von Werder, K. (1980). Growth of prolactinomas during pregnancy. In Faglia, G., Giovanelli, M. A. and Macleod, R. M. (eds.) *Pituitary Microadenomas*. pp. 535–41. (London: Academic Press)

12. Jacobs, H. S. (1981). Abnormal prolactin secretion in men and women. In Crosignani, P. G. and Rubin, B. L. (eds.) *Endocrinology of Human Infertility: New Aspects*. pp. 129–38. (London: Academic Press)

13. Randall, S., Lang, I., Chapman, A. J., *et al.* (1982). Pregnancies in women with hyperprolactinaemia: obstetric and endocrinological management of 50 pregnancies in 37 women. *Br. J. Obstet. Gynaecol.*, **89**, 20

14. Glass, M. R., Shaw, R. W., Butt, W. R., Logan Edwards, R. and London, D. R. (1975). An abnormality of oestrogen feedback in amenorrhoea–galactorrhoea. *Br. Med. J.*, **3**, 274

15. Jacobs, H. S., Franks, S., Murray, M. A. F., Hull, M. G. R., Steele, S. J. and Nabarro, J. D. N. (1976). Clinical and endocrine features of hyperprolactinaemic amenorrhoea. *Clin. Endocrinol.*, **5**, 439

16. Aono, T., Miyake, A., Schioji, T., Kinugasa, T., Onishi, T. and Kurachi, K. (1976). Impaired LH release following exogenous estrogen administration in patients with amenorrhoea galactorrhoea syndrome. *J. Clin. Endocrinol. Metab.*, **42**, 696

17. Bohnet, H. G., Dahlen, H. G., Wuttke, W. and Schneider, H. P. G. (1976). Hyperprolactineamic anovulatory syndrome. *J. Clin. Endocrinol. Metab.*, 132

18. Moult, P. J. A., Rees, L. H. and Besser, G. M. (1982). Pulsatile gonadatrophin secretion in hyperprolactinaemic amenorrhea and the response to bromocriptine therapy. *Clin. Endocrinol.*, **16**, 153

19. Leyendecker, G., Struve, T. and Plotz, E. J. (1980). Induction of ovulation with chronic intermittent (pulsatile) administration of LHRH in women with hypothalamic and hyperprolactinaemic amenorrhoea. *Arch. Gynaecol.*, **229**, 172

56
Surveillance of Parlodel (bromocriptine) in pregnancy and offspring

P. KRUPP and I. TURKALJ

Hyperprolactinaemic conditions often lead to infertility, particularly in female patients. Before the therapeutic potential of Parlodel (bromocriptine) was investigated in women suffering from such endocrinological disorders, the drug was carefully studied in animals. The results of the comprehensive toxicological studies, which were performed in various animal species including the stump-tailed monkey, indicate that Parlodel is neither mutagenic, embryotoxic or teratogenic[1]. This information is important in so far as women with infertility secondary to hyperprolactinaemia may become pregnant when treated with Parlodel[2,3] and medication is likely to continue after conception, if only until the patient becomes aware that she is pregnant or the diagnosis is confirmed. It was, therefore, essential to ascertain in humans whether this drug does not affect the course and the outcome of pregnancy or the postnatal development of the offspring when continued after conception. To investigate this problem, a stepwise procedure consisting of three surveys was set up. The first two surveys were aimed at gathering information on the progress and outcome of pregnancies in women treated with Parlodel during gestation. The data collection of the first study was based on spontaneous reporting. The results of this survey have already been published[4]. The second survey consisted of an intensive monitoring project; with this approach it was possible to obtain information from the participating clinics about all pregnant women being treated with Parlodel. The third step was a follow-up survey of the postnatal development of infants exposed to Parlodel *in utero*. This investigation was performed because bromocriptine, the active ingredient of Parlodel, crosses the placental barrier.

SPONTANEOUS REPORTING

Clinicians known to treat women suffering from hyperprolactinaemic conditions with Parlodel were invited to cooperate in a pregnancy survey. Special report forms were provided for obtaining the relevant information about the indication and dosage of bromocriptine, on the course, duration and outcome of pregnancy as well as on the status of the newborn babies, including sex, weight and length. At first, most reports came from clinicians who had been involved in the clinical evaluation of Parlodel before the product was marketed; the standard of record keeping was high, as virtually every patient could be followed up on an individual basis. Later, when the survey was extended and physicians of more than 30 countries participated, individual monitoring was no longer possible. Consequently, in some cases the reports were incomplete. For obvious reasons a control group could not be included.

Information was obtained on 1410 pregnancies in 1335 patients treated with Parlodel after conception, from 1973 to 1980. In 82% of the cases, Parlodel was given for the treatment of amenorrhoea or luteal insufficiency, while in 18% pituitary tumours, including acromegaly, were reported as the primary diagnosis.

The median age of the patients was 29 years, the oldest being 42 years. The daily dose of Parlodel ranged from 1.25 to 40 mg, the median daily dose being 5 mg. The median duration of Parlodel medication after conception amounted to 21 days. However, in a few patients the drug was already discontinued 1 day after conception. Nine patients were treated throughout the period of gestation. The course of pregnancy was uneventful in these patients; all were delivered healthy babies with no abnormalities.

Spontaneous abortion occurred in 11.2% of the pregnancies; this figure includes nine missed abortions. This percentage compares favourably with those of 10–15% quoted in the literature for a normal population[5]. There was no evidence that the occurrence of spontane-

522

ous abortion was influenced by the Parlodel dosage, the duration of treatment after conception or withdrawal of the drug. Moreover, no consistency could be found with respect to the interval between discontinuation of Parlodel and the occurrence of abortion such as might be expected if cessation of therapy was associated with hormonal changes, leading to abortion.

Of the 1410 pregnancies 86% resulted in births, 97.8% were single births. Twenty-four patients delivered twins and two patients triplets. Two mothers with twins and one mother with triplets were receiving concomitant treatment with clomiphene or gonadotrophin. If these multiplets are disregarded, the corrected incidence of twin births (1.8%) is somewhat but not significantly increased when compared with a normal population[6]. Likewise, in two other surveys of babies born to Parlodel-treated mothers, multiplets were observed only when clomiphene or gonadotrophins had also been prescribed concurrently[7,8]. The mean birth weights of both, single births and twins, were comparable with those in a normal population.

Minor congenital malformations or abnormalities were noted in 2.5% of the babies. Most often they consisted of congenital dislocation of the hip or talipes. In addition to certain organ deficiencies such as hydrocephalus, pulmonary atresia or renal agenesis, the major malformations, observed in 1% of the babies, included two cases of Down's syndrome. However, in a special study performed in babies born to Parlodel-treated mothers, no drug-induced chromosomal defects could be found[9]. Moreover, exploratory data analysis revealed no difference with respect to the daily dose, the duration of treatment after conception, or the total intake of Parlodel between mothers who gave birth to normal children and those who had children with malformations.

INTENSIVE MONITORING

The second survey of Parlodel in pregnancy, which was started in 1979, is still ongoing and is scheduled to last until the end of September 1983. This intensive monitoring project is being conducted in 35 clinics in 12 different countries. In these clinics each patient receiving Parlodel after conception was registered and followed up until delivery. Therefore, under-reporting and other drawbacks of the first survey, based on spontaneous reporting, could be prevented. Again, special patient sheets were designed for data collection. The survey included a comparative group consisting of babies with malformations, who were born at the participating clinics to mothers not treated with Parlodel during the monitoring period. However, at some of the clinics in one country the information on the babies, serving as controls, could be obtained only via the national malformation register and not with the special design forms. During the progress of the study it also became evident that at some clinics, the control babies were not examined by the same physician and not as carefully as the babies exposed to Parlodel *in utero*. Therefore, only a limited comparison between the two groups is possible, and in particular, with respect to minor malformations and abnormalities.

The available information on 563 pregnancies in Parlodel-treated mothers confirmed the results obtained in the first survey: the main indication for Parlodel medication was amenorrhoea; only about 19% of the patients received the drug for a pituitary tumour or for acromegaly. The median age of the mothers was 28 years, the daily dose of Parlodel 5 mg and the median duration of medication after conception 24 days. However, the incidence of spontaneous abortion and the corrected incidence of twin births were 8.8% and 1.4% respectively, somewhat lower than in the first survey. No triplets were reported. Likewise, the malformation rate, calculated for the babies born to Parlodel-treated mothers, was also lower in this intensive monitoring study. The incidence for major malformations was 1.7% and that for minor malformations 0.8%. No clustering of a special type of birth defect could be recognized. With the exception of three babies with talipes and two babies with ventricular septal defects – malformations relatively often seen in the normal population – the other types of birth defects noted in the exposed babies were observed just once each, and no organ system was preferentially affected.

POSTNATAL DEVELOPMENT

In the third survey, which consisted of a follow-up investigation, children exposed to Parlodel *in utero* were examined by paediatricians according to a defined questionnaire. The main difficulty encountered was the enrolment of these children, as many lived far away from the clinics where their mothers had been treated; others had moved with their families and they could no longer be traced.

Up to now information on 212 Caucasian children is available.

Their age at examination ranged from 5 to 63 months. Most had been exposed to Parlodel *in utero* during the first 4 weeks after conception. One child was exposed throughout gestation. In 82% of this cohort weight and height were within the normal range; 12 and 10%, respectively, exceeded the 95th percentile. The clinical findings noted in some of these children were scattered throughout all organ systems; they included abnormalities already present at birth, functional disorders such as constipation, conditions such as atopic dermatitis or viral infections such as varicella. Findings of these types are frequently observed in children of this age. No specific pattern of abnormal postnatal development could be recognized. These results have recently been confirmed with a follow-up study on 134 Japanese infants born to Parlodel-treated mothers[8].

DISCUSSION AND CONCLUSION

The results obtained in the first two surveys are similar and indicate that there is no special risk for the fetus inherent in Parlodel therapy during pregnancy, as the rates of spontaneous abortion, multiple pregnancy and, in particular, of malformations were not increased in patients treated with this drug during gestation.

According to a recent comprehensive review of the literature, the congenital malformation rates published ranged from 1 to 9%[10]. The rates of 3.5 and 2.5% observed in this surveillance lie well within these limits. Moreover, the classification of malformations encountered, according to the organ systems affected, shows a distribution similar to that described by Heinonen *et al.*[11]. The data gleaned from the intensive monitoring study is probably more realistic, as in this survey every patient treated with Parlodel after conception was recorded. The information based on spontaneous reporting – the method used in the first survey – tended to overestimate negative effects.

The results obtained in the follow-up study indicate that exposure to Parlodel *in utero* does not influence postnatal development.

Summing up, no adverse effect of Parlodel medication during pregnancy could be recognized by this comprehensive surveillance which was conducted over a decade. However, as Parlodel diminishes prolactin secretion in the fetus and as the occurrence of spontaneous abortion is not enhanced by interruption of treatment, it is recommended that Parlodel be stopped as soon as pregnancy is confirmed unless there is a definite indication for it to be continued.

References

1. Richardson, B. P., Turkalj, I. and Flückiger, E. (1983). Bromocriptine. In Lawrence, D. R. (ed.) *Safety and Testing of New Drugs, Prediction and Performance*. (In press)
2. Thorner, M. O., Besser, G. M. and Jones, A. (1975). Bromocriptine treatment of female infertility: Report of 13 pregnancies. *Br. Med. J.*, **iv**, 964
3. Franks, S., Jacobs, H. S. and Hull, M. G. (1977). Management of hyperprolactin-aemic amenorrhoea. *Br. J. Obstet. Gynaecol.*, **84**, 241
4. Turkalj, I., Braun, P. and Krupp, P. (1982). Surveillance of bromocriptine in pregnancy. *J. Am. Med. Assoc.*, **247**, 1589
5. Helbing, W. (1966). Pathologie der Frühschwangerschaft. In Döderlein, G. and Wulf, K.-H. (eds.) *Klinik der Frauenheilkunde und Geburtshilfe*. Vol. 5, p. 22. (Munich: Urban and Schwarzenberg)
6. Deutsche Forschungsgemeinschaft (German Research Council) (1977). *Schwanger-schaftsverlauf und Kindsentwicklung*. p. 86. (Boppard, W. Germany: Harald Boldt.)
7. Thorner, M. O., Edwards, C. R. W., Charlesworth, M., Dacie, J. E., Moult, P. J. A., Rees, L. H., Jones, A. E. and Besser, G. M. (1979). Pregnancy in patients presenting with hyperprolactinaemia. *Br. Med. J.*, **2**, 771
8. Kurachi, K. (1983). A follow-up of infants born to mothers treated with bromocrip-tine: Results obtained by the Japanese Study Group on Hyperprolactinaemia. (In press)
9. Schellekens, L. A., Snuiverink, H. and van den Berghe, H. (1977). Chromosomal pattern of children born after induction of ovulation with bromocriptine. *Drug Res.*, **27**, 2151
10. Hauser, G. A. (1980). Bromocriptine in pregnancy: No teratogenic risk. *Med. Trib.*, **15**, 45
11. Heinonen, O. P., Slone, D. and Shapiro, S. (1977). *Birth Defects and Drugs in Pregnancy*. (Littleton, Ill.: Publishing Sciences Group)

57
Prolactinomas in pregnancy

T. BERGH AND S. J. NILLIUS

It is well known that women with pituitary tumours may develop symptoms from tumour enlargement during pregnancy[1]. To decrease the risk of pregnancy-induced tumour growth some authorities recommend that women with prolactinomas should have their tumour treated by irradiation or surgery before pregnancy. However, the effect of X-ray therapy on prolactinomas is slow and often ineffective[2]. Furthermore, irradiation does not completely prevent the risk of tumour growth during pregnancy[1]. Pituitary microsurgery has to be performed by very experienced neurosurgeons; and in inexpert hands it can have disastrous results[2]. Because of the poor outcome of pituitary microsurgery in women with prolactinomas, Nabarro[2] in a recent review concluded that bromocriptine should be used as much as possible. The risk for serious irreversible complications due to growth of prolactinomas during pregnancy induced by bromocriptine has been exaggerated[1]. Today primary medical therapy with dopamine agonists is given to most infertile women with prolactin-secreting pituitary adenomas.

PRIMARY BROMOCRIPTINE TREATMENT OF INFERTILE WOMEN WITH PROLACTINOMAS

The risk that women with prolactinomas develop symptoms from tumour enlargement during pregnancy has previously been estimated to vary between 5 and 25%[1]. In nine recent studies 268 hyperprolactinaemic women with untreated prolactinomas experienced a

Table 1 Number of pregnancies and tumour complication in nine series of hyperprolactinaemic infertile women given primary dopamine agonist therapy. Patients who have had tumour therapy with surgery or irradiation are not included

			Prolactinoma complications during pregnancy			
Reference	No. of patients	No. of pregnancies	Visual impairment	Radiologic progression	Total no. of patients	Comments
3,4	30	33	1	4	5	14 patients with macroadenomas
5	38	38	1	4	4	
6	25	25	0	0	0	Macroadenomas not treated
7	15	17	0	1	1	
8	61	79	1	0	1	
9	30	40	0	1	1	
10	48	47	0	0	0	Macroadenomas not treated
11	19	19	1	7	7	
Total	268	300	4	17	19	

total of 300 term pregnancies after treatment with dopamine agonists, mostly bromocriptine (Table 1). In only four of these pregnancies were there severe complications that had to be treated. All four patients were successfully treated by bromocriptine or surgery during the pregnancy. No evidence of tumour growth was found during pregnancy or at the postpartum evaluation in 281 of the 300 pregnancies (94%).

We have given primary bromocriptine therapy to 68 infertile women with hyperprolactinaemia. Forty-eight had an asymmetric pituitary fossa. The sellar asymmetry was pronounced in 24 of the women (asymmetry > 3 mm). None of the patients had received prior tumour therapy with irradiation or surgery. Empty sella or suprasellar extension of the pituitary tumour was excluded by computerized tomography (CAT scan). The mean prolactin level before treatment was $65 \mu g \, l^{-1}$ (range 24–$144 \mu g \, l^{-1}$) in the women with a normal sella and $101 \mu g \, l^{-1}$ (range 30–$1470 \mu g \, l^{-1}$) in the women with radiological changes of the pituitary fossa. The bromocriptine treatment resulted in 90 pregnancies in the 68 women (69 term pregnancies, 11 induced and 10 spontaneous abortions).

Evidence of tumour growth during pregnancy was found in five women. One woman developed visual field defects in the last trimester of the pregnancy. Reinstitution of bromocriptine restored normal vision and the pregnancy could continue to term. Postpartum sellar X-ray showed destruction of the sella[12]. In four other women the sellar X-ray had changed during the pregnancy. One of the women complained of headache from the second trimester but had normal visual fields. The other three women had clinically uneventful pregnancies. The subtle radiographic changes in these four women were probably caused by tumour growth during pregnancy. However, it is not known whether similar changes may occur during pregnancy in healthy women. In three of the four women, radiological regression occurred within 2 years after the delivery[3]. One of the patients in our series had radiological signs of tumour enlargement despite a normal sellar X-ray before pregnancy. There are other case reports in the literature indicating that patients with normal sellar X-rays might develop severe tumour complications during pregnancy[1]. Such a patient was recently referred to us. Before pregnancy her sellar X-ray was judged to be normal. In the last trimester of pregnancy she developed visual field defects and decreased visual acuity. Vision rapidly returned to normal when bromocriptine was reinstituted during the pregnancy. The tumour regression was verified by CAT scan[13]. Thus, a normal pituitary fossa X-ray does not exclude the risk of pregnancy-induced pituitary tumour growth. A pretreatment CAT scan should be performed in all infertile women with hyperprolactinaemia.

MANAGEMENT OF WOMEN WITH PROLACTINOMAS DURING PREGNANCY

The infertile woman with hyperprolactinaemia should be fully informed about the possibility of tumour enlargement during pregnancy. If she develops symptoms that may be associated with tumour growth, she should be referred to a specialist familiar with the rare complications. During pregnancy, the patient should be followed up with monthly visual field examinations for earliest possible detection of visual impairment.

If symptoms of rapid tumour enlargement occur during pregnancy they can be treated with favourable outcome for mother and child. The two patients we have seen with visual field defects during pregnancy have both rapidly responded to bromocriptine with normalization of vision. In the literature there are other case reports in which prolactinoma complications during pregnancy have been successfully treated with bromocriptine[14]. Reinstitution of bromocriptine should therefore be the treatment of choice, if symptoms of tumour expansion occur. Should this therapy fail other treatment alternatives are available[1].

It has been suggested that bromocriptine treatment should be maintained throughout pregnancy to prevent tumour enlargement. Bromocriptine has not been shown to have any adverse effects on the pregnancy or the fetus[15]. However, the incidence of serious tumour complications during pregnancy is very low. We therefore do not think that it is justified to give prophylactic medical treatment with bromocriptine to all pregnant women with hyperprolactinaemia.

POSTPARTUM MANAGEMENT OF PATIENTS WITH PROLACTINOMAS

Some authors have discouraged patients with prolactinomas from breast feeding in order to decrease the stimulatory effect on the pituitary lactotrophs[11]. All our patients with prolactinoma have breast fed without any untoward effects being observed. One of the patients with visual field defects during pregnancy could breast feed normally when bromocriptine therapy was discontinued 2 days postpartum[13]. In this patient further tumour regression could be verified radiologically during the period of lactation. In our opinion there is therefore no reason to withhold hyperprolactinaemic women from the advantages of breast feeding.

After pregnancy and lactation many hyperprolactinaemic patients have decreased serum prolactin levels in comparison with the pretreatment values. In some women spontaneous ovulatory menstruations have even returned[7,14]. In our present series 31 of the women with sellar asymmetries have had their prolactin levels measured after the bromocriptine-induced pregnancies. In these women the mean prolactin level decreased from 110 to $76 \mu g l^{-1}$ (p < 0.05). Only three of the women had a higher prolactin level after pregnancy than before. Thus it is very uncommon for pregnancy to make the hyperprolactinaemic condition worse.

CONCLUDING REMARKS

The incidence of complications caused by growth of prolactinomas during pregnancy is low. The risk that pregnancy-induced tumour expansion leads to severe and permanent sequelae is very small in carefully supervised patients. In infertile hyperprolactinaemic patients without evidence of extrasellar growth of a prolactinoma, primary medical therapy with dopamine agonists is the treatment of choice.

References

1. Nillius, S. J., Bergh, T. and Larsson, S.-G. (1980). Pituitary tumours and pregnancy. In Derome, P. J., Jedynak, C. P. and Peillon, F. (eds.) *Pituitary Adenomas. Biology, Physiopathology and Treatment*, pp. 103–11. (France: Asclepios Publishers)
2. Nabarro, J. D. N. (1982). Pituitary prolactinomas. *Clin. Endocrinol.*, **17**, 129
3. Bergh, T., Nillius, S. J., Larsson, S.-G. and Wide, L. (1981). Effects of bromocriptine-induced pregnancy on prolactin-secreting pituitary tumours. *Acta Endocrinol.*, **98**, 333
4. Bergh, T., Nillius, S. J., Enoksson, P., Larsson, S.-G. and Wide, L. (1982). Bromocriptine-induced pregnancies in women with large prolactinomas. *Clin. Endocrinol.*, **17**, 625
5. Crosignani, P. G., Ferrari, C., Scarduelli, C., Picciotti, M. C., Caldara, R. and Malinverni, A. (1981). Spontaneous and induced pregnancies in hyperprolactinemic women. *Obstet. Gynecol.*, **58**, 708
6. Jewelewicz, R. and Van de Wiele, R. L. (1980). Clinical course and outcome of pregnancy in twenty-five patients with pituitary microadenomas. *Am. J. Obstet. Gynecol.*, **136**, 339
7. Nyboe Andersen, A., Starup, J., Tabor, A., Kålund Jensen, H. and Westergaard, J. G. (1983). The possible prognostic value of serum prolactin increment during pregnancy in hyperprolactinaemic patients. *Acta Endocrinol.*, **102**, 1
8. Pepperell, R. J. (1981). Prolactin and reproduction. *Fertil. Steril.*, **35**, 267
9. Randall, S., Laing, I., Chapman, A. J., Shalet, S. M., Beardwell, C. G., Kelly, W. F. and Davies, D. (1982). Pregnancies in women with hyperprolactinaemia: obstetric and endocrinological management of 50 pregnancies in 37 women. *Br. J. Obstet. Gynaecol.*, **89**, 20
10. Rjosk, H.-K., Fahlbusch, R. and von Werder, K. (1982). Influence of pregnancies on prolactinomas. *Acta Endocrinol.*, **100**, 337
11. Shewchuck, A. B., Adamson, G. D., Lessard, P. and Ezrin, C. (1980). The effect of pregnancy on suspected pituitary adenomas after conservative management of ovulation defects associated with galactorrhea. *Am. J. Obstet. Gynecol.*, **136**, 659
12. Bergh, T., Nillius, S. J. and Wide, L. (1978). Clinical course and outcome of pregnancies in amenorrhoeic women with hyperprolactinaemia and pituitary tumours. *Br. Med. J.*, **i**, 875
13. Bergh, T., Nillius, S. J., Enoksson, P. E. and Wide, L. (1983). Bromocriptine regression of suprasellar extension of a prolactinoma during pregnancy. (Submitted for publication)
14. Bergh, T. and Nillius, S. J. (1982). Prolactinomas – follow-up of medical treatment. In Molinatti, G. M. (ed.) *A Clinical Problem: Microprolactinoma. Diagnosis and Treatment.* pp. 115–30. (Amsterdam: Excerpta Medica)
15. Turkalj, I., Braun, P. and Krupp, P. (1982). Surveillance of bromocriptine in pregnancy. *J. Am. Med. Assoc.*, **247**, 1589

Part III

Section 2

Advances in Fertility Control and the Treatment of Sterility*

* This special symposium was sponsored by Schering AG

58
Pre-treatment evaluation of ovarian infertility

G. BETTENDORF

ABSTRACT

Pretreatment evaluation of a disease means to evaluate a diagnosis in the individual patient according to which a proper selection of the type of treatment is indicated.

In respect to ovarian dysfunction as a cause for infertility, the endocrine status has to be evaluated. Patients can be divided into oestrogen positive and oestrogen negative. In the last mentioned group further sub-grouping has to be done according to the FSH and LH concentration. For both oestrogen positive and oestrogen negative patients the prolactin and the androgen status as well as the thyroid function has to be tested.

Having the information on the oestrogen, the gonadotrophin, the prolactin, the androgen and the thyroid status of the individual patient the basis for the selection of the type of stimulation therapy can be given.

Infertility is a diagnosis applied to a couple. Clinical examination with endocrinological tests in both partners will enable the physician to evaluate defects in the reproductive functions: ovarian dysfunction associated with amenorrhoea, oligomenorrhoea, polymenorrhoea or anovulatory cycles and luteal insufficiency.

535

There is a continuous transition between normal ovulatory cycles, luteal insufficiency and anovulatory cycles to amenorrhoea. There is insufficient follicular maturation followed by ovulation and defective luteal function or no ovulation and luteinization. The *corpus luteum insufficiency* is a distinct and common form of infertility. Irregular patterns of the menstrual cycle are common.

Anovulatory cycles mostly are combined with irregular cycles, there is follicle growth and steroid production but no ovulation and no luteal function. In many women a gamut of different functional patterns may be observed in consecutive cycles. Cycles with obvious luteal insufficiency may be interspersed between perfectly normal ovulatory ones which, in turn, may be replaced by anovulatory cycles.

In amenorrhoea there is no follicle growth and no oestrogen production which leads to endometrium proliferation and bleeding. The causes of these different symptoms of ovarian dysfunction are as follows:

(1) Insufficient stimulation.
(2) Primary ovarian dysfunction.
(3) Elevated androgens (ovary or adrenal).
(4) Elevated prolactin.
(5) Thyroid dysfunction
(6) Diabetes.
(7) Nutritional (starvation or obesity).
(8) Drug induced.
(9) Psychogenic.

For the examination of the functional state the activity of ovarian hormones (oestrogen) and of those hormones that influence ovarian activity (gonadotrophins, prolactin, androgens, corticoid and thyroid hormones) have to be tested, either by clinical methods or by assays.

The oestrogen activity is a measure of ovarian activity which is dependent on hypothalamo-pituitary stimulation. By simple clinical methods the oestrogen situation can be tested. In patients with spontaneous bleedings there must be an oestrogen activity; the same applies in those who respond with a bleeding following progestin medication. The cervical gland is a very sensitive target and reacts with mucus production under the influence of oestrogens; the vaginal epithelium shows maturation. All these parameters can be checked very easily and give good information on the oestrogen activity. Only in special situations (e.g. during HMG therapy) do analytical procedures have to be taken for exact measurement of oestrogen concentration, either by chemical procedures or by immunoassays:

(1) Clinical tests:
    (a) Endometrium – (i) spontaneous bleeding; (ii) progesterone-induced bleeding (progestin test).
    (b) Cervix – (i) spontaneous secretion; (ii) oestrogen-induced secretion.
    (c) Vaginal cytology.
(2) Analytical tests: serum oestradiol levels and total urinary oestrogens.

Androgens are produced in the ovary and in the adrenal gland. Hyperandrogenism clinically is diagnosed by symptoms such as acne, hirsutism and virilization. The blood concentration of testosterone, androstenedione and dehydroepiandrosterone can be measured. A normal adrenal and thyroid function is essential for a physiological ovarian activity; in functional disturbances therefore the adrenal and thyroid hormones have to be tested:

(1) Clinical tests – virilization, acne and hirsutism.
(2) Analytical tests – testosterone and androstenedione levels.

The status of the pituitary cannot be tested clinically. But there is a strong correlation to the oestrogen activity: when there are oestrogens there must be a stimulation of the ovaries by the pituitary and direct measurement of FSH and LH will not give further information. In those cases where no oestrogen activity is found, pituitary function can only be evaluated by measurement of FSH and LH, which will result either in elevated or in subnormal values. In addition the pituitary reactivity can be tested by the LH-RH test, but this will not give additional information for further clinical procedures. A circhoral fluctuation of the LH concentration is found in normal ovarian function. In hypothalamic amenorrhoea this fluctuation is seized. In cyclic ovarian insufficiency changes in the LH fluctuation, either in frequency or in amplitude, can be found:

(1) Clinical test – correlation to oestrogen activity.
(2) Analytical tests – FSH, LH, LH-RH and LH fluctuation.

It is well known that *prolactin* is involved in ovarian function. Elevated prolactin leads to ovarian insufficiency. Clinically galactorrhoea is mostly combined with hyperprolactinaemia. But for proper evaluation prolactin has to be measured. Several stimulation tests are of questionable value:

(1) Clinical tests – galactorrhoea.
(2) Analytical tests — prolactin, TRH, metoclopramide and sulpiride stimulation.

Various proposals for pre-treatment evaluation of ovarian dysfunction and for their classification have been made. The first WHO classification (1973) was based on the endogenous oestrogen activity and the level of gonadotrophins. Group I comprised patients with amenorrhoea and with little or no evidence of endogenous oestrogen activity. Group II comprised women with a variety of menstrual cycle disturbances including amenorrhoea, who exhibited distinct endogenous activity and gonadotrophins in the normal range. Group III comprised women with primary ovarian failure associated with low endogenous oestrogen activity and elevated gonadotrophins. This classification was revised in 1976 and the prolactin status was added to the above-mentioned groups. The androgen, corticoid and thyroid hormones were not considered.

A pre-treatment classification in particular should meet therapeutic aspects. The diagnosis, as correct as possible, should be found within a short period of time with a minimum of expenses.

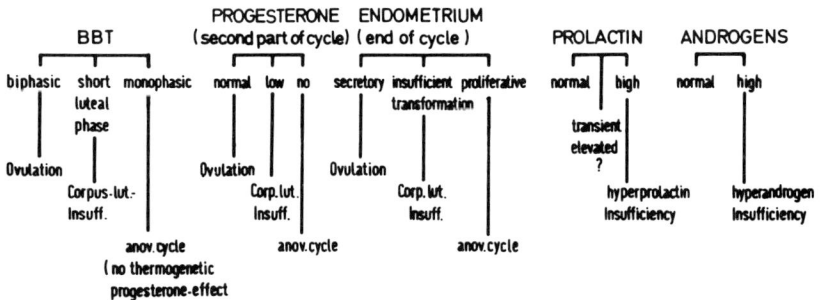

Figure 1 Diagnostic evaluation of ovarian dysfunction in patients with spontaneous bleedings

Diagnostic tools for evaluation of ovarian dysfunction are:

(1) Clinical tests – history, general examination, gynaecological examination, cervical factor, vaginal smear, endometrium biopsy, progestin level and ovarian biopsy.
(2) Analytical tests – oestrogens, progesterone, androgens, gonadotrophic (basic level, ratio, fluctuations), prolactin and thyroid hormones.

In patients with menstrual-cycle disturbances ovarian function can be mainly checked by clinical methods. The pattern of the basal body temperature indicates a biphasic or ovulatory cycle, a short hyperthermic phase means luteal insufficiency and a monophasic pattern suggests an anovulatory cycle. The results can be supported by testing of progesterone levels either by direct measurement in the second part of the cycle and/or by the histology of the endometrium at the beginning of bleeding. For further evaluation prolactin and androgen estimations are necessary (Figure 1).

In amenorrhoea clinical tests enable the physician to differentiate between those patients with endogenous oestrogen activity and those who have none. This can be done by examination of the cervical factor, by the progestin test, by the endometrium biopsy or by the vaginal cytology. By additional analytical procedures FSH/LH measurement can characterize patients in those with high, normal or low gonadotrophins. The frequent measurement of LH shows if the LH fluctuation is normal, irregular in frequency or amplitude or if there is no fluctuation. Of further importance is the LH:FSH ratio and, as in spontaneous bleeders, the prolactin and androgen situation (Figure 2).

The diagnostic work-up results in a treatment-orientated classification of ovarian insufficiency. It should be emphasized that this in particular is possible by a careful clinical and gynaecological examination, which is supplemented by a few laboratory parameters.

The ovulation-induction era started 23 years ago. At first gonadotrophins became available followed by clomiphene, LH-RH and prolactin inhibitors. Direct stimulation of ovarian function is possible by FSH-LH preparations. Pituitary stimulation is possible by pulsatile LH-RH administration. Clomiphene acts via hypothalamo-pituitary stimulation and leads to normalization of ovarian function. Prolactin inhibitor normalizes the prolactin levels; corticoids can normalize the androgen levels in this way leading to improvement of ovarian

CERVICAL FACTOR   PROGESTIN-TEST   ENDOMETRIUM BIOPSY   VAGINAL CYTOLOGY

good   poor   +   Ø   proliferative   atrophic   mature   atrophic

Estrogens   Estrogens   Estrogens   Estrogens

present   absent   present   absent   present   absent   present   absent

FSH LH normal   low or high   =   =   =   =

CLINICAL

FSH – LH   LH:FSH   PROLACTIN   ANDROGENS

high   normal   low   high   normal   low   high   normal   high   normal

Fluctuation

normal +/Ø   +/Ø

hyper- normo- hypo-

WHO III   II   I   V / VI

ANALYTICAL

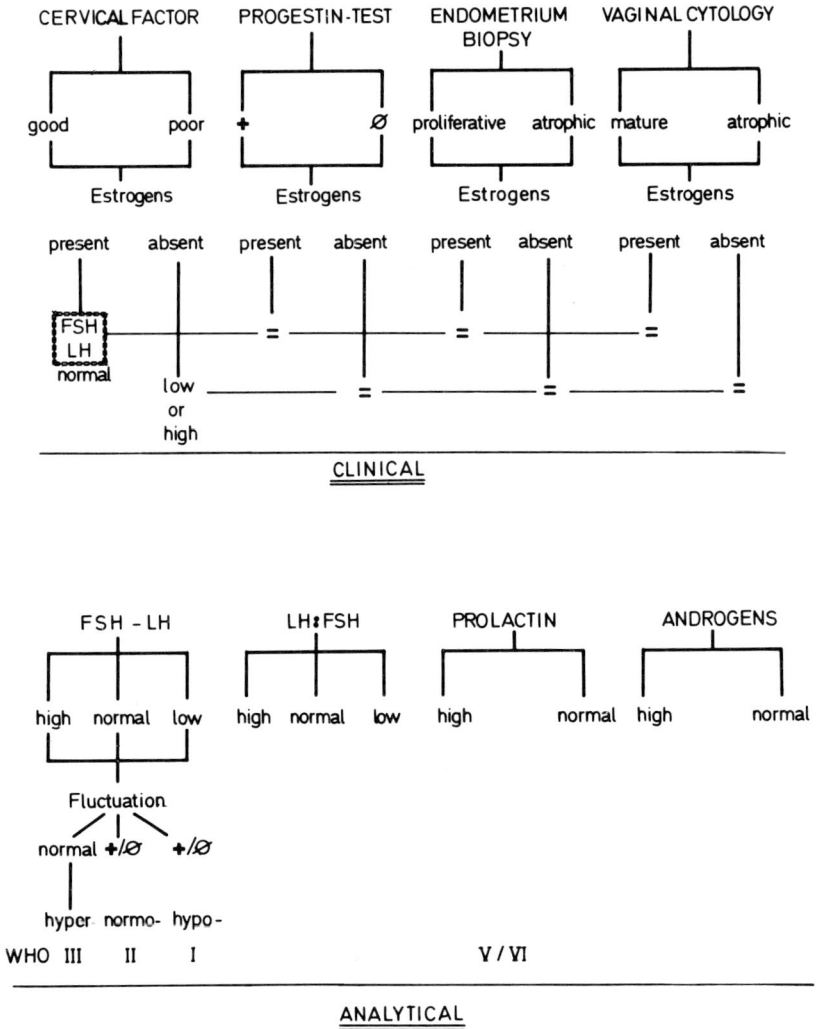

Figure 2 Diagnostic evaluation of ovarian dysfunction in patients with amenorrhoea (+/Ø = LH fluctuation irregular in frequency or in amplitude, or no fluctuation)

540

function. In addition it should be mentioned that the nutritional factors, psychic conditions and the whole environment are involved in normal ovarian or better reproductive function. The factors entailed can be summarized as follows:

(1) Direct – FSH/LH (hMG/hCG)
(2) Via pituitary stimulation (LH-RH)
(3) Via hypothalamo-pituitary stimulation (clomiphene)
(4) Via normalization of:
    (a) Prolactin status – prolactin inhibitor
    (b) Androgen status – corticoids
    (c) Thyroid function – thyroid hormones
(5) Via normalization of nutritional factors, psychic condition (psychotherapy) or environment (psychosocial)

After performing the pre-treatment examination of the patients, the physician comes to a diagnosis, which enables him to select the type of treatment and to be of prognostic value (Figures 3 and 4).

Pulsatile LH-RH is effective in patients with no oestrogen activity,

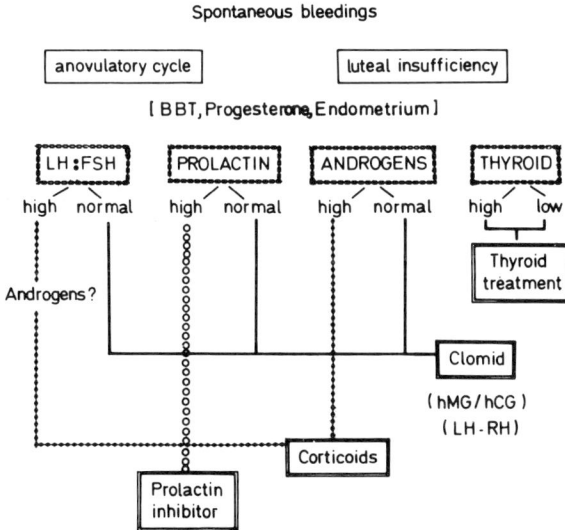

Figure 3 Treatment-oriented classification of ovarian dysfunction in patients with spontaneous bleeding

541

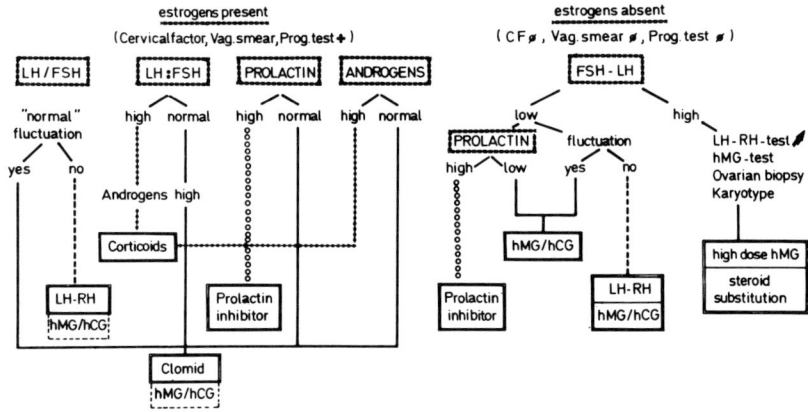

Figure 4 Treatment-oriented classification of ovarian dysfunction in patients with amenorrhoea

Figure 5 Indications for treatment with LH-RH (hatched area those in which the indication for this type of treatment is given)

low and stable LH levels and no or irregular LH fluctuation (Figure 5). hMG/hCG is effective in patients with no oestrogen activity, low FSH/LH levels and clomiphene failure (Figure 6). Clomiphene is effective in patients with oestrogen activity, or with low-to-normal FSH/LH values in luteal insufficiency, anovulatory cycles or amenorrhoea (Figure 7). Prolactin inhibitors are effective in patients with hyperprolactinaemia (Figure 8) and corticoids with elevated androgens (Figure 9).

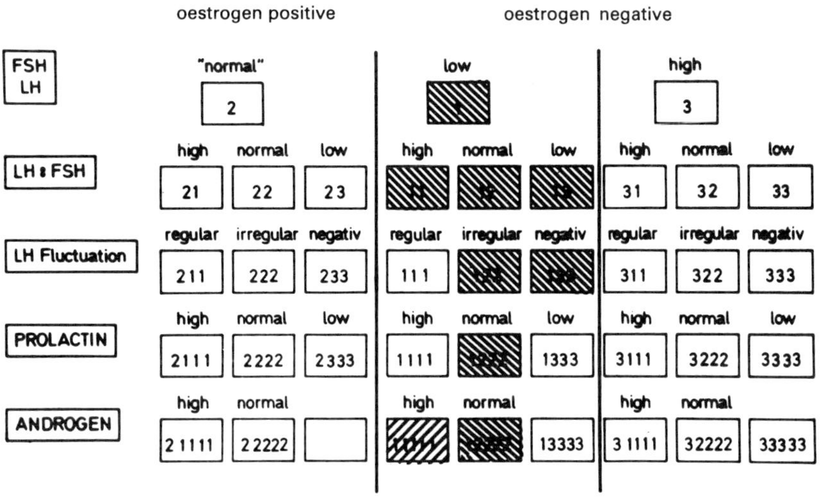

Figure 6   Indications for treatment with hMG/hCG

The most effective and most intensively studied treatment is that with hMG/hCG. With this ovarian stimulation in nearly all patients with ovarian dysfunction, stimulation with ovulation is possible. In the other types of treatment there is always a group of patients in whom ovarian function cannot be normalized; mostly the reason cannot be found. Sometimes combination therapy is effective in those patients; for example, clomiphene plus hCG, prolactin inhibitor plus clomiphene, and corticoids with clomiphene.

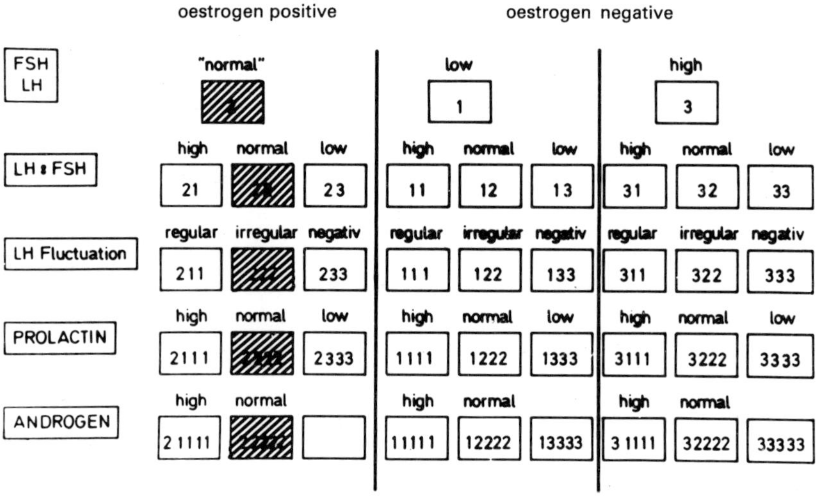

Figure 7 Indication for treatment with clomiphene

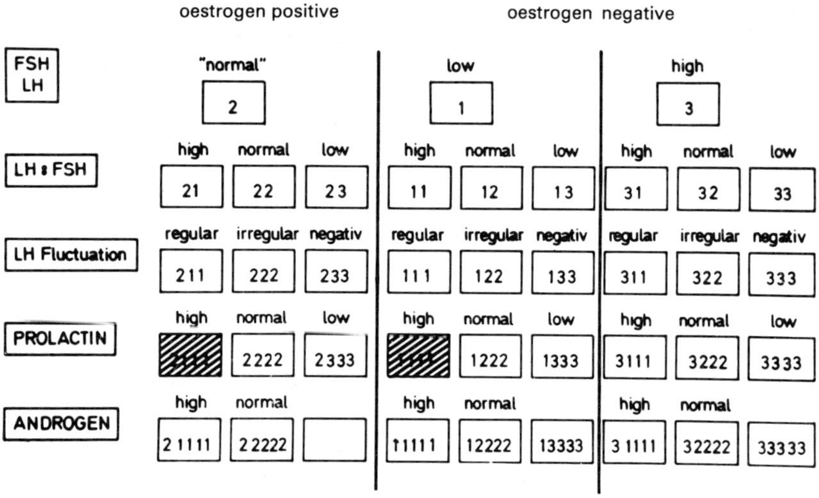

Figure 8 Indication for treatment with prolactin inhibitors

oestrogen positive   oestrogen negative

FSH LH	"normal"	low	high
	2	1	3

LH : FSH	high	normal	low	high	normal	low	high	normal	low
	▨	22	23	11	12	13	31	32	33

LH Fluctuation	regular	irregular	negativ	regular	irregular	negativ	regular	irregular	negativ
	211	222	233	111	122	133	311	322	333

PROLACTIN	high	normal	low	high	normal	low	high	normal	low
	2111	2222	2333	1111	1222	1333	3111	3222	3333

ANDROGEN	high	normal		high	normal		high	normal	
	▨	2 2222		▨	12222	13333	3 1111	32222	33333

Figure 9   Indications for treatment with corticoids

Mostly pregnancy occurs during the first three treatment cycles in all therapeutic trials and it is obvious that the results after five or six treatment cycles are markedly reduced. Dealing with the infertile couple, one always should remember that there may be additional factors and that after some time treatment should be stopped and the diagnosis re-evaluated.

59
Hyperprolactinaemic infertility: some considerations on medical management

M. O. THORNER, M. L. VANCE and R. M. MACLEOD

ABSTRACT

Hyperprolactinaemia is a common cause of infertility in women. The most common cause for hyperprolactinaemia (after excluding ingestion of medications which elevate prolactin) is a pituitary tumour. These tumours can either be small (diameter less than 10 mm) = microadenomas, or, if greater than 10 mm, are termed macroprolactinomas. Although this distinction is arbitrary, it is often useful in predicting the outcome of transsphenoidal surgery, although the basal serum prolactin is a better predictor.

Irrespective of the size of the tumour or the pretreatment prolactin level, medical treatment with dopamine agonist drugs (e.g. bromocriptine, lisuride and pergolide) is effective in >80% of cases in lowering prolactin levels and in restoring gonadal function. The large tumours undergo volume reduction under this form of therapy. The potential problem of tumour expansion during pregnancy which is a function of the pre-existing tumour is reviewed. This risk appears extremely small in microadenomas but may be clinically significant in 10–25% of macroadenoma patients. The dilemmas of the management of this controversial problem are discussed.

INTRODUCTION

Since human prolactin was isolated and characterized 13 years ago, the study of the control of prolactin secretion has been intensive. Hyperprolactinaemia is the most commonly identifiable hypothalamic pituitary disorder[1,2]. The dominant inhibitory nature of hypothalamic control of prolactin secretion may be the reason that hyperprolactinaemia is such a common condition. During the past decade two separate therapeutic approaches to the management of hyperprolactinaemia have been introduced: transsphenoidal selective pituitary microsurgery and medical therapy to suppress prolactin secretion with orally active long-acting dopamine agonist drugs. Small prolactin-secreting tumours are treated extremely satisfactorily both with medical and with surgical therapy, both in terms of lowering serum prolactin levels to normal and in restoring gonadal function. However, for the larger tumours, either where the tumour is invasive or the pretreatment serum prolactin level is greater than $250\,ng\,ml^{-1}$ the results of surgery are poor in terms of restoring to normal circulating prolactin levels and gonadal function[3-5]. We now discuss the medical management of hyperprolactinaemia, potential problems during pregnancy and the management of large prolactin-secreting pituitary tumours.

Although hyperprolactinaemia can occur in adolescence, during the middle years and old age, it is usually recognized in patients between the ages of 20 and 35. The presentation of hyperprolactinaemia varies between women and men. Women usually present with menstrual abnormalities, amenorrhoea, oligomenorrhoea, and menorrhagia, or regular cycles with infertility. In addition, women often note a decrease in libido and dyspareunia due to oestrogen deficiency. There are often no characteristic findings on physical examination; however, the breast tissue is well preserved, Montgomery tubercles are prominent and galactorrhoea is sometimes present. Galactorrhoea is a poor discriminator for the presence or absence of hyperprolactinaemia, as it may occur in women with normal prolactin levels and may be absent in patients with extremely high serum prolactin levels[6]. The reason for this is that galactopoiesis is dependent on a complex interaction of many hormones, of which prolactin is only one, albeit an essential one. The incidence of galactorrhoea in women with hyperprolactinaemia varies from 30 to 82%[1,7] and in men it is present in 20–30%[8-10]. In men the usual presentation is with symptoms due to expansion of the tumour giving rise to headache, and/or visual field defects due to compression of the optic chiasm. In addition men often suffer from impotence and loss of libido and have a hypogonadal appearance, being overweight and demonstrating reduced beard growth. The circulating testosterone levels are low, thus providing biochemical documentation of the hypogonadal state that is suspected clinically.

EVALUATION OF HYPERPROLACTINAEMIA

The major prolactin-inhibiting hormone is the catecholamine dopamine. Hyperprolactinaemia may, therefore, result from ingestion of drugs that either prevent the synthesis of dopamine or deplete its stores (e.g. α-methyl-dopa and reserpine, respectively) or block dopamine receptors on lactotrophs (e.g. phenothiazines, butyrophenones, or benzamides). Oestrogens act directly at the pituitary to stimulate lactotrophs and increase prolactin synthesis; this is associated with lactotroph hypertrophy. Occasionally primary hypothyroidism may be associated with mild hyperprolactinaemia and hence thyroid function tests should always be performed in these patients[11]. In young women hypothyroidism may present only with menstrual problems, without any of the usual symptoms or clinical stigmata. Drug-induced hyperprolactinaemia and that due to hypothyroidism usually results in relatively minor elevations of serum prolactin level, rarely to greater than $100 \, ng \, ml^{-1}$. Pituitary tumour is the most common cause of hyperprolactinaemia. Such tumours are often subdivided into microadenomas or macroadenomas[3]. The microadenoma is defined as a tumour found at surgery with a diameter of less than 10 mm and associated serum prolactin levels are usually less than $200 \, ng \, ml^{-1}$. It is now, with the advent of the high-resolution CT scanner, possible for these tumours to be diagnosed prior to surgery[12]. In the past there was considerable controversy about the radiological appearance of microadenomas, based on changes in the contour in the pituitary fossa seen on polytomography. It is now clear that many of the 'specific' changes were probably non-specific and represented normal variants. Although these problems have been circumvented with the later generations of CT scanners, a new problem has now arisen. Since microadenomas probably are found in a proportion of the 'normal' population the radiographic presence of a microadenoma may not necessarily be synonymous with the lesion responsible for the hyperprolactinaemia.

We evaluate our patients with hyperprolactinaemia by taking a full history and performing a thorough physical examination. Particular emphasis is placed on looking for signs of hypothyroidism, evaluating the visual fields, and examining for signs of gonadal dysfunction. The most useful single investigation is the measurement of serum prolactin in the basal state on two or three independent visits. Repeated measurement is obviously not necessary if the first value is found to be extremely high (e.g. greater than $500 \, \text{ng ml}^{-1}$). We also evaluate thyroid function by measuring a serum thyroxine, T_3 resin uptake, and a serum TSH. To determine whether there is any structural lesion in the pituitary we perform a high-resolution CT scan. We normally perform a visual field assessment using the Goldmann apparatus. Other endocrine testing of ACTH, GH, and gonadotrophin reserve is performed only if indicated.

DOPAMINE AGONIST THERAPY

The dopamine agonist ergot derivatives are effective when given by mouth. These drugs include bromocriptine, lergotrile, lisuride and pergolide. They act by binding to specific dopamine receptors on the lactotrophs. Each of these compounds appears to be long-acting and thus can suppress prolactin secretion throughout a 24-hour period. After a single 2.5 mg dose of bromocriptine prolactin levels are suppressed by approximately 80% in hyperprolactinaemic subjects

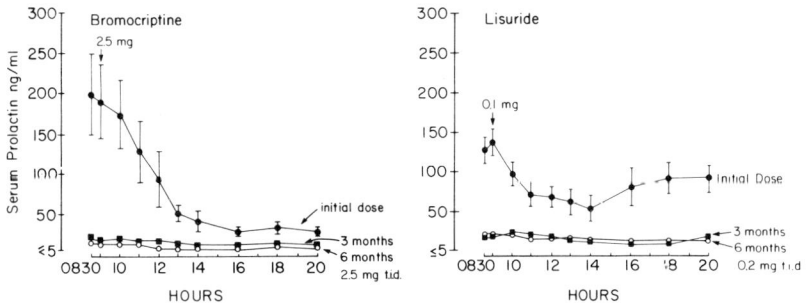

Figure 1 Serum prolactin levels in seven hyperprolactinaemic women after bromocriptine administration (left) and in six hyperprolactinaemic women after lisuride administration (right). The effects of a single acute dose and chronic therapy for 3 and 6 months are shown. Note that during chronic therapy suppression of prolactin with both drugs is similar

within 4 hours of administration and remain suppressed for at least 11 hours. Similar observations have been made after a single 0.1 mg dose of lisuride. Figure 1 compares serum prolactin levels in hyperprolactinaemic subjects after bromocriptine and lisuride administration. The normal dose of bromocriptine (2.5 mg three times daily) or lisuride (0.2 mg three times daily) maintains the suppression of prolac-

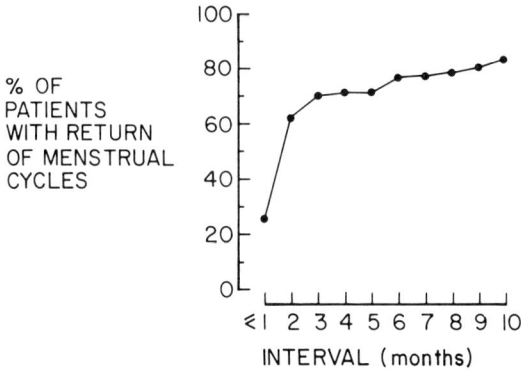

Figure 2 Cumulative percentage of 58 amenorrhoeic hyperprolactinaemic women with return of regular menstrual cycles related to months on bromocriptine therapy. Reproduced with permission from reference 14

tin secretion. Pergolide appears to be longer acting[13]. Figure 2 shows the percentage of amenorrhoeic patients in whom normal menstrual cycles returned plotted against the duration of bromocriptine therapy. It is apparent that within 1 month of initiation of therapy 25% of patients had a return of regular menstrual cycles; within 6 months this percentage rose to greater than 60%; at the end of 10 months 83% had a return of regular menstrual cycles. Of the 17% who did not have a return of normal cycles, all but one patient had previously been treated with either external pituitary irradiation, surgery or both[14]. The result in terms of return of gonadal function is similar in the men. Thus, irrespective of whether the patient has a microadenoma or a macroadenoma the suppression of prolactin, with medical therapy, restores gonadal function in the vast majority of these patients. At the present time bromocriptine, lisuride and pergolide appear to have similar efficacy. Pergolide has the practical advantage that it only needs to be given once daily.

551

HYPERPROLACTINAEMIA AND PREGNANCY

Many women present with infertility but wish to become pregnant once their ovarian function has been restored. Certain potential problems of pregnancy need recognition. During pregnancy the normal pituitary gland increases in size and it has been observed that some patients with pituitary tumours, meningiomas and other parasellar diseases develop symptoms from growth of these neoplasms during pregnancy. Therefore, the tumour expansion during pregnancy is not a result of the therapy, but instead is intrinsic to the basic disease which is aggravated by the pregnancy.

The incidence of pituitary tumour expansion during pregnancy is unknown. As a rough estimate between 10 and 25% of macroadenomas may enlarge during pregnancy and thus give rise to symptoms. For microadenomas the incidence is probably less than 1% and possibly less than 0.1%[15,16].

Our policy is to discuss thoroughly these risks with our patients and then to recommend to all patients (except those who have pre-existing visual field defects) medical treatment with dopamine agonist drugs. We consider it vital to have excellent baseline neuroradiological and neuro-ophthalmological data before the patient becomes pregnant. This obviates serious management problems if the patient develops symptoms and minor field defects are detected for the first time during pregnancy. The number of women who have large tumours with field defects prior to therapy is very small. In these patients the risks have to be carefully evaluated and the question of surgical decompression of the tumour prior to pregnancy needs serious consideration.

The patients are asked to use mechanical contraception during the early months of therapy, so that they do not become pregnant and their menstrual cycles can be documented. If the patient wishes to become pregnant after three regular menstrual cycles and documentation of a biphasic basal body temperature chart, we advise her to discontinue contraceptive precautions. As soon as a period is 48 hours overdue the dopamine agonist therapy is stopped and a serum β-HCG level is measured. The patient is closely followed up throughout the pregnancy and, if there is any sign of the development of compressive symptoms, the patient is re-started on medical therapy. We do not recommend routinely continuing the dopamine agonist therapy throughout the pregnancy since it is clear that these drugs cross the placenta and prolactin levels in both the mother and the fetus are suppressed. It is of interest that the amniotic fluid prolactin levels remain extremely high and this presumably reflects production of prolactin by the decidua which is not under dopaminergic control.

Extensive studies have been performed to determine whether there is teratogenic effect of bromocriptine[17]. All studies to date indicate that bromocriptine is safe to use to induce fertility, but the oldest child born to a women who took bromocriptine to induce fertility is now only 10 years old. Therefore, the full development of the children has not yet been documented. The teratogenicity studies of lisuride are discussed in Chapter 60.

MACROADENOMAS SECRETING PROLACTIN

Surgery rarely cures the large prolactin-secreting pituitary adenoma. Patients with pretreatment prolactin levels of greater than 250 ng ml^{-1} or patients with invasive prolactin-secreting pituitary tumours stand less than a 30% chance of being cured by surgery alone[3-5]. An alternative treatment is needed.

The objectives of both medical and surgical treatment are: (1) to reduce the size of the pituitary tumour, particularly if it is producing compressive symptoms; (2) to restore or maintain normal anterior pituitary function; (3) to reduce the serum prolactin level to normal; and (4) to prevent recurrence of the disease. Multicentre studies suggest that some patients with prolactin-secreting pituitary tumours demonstrate rapid improvement in visual fields and resolution of headaches after starting bromocriptine, lisuride, or pergolide therapy[19-27]. This is associated with the reduction of prolactin levels usually by greater than 80% and into the normal range on many occasions. Of greater significance is the improvement of visual field abnormalities in most patients and the radiological evidence of a decrease in tumour size during bromocriptine, lisuride and pergolide therapy. Some investigators advocate medical therapy as primary treatment of patients who present with visual field abnormalities. Indeed the dramatic clinical improvement as a result of reduction in tumour size without the risk of development of hypopituitarism is strong supportive evidence for this recommendation. However, withdrawal of dopamine agonist therapy usually results in a return of hyperprolactinaemia and tumour re-expansion with the attendant risk of visual compromise[25]. In this context, these drugs may be

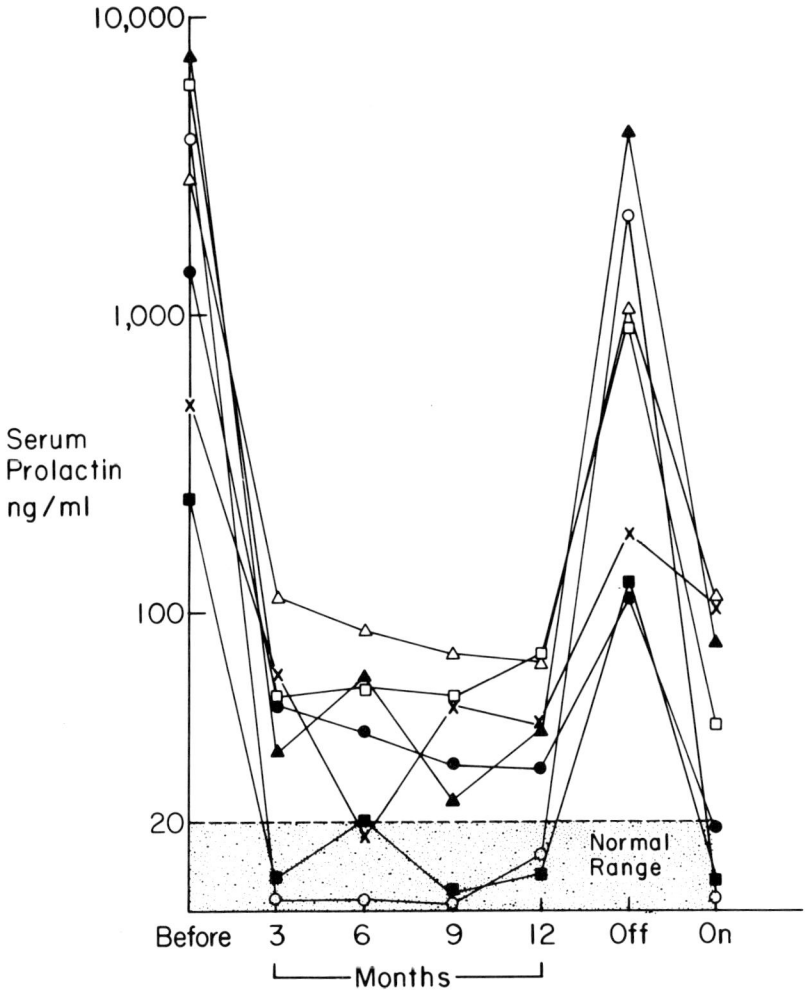

Figure 3 Mean serum prolactin of 10 samples drawn at fixed intervals through the day in seven patients with prolactin-secreting macroadenomas. The results are shown before, at the end of 1 year, after withdrawal, and after re-starting therapy. Note the reduction in the serum prolactin levels during bromocriptine therapy, the increase in the levels when therapy was stopped, and further suppression when therapy was reinitiated. Reproduced with permission from reference 28

viewed as 'replacement' therapy. Thus, a functional dopamine deficiency at the level of the tumour is reversed by dopamine agonists and chronic therapy is required. The size reduction of these tumours can be explained by a reduction in the volume of the individual cells[18]. Diminished cytoplasmic and to a lesser extent nuclear volumes are responsible for these changes. The cell undergoes transformation from an active to a relatively quiescent state with little rough endoplasmic reticulum and decreased nuclear size.

Our major experience has been with bromocriptine. However, in the patients whom we have treated with lisuride the results appear similar. In our series of seven men and six women with hyperprolactinaemia and radiologically documented suprasellar extension, who have had no other antecedent therapy, bromocriptine therapy (2.5mg three times daily) resulted in suppression of serum prolactin levels by 86–99% after 12 months; two of the six men and four of the seven women achieved normal serum prolactin levels. Gonadal function was restored or improved in 12 of the 13 patients. Six of seven women had return of cyclic menses. One woman who had been amenorrhoeic for 16 years has not yet had return of menses; her pretreatment serum prolactin value was 770 ng ml^{-1} and decreased to 110 ng ml^{-1} after 12 months of therapy. Initially, visual fields were normal in the women and abnormal in five of the six men. After institution of bromocriptine therapy, visual fields improved or became normal in all five men. All patients had a radiologically demonstrated (either by CT scan or pneumocisternography) reduction in tumour size. Bromocriptine was withdrawn in seven patients, and Figure 3 illustrates the changes in serum prolactin level in these seven patients during treatment with, after withdrawal of, and re-institution of bromocriptine. In one patient withdrawal of therapy resulted in return of visual field abnormalities which promptly improved 3 days after re-institution of bromocriptine (Figure 4). Figure 5 shows the changes seen in the CT scans of a woman who was treated for 1 year with bromocriptine. Serum prolactin level decreased from 7340 to 40 ng ml^{-1}. 6 days after withdrawal of bromocriptine at 1 year the serum prolactin level was 3960 ng ml^{-1} and the tumour was clearly larger. Within 8 days of re-starting bromocriptine, the tumour decreased towards the pre-withdrawal size; after 1 month of therapy the serum prolactin value was 77 ng ml^{-1}.

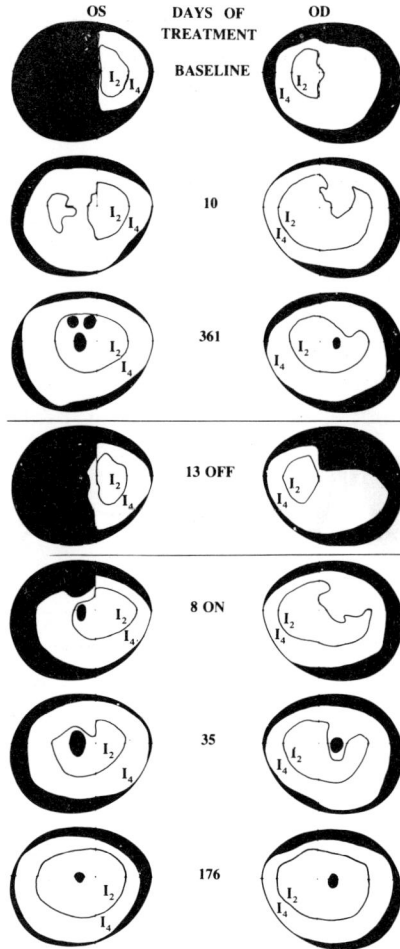

Figure 4 Diagrammatic representation of visual field plot in a 24-year-old man before, during, after withdrawal, and after reinstitution of bromocriptine therapy. The visual fields were plotted using the Goldmann apparatus under light intensive, 1000 apostilb (I_4) and 100 apostilb (I_2). The black periphery indicates a normal visual field for comparison. Before therapy (baseline) a bitemporal hemianopsia, complete in the left eye and incomplete in the right eye, was present. The visual fields were greatly improved at 10 days, and only an equivocal superior bitemporal quadrantic defect to the low intensity object was present on the 361st day. On the 13th day after withdrawal of medical therapy, the field defects recurred; an almost complete temporal hemianopsia in the left eye and an incomplete temporal hemianopsia in the right eye were present. Progressive improvement in the visual fields was again observed over 6 months after reintroduction of therapy. Reproduced with permission from reference 25

CONCLUSIONS

Hyperprolactinaemia is an important cause of infertility in women. Its recognition in an individual patient is important since specific, simple, and reliable therapy is available with dopamine agonist drugs. Problems of potential pituitary tumour expansion during pregnancy exist but are minor in patients with microadenomas, who make up greater than 80% of such patients. The recognition of the hyperprolactinaemic syndromes and the advent of dopamine agonist drugs offer a major advance in the treatment of infertility.

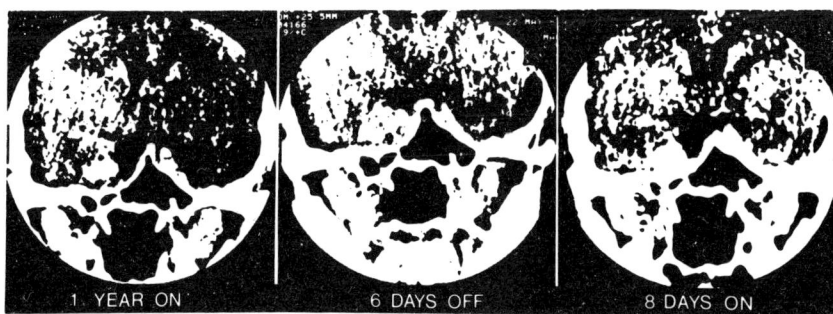

Figure 5 Coronal sections of CT scan through the sella turcica; at 1 year of bromocriptine treatment (left) in a young woman with a prolactin-secreting macroadenoma. There is a partially empty fossa and some residual tumour in the cavernous sinus. 6 days after bromocriptine withdrawal (centre) the tumour has re-expanded to fill the pituitary fossa, and 8 days after re-starting therapy (right) the tumour size had decreased towards the pre-withdrawal value. Reproduced with permission from reference 28

References

1. Franks, S., Murray, M. A. F., Jequier, A. M., Steele, S. J., Nabarro, J. D. N. and Jacobs, H. S. (1975). Incidence and significance of hyperprolactinemia in women with amenorrhea. *Clin. Endocrinol.*, **4**, 597
2. Franks, S., Nabarro, J. D. N. and Jacobs, H. S. (1977). Prevalence and presentation of hyperprolactinemia in patients with 'functionless' pituitary tumours. *Lancet*, **1**, 778
3. Hardy, J. and Mohr, G. (1981). Le prolactionome aspects chirurgicaux. *Neurochirurgie*, **27**, (Suppl. 1), 41
4. Randall, R. V., Laws, E. R., Abboud, C. F., Ebersold, M. J., Kao, P. C. and

557

Scheithauer, B. W. (1983). Transsphenoidal microsurgical treatment of prolactin-producing pituitary adenomas. Results in 100 patients. *Mayo Clin. Proc.*, **58**, 108

5. Tindall, G. T., McLanahan, S. and Christy, J. H. (1978). Transsphenoidal microsurgery for pituitary tumors associated with hyperprolactinemia. *J. Neurosurg.*, **48**, 849

6. Kleinberg, D. L., Noel, G. L. and Frantz, A. G. (1977). Galactorrhea: 235 cases including 48 with pituitary tumors. *N. Engl. J. Med.*, **296**, 589

7. Hardy, J., Beauregard, H. and Robert, F. (1978). Prolactin-secreting pituitary adenomas: Transsphenoidal microsurgical treatment. In Robyn, C. and Harter, M. (eds.). *Progress in Prolactin Physiology and Pathology*, pp. 261–70. (New York: Elsevier)

8. Carter, J. N., Tyson, J. E., Tolis, G., Van Vliet, S., Faiman, G. and Friesen, H. G. (1978). Prolactin-secreting tumors and hypogonadism in 22 men. *N. Engl. J. Med.*, **299**, 847

9. Segal, S., Yaffee, H., Laufer, N. and Ben-David, M. (1979). Male hyperprolactinemia: effects on fertility. *Fertil. Steril.*, **32**, 556

10. Thorner, M. O., Edwards, C. R. W., Hanker, J. P., Abraham, G. and Besser, G. M. (1977). Prolactin and gonadotropin interaction in the male. In Troen, P. and Nankin, H. (eds.) *The Testis in Normal and Infertile Men.* pp. 351–66. (New York: Raven Press)

11. Molitch, M. E. and Reichlin, S. (1982). Hyperprolactinemia. In Cotsonas, N. J. (ed). *Disease-A-Month*, **28**, 1

12. Hemminghytt, S., Kalkhoff, R. K., Daniels, D. L., Williams, A. L., Grogan, J. P. and Haughton, V. M. (1983). Computed tomographic study of hormone-secreting microadenomas. *Radiology*, **146**, 65

13. Perryman, R. L., Rogol, A. D., Kaiser, D. L., MacLeod, R. M. and Thorner, M. O. (1981). Pergolide mesylate: Its effects on circulating anterior pituitary hormones in man. *J. Clin. Endocrinol. Metab.*, **53**, 772

14. Thorner, M. O. and Besser, G. M. (1978). Bromocriptine treatment of hyperprolactinemic hypogonadism. *Acta Endocrinol.*, **88**, Suppl. **216**, 131

15. Gemzell, C. and Wang, C. F. (1979). Outcome of pregnancy in women with pituitary adenoma. *Fertil. Steril.*, **31**, 363

16. Skrabanek, P., McDonald, D., Meagher, D. et. al. (1980). Clinical course and outcome of thirty-five pregnancies in infertile hyperprolactinemic women. *Fertil. Steril.*, **33**, 391

17. Turkalj, I., Braun, P. and Krupp, P. (1982). Surveillance of bromocriptine in pregnancy. *J. Am. Med. Assoc.*, **247**, 1589

18. Tindall, G. T., Kovacs, K., Horvath, E. and Thorner, M. O. (1982). Human prolactin-producing adenomas and bromocriptine: A histological, immunocytochemical, ultrastructural, and morphometric study. *J. Clin. Endocrinol. Metab.*, **55**, 1178

19. Chiodini, P., Luizzi, A., Cozzi, R., et al. (1981). Size reduction of macroprolactinomas by bromocriptine or lisuride treatment. *J. Clin. Endocrinol. Metab.*, **53**, 737

20. George, S. R., Burrow, G. N., Zinman, B. and Ezrin, C. (1979). Regression of pituitary tumors, a possible effect of bromergocryptine. *Am. J. Med.*, **66**, 697

21. Grisoli, F., Vincentelli, F., Jaquet, P., Guilbout, M., Hassoun, J. and Farnarier, P. (1980). Prolactin secreting adenomas in 22 men. *Surg. Neurol.*, **13**, 241

22. Hamilton, D. J., George, B., Sommers, C., Zaniewski, M., Bryan, J. and Boyd, A. E. (1983). Comparison of pergolide and bromocriptine in prolactin disorder. Presented at the *64th Annual Meeting, The Endocrine Society, San Francisco*, abstract 564

23. McGregor, A. M., Scanlon, M. F., Hall, K., Cook, D. B. and Hall, R. (1979). Reduction in size of a pituitary tumor by bromocriptine therapy. *N. Engl. J. Med.*, **300**, 291

24. Thorner, M. O., Martin, W. H., Rogol, A. D. et. al. (1980). Rapid regression of

pituitary prolactinomas during bromocriptine treatment. *J. Clin. Endocrinol. Metab.*, **51,** 438

25. Thorner, M. O., Perryman, R. L., Rogol, A. D., *et al.* (1981). Rapid changes of prolactinoma volume after withdrawal and reinstitution of bromocriptine. *J. Clin. Endocrinol. Metab.*, **53,** 480

26. Vaidya, R. A., Allorkar, S. D. and Rege, N. R. (1978). Normalization of visual fields following bromocriptine treatment in hyperprolactinemic patients with visual field constriction. *Fertil. Steril.*, **29,** 632

27. Wollesen, F., Andersen, T. and Karle, A. (1982). Size reduction of extrasellar pituitary tumors during bromocriptine treatment: Quantitation of effect on different types of tumors. *Ann. Intern. Med.*, **96,** 281

28. Vance, M. L., Evans, W. S. and Thorner, M. O. (1983). Drugs five years later: bromocriptine. *Ann. Intern. Med.* (In press.)

60
Lisuride – a new drug for treatment of hyperprolactinaemic disorders

R. HOROWSKI, R. DOROW, A. SCHOLZ, L. DE CECCO
and W. H. F. SCHNEIDER

SUMMARY

Lisuride (Dopergin®), a highly active dopaminergic ergot derivative with prolactin-lowering properties, has an outstanding affinity as an agonist for dopamine receptors. It is concentrated by a factor of 5–10 above lisuride plasma levels within the pituitary where it acts on dopamine receptors which inhibit prolactin release. In rats, oral lisuride is 10–30 times more active on a weight basis as a prolactin-lowering agent than bromocriptine. In carcinogenicity studies in rodents, no endometrial carcinomas could be found after 2 years of treatment; on the contrary, development of pituitary tumours was prevented almost completely and there was a dose-dependent reduction in the incidence of mammary tumours. Studies in rats, rabbits and monkeys revealed no teratogenic potential of the drug. On acute administration, doses as low as 0.1 mg of lisuride p.o. decrease prolactin plasma levels in humans; this effect is enhanced and prolongated on repeated administration. Its effect is highly specific and no other hormonal systems are affected with the exception of growth hormone. Lisuride can be used in all clinical conditions where a dopaminergic or prolactin-lowering effect is needed, and its activity is unsurpassed by any other form of treatment. In the prevention of post-partum lactation, controlled studies point to a lower incidence of rebound lactation than observed with other treatments. Lisuride effectively restores normal cycles and fertility in hyperprolactinaemic women. In the pregnancies documented so far, which were induced by lisuride treatment, no evidence for any particular abnormality was observed. In healthy males, lisuride treatment did not affect spermatogenesis. In hyperprolactinaemic men suffering from prolactin-producing tumours, testosterone synthesis as well as libido, potency and fertility can be restored with lisuride. In the case of macroprolactinomas, treatment with lisuride not only lowered prolactin levels but also led to a sometimes dramatic reduction of tumour volume.

All these data suggest that lisuride is a highly effective drug in the treatment of menstrual cycle and fertility disorders and related situations, and a valuable alternative to bromocriptine.

Lisuride (Dopergin®; 8-(9,10-didehydro-6-methyl-ergolin-8α-yl)-1,1-diethyl-urea hydrogen maleate; Figure 1) is a semi-synthetic ergot derivative with an outstanding affinity for central monoamine receptors.

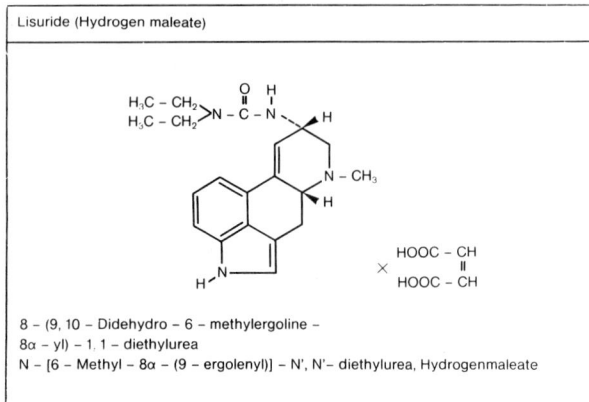

Figure 1   The structure of lisuride

In numerous pharmacological experiments lisuride has been shown to be a potent direct dopamine agonist as well as a serotonin partial agonist[1–3]; at much higher dosages, it has also α-adrenolytic and even β-receptor blocking activity (Table 1). In biochemical *in vitro* and *in vivo* investigations lisuride has been shown to be one of the most potent dopamine receptor agonists. The compound displays a very high affinity for D_1 and D_2 dopamine receptors as well as for 5-HT_1 and 5-HT_2 receptors[4,5].

Table 1 Pharmacological profile of lisuride

LOW DOSES

High-affinity binding to serotonin (5-HT_1 and 5-HT_2) receptors

Functional inhibition of serotoninergic neurones of raphe dorsalis and inhibition of peripheral effects of serotonin	Prevention of migraine attacks (daily dose 0.075 mg by mouth)

High-affinity binding to dopamine receptors of the anterior pituitary

Inhibition of prolactin release (acute effect) and synthesis	Prevention of lactation, treatment of galactorrhoea, amenorrhoea and other cycle and fertility disorders (daily dose 0.4–4 mg by mouth)

INTERMEDIATE DOSES

High-affinity binding to dopamine receptors of the striatum

Postsynaptic activation of dopamine receptors (particularly in supersensitive states, e.g. dopamine-depleted animals)	Treatment of Parkinsonism and related diseases (daily dose 0.6–10 mg by mouth)

HIGH DOSES

Binding to α- and β-receptors

α-adrenolytic and β-blocking effects	No clinical correlations

---

When given to rats, dosages in the microgram range inhibit the firing rate of raphe dorsalis neurones – an effect that seems to be due to an activation of 5-HT autoreceptors which results in a functional inhibition of serotonin effects[6]. The interaction of lisuride with serotoninergic systems is believed to be the pharmacological basis for the high efficacy of lisuride in the prevention of migraine attacks[7].

Doses of lisuride in a similar range reduce reserpine-induced rigidity and, at higher doses, also akinesia and hypothermia[8,9]. In rats that were not pretreated with reserpine, lisuride inhibited the neuronal firing rate of dopaminergic neurones in the substantia nigra[6]. This phenomenon is interpreted as being due to a negative feedback mechanism as a consequence of the stimulation of dopamine receptors by lisuride. The very potent dopamine agonist activity of lisuride in these systems is the basis for the use of this drug in the treatment of Parkinson's disease, which is defined by a deficit of dopamine in the nigroneostriatal pathway[10].

The unique combination of dopaminergic activity and functional serotonin antagonism is the cause of the occurrence of pronounced, stereotyped and long-lasting mounting behaviour which can be observed in rats treated with high doses of lisuride. This behavioural phenomenon which mimics male sexual activity seems to be independent from the hormonal situation of the animals because it can be produced also in female, juvenile or castrated animals[11]. In castrated male rats, lisuride restores in a dose-dependent way not only mounting behaviour, but also penile erection, intromission and ejaculation. These effects confirm that in rats, sexual activity can be restored or enhanced by a combination of serotonin antagonistic and dopaminergic activity[12].

Since dopamine plays a crucial role in preventing prolactin release from anterior pituitary prolactin cells, it is not surprising that extremely low oral doses of lisuride 10 μg (kg body weight)$^{-1}$ significantly lower serum prolactin levels in rats. In this respect, lisuride is at least 10 times more active than bromocriptine. Amongst all dopamine agonists used clinically lisuride has the highest affinity for dopamine receptors located on pituitary prolactin cells (Table 2). Furthermore,

Table 2 Competition by various agents for [^{3}H]-spiperone binding to 7315a pituitary tumour*

Agonist	K_i $(nmol\,l^{-1})$†
Lisuride	0.39±0.18
Bromocriptine	10±4
Pergolide	45±7
6,7-ADTN	236±66
Apomorphine	250±70
DA	2 900±1 200
1-Epinephrine	17 000±1 000
1-Norepinephrine	29 000±8 000
Serotonin	83 000±30 000

*Modified from reference 13.
†Means ±SE.

lisuride prevents prolactin-dependent function in rats, such as lactation, mammary development and luteolysis[14]. In carcinogenicity studies where female rats and mice were treated with various doses of lisuride over a period of 2 years, lisuride prevented in a dose-dependent way the development of pituitary and mammary tumours

Table 3 Tumour incidence (%) in female rats treated with lisuride for 104 weeks*

Dosage (mg kg^{-1} by mouth)	Surviving animals (n)	Mammary adenomas	All pituitary tumours	(males)
Controls	29	32	48	(40)
0.02	39†	16	49	(18)†
0.2	44†	6†	12†	(16)†
1.0	39†	2†	4†	(10)†

*From G. Schuppler (personal communication).
†Difference between control value and incidence significant at $p \leqslant 0.05$
Also dose-dependent decrease in tumour incidence: adrenal tumours (phaeochromocytomas and cortical adenomas) and thyroid C-cell adenomas.
There was no significant increase in tumour incidence (in particular no increase in endometrial tumours).

(Table 3) as well as of tumours of other organs (G. Schuppler, personal communication). No increase in the number of endometrial tumours was observed in the lisuride studies. In these as well as in other studies, where the development of pituitary tumours was prevented by treatment with lisuride the life-span of the animals was increased.

Extensive studies in rodents and monkeys failed to give any evidence of a teratogenic effect; lisuride was embryotoxic only at doses where also some of the adult animals died. The compound crosses the blood–placenta barrier and the blood–brain barrier and seems to achieve higher levels in brain areas with larger numbers of dopamine receptors. In the pituitary, its target organ, radioactivity after treatment with [³H]lisuride is 5–10 times higher than in the blood. This accumulation may be the reason why the prolactin-lowering effect of lisuride is enhanced on repeated administration[15].

In humans lisuride is completely absorbed but undergoes, like most ergots including bromocriptine, a variable first-pass effect. Prolactin-lowering activity does not seem to correlate with lisuride plasma levels as measured by specific RIA but side-effects seem to be more likely with higher concentrations in the blood. The variability in plasma levels may be the reason why – again as with other ergots – the dosage needs to be adjusted individually in all indications except prevention of postpartum lactation (where dopamine agonists are tolerated particularly well, possibly because of altered pharmaco-kinetics or to a cross-tolerance with oestrogens as regards nausea and other side-effects).

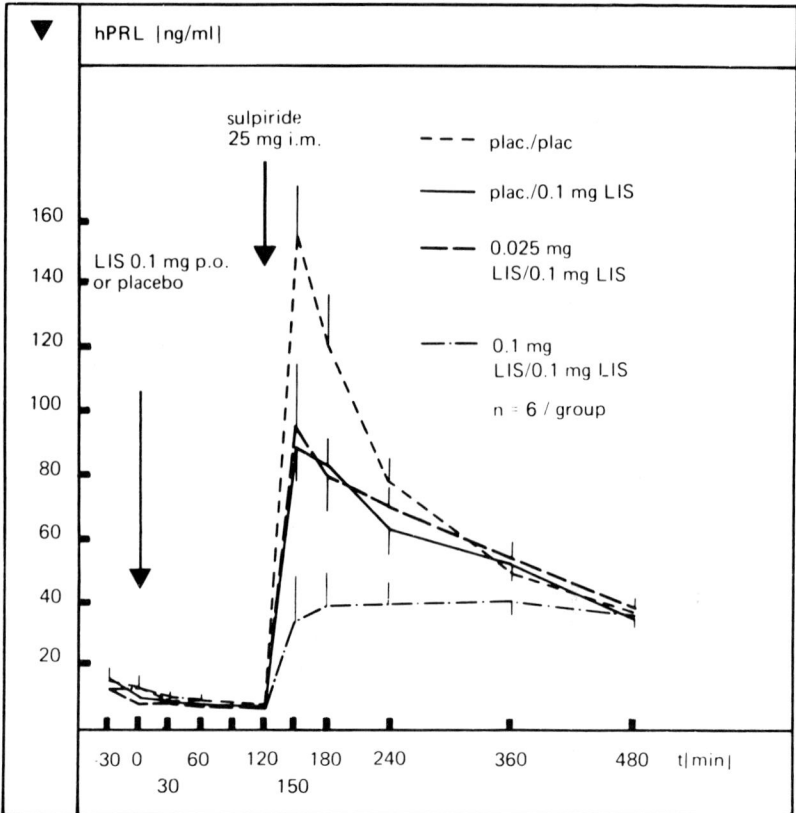

Figure 2 Influence of treatment for 2 weeks with placebo, 0.025 mg lisuride (LIS) three times daily or 0.1 mg lisuride three times daily on the acute effect of 0.1 mg lisuride on sulpiride-induced hyperprolactinaemia in healthy female volunteers. From reference 15

Lisuride is excreted from plasma and has a half-life of 2–3 hours[16]. Again, there is no correlation with its effects on prolactin levels which are lowered by a single dose of lisuride for 8–12 hours. This observation points again to a pituitary accumulation, as well as the observation that the prolactin-lowering effect is clearly enhanced on repeated administration (Figure 2), and plasma prolactin levels remain low for days or even weeks after cessation of treatment in patients with prolactin-producing adenomas. The prolactin-lowering effect of lisuride is dose and time dependent. A dose of 0.2 mg lisuride is equipotent to a dose of 2.5 mg bromocriptine. Similar dose-dependent effects were observed in the inhibition of postpartum lactation: whilst 3×0.05 mg failed to be better than placebo, 3×0.1, 3×0.2 and 3×0.3 mg daily lowered prolactin and prevented lactation in postpartum women in a dose-dependent way[17]. In two controlled comparative studies vs. bromocriptine, similar clinical effects could be achieved by doses of 0.2 mg lisuride and 2.5 mg bromocriptine; in both studies, however, there was less rebound lactation after a fortnight's duration of treatment in the lisuride group[18,19] (Table 4). This difference, too, can be interpreted in terms of a higher affinity of lisuride for dopamine receptors within the pituitary and its accumulation there.

Treatment with dopamine agonists has been shown recently to be very useful also in lactating women with beginning or fully established mastitis. By reducing the breast congestion immediately after application, it is even possible in some cases to avoid use of antibiotics and to maintain breast feeding.

Dopamine agonists are also able to inhibit galactorrhoea, whether associated with elevated prolactin levels or not, and they can also effectively reduce mastodynia and other symptoms of pathological forms of the so-called premenstrual syndrome, as shown for lisuride in one extensive controlled double-blind study using 2×0.1 mg daily[20]. Beneficial effects of this treatment on psychic and EEG alterations in this syndrome are possibly not caused by the prolactin-lowering effect of this compound, but may also reflect interaction with other dopaminergic or serotoninergic systems in the brain, as is the case in the preventive treatment of migraine with lisuride[7]. It may be relevant that this condition is often influenced by hormonal changes and can occur during the premenstrual phase.

It is still unclear whether prolactin-lowering drugs are also of clinical use in other breast diseases, e.g. cystic mastopathy, or whether even the incidence of mammary tumours might be reduced by long-term treatment with those compounds, as has been observed in animal studies.

Table 4 Overall clinical evaluation of effects of bromocriptine and lisuride on sulpiride-induced hyperprolactinaemia[†]

Lisuride

Patient No.	Secretion A*	Secretion B**	Congestion A	Congestion B	Pain A	Pain B
1	0	0	0	1	0	0
3	2	1	0	0	0	0
4	0	0	0	0	0	0
5	0	0	0	0	0	0
7	0	0	1	0	1	0
8	0	0	0	0	0	0
10	0	0	0	0	0	0
11	0	0	0	0	0	0
12	Dropped out – dizzyness on day 10					
15	2	1	4	1	2	1
18	0	0	0	0	0	0
19	0	0	0	0	0	0
22	0	0	0	0	0	0
23	10	0	0	0	0	0
26	0	0	1	1	0	0
28	0	0	1	0	0	0
29	4	0	2	0	0	0
31	0	0	0	0	0	0
33	0	0	0	0	0	0
37	2	0	2	0	2	0
38	0	0	0	0	0	0
Total	**20**	**2**	**11**	**3**	**5**	**1**

Bromocriptine

Patient No.	Secretion A	Secretion B	Congestion A	Congestion B	Pain A	Pain B
2	3	2	4	2	3	1
6	4	0	0	0	0	0
9	0	0	0	0	0	0
13	0	0	1	0	0	0
14	Dropped out – dizzyness on day 10					
16	0	0	0	0	0	0
17	0	2	0	2	0	0
20	0	0	0	0	0	0
21	0	0	0	0	0	0
24	0	5	0	4	0	4
25	Dropped out – headache on day 10					
27	0	0	0	0	0	0
30	0	0	0	0	0	0
32	0	4	0	3	0	3
34	0	0	2	0	0	0
35	0	0	0	0	0	0
36	Dropped out – stomach ache on day 6					
39	0	0	0	0	0	0
40	3	6	3	6	3	6
41	2	0	1	1	0	0
42	0	0	0	0	0	0
Total	**12**	**19**	**11**	**18**	**6**	**14**

*A is the sum of the scores for the first 15 days (treatment).
**B is the sum of the scores for the last 10 days (rebound).

Score	Milk secretion	Congestion	Pain
0	No milk	None	None
1	Few drops on expression	Mildly or slightly indurated	Mild
2	Abundant on manual expression	Moderately indurated	Moderate
3	Spontaneous stream of milk	Severe	Severe, . requiring analgesics

[†]From reference 19.

According to its direct effect on the prolactin-producing cell, lisuride can lower prolactin levels in all situations, and thereby change or restore biological function. Elevated prolactin levels in women may cause anovulation, premenstrual symptoms, short luteal phases or, at higher levels, amenorrhoea with or without associated galactorrhoea. Prolactin may influence steroid production at the gonadal level, but the most important mechanism by which elevated prolactin levels inhibit gonadal function seems to be due to a change in the pulsatile LHRH secretion from the hypothalamus possibly associated with an altered dopamine turnover. This can be demonstrated by the observation that pulsatile administration of exogenous LHRH is able to restore normal ovulatory cycles and thereby achieves pregnancies even in the presence of greatly elevated prolactin levels. A similar result, however, can better be obtained by lowering elevated prolactin levels using dopamine agonists such as lisuride. Here, within months, normal menstrual cycles and thus pregnancies can be ob-

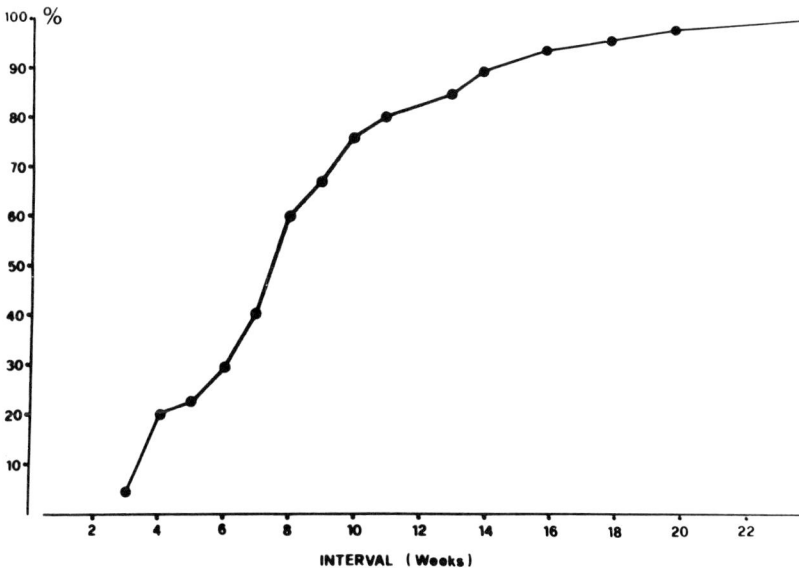

Figure 3 Percentage of 45 amenorrhoeic, hyperprolactinaemic women with return of regular cycles relative to weeks of lisuride treatment. From reference 19

tained (Figure 3)[19]. Owing to the high specificity of lisuride for dopamine receptors, no other hormones are affected by treatment with it.

569

In the treatment of hyperprolactinaemic disorders, one can expect higher prolactin levels (above 100 and particularly above 500 ng ml^{-1}) to be caused by larger pituitary adenomas, which, as a rule, need higher doses of lisuride. Since there are, however, exceptions, and since bioavailability of dopamine agonists varies sometimes considerably, it has become clinical practice to start with low, slowly increasing doses which are given at meals (this also helps to avoid initial side-effects such as nausea) and preferentially in the evening in order to minimize risks caused by orthostatic hypotension which, if it occurs, most often is seen only once after the first effective dosage. If with the standard daily dose of 2–3 × 0.2 mg no sufficient effect on symptomatology and prolactin levels has been achieved, the dosage can be increased at weekly to monthly intervals until prolactin levels and biological function are normalized. Daily doses of lisuride as high as 5.0 mg may be necessary in rare cases of pituitary macroadenomas.

However, in spite of the high success rate of treatment with dopamine agonists in hyperprolactinaemic disorders, treatment should not be started at once when elevated prolactin levels have been detected. A differential diagnosis is necessary which may rule out physiological causes (including lactation, stress, etc.) or, for example, hypothyroidism. In this disease, low peripheral thyroxin levels can result in an enhanced TRH function which not only acts on TSH but also releases prolactin from the anterior pituitary. This type of hyperprolactinaemia, therefore, responds well to thyroid hormone substitution therapy. In addition, drugs that are known to increase prolactin levels (such as metoclopramide, sulpiride, neuroleptics, cimetidine, reserpine and α-methyl-dopa) must be identified and, if possible, withdrawn. Great care must be taken in identifying a pituitary tumour as the cause of hyperprolactinaemia by use of a skull X-ray and, if necessary, CAT scanning. Even if most experts today agree that medical treatment with the dopamine agonists bromocriptine or lisuride is the treatment of choice, there are rare but well-documented cases in the literature where a pregnancy with high oestrogen levels has caused a considerable increase of some of these tumours resulting even in blindness or death. Therefore, particular care has to be taken in women who desire to become pregnant and who have evidence of large adenomas. Monthly visual field examination and prolactin measurements are necessary during pregnancy and women should be advised to refer to a hospital at the earliest clinical signs indicating re-growth of a tumour (e.g. head-aches and visual disturbances), in order to undergo medical treatment or neurosurgical intervention.

No such events, however, have been seen in the more than 100 pregnancies induced by lisuride treatment. Similarly, no adverse effects of lisuride on pregnancy development and outcome have been observed, and particularly no malformations have been reported so

Table 5 Outcome of 118 pregnancies obtained by treatment with lisuride*

Early abortion	21 (17.8%)
Tubal pregnancy	1
Healthy infants	97

*Data on file (Schering).
There were no malformations and the sex ratio was normal.

far (Table 5). Although this number is still too low to draw definite conclusions from, the likelihood of an increased risk is already very low, and the results of the animal studies with lisuride as well as the experience obtained with bromocriptine as the other prolactin-lowering drug of ergot structure seem reassuring. The relatively high percentage of stillbirths observed in our consecutive 118 pregnancies seems to be not too unusual in women with fertility problems, particularly if one considers that treatment with lisuride was, for many of them, a last chance.

Whilst oestrogens rarely may enhance tumour growth, dopamine agonists have been reported to reduce the volume of macroprolactin-omas in a high percentage of cases treated; in agreement with this, and also in confirming animal data as reported above, chronic treatment with lisuride has been shown to lower prolactin levels in patients with pituitary tumours and to restore normal ovulatory cycles, or, in males, libido and potency[21]; clear evidence for tumour shrinkage has also been obtained[22]. It has therefore been proposed to use medical treatment by dopamine agonists in patients with prolactin-producing tumours. However, if neurosurgery is to be performed, pretreatment with lisuride or bromocriptine is quite help-ful and seems to improve the results of surgery. In these as in other conditions, the use of intravenous lisuride may be of value both for treatment and for diagnosis.

In conclusion, lisuride is the most potent dopamine agonist for clinical use that can be used as a prolactin-lowering compound whenever prolactin is involved in the pathophysiology of symptoms and diseases. It is well tolerated and no particular toxicity has been reported. Lisuride (Dopergin) thus can be used as an effective and safe prolactin-lowering and dopamine agonist drug.

References

1. Horowski, R. and Wachtel, H. (1976). Direct dopaminergic action of lisuride hydrogen maleate, an ergot derivative, in mice. *Eur. J. Pharmacol.*, **36**, 373
2. Podvalovà, I. and Dlabac, A. (1972). Lysenyl, a new antiserotonin agent. *Res. Clin. Stud. Headache*, **3**, 325
3. Pieri, L., Keller, H. H., Burkard, W. and Da Prada, M. (1978). Effects of lisuride and LSD on cerebral monoamine systems and hallucinosis. *Nature (Lond.)*, **272**, 278
4. Reynolds, G. P. and Riederer, P. (1981). The effects of lisuride and some other dopaminergic agonists on receptor binding in human brain. *J. Neural Transm.*, **51**, 107
5. Peroutka, S. J., Lebovitz, R. M. and Snyder, S. H. (1981). Two distinct central serotonin receptors with different physiological functions. *Science*, **212**, 827
6. Rogawski, M. A. and Aghajanian, G. K. (1979). Response of central monoaminergic neurons to lisuride: comparison with LSD. *Life Sci.*, **24**, 1289
7. Horowski, R. (1982). Role of monoaminergic mechanisms in the mechanism of action of ergot derivatives used in migraine. In Rose, F. C. (ed.). *Advances in Migraine*, pp. 187–198. (New York: Raven Press)
8. Loos, D., Halbhübner, K. and Herken, H. (1977). Lisuride, a potent drug in the treatment of muscular rigidity in rats. *Naunyn-Schmiedeberg's Arch. Pharmacol.*, **300**, 195
9. Horowski, R. (1978). Differences in the dopaminergic effects of the ergot derivatives bromocriptine, lisuride and d-LSD as compared with apomorphine. *Eur. J. Pharmacol*, **51**, 157
10. Calne, D., Horowski, R., McDonald, R. J. and Wuttke, W. (eds.) (1983). *Lisuride and Other Dopamine Agonists*. (New York: Raven Press)
11. Horowski, R. and Dorow, R. (1981). Influence of estradiol and other gonadal steroids on central effects of lisuride and comparable ergot derivatives. In Wuttke, W. and Horowski, R. (eds.). *Gonadal Steroids and Brain Function*, pp. 169–181. (Berlin: Springer Verlag)
12. Ahlenius, S., Larsson, K. and Svensson, L. (1980). Stimulating effects of lisuride on masculine sexual behaviour of rats. *Eur. J. Pharmacol.*, **64**, 47
13. Cronin, M. J., Valdenegro, C. A., Perkins, S. N. and MacLeod, R. M. (1981). The 7315a pituitary tumor is refractory to dopaminergic inhibition of prolactin release but contains dopamine receptors. *Endrocrinology*, **109**, 2160
14. Ausková, M., Rezábek, K., Zikán, V. and Semonský, M. (1974). Suppression of lactation in rats with lysenyl(R) SPOFA (N-(D-6-methyl-8-isoergolenyl) N', N'-diethylcarbamide hydrogen maleate). *Endocrinol. Exp.*, **8**, 51
15. Horowski, R. (1982). Some aspects of the dopaminergic action of ergot derivatives and their role in the treatment of migraine. In Critchley, M., *et al.* (eds.). *Advances in Neurology*, Vol. **33**, pp. 325–340. (New York: Raven Press)
16. Hümpel, M., Nieuweboer, B., Hasan, S. H. and Wendt, H. (1981). Radioimmuno-

assay of plasma lisuride in man following intravenous and oral administration of lisuride hydrogen maleate; effects on plasma prolactin level. *Eur. J. Clin. Pharmacol.*, **20,** 47

17. Hardt, W., Schmid-Gollwitzer, M. and Horowski, R. (1979). Suppression of lactation with lisuride. *Gynecol. Obstet. Invest.*, **10,** 95
18. van Dam, L. H. and Rolland, R. (1981). Lactation-inhibiting and prolactin-lowering effect of lisuride and bromocriptine: A comparative study. *Eur. J. Obstet. Gynecol. Reprod. Biol.*, **12,** 323
19. De Cecco, L., Venturini, P. L., Ragni, N., Valenzano, M., Constantini, S. and Horowski, R. (1983). Dopaminergic ergots in lactation and cycle disturbances. In Calne, D. B., Horowski, R., McDonald, R. J. and Wuttke, W. (eds.). *Lisuride and Other Dopamine Agonists*, pp. 291–299. (New York: Raven Press)
20. Schwibbe, M., Becker, D. and Wuttke, W. (1983). EEG and psychological effects of lisuride in women with premenstrual tension. In Calne, D. B., Horowski, R., McDonald, R. J. and Wuttke, W. (eds.). *Lisuride and Other Dopamine Agonists*, pp. 345–355. (New York: Raven Press)
21. Verde, G., Chiodini, P. G., Liuzzi, A., *et al.* (1980). Effectiveness of the dopamine agonist lisuride in the treatment of acromegaly and pathological hyperprolactinemic states. *J. Endocrinol. Invest.*, **4,** 405
22. Chiodini, P., Liuzzi, A., Cozzi, R., *et al.* (1981). Size reduction of macroprolactinomas by bromocriptine or lisuride treatment. *J. Clin. Endocrinol. Metab.*, **53,** 737

61
Benefits and risks of hormonal contraception – interpretation

M. SMITH

ABSTRACT

The pill is undoubtedly one of the greatest and most efficient of medical advances. In 1976 in the UK 3.5 million women took the pill but following adverse publicity linked to often misinterpreted findings of the report from the RCGP this number decreased by 600 000. Caution should certainly be taken in those over 35 years who smoke but general acceptance of all possible side-effects without informed interpretation is not in the best interests of patients. Happily, recent advances in pill dosage and formulation together with follow-up studies from the RCGP, have suggested there is no new overall increased risk in the long term and that there may be benefits due to the pill decreasing the incidence of benign breast disease, cancer, cysts of the ovary and PID. From the low level of up-take of 2.8 million in 1979, by 1982 approximately 3.3 million in the UK are again taking the pill. The lost 500 000 have returned and it is likely that 3.35 million women will be taking it in 1983. This trend can, however, only continue where there is a forward looking family planning service particularly among the young and deprived. Patients must be actively sought out and walk-in service for all methods currently used must be provided. We must continue to restore confidence in the pill as we are unlikely to have anything better as a contraceptive agent if at all until the next century.

In the relatively minor controversies that occur concerning what must undoubtedly be one of the greatest medical advances ever – the birth pill – it is the daily practice of clinicians on being consulted by women taking the pill that provides clinicians with their confidence in the method.

We should never forget that interpretation is the key word that may be vital for the well-being of our patients. It is the clinicians who put the latest scientific report into perspective.

The pill is a topical subject. In my office at home, in the space of a few months, photocopies of articles written both 'for' but slightly more often 'against' the pill and other birth-control methods that have appeared in the national and local press and women's magazines have produced a pile, inches high. To read some of the more sensational articles gives me cause to wonder whether the writer has discovered new methods, since they often do not sound like those used by the vast majority of people that I deal with; but they are. The writer's interpretation, however, is different.

The fact is that the pill is probably the most efficient medicine we have ever known. That is easy to interpret. It is virtually 100% effective in preventing pregnancy, but this rarely gets mentioned.

The often finer effects of the pill that are discussed in the following chapters are based on the author's precise scientific research and observations. The interpretation of these results and their practical effect, or the lack of it upon women, needs to be interpreted by others with specialist knowledge – both epidemiological and practical.

Later chapters will be describing the effect that the pill has upon the levels of fat in a woman's blood. It will be explained, where relevant, that most often what we are really dealing with is the significance of these biochemical findings.

If misinterpreted, these findings can have an unnecessary and alarming effect upon the confidence of the users, not to mention the destruction it may cause to their personal relationships. It may lead them to change from one method to another, away from the one they really want to use, to a method that they may not be motivated towards and will therefore use less effectively, with possibly disastrous results in terms of an unwanted pregnancy at worst, and at best a lessening in the quality of their lives.

To see the magnitude of such effects I would like to point out a few basic facts. In retrospect, the cause and effect seem obvious though the details will always be open to discussion. In 1976 there were in the United Kingdom 3½ million women taking the pill. In 1977 a respected body of researchers from the Royal College of General Practitioners published a report, the most notable and practical conclusions of which were that the excess mortality due to the pill increased with age, cigarette smoking and duration of pill usage. By 1979 there were 600 000 fewer women taking the pill. I remember that, together with colleagues from the Family Planning Association, I did some sums at the time and concluded that if women over 35 years of age alone had been advised to take heed of the signposts to safer pill taking that the RCG Report offered, then almost one half of the women who fled from the pill having had their confidence shaken need not have done so. There were only some 350 000 women at most who were taking the pill and who were over 35. If personal symptoms suffered were the reasons why the others stopped taking the pill, then it is understandable that the women would want to change. But as those of us with chemical experience know, those symptoms, too, vary with the confidence that a women has in her chosen method. Caution on the part of the doctor prescribing for those who are over 35 and who smoke is the main and justifiable inference to be taken from those RCGP findings which were published in a journal aimed at the medical profession, the *Lancet*. In medical affairs, such statistically based facts will usually require personal articulation for the person most concerned – the patient – if she is to be best served. A general acceptance of facts, without informed interpretation, will not be in the best interests of a minority of patients.

One small but definite example of my message is presented in the *Lancet* on October 30th 1982, again by the RCGP, based on their oral contraceptive study. In summary it reads 'previous studies of gall bladder disease provided strong evidence of increased incidence associated with the use of oral contraceptives.' This present study suggests that there is no overall increased risk in the long term and that the previously demonstrated disease occurs *only* in women who are susceptible to it. The acceleration may be associated with the dose of oestrogen in the oral contraceptive. It is perhaps unfortunate that women who would be happy to take the pill were it not for the diminished confidence medical reports can induce when they are given inappropriate publicity, regard themselves as unhappy contraceptors. They are worried women, or worse still they are forced, unwantedly, into motherhood. In both instances it is more often the other methods of contraception that wrongly get the blame. The

577

woman is understandably less happy with them than she would be with the method she really wants to use. The wisest interpretation of that report might have been to follow the implied advice in favour of using the lowest effective dose.

But what about the benefits of the pill? I am going to expand a little on a few of them and largely quote from an article by Howard Ory – the epidemiologist – in the July/August 1982 issue of *Family Planning Perspectives*. He points out that in the United States alone 50 000 hospital admissions are prevented each year due to the beneficial effects the pill has on women taking it. Benign breast diseases are prevented as well as cancer that would otherwise have occurred in the reproductive systems of those women. 50 000 women: if only those individuals were able to know that it was the pill that could have saved them surgery, we might be witnessing a rise in pro-pill pressure groups!

Those of us who have seen the anxieties caused to women with a breast lump in the days they have to wait to consult a surgeon, with the fear of an operation heavy on their minds, can take heart from the fact that of those of our patients who are on the pill, three out of four will not have to suffer that experience.

Cysts of the ovary, too, are affected beneficially by taking the pill, reducing again the need for surgical operations that would otherwise have been necessary. It is estimated that some 3000 such operations are prevented in the United States each year among women who are taking the pill. Further, pill-users have only half the chance of suffering from anaemia, as well as pelvic inflammatory disease which causes pelvic pain and often continual suffering. The pill may prevent pelvic inflammatory disease in two out of three women who would otherwise get it.

The low-dose pills including the pill with three different dose phases throughout a woman's cycle – the triphasics – together with others first introduced around 1980 allow a woman, these days, to take in a whole month less hormone than she would have taken in a day 20 or more years ago and still afford almost 100% protection against pregnancy. A 95% reduction in dosage while still maintaining efficiency; I find that quite amazing.

The outcome of much misinterpretation about the scientific data on the pill has happily not influenced the pill-taking habits of the bulk of the women in the UK for too long. They have been flocking in their hundreds of thousands back to the pill. From the low level of uptake, 2.8 million women in 1979, and with the introduction and rapidly growing popularity of triphasic pills in 1980 as well as other low-dosed pills, we are now able to see that about 3.3 million women have again taken the pill during 1982. The lost 500 000 have returned. It is likely that 3 350 000 women will be taking it in 1983, another 50 000.

On behalf of our patients, what we ask of our research colleagues is that in the more open medical climate in which we now live, we all work towards communicating clearly those results that justifiably call for a change in practice, noting specifically, for instance, that the older woman who smokes is especially at risk, so that we can try to protect her from the harm that her smoking habit may cause.

The real risks of not taking the pill when nothing else is acceptable is of course the risk of an unwanted pregnancy. This single risk can make biochemical discussions like those given in the rest of this book, which enlarge upon the potential, theoretical, risks of taking the pill, seem so thin as not to be in the same league at all.

In April last year the Chairman of the Family Planning Association, John Dunwoody, himself a general practitioner as well as being a Chairman of a Health Authority, wrote to all the chairmen of the health authorities and pointed out that despite very marked improvements in the introduction of free family planning, there is still a long way to go. And this is in the UK where we don't face the cultural difficulties of our colleagues in Ireland.

High levels of unwanted pregnancies and abortions continue to be acknowledged as a severe problem. The huge costs of unwanted social and other services including education and housing are often hidden and therefore generally unacknowledged. None the less, with an estimated 200 000 unwanted pregnancies annually in the UK spread across some 300 health authorities, financial as well as health implications for each district cannot be ignored. In particular it is among the young and the deprived that a forward-looking family planning service can do most to help prevent the unwanted pregnancies and abortions that otherwise follow. Recent US research shows that family planning provision can save twice its cost in related health and welfare services every year.

The advantages of providing a contraceptive service are well covered in a series of articles published between October 1981 and October 1982 in the *British Journal of Family Planning*.

Dr Moulds, from general practice in the UK points out that the

NHS family planning service is mainly attracting patients who are highly motivated. He believes it will not be a successful service until it attracts a considerable proportion of those who are at present unmotivated. He suggests that as well as providing a comprehensive and up-to-date family planning service, a general practitioner must actively seek out patients. From the consumer point of view it is a walk-in service rather than an appointment system that attracts them to the clinics in preference to the modern-day general practice surgery. Obviously, women with unwanted conceptions will frequently be referred to hospital, so it is vitally important perhaps that there the first opportunity for a discussion about contraception with a doctor who is motivated and well versed in the subject should be available.

My main plea is that we should continue to restore confidence in the pill, the greatest method of contraception we have ever had. We are most unlikely to have anything appreciably better, if at all, before the next century. Confidence should be expressed also in the other methods currently used. Motivation, that most important aspect of contraception, needs to exist amongst the professionals and other staff themselves and be passed on to the user. In recent years Governments have constantly put forward the philosophy that prevention is better than cure. A case can be made that family planning is fundamental to preventive medicine and is the foundation upon which any health programme will rest if it is to succeed.

62
Towards safer oral contraception

C. R. KAY

ABSTRACT

The large size of the Royal College of General Practitioners' Oral Contraception Study enables the risk to users to be estimated with increased precision. It is now clear that non-smokers may safely use oral contraceptives beyond the age of 40 years, especially if brands with low-progestogen activity are prescribed. There is no longer convincing evidence that duration of use contributes materially to the risk. However, for cigarette smokers it would normally be unwise to continue use after the age of 35 years, unless they stop smoking.

Recent publications from the Royal College of General Practitioners' Oral Contraception Study have analysed the association of oral contraceptive (OC) usage with vascular diseases – both total[1] and fatal[2]. These data support and extend similar observations from other studies[3].

All analyses show that the risk is substantially confined to cigarette smokers over the age of 35 years. Thus, in the age group 35–44 years the excess mortality risk is 1 in 2000 users each year in smokers (a statistically significant excess) while in non-smokers the risk is much less at 1 in 6700 users per annum, and this estimate does not differ significantly from the risk in non-pill users.

Unlike previous analyses of mortality published in 1977[4], there is now no evidence of a relationship to duration of use. There is a suggestion from the mortality data that the increased risk of vascular disease may persist after OCs have been stopped. The analyses of total incidence of arterial disease show that this apparent risk in former users is confined to cerebrovascular disease and that the increased occurrence persists for at least 6 years. However, the risk is small and since it has not been observed in other studies it must be regarded as a hypothesis that requires confirmation. There is also weak evidence that the occurrence of cerebrovascular disease in OC users may be related to duration of use, but the trend is not statistically significant and also requires confirmation in other studies. The study was unable to confirm the observation of Slone and colleagues[5] that the risk of myocardial infarction was related to duration of OC use.

Because relative risks of vascular disease mortality in OC users were generally higher than for vascular disease incidence, there is an implication that case-fatality rates may be higher in OC users. This was shown to be true, but is entirely due to the high case-fatality rate in OC users who smoke cigarettes. This rate is double that in OC users who do not smoke, and in non-OC users whether they smoke or not. This further demonstrates the crucial influence of cigarette smoking on the safety of oral contraception.

All these estimates of risk are based on a population of women who have used a wide range of OCs, many containing higher doses of steroids than are currently used. The demonstration of the progestogen dose dependency of the risk of arterial disease associated with OC usage[6–10] means that if brands are used with a low level of progestogen activity, the risks are likely to be materially lower. Thus, the use of low-dose progestogen brands and the careful exclusion from oral contraception of the small minority of women who have an increased risk of vascular disease will allow the great majority of women to use the pill with remarkable safety.

References

1. Royal College of General Practitioners' Oral Contraception Study. (1983). Incidence of arterial disease among oral contraceptive users. *J. R. Coll. Gen. Pract.*, **33**, 75
2. Royal College of General Practitioners' Oral Contraception Study. (1981). Further analyses of mortality in oral contraceptive users. *Lancet*, **1**, 541
3. Vessey, M. P. (1980). Female hormones and vascular disease – an epidemiological overview. *Br. J. Fam. Plan.*, Suppl. **6**, 1

4. Royal College of General Practitioners' Oral Contraception Study. (1977). Mortality among oral contraceptive users. *Lancet*, **2**, 727

5. Slone, D., Shapiro, S., Kaufman, D. W. and Rosenberg, L. (1981). Risk of myocardial infarction in relation to current and discontinued oral contraceptive use. *N. Engl. J. Med.*, **305**, 420

6. Royal College of General Practitioners' Oral Contraception Study. (1977). Effect on hypertension and benign breast disease of progestogen component in combined oral contraceptives. *Lancet*, **1**, 624

7. Khaw, K-T. and Peart, W. S. (1982). Blood pressure and contraceptive use. *Br. Med. J.*, **285**, 403

8. Kay, C. R. (1980). The happiness pill? *J. R. Coll. Gen. Pract.*, **30**, 8

9. Meade, T. W., Greenberg, G. and Thompson, S. G. (1980). Progestogens and cardiovascular reactions associated with oral contraceptives and a comparison of the safety of 50- and 30-μg oestrogen preparations. *Br. Med. J.*, **280**, 1157

10. Kay, C. R. (1982). Progestogens and arterial disease – evidence from the Royal College of General Practitioners' study. *Am. J. Obstet. Gynecol.*, **142**, 762

63

The influence of the triphasic pill and a desogestrel-containing combination pill on some physical, biochemical and hormonal parameters: a preliminary report

C. P. Th. SCHIJF, C. M. G. THOMAS, P. N. M. DEMACKER, W. H. DOESBURG and R. ROLLAND

SUMMARY

The triphasic pill contains the lowest dose of progestogens given per cycle. The recently introduced desogestrel-containing combination pill is claimed to have less androgenic side-effects than combination pills containing levonorgestrel. A better comparison would be between the triphasic pill and the desogestrel-containing pill. This is the purpose of this report. The following items were measured during the follicular and luteal phase of a control cycle and during the third week of pill intake of both the third and sixth pill cycle: body-weight, blood pressure, total cholesterol, HDL-cholesterol, fasting triglycerides and testosterone. Blood glucose and insulin levels were measured during a glucose tolerance test at the beginning and the end of the study. Body-weight increased and blood pressure remained unchanged during the control cycle. Both pill types had no influence on these parameters. Total cholesterol, HDL-cholesterol and fasting triglycerides showed no significant changes during the control cycle or during pill intake except for a significant decrease of total cholesterol in the desogestrel group. The triphasic pill did not alter the glucose or insulin response to glucose. In the desogestrel group both these responses increased significantly. Testosterone increased significantly during the control cycle but no significant changes were observed during pill intake in both groups. It is concluded that the observed changes in biochemical and hormonal parameters are minor and only reach the level of significance in the desogestrel group.

INTRODUCTION

Since the introduction of oral contraceptives continuous efforts have been made to reduce both the oestrogen and progestogen content per pill. Also, more specific progestogens have been introduced like levonorgestrel. A drawback of the low-dose oral contraceptives has been the decreased cycle control, with increased intermenstrual bleeding.

The recently introduced triphasic formula with 40% less levonorgestrel as compared with sub-50 oral contraceptives containing this progestogen does not have this disadvantage: despite the low dose of progestogens its cycle control and overall tolerance are excellent[1].

In 1981 Marvelon was introduced. This sub-50 oral contraceptive contains desogestrel – a new progestogen, which has been claimed to be a more specific progestogen than levonorgestrel with less androgenic residual effects[2].

From the data presented so far it can be questioned whether these findings, often based on receptor studies, have any significant clinical relevance. Futhermore, a comparison between Marvelon and a triphasic formula like Trigynon would be more appropriate since the triphasic formula can be considered as a breakthrough in the search for the best oral contraceptive.

Finally, many reports in the literature are uncritical in the definition of the control group. The aim of the present, preliminary report is to evaluate very carefully in a limited number of healthy women physical, hormonal and biochemical findings during the normal menstrual cycle and then to compare these with the same findings during intake of either Trigynon or Marvelon.

MATERIALS AND METHODS

Women who visited the outpatient department asking for oral contraception were informed about the study design. If no contraindications for the use of oral contraceptives were found and if the woman gave informed consent, she was selected for the study. During a control cycle during the early follicular and late luteal phases body-weight, blood pressure, total cholesterol, HDL-cholesterol, fasting triglycerides, serum testosterone and testosterone in saliva values were measured. Then at random each women received either Trigynon or Marvelon which was continued for at least 6 months. During the third week of pill intake (maximal effect of the pill) in the third and sixth cycle the above-mentioned measurements were repeated. A glucose tolerance test was also performed in each woman during the early follicular phase of the cycle and repeated during the third week of the sixth pill cycle. 50 g of glucose were given and at 0, 10, 20, 30, 60 and 90 minutes both glucose and insulin were measured. All blood and saliva samples were taken at 09.00 a.m. (fasting) and the glucose tolerance tests also started at 09.00 a.m. All hormonal and biochemical measurements were performed by specific, precise and accurate means[3,4]. Statistical evaluation of the data was performed with Student's t test for the paired case comparing data from the early follicular phase of the cycle with those obtained in the same woman during the late luteal phase or during pill intake. Although it is our intention to study 30 women, 15 in each group, so far only 11 cases are ready for complete evaluation and their results will be presented.

Table 1 Body-weight (in kg) during the early follicular (EF) and late luteal (LL) phases of the menstrual cycle and during the third week of pill intake in the third and sixth pill cycle (3 OAC, 6 OAC). Control is the two subgroups together during the menstrual cycle

Regimen	EF	LL	3 OAC	6 OAC
Trigynon*	60.8±3.2	61.1±3.2	60.3±3.7	61.3±3.4
Marvelon*	62.0±1.1	62.4±1.3	61.6±1.3	61.2±1.4
Control**	61.4±5.8[+]	61.7±5.8[+]		

*Mean ±SE.
**Mean ±SD.
[+]Values significantly different at $p = 0.005$.

RESULTS

Table 1 depicts body-weight during the control cycle and during the intake of either Trigynon or Marvelon. Body-weight increases significantly during the cycle. However, no influence on this parameter can be seen during pill intake compared with the early follicular phase. Table 2 shows systolic and diastolic blood pressure: no

Table 2 Blood pressure (in mmHg) during a control cycle and during intake of either Trigynon or Marvelon. Results are given as means ±SE

Phase of cycle	Trigynon		Marvelon	
	Systolic	Diastolic	Systolic	Diastolic
Early follicular	115 ±3.5	79.5±2.7	112 ±2.4	63 ±4.0
Late luteal	118 ±2.7	77.7±3.2	111.6±3.2	64 ±4.0
3 OAC*	114.6±6.0	72.4±4.1	112.0±2.3	63.2±3.4
6 OAC*	120 ±6.6	77.2±3.9	117 ±4.8	67.8±2.7

*Values determined during third week of pill intake in third (3 OAC) and sixth pill (6 OAC) cycle.

significant changes were observed during the normal cycle, nor during pill intake. Table 3 gives fasting triglyceride, total cholesterol, and HDL-cholesterol concentrations during the normal cycle and during pill intake. Fasting triglyceride values are significantly increased during the third Marvelon cycle. Both Trigynon and Marvelon tend to decrease total cholesterol value whereas no influence on

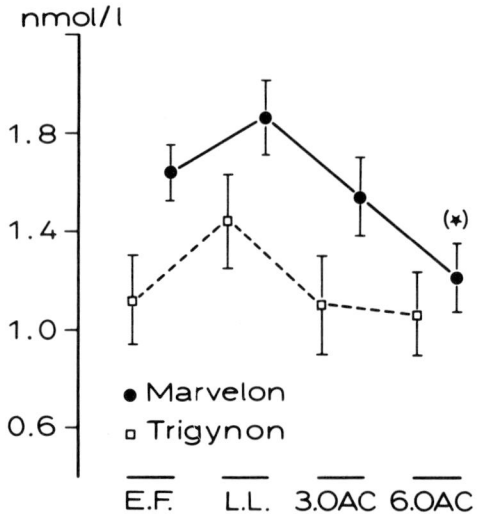

Figure 1 Serum testosterone levels (in nmol l^{-1}) in women using Trigynon or Marvelon during a control cycle and during pill intake. Values are shown as means ±SE. (*) Difference between values significant: $0.1 > p > 0.05$.
EF = Early follicular phase; LL = late luteal phase; 3 OAC = value during third week of third cycle; 6 OAC = value during third week of sixth cycle

Table 3 Fasting triglyceride, total cholesterol and HDL-cholesterol values during the control cycle and during intake of either Trigynon or Marvelon. Results are given as means ±SE. Control is the two subgroups together

Regimen	I Early follicular	II Late luteal	III 3 OAC*	IV 6 OAC*	p value I-II	I-III	I-IV
Triglyceride (mmol l⁻¹)							
Trigynon	0.66±0.18	1.09±0.20	0.84±0.15	0.98±0.38	0.06	0.21	0.52
Marvelon	1.22±0.13	1.02±0.21	1.82±0.12	1.31±0.19	0.36	0.002	0.55
Control	0.92±0.14	1.33±0.12			0.32		
Total cholesterol (mmol l⁻¹)							
Trigynon	4.56±0.34	4.42±0.30	4.02±0.22	3.91±0.34	0.57	0.27	0.07
Marvelon	5.11±0.34	4.47±0.24	4.81±0.24	4.43±0.33	0.38	0.30	0.04
Control	4.81±0.24	4.44±0.22			0.26		
HDL-cholesterol (mmol l⁻¹)							
Trigynon	1.62±0.18	1.49±0.18	1.53±0.14	1.48±0.15	0.05	0.04	0.15
Marvelon	1.09±0.11	1.14±0.12	1.17±0.06	1.21±0.05	0.30	0.46	0.28
Control	1.38±0.13	1.33±0.12			0.31		

* Values determined during third week of pill intake in third (3 OAC) and sixth pill (6 OAC) cycle.

HDL-cholesterol is seen. No cyclic changes in these parameters are found.

Figure 1 shows the serum testosterone values. In both groups there is a tendency to higher testosterone levels during the late luteal phase. If the control cycles of the two groups are combined this difference is highly significant ($p = 0.003$). During the sixth month of Marvelon serum testosterone level is somewhat lower than during the early follicular phase ($p = 0.08$). All testosterone levels during pill intake are within the normal cyclic range and in general lower than during the late luteal phase of the cycle.

Testosterone in saliva gives much the same picture as testosterone in serum does: lower levels are obtained during pill intake in both

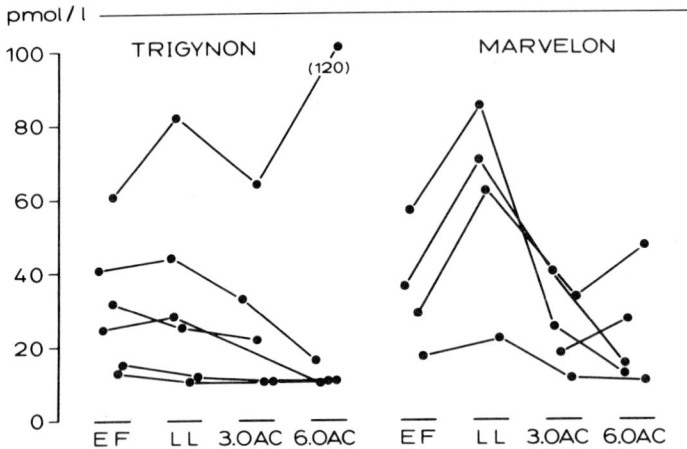

Figure 2 Saliva testosterone levels (in pmol l^{-1}) in women using Trigynon or Marvelon during a control cycle and during pill intake. Individual values are given.
EF = Early follicular phase; LL = late luteal phase; 3 OAC = value during third week of third cycle; 6 OAC = value during third week of sixth cycle

the Marvelon and the Trigynon groups (Figure 2). Since in both groups some values are missing, no statistical evaluation has been carried out between cyclic and pill results. If the data from all the control cycles until so far are combined ($n = 15$) then a highly significant increase ($p = 0.003$) is seen in the late luteal as compared with the early follicular phase of the cycle.

Figures 3 and 4 depict the serum glucose and insulin responses to 50 g glucose orally. In the Trigynon group there was a small ($p = 0.06$) increase in fasting glucose levels. In the Marvelon group this is less obvious, whereas the glucose response as calculated as the area under the curve in this group increases significantly ($p = 0.04$). Also, fasting insulin levels ($p = 0.001$) and the insulin responses to glucose ($p = 0.005$) deteriorate during Marvelon use. However, the observed changes are still well within the normal range for healthy women.

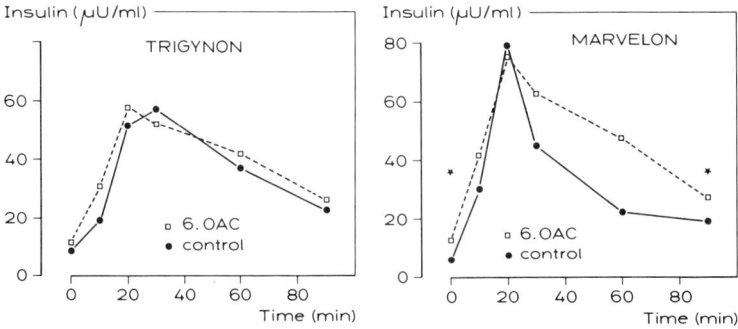

Figure 3 Blood glucose levels (mean ±SE) after 50 g glucose load (by mouth) during early follicular phase of control cycle and during treatment with Trigynon or Marvelon (third week of the six cycle 6 OAC). Difference between control and experimental values significant: (*)$0.1 > p > 0.05$; *$p < 0.05$

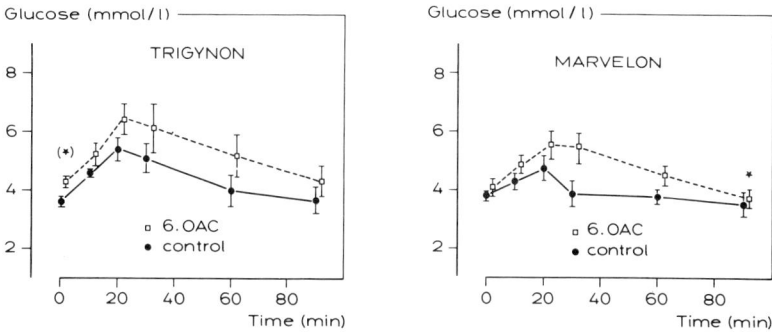

Figure 4 Mean serum insulin levels after 50 g glucose load (by mouth) during a control cycle and during intake of Trigynon or Marvelon (in third week of sixth cycle). * Difference between control and experimental values significant at $p < 0.05$. For further details, see the text

DISCUSSION

This study has so far demonstrated that all studies dealing with physical, biochemical and hormonal effects of oral contraceptives should have a well-defined group of normal, cyclic women as control.

Both body-weight and testosterone change during the cycle and if the late luteal phase is taken as reference point, most pill types will show a decrease both in serum testosterone and in testosterone in saliva.

Both total cholesterol and HDL-cholesterol do not change significantly during the normal cycle or during Trigynon – or Marvelon administration. Although no changes in HDL-cholesterol are seen during the cycle, this parameter does show significant changes in women used to physical exercise as compared with values in controls. This fact must also be taken into account when studies dealing with effects brought about by the intake of oral contraceptives are evaluated. The observed increase in fasting triglycerides during the third month of Marvelon use should be regarded with caution. Especially this parameter shows an intraindividual variation of 30% and the observed difference may very well be accidental[5].

Serum testosterone (total testosterone) and saliva testosterone (more a measure for free testosterone) values do not change during Trigynon or Marvelon intake if compared with the early follicular phase of the normal cycle, whereas the values are decreased if compared with the late luteal phase. Therefore, little or no differences are present between the examined pill types concerning influence on androgen metabolism.

Trigynon has little or no influence on glucose metabolism, whereas both glucose and insulin responses deteriorate significantly during Marvelon use. This has also been observed by others[6]. Although the change in the glucose response in general is thought to be brought about by oestrogens, the change in the insulin response is more complex and is also to be seen as an effect brought about by progestogens.

In conclusion, therefore, it cannot be decided solely from this study or studies measuring the same parameters which of these two pill types should be preferentially prescribed since all induced changes are well within the normal range. The triphasic pill, however, gives a significantly better cycle control as compared with combination pills like Marvelon (see Chapter 7) and this fact in general favours the use of this oral contraceptive.

Acknowledgements

We are grateful to Miss M. de Groot for her secretarial assistance. The insulin levels were measured in the laboratory for chemical and experimental endocrinology (head Professor Th. Benraad), St. Radboud University Hospital.

References

1. Zador, G. (1982). Clinical performance of a triphasic administration of ethinyl estradiol and levonorgestrel in comparison with the 30 + 150 μg fixed-dose regime. In Haspels, A. A. and Rolland, R. (eds.). *Benefits and Risks of Hormonal Contraception*, pp. 43–55. (Lancaster: MTP Press)
2. Viinikka, L. (1978). Biological effects and metabolism of ORG 2969, a new synthetic progestagen, in man. Acta Universitatis Ouluensis Series D, Medica no. 38, Clinica Chemica nr. 3.
3. Demacker, P. N. M., Schade, R. W. B., Jansen, R. T. P. and van 't Laar, A. (1982). Intra-individual variation of serum cholesterol, triglycerides and high density lipoprotein cholesterol in normal humans. *Atherosclerosis*, **45**, 259
4. Thomas, C. M. G. and Rolland, R. (1983). Methods of measurements of testosterone in serum and saliva as performed in our laboratory will be published in the final report.
5. Demacker, P. N. M., Hijmans, A. G. M., Vos-Jansen, H. E., van 't Laar, A. and Jansen, A. P. (1980). A study of the use of polyethylene glycol in estimating cholesterol in high density lipoprotein. *Clin. Chem.*, **26/13**, 1775
6. Briggs, M. H. (1982). Comparative investigation of oral contraceptives using randomized, prospective protocols. In Haspels, A. A. and Rolland R. (eds.). *Benefits and Risks of Hormonal Contraception*, pp. 115–30. (Lancaster: MTP Press)

64
Clinical comparison between a monophasic preparation and a triphasic preparation

U. LACHNIT-FIXSON, S. AYDINLIK and J. LEHNERT

ABSTRACT

The triphasic preparation containing 6 coated tablets of 0.05 mg levonorgestrel (LN) + 0.03 mg ethinyloestradiol (EE), 5 coated tablets of 0.075 mg LN + 0.04 mg EE and 10 coated tablets of 0.125 mg LN + 0.03 mg EE (Triquilar®/Logynon®) was compared in a randomized multicentre trial with a monophasic combined pill composed of 0.15 mg desogestrel + 0.03 mg ethinyloestradiol (Marvelon®).

The main purpose of this study – planned for 6 treatment cycles – was to elucidate possible differences in cycle stability, i.e. the incidence of spotting and breakthrough bleeding episodes and failure of withdrawal bleeding to occur. A total of 555 women were enrolled and completed 3060 cycles. In a randomized fashion 278 of the volunteers were assigned to the triphasic preparation (preparation 1), and 277 to the monophasic combination (preparation 2). 84.5% of the women completed the six months treatment period on both preparations. However, whereas only 6.1% of triphasic takers discontinued medication prematurely because of medical reasons (side-effects), 11.9% of the women on the monophasic preparations did so, mainly because of bleeding irregularities. Calculated in terms of the total number of triphasic cycles the spotting rate was 6.4%, the BTB rate 1.2%. In 0.4% of all cycles spotting + BTB were recorded in the

same cycle. The corresponding figures for the monophasic preparation are as follows: spotting 16.5%, BTB 2.8% and spotting + BTB for
the same cycles 1.1%. The amenorrhoea rate was 0.2% for the triphasic
and 0.9% for the monophasic preparation.

All differences were statistically highly significant (Chi-square
test) and not only confined to the beginning of medication, but also
present in the 6th treatment cycle. Spotting rates in cycles 1 + 2 for
preparation 1 = 10.9%, for preparation 2 = 28.5%; in cycle 6 for
preparation 1 = 2.6%, for preparation 2 = 10.3%. BTB rates in cycles
1 + 2 for 1 = 2.0%, for 2 = 6.7%; in cycle 6 for 1 = 0.4%, for 2 =
2.2%.

Another interesting difference between the two preparations concerned body-weight, which remained constant in 75.2% of the triphasic users, but in only 61.1% of the monophasic users. Minor
weight gains (+<2 kg) occurred in 11.3% of women taking preparation 1 and in 15.4% of women on preparation 2. Only 5.2% of
the triphasic users versus 16.7% of the women on the monophasic
combination had gained more than 2 kg after 6 months. These differences were also statistically highly significant.

Conclusion

Though it has been claimed that desogestrel has a higher progestogenic activity than levonorgestrel the triphasic levonorgestrel-
contraceptive – which contains 40% less progestogen (1.925 mg) than
the monophasic desogestrel-combination (3.15 mg) – provides a much
better cycle control. Increase in body-weight occurs significantly
more often in users of the desogestrel combination.

INTRODUCTION

There can no longer be any doubt that oral contraceptives containing
low amounts of oestrogen *and* progestogen have less influence on
parameters of the haemostatic system and metabolic functions than
do high-dose preparations[1-3]. Therefore, their use is to be recommended, as WHO already have in 1978[4].

However, it is well known that a high rate of spotting and breakthrough bleeding may limit the acceptability of low-dose
contraception. The triphasic approach seems to avoid this dilemma. It
has been clearly demonstrated in two carefully conducted controlled

trials that the triphasic preparation Logynon provides significantly better cycle stability than Microgynon 30 though this monophasic preparation contains 40% more levonorgestrel than the triphasic product[5,6].

In 1981 Marvelon, a monophasic preparation containing 150 μg of the new progestogen desogestrel and 30 μg ethinyloestradiol was introduced in several European countries. Desogestrel has been claimed[7] to have higher progestational activity and fewer androgenic residual effects than levonorgestrel.

The aim of the present study was to assess the overall tolerance, principally in terms of cycle control, of this new monophasic preparation in comparison with the triphasic levonorgestrel-containing pill (Table 1).

Table 1 Composition of trial preparations

Marvelon	Triquilar (Logynon)
0.150 mg desogestrel 0.03 mg ethinyloestradiol	6 coated tablets: 0.05 mg levonorgestrel 0.03 mg ethinyloestradiol
	5 coated tablets: 0.075 mg levonorgestrel 0.04 mg ethinyloestradiol
	10 coated tablets: 0.125 mg levonorgestrel 0.03 mg ethinyloestradiol

In order to establish statistically significant differences between the two preparations the planning design for the study required the inclusion of a minimum of 200–250 women per trial group for a period of six cycles.

MATERIALS AND METHODS

The multicentre comparative trial between the two preparations was conducted in Austria, Germany, the Netherlands and the UK. Both clinics and gynaecologists in private practice participated in the trial. A total of 555 women were enrolled and followed up for six treatment cycles. The participants were allocated to the two treatment groups in a randomized fashion, 278 to the triphasic and 277 to the monophasic preparation. More than 60% of the women were below the age of 30 in both groups. Also, there was no difference with regard to parity, number of miscarriages or intermenstrual bleeding.

Identical protocols suitable for computer analysis were used. After careful instruction about the purpose of the study each woman was asked to note details concerning cycle length, duration and intensity of withdrawal bleeding, abnormal bleeding episodes and other items on a special chart. A routine examination including blood pressure and body-weight and a detailed gynaecological check-up was done at admission. Follow-up visits were done after one, three and six cycles. Then body-weight and blood pressure were checked and the data from the individual bleeding charts transferred to the computer protocols. Spontaneously mentioned or obvious side-effects were also recorded.

RESULTS

The 555 women completed a total number of 3060 cycles, 1536 cycles on Logynon and 1524 cycles on Marvelon.

The number of women completing each cycle ($n = 278$ for Logynon

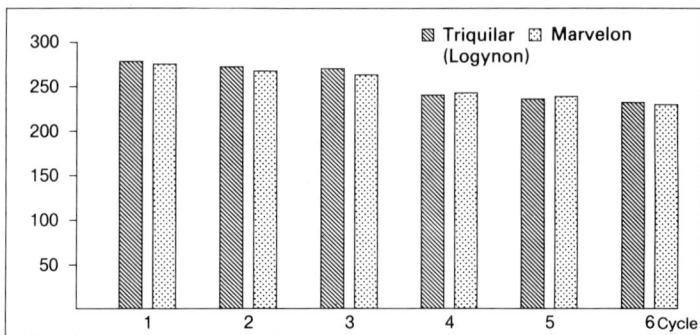

Figure 1 Number of women completing treatment cycles in both experimental groups

and $n = 277$ for Marvelon) is shown in Figure 1. 84.5% of the women finished the 6-month treatment period on the two preparations. However, whereas only 6.1% of triphasic takers discontinued medication prematurely for medical reasons, 11.9% of the women on the

598

monophasic combination did so, mainly because of bleeding irregularities and headaches.

Efficacy

Omission of tablets was admitted in 23 Logynon and in 19 Marvelon cycles. One pregnancy occurred in the triphasic group, none in the monophasic group. This one pregnancy was classified by the attending physician as clearly due to patient failure: a young girl of 15 years had omitted two consecutive tablets during the first days of the third cycle.

Cycle control

Both formulations exerted a normalizing effect on cycle length and duration of bleeding, especially in women with previously prolonged bleeding episodes.

Equally, the two preparations reduced previously heavy bleedings to the same extent. However, 'scanty' bleeding was reported more frequently by women on the monophasic combination than by

Table 2 Percentage of patients with intensity of menstrual flow before and during treatment

Intensity	Before treatment	6th Logynon cycle	6th Marvelon cycle
Scanty	7.3	18.3	32.3
Normal	82.9	79.6	65.5
Heavy	9.8	2.1	2.2

women using the triphasic formulation, as can be seen in Table 2. Failure of withdrawal bleeding to occur was comparatively rare in both groups. The rate was 0.2% for the triphasic and 0.9% for the monophasic preparation; the difference was statistically significant ($p < 0.01$).

Of special interest were possible differences in the incidence of spotting and breakthrough bleeding: calculated in terms of the total number of triphasic cycles the spotting rate was 6.4%, the BTB rate 1.2%. In 0.4% of all cycles spotting and BTB were recorded in the same cycle. The corresponding figures for the monophasic preparation are much higher: spotting 16.5%, BTB 2.8% and both episodes in the same cycle 1.1%. Applying the Chi-square test these differences are highly significant ($p < 0.001$).

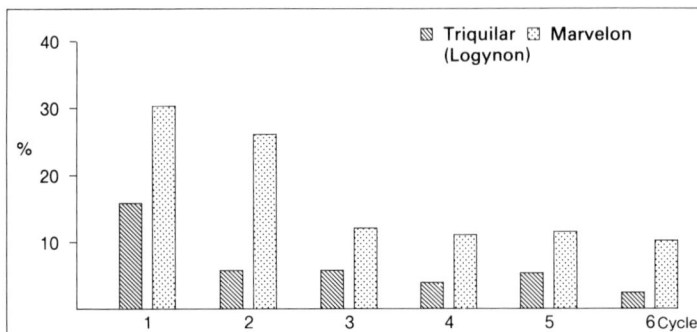

Figure 2 Percentage of spotting episodes in women completing treatment cycles in both experimental groups

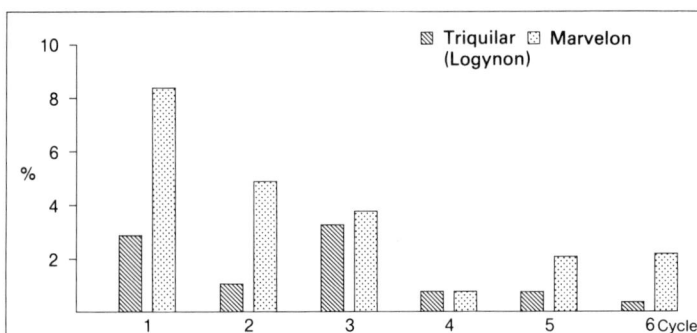

Figure 3 Percentage of breakthrough bleeding episodes in women completing treatment cycles in both experimental groups

Even more informative are Figures 2 and 3 which clearly demonstrate that – though most evident in the first two cycles – differences persisted during the whole treatment period.

Body-weight and blood pressure

Another interesting difference between the two preparations concerned body-weight, which remained constant in 75.2% of the triphasic users, but in only 61.1% of the monophasic users. Minor weight gains (+ < 2 kg) occurred in 11.3% of women on Logynon and in 15.4% of women on Marvelon. Only 5.2% of the triphasic users, as against 16.7% of the women on the monophasic combination, had

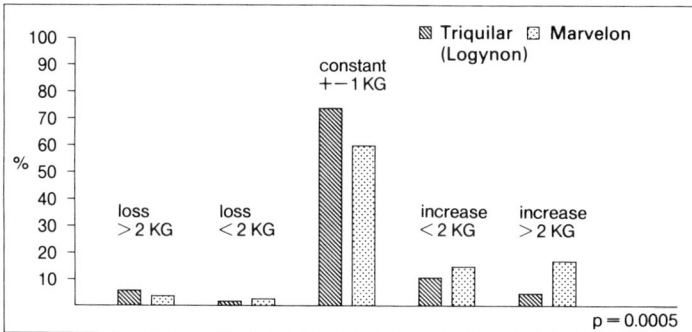

Figure 4 Percentage of experimental groups showing changes in body-weight after 6 months' treatment. * Difference between groups significant at $p = 0.0005$

gained more than 2 kg after 6 months (Figure 4). These differences are also statistically highly significant. Minor and major weight losses were similar with both preparations.

Blood pressure remained constant in the vast majority of women on both products. After 6 months Logynon a fall was recorded in four of five cases with RR values over 140/90 mmHg at start of therapy, while of 219 women with normal blood pressure, increases to values over 140/90 mmHg were recorded in four. With Marvelon normalization took place in two out of three women with RR values over 140/90 mmHg. From 222 women with normal blood pressure seven developed values over 140/90 mmHg within 6 months (Table 3).

Side-effects

Both low-dose products were well tolerated. Only few women reported the subjective side-effects commonly associated with oral contraceptive use under the two preparations. Headaches, including the migrainous type, and complaints about breast tenderness were somewhat more frequent in the Marvelon group (Table 4).

601

Acne developed in four women on Marvelon, but in only one woman on Logynon.

DISCUSSION

The triphasic levonorgestrel contraceptive provides a much better cycle control than the monophasic desogestrel combination. The differences in intracyclical bleeding episodes between the triphasic levonorgestrel preparation and the monophasic $150 \mu g$ desogestrel combination are even more pronounced than those observed in other comparative studies between the triphasic product and a monophasic $150 \mu g$ levonorgestrel combination[5,6].

Table 3 Blood pressure changes in four subjects using Logynon and in seven subjects using Marvelon

Triphasic (Logynon) Last cycle before medication	6th cycle	Monophasic (Marvelon) Last cycle before medication	6th cycle
1. 125/85	135/110	1. 125/70	150/95
2. 140/90	145/90	2. 130/90	145/80
3. 140/80	160/70	3. 120/70	145/75
4. 110/60	150/80	4. 130/70	145/90
		5. 130/70	140/100
		6. 140/85	150/90
		7. 140/90	160/100

Table 4 Percentage of women suffering subjective side-effects

Side-effect	Triphasic group	Monophasic group
Nausea	4.3	4.0
Headache	4.6	5.4
Migraine	0.7	1.4
Breast tenderness	2.2	5.4

Since it has been claimed that desogestrel has higher progestogenic activity[7], this is a rather unexpected finding. The results of our comparative clinical study once more clarify that in oral contraception one normally deals with combined oestrogen–progestogen effects.

An optimal oestrogen–progestogen ratio, for instance, may be more important for the overall effect of the preparation than partial qualities of the hormonal components.

Also, androgenic residual effects of progestogens are clinically almost irrelevant in modern low-dose preparations. Weight gain and skin problems like acne and seborrhoea are said to be clinical signs of androgenic activity of oral contraceptives. There is no evidence for a higher incidence of weight gain and acne with the triphasic levonorgestrel preparation in comparison with the desogestrel combination. On the contrary, increase in body-weight occurred significantly more often in users of the desogestrel combination. Likewise acne – though very rare with both products – occurred in four cases as opposed to only one with the triphasic preparation.

References

1. Larsson-Cohn, U. (1982). Lipoproteins and the estrogenicity of oral contraceptives. In Haspels, A. A. and Rolland, R. (eds.). *Benefits and Risks of Hormonal Contraception*, p. 95. (Lancaster: MTP Press)
2. Briggs, M. H. (1982). Comparative investigation of oral contraceptives using randomized, prospective protocols. In Haspels, A. A. and Rolland, R. (eds.). *Benefits and Risks of Hormonal Contraception*, p. 115. (Lancaster: MTP Press)
3. Winckelmann, G., Kaiser, E. and Christl, H. L. (1982). Effects of a triphasic and a biphasic oral contraceptive on various hemostatic parameters. In Haspels, A. A. and Rolland, R. (eds.) *Benefits and Risks of Hormonal Contraception*, p. 104. (Lancaster: MTP Press)
4. World Heath Organization (1978). Steroid contraception and the risk of neoplasia. *WHO Tech. Rep. Ser.*, **619**
5. Zador, G. (1982). Clinical performance of a triphasic administration of ethinyl estradiol and levonorgestrel in comparison with the 30 + 150 μg fixed-dose regime. In Haspels, A. A. and Rolland, R. (eds.). *Benefits and Risks of Hormonal Contraception*, p. 43. (Lancaster: MTP Press)
6. Carlborg, L. (1982). Acceptability of low-dose oral contraceptives: results of a randomized Swedish multicenter study comparing a triphasic (Trionetta®) and a fixed-dose combination (Neovletta®). In Haspels, A. A. and Rolland, R. (eds.). *Benefits and Risks of Hormonal Contraception*, p. 78. (Lancaster: MTP Press)
7. Bergink, E. W., *et al.* (1981). Binding of a contraceptive progestogen Org 2969 and its metabolites to receptor proteins and human sex hormone binding globulin. *J. Ster. Biochem.*, **14**, 175

65
Comparative study of lipid metabolism and endocrine function in women receiving levonorgestrel- and desogestrel-containing oral contraceptives

U. J. GASPARD, M. A. ROMUS and D. GILLAIN

SUMMARY

The aim of this randomized study was to evaluate potential altera-tions of the lipid profile and endocrine function in carefully matched healthy female volunteers investigated before and at 6 months' use of three new oral contraceptives (OCs): Logynon ($n=13$), a triphasic OC containing low doses of ethinyloestradiol (EE) + levonorgestrel (LNg), Marvelon ($n=14$), a monophasic OC containing low doses of EE + desogestrel (DOG, a new progestogen derived from LNg) and Ovidol ($n=11$), a sequential OC containing higher doses ($50\,\mu g$) of EE + DOG.

At the 6th month of OC use, results were as follows: *(1) Lipid profile:* Total-C, HDL-C, LDL-C and their ratios were unchanged; Apo AI/Apo B ratio was somewhat increased with all three OCs. VLDL + total triglycerides were significantly increased with Ovidol only. *(2) Hormones:* PRL levels were unchanged. FSH, LH, E2 and P were low, indicating effective ovulation inhibition in all individuals. Free T levels were equally well inhibited by all three OCs due to increased SHBG (Ovidol + 397% from basal, Marvelon + 352%, Logynon + 127%). PRA was significantly increased with Ovidol only. Free F was unchanged.

In conclusion, Marvelon, and particularly Ovidol (marked increase in VLDL, TG, SHBG, CBG, PRA) are distinctly more oestrogenic than Logynon.

INTRODUCTION

Laboratory findings indicate that the amount and chemical nature of oestrogens and progestogens contained in oral contraceptives (OCs) are correlated with alterations in blood coagulation factors, glucose and lipid metabolism, probably resulting in clinical problems for the OC users[1].

Progestogens contained in the OCs are derived mainly from 19-nortestosterone and may exert metabolic actions depending not only on their progestagenic but also on their androgenic and anti-oestrogenic properties. In this study, we compared the influence on serum lipids and on various hormonal parameters of a triphasic OC containing particularly low doses of a well-known 19-nortestosterone-derived progestogen, levonorgestrel (LNg) with a sequential and a monophasic preparation containing low doses of desogestrel (DOG), a new 3-deoxo-11-methylene derivative of LNg. We tried to assess whether the metabolic and hormonal alterations observed indicated any difference of action between DOG and LNg.

SUBJECTS AND METHODS
Subjects

All women studied (*n*=37) were healthy, young medical students (mean age 22.75 years, mean ideal body-weight 101%), who had never used oral contraception previously or had stopped OCs for at least 8 weeks prior to the study.

In each individual, a fasting blood sample was obtained at 08.30 a.m. 7 days before menstruation during a spontaneous cycle (control cycle). After exclusion of any contraindication to OC use and following a normal gynaecological examination, three groups of, respectively 13, 10 and 14 women were constituted at random. All subjects from group I received Trigynon for six cycles, beginning on day 1 of the first treatment cycle, with a 7-day free interval between each treatment cycle. The subjects from group II were assigned Ovidol in a similar way and women from group III received Marvelon. A second blood sample was obtained the last 3 days of the sixth cycle of OC use in each individual. Composition of the OCs is given in Table 1.

Table 1 Oral contraceptives used

Nature of the preparation	Triphasic	Sequential	Monophasic
Trade names	Trigynon	Ovidol	Marvelon
Components	1. EE 0.03 mg + LNg 0.05 mg (days 1–6) 2. EE 0.04 mg + LNg 0.075 mg (days 7–11) 3. EE 0.03 mg + LNg 0.125 mg (days 12–21)	1. EE 0.05 mg (days 1–7) 2. EE 0.05 mg + DOG 0.125 mg (days 8–21)	EE 0.03 mg + DOG 0.150 mg (days 1–21)

EE = Ethinyloestradiol; LNg = Levonorgestrel; DOG = Desogestrel.

Methods

FSH, LH, PRL, progesterone (P), oestradiol (E_2), total testosterone (T), total cortisol (F), aldosterone (Aldo) and plasma renin activity (PRA), were measured by radioimmunoassay, and estimations of sex hormone binding globulin (SHBG), transcortin (CBG), free T and free F were made according to procedures previously described[2]. Serum lipids and lipoproteins were determined by enzymatic, chemical and electroimmunoassay methods reported elsewhere[3].

RESULTS

Lipids

Changes in serum lipid and lipoprotein concentrations after 6 months of use of each OC are detailed in Table 2.

Starting values of lipid concentrations were similar in the three groups of patients before treatment. After 6 months of OC use, total TG were significantly more elevated in the Ovidol group, apoprotein

607

B levels were significantly reduced in the Marvelon group and accordingly Apo AI/Apo B ratio was increased.

Table 2 Serum lipid profile at 6 months of oral contraceptive use

Variable	Group mean values (pretreatment = 100%)		
	Triphasic, Trigynon (EE+LNg)	Monophasic, Marvelon (EE+DOG)	Sequential, Ovidol (EE+DOG)
Total triglycerides	+ 29 (%)	+ 21	+ 90**
Total phospholipids	+ 8.8	+ 7.2	+ 16.3**
Total cholesterol	+ 4.6	+ 1.8	+ 9.6
HDL cholesterol	0	+ 5.3	+ 1.7
LDL cholesterol	+ 1	− 4	+ 4
HDL cholesterol: total cholesterol	− 2	+ 3.8	− 6
LDL cholesterol: HDL cholesterol	+ 4	− 7.7	− 1.1
Apoprotein A_I	+ 13.2*	+ 14.5*	+ 18.5*
Apoprotein B	+ 2.2	− 19*	+ 11.7
Apo A_I:Apo B	+ 18.4	+ 40.9**	+ 22

*$p < 0.05$; **$p < 0.001$ (paired t test for comparison of pretreatment and 6-month values).
EE = Ethinyloestradiol; LNg = Levonorgestrel; DOG = Desogestrel.

Hormones

Alterations of hormone levels after 6 months of OC use are given in Table 3. All hormone and carrier protein levels were similar in the three groups before treatment. After 6 months of OC use FSH and LH levels were significantly more inhibited in the Marvelon group; SHBG levels were significantly more elevated in the Ovidol and Marvelon groups; and CBG levels were more elevated in the Ovidol group.

DISCUSSION AND CONCLUSIONS

Lipids

This study clearly shows, as indicated already by Larsson-Cohn et al.[4], that the triphasic formulation provides a favourable EE:LNg ratio which allows the androgenic–antioestrogenic properties of LNg to be appropriately balanced by the oestrogen content for effects on

Table 3 Influence of oral contraceptives on plasma hormone levels before and after 6 months of use. Results are given as means ±SE*

Plasma hormones	Trigynon (n = 13)		Ovidol (n = 10)		Marvelon (n = 14)	
	Pretreatment	6th month	Pretreatment	6th month	Pretreatment	6th month
FSH (mIU ml⁻¹)	4.23±0.67	2.65±0.57 NS	4.14±0.62	2.84±0.67 NS	3.60±0.48	1.97±0.35 0.001
LH (mIU ml⁻¹)	6.61±0.93	4.81±1.08 NS	9.30±3.66	5.30±1.32 NS	6.84±1.35	3.09±0.45 0.01
PRL (μU ml⁻¹)	463±111	428±71 NS	430±68	442±63 NS	482±99	320±81 NS
E2 (pg ml⁻¹)	152±29	34±5 0.006	124±27	33±7 0.02	163±24	57±30 0.02
P (ng ml⁻¹)	8.10±1.64	0.31±0.26 0.01	6.61±1.40	0.17±0.02 0.006	9.59±2.33	0.20±0.04 0.001
Total T (pg ml⁻¹)	486±34	324±50 0.02	507±64	393±49 NS	429±66	312±46 0.07
Free T (pg ml⁻¹)	5.08±1.06	1.90±0.31 0.002	5.99±1.36	1.60±0.22 0.002	4.90±1.47	1.50±0.20 0.005
SHBG (nmol l⁻¹)	84±14	191±25 0.000	70±7	348±37 0.000	59±8	267±22 0.000
Total F (ng ml⁻¹)	193±10	405±34 0.000	173±12	460±37 0.000	176±11	393±24 0.000
Free F (ng ml⁻¹)	11.7±1.0	13.1±1.7 NS	10.5±1.1	15.7±1.8 NS	10.6±1.2	14.2±2.4 NS
CBG (mg l⁻¹)	43.4±2.6	80.1±2.0 0.000	40.8±1.7	94.5±4.5 0.000	40.8±2.6	83.7±2.6 0.000
Aldo (pg ml⁻¹)	248±31	241±59 NS	220±28	274±29 NS	240±40	304±43 NS
PRA (ng ml⁻¹ h⁻¹)	2.10±0.30	4.38±1.07 NS	2.06±0.29	6.15±1.58 0.01	3.05±1.58	3.51±0.77 NS

*Paired Student's t test used for comparison of pretreatment and 6th month values and result given in italics; NS = not significant.

609

metabolic end-points such as HDL-C, apolipoprotein A_I concentrations, etc. The triphasic preparation containing LNg and the two other preparations containing DOG had no influence on total-C, HDL-C or LDL-C. HDL-C/total-C and LDL-C/HDL-C ratios were unchanged while Apo A_I/Apo B ratio was slightly increased (mainly during Marvelon treatment). These observations are corroborated by other studies[5,6] and confirm an apparent lack of atherogenic effect of these preparations on the lipid profile. However, marked oestrogenic dominance of Ovidol is abided by a very important increase in VLDL and TG, not found with the other preparations tested.

Hormones and carrier proteins[2]

All three OCs inhibited pituitary gonadotrophin secretion and gonadal function in all the cases studied. All three OCs exerted dominant oestrogenic effects as exemplified by marked and significant increases in CBG (Ovidol >> Marvelon > Trigynon). Free F levels are, however, unchanged.

The lower antioestrogenic activity of DOG *vs.* LNg is best exemplified in our study by a significantly greater rise in SHBG during Marvelon and Ovidol treatment (Ovidol > Marvelon >> Trigynon). However, free T levels are equally effectively suppressed by all three preparations.

In summary, oestrogen dominance is slightest in Trigynon but sufficient to balance the antioestrogenic properties of LNg and the triphasic preparation seems well equilibrated. Marvelon and especially Ovidol are more oestrogenic (less antioestrogenic) preparations. The administration of the latter one is accompanied by an excessive increase in VLDL, TG, SHBG, CBG and PRA.

References

1. Briggs, M. H. and Briggs, M. (1982). Randomized prospective studies on metabolic effects of oral contraceptives. *Acta Obstet. Gynecol. Scand.*, **105**, (suppl.), 25
2. Gaspard, U. J., Romus, M. A., Gillain, D., Duvivier, J., Demey-Ponsart, E. and Franchimont, P. (1983). Plasma hormone levels in women receiving new oral contraceptives containing ethinyl estradiol plus levonorgestrel or desogestrel. *Contraception*, **27**, 577
3. Gaspard, U. J., Romus, M. A., Plomteux, G., Buret, J. and Luyckx, A. S. (1983). Serum lipid profile and liver function tests in women receiving oral contraceptives containing levonorgestrel or desogestrel (In preparation)
4. Larsson-Cohn, U., Fåhreus, L., Wallentin, L. and Zador, G. (1981). Lipoprotein

changes may be minimized by proper composition of a combined oral contraceptive. *Fertil. Steril.*, **35,** 172

5. Cullberg, G., *et al.* (1982). Two oral contraceptives, efficacy, serum proteins, and lipid metabolism. *Contraception,* **26,** 229
6. Briggs, M. H. and Briggs, M. (1983). Comparative metabolic effects of oral contraceptives containing levonorgestrel or desogestrel. In the Elstein, M. (ed.) *Update on Triphasic Oral Contraception* (Amsterdam: Excerpta Medica)

Part III

Section 3

Trends in Oral Contraception*

* This special symposium was sponsored by Organon BV

66
Serum glycosylated proteins as a measure of carbohydrate metabolism in users of oral contraceptives

H. J. KLOOSTERBOER, G. J. BRUINING, P. LIUKKO,
S. NUMMI and L. LUND

SUMMARY

Women using oral contraceptives may display minor alterations in carbohydrate metabolism. Using the oral glucose tolerance test (oGTT) it has been demonstrated that currently used low-dose combination pills induce an increase in the insulin response. In addition it has been suggested that during long-term use of low-dose combination pills glucose tolerances deteriorate. The oGTT is not performed under physiological conditions, and so it is questionable as to whether such a test truly reflects the glucose metabolic state. Moreover, the results are often influenced by factors such as stress and diet. The amount of glycosylated protein in serum is at present considered a good index of glucose homeostasis during the fourteen days preceding blood sampling.

A reliable method for the determination of serum glycosylated proteins, which allows assessment of carbohydrate metabolism under more physiological conditions than those found in the oGTT, has been developed in our laboratory.

This method was applied for the estimation of the effect of a new progestational compound, desogestrel, on carbohydrate metabolism. Glycosylated serum proteins, measured as the amount of hydroxymethylfurfural released per gram of protein, was estimated in (a) women receiving 0.125 mg desogestrel per day for 2 months and (b) women receiving the new oral contraceptive combination 0.150 mg desogestrel + 0.030 mg ethinyloestradiol (EE) for 3, 18 or 24 months.

It can be concluded from these studies that neither desogestrel alone nor the 150/30 combination of desogestrel and EE have any effect on carbohydrate metabolism.

INTRODUCTION

A decrease in the hormonal content of combined oral contraceptives (OCs) considerably reduces their effect on carbohydrate metabolism using the oral glucose tolerance test[1-3]. This test demonstrates a minor decrease in glucose tolerance and a small increase in insulin response in users of low-dose OCs. However, the results of an oral glucose tolerance test can be influenced by a number of factors such as stress and diet. This may partly explain the large variations found with a glucose loading test and makes it unsuitable for the detection of small alterations in carbohydrate metabolism as observed in OC users. Furthermore, the test is carried out with an amount of glucose that is normally not consumed in a single meal. It is therefore questionable whether the results of the glucose tolerance test truly reflect the actual glucose metabolic state.

-Apart from the oral glucose tolerance test, the extent of glycosylation of haemoglobin (measured as per cent HbA_1) is used as an index of glucose control in diabetic patients[4]. The per cent HbA_1 may increase 2–3 fold in diabetic patients[4]. The value is already considerably increased in non-diabetic subjects with slightly impaired glucose tolerance[5]. Glycosylation of haemoglobin is a non-enzymatic process, which can occur with proteins in various tissues and with all blood proteins. In addition to HbA_1 the estimation of the level of glycosylated serum proteins is a good method for the assessment of glucose homeostasis[6]. The amount of glucose bound to serum proteins is determined by the time the proteins circulate in the blood and by the glucose concentration during that time. The value is 2–3 fold increased in diabetic patients.

In the present study, the glycosylation of serum proteins was measured in women receiving the new progestational compound desogestrel alone, and in women taking a new oral contraceptive combination containing 0.15 mg desogestrel and 0.03 mg ethinyloestradiol (EE). The results of the studies with desogestrel + EE were compared with those from another OC preparation containing 0.15 mg levonorgestrel and 0.03 mg EE or from a control group without oral contraception.

MATERIALS AND METHODS

Young healthy women, aged 21–35 years, who had not taken hormonal medication for at least 2 months, participated in the studies. Blood samples were drawn after overnight fasting at the times indicated in the tables. Blood was allowed to clot for 45 min at room temperature and was subsequently centrifuged ($10^4 \, \mathrm{N \, kg^{-1}}$, 15 min) for preparation of serum. Serum was stored at $-20°\mathrm{C}$ until use.

The following clinical studies were performed.

Desogestrel alone

A group of 10 women took one tablet containing 0.125 mg desogestrel per day for 2 months followed by 1 month without treatment.

Desogestrel + EE

Prospective comparative studies – Women received tablets containing either 0.15 mg desogestrel and 0.03 mg EE or 0.15 mg levonorgestrel and 0.03 mg EE. The treatment was started on the first day of the cycle. Each cycle consisted of 21 days of tablet taking followed by a 7-day tablet-free period. In one study the treatment period lasted 3 months and in the other 24 months. In both cases the treatment was followed by a control period of 2 months.

A retrospective study – The women came from an ordinary medical practice in the Netherlands. One group of women had taken the combination 0.15 mg desogestrel and 0.03 mg EE for 1.5 years and another comparable group of women had not used hormonal contraception.

Estimation of glycosylated proteins

The thiobarbituric assay was used for the estimation of the amount of glucose released as hydroxymethylfurfural (HMF) from the proteins during hydrolysis at high temperatures. In comparison with other described methods[6,7] the procedure for hydrolysis of glucose from the proteins was modified with respect to three points. Firstly, hydrolysis was performed after removal of sialic acid; secondly, hydrolysis was carried out with acetic acid instead of oxalic acid; and thirdly, hydrolysis was done under anaerobic conditions. These alterations improved the sensitivity and reduced the variation of the method. The method will be described in detail elsewhere. The extent of glycosylation is expressed as μmol HMF released per gram of protein. For validation purposes, the method was also applied to haemolysates of diabetic patients on which an estimation of the % HbA_1 had been carried out by a standard chromatographic procedure. An excellent correlation was found between these methods.

RESULTS

The amount of HMF released per gram proteins in serum samples of 10 women receiving 0.125 mg desogestrel per day for 2 months was not influenced by treatment. The mean ($\pm$SD) pretreatment value was $0.79\pm0.11\,\mu$mol HMF (g protein)$^{-1}$; values after 1 and 2 months' treatment were 0.75 ± 0.13 and $0.75\pm0.17\,\mu$mol HMF (g protein)$^{-1}$, respectively. The post-treatment value was $0.7\pm0.15\,\mu$mol HMF (g protein)$^{-1}$.

Table 1 Mean ($\pm$SD) values of glycosylated serum proteins (in μmol HMF (g protein)$^{-1}$ in 10 women treated with 0.15 mg desogestrel + 0.03 mg EE or 0.15 mg levonorgestrel + EE for 3 months

Sample	Desogestrel + EE	Levonorgestrel + EE
Pretreatment	0.79±0.14	0.76±0.14
3 months' treatment	0.79±0.10	0.75±0.12
2 months' post treatment	0.78±0.14	0.70±0.14

Table 1 shows the results of a comparative study between two groups of women receiving 0.15 mg desogestrel and 0.03 mg EE or 0.15 mg levonorgestrel and 0.03 mg EE for 3 months. The amount of HMF per gram of protein was unchanged and no statistically significant difference was observed between the two groups. A similar result was found with both combinations after treatment for 2 years (Table 2).

Table 2 Mean (±SD) values of glycosylated serum proteins (in μmol HMF (g protein)$^{-1}$) in 10 women treated with 0.15 mg desogestrel + 0.03 mg EE or 0.15 mg levonorgestrel + 0.03 mg EE for 2 years

Sample	Desogestrel + EE	Levonorgestrel + EE
Pretreatment	1.05±0.14	0.97±0.10
3 months' treatment	1.14±0.16	1.03±0.09
6 months' treatment	1.07±0.12	1.01±0.10
12 months' treatment	1.05±0.10	0.96±0.12
18 months' treatment	0.97±0.13	0.86±0.12
24 months' treatment	0.99±0.16	0.85±0.10
2 months' post treatment	0.91±0.15	0.83±0.13

In the retrospective study it was found that treatment for 1.5 years with 0.15 mg desogestrel and 0.03 mg EE gave similar values for the extent of glycosylation of serum proteins to those observed in untreated controls: mean (±SD) values for glycosylated protein were $0.6\pm0.05\,\mu$mol HMF (g protein)$^{-1}$ in the treated group ($n = 27$) and $0.56\pm0.07\,\mu$mol HMF (g protein)$^{-1}$ in the controls ($n = 28$).

DISCUSSION

The estimation of glycosylated proteins as a measure for glucose homeostasis has a number of advantages over the generally used oral glucose tolerance test. The amount of glucose irreversibly bound to proteins is an indication of the status of carbohydrate metabolism over a longer period of time under physiological conditions.

The extent of glycosylation of serum proteins reflects carbohydrate metabolism in the one or two weeks before blood sampling since it is determined mainly by the half-life of albumin, which is 15 days.

In contrast, the oral glucose tolerance test is carried out with an unphysiological high glucose load and gives only an impression of glucose tolerance at any one moment. Glucose tolerance is influenced by several factors which may increase the variation of the test and makes it less reliable for detecting small alterations in carbohydrate metabolism. In our view the estimation of glycosylated proteins is a better alternative for assessing glucose homeostasis in pill users.

Small effects of low-dose combination pills on carbohydrate metabolism are observed using the oral glucose tolerance test. The test indicates a minor alteration in the glucose tolerance and a small increase in the insulin response[1-3,8]. The effects of progestogens alone at doses lower than those used in combined preparations on these variables are stronger than with low-dose OCs[9-11].

Desogestrel when tested for 2 months at a dose of 0.125 mg per day does not have an effect on the extent of glycosylation of serum proteins. The 150/30 combination of desogestrel + EE also does not influence the amount of glucose bound to serum proteins even after long-term use. Similar results were observed with the 150/30 levonorgestrel + EE combination. It can be concluded that glucose metabolism is not influenced by desogestrel alone or in combination with EE at the doses tested in the present study.

References

1. Wynn, V., Godsland, I., Nithyananthan, R., Adams, P. W., Melrose, J., Oakley, N. W. and Seed, M. (1979). Comparison of effects of different combined oral-contraceptive formulations on carbohydrate and lipid metabolism. *Lancet*, **1**, 1045
2. Briggs, M. H. (1979). Biochemical basis for the selection of oral contraceptives. *Int. J. Gynecol. Obstet.*, **16**, 509
3. Spellacy, W. N. (1982). Carbohydrate metabolism during treatment with estrogen, progestogen, and low-dose oral contraceptives. *Am. J. Obstet. Gynecol.*, **142**, 732
4. Abraham, E. C., Huff, T. A., Cope, N. D., Wilson, J. B. Jr., Bransome, E. D. and Huisman, T. H. J. (1978). Determination of the glycosylated hemoglobins (HbA₁) with a new microcolumn procedure. *Diabetes*, **27**, 931
5. Verrillo, A., de Teresa, A., Golia, R. and Nunziata, V. (1983). The relationship between glycosylated haemoglobin levels and various degrees of glucose intolerance. *Diabetologia*, **24**, 391
6. McFarland, K. F., Catalano, E. W., Day, J. F., Thorpe, S. R. and Baynes, J. W. (1979). Non-enzymatic glucosylation of serum proteins in diabetes mellitus. *Diabetes*, **28**, 1011
7. Yue, D. K., Morris, K., McLennan, S. and Turtle, J. R. (1980). Glycosylation of plasma protein and its relation to glycosylated hemoglobin in diabetes. *Diabetes*, **29**, 296

8. Vermeulen, A. and Thiery, M. (1982). Metabolic effects of the triphasic oral contraceptive Trigynon. *Contraception*, **26**, 505

9. Spellacy, W. N., Buhi, W. C. and Birk, S. A. (1981). Prospective studies of carbohydrate metabolism in 'normal' women using norgestrel for eighteen months. *Fertil. Steril.*, **35**, 167

10. Spellacy, W. N., Buhi, W. C. and Birk, S. A. (1976). Carbohydrate and lipid metabolic studies before and after one year of treatment with ethynodiol diacetate in 'normal' women. *Fertil. Steril.*, **27**, 900

11. Spellacy, W. N., Buhi, W. C. and Birk, S. A. (1975). Effects of norethindrone on carbohydrate and lipid metabolism. *Obstet. Gynecol.*, **46**, 560

67
Androgenic, oestrogenic and antioestrogenic effects of desogestrel and lynestrenol alone: effects on serum proteins, sex hormones and vaginal cytology

G. CULLBERG and L.-Å. MATTSSON

SUMMARY

Desogestrel (Dgl)/ ethinyloestradiol (Marvelon, Organon) has a pronounced increasing effect on sex hormone binding globulin (SHBG). This can be due to an oestrogenic effect of Dgl or lack of androgenicity. These possibilities were evaluated using the effects on serum proteins and vaginal cytology. 0.125, 0.250 and 0.500 mg Dgl daily was given orally in a randomized order to eight healthy fertile women and also, in comparison 5 mg lynestrenol (Lyn). Each treatment lasted 6 weeks. The methods used were electroimmunoassay for SHBG, ceruloplasmin, cortisol binding globulin (CBG), thyroxin binding globulin (TBG) and prealbumin, radioimmunoassay for 17β-oestradiol (E_2), testosterone and vaginal cytology as maturation value (MV). Results found indicated a dose-dependent depression of E_2, SHBG and MV. The correlation was however much stronger for Dgl dose versus SHBG decrease ($r=0.97$) than for E_2 decrease versus SHBG ($r=0.54$) indicating an *hepatocyte blocking effect* by Dgl rather than a lowered E_2-stimulation of SHBG production. No *androgenic effects* such as increases in prealbumin or depression of TBG were seen after Dgl but a small significant increase in prealbumin was found for Lyn. No *oestrogenic effects* such as increases in CBG, ceruloplasmin or MV were seen for Dgl or Lyn but an antioestrogenic effect on NV was seen.

INTRODUCTION

During the past 5 years it has been shown that some of the most widely used gestogens behave in many ways metabolically as androgens[1]. Epidemiological studies suggest that lipid patterns, for example low HDL cholesterol values are correlated with increased risk for coronary heart disease[2]. The androgenic side-effects of oral contraceptives such as weight gain, hirsutism and acne, are common causes of withdrawal.

It is thus important to find gestogens with less androgenicity. Starting from lynestrenol, the desogestrel was synthesized (Figure

LYNESTRENOL   DESOGESTREL

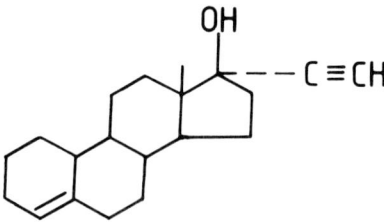 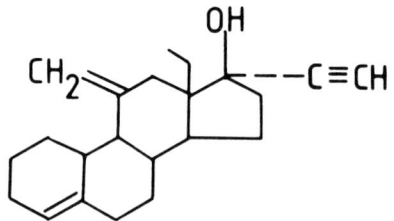

Figure 1   Structural formulae of lynestrenol and desogestrel

1). When combined with ethinyloestradiol it appeared to be devoid of androgenicity in spite of being a 19-nor-testosterone derivate[3]. It allows increases in sex hormone binding globulin (SHBG) and HDL-cholesterol values in contrast to the other gonane, levonorgestrel. But interesting questions arise; does it have any oestrogenic, antioestrogenic or androgenic properties when given alone in comparison with, for example, lynestrenol?

To find out, we performed a study evaluating vaginal cytology and serum proteins from eight regularly menstruating women who were healthy apart from endometriosis. They had not taken any hormones during the last 3 months. A blood sample was taken before treatment.

The women were then given 0.125, 0.25 or 0.5 mg desogestrel and 5 mg lynestrenol in daily doses (Table 1). The treatments were given in a randomized order, i.e. one women starting with lynestrenol

Table 1 Examples of experimental protocol. The other four women had similar cycles of drug intake. Each treatment was taken for 6 weeks and samples taken at 0, 6, 12, 18 and 24 weeks

Patient	Treatment*			
	1	2	3	4
1	L	0.125 D	0.25 D	0.5 D
2	0.125 D	L	0.5 D	0.25 D
3	0.125 D	0.5 D	0.25 D	L
8	0.5 D	0.25 D	L	0.125 D

*Figures are mg taken daily.
D = Desogestrel; L = 5 mg lynestrenol.

and then going on with the desogestrel and another starting with desogestrel, etc. Each dose was given for 6 weeks without any treatment-free intervals.

Serum was analysed for SHBG, cortisol binding globulin (CBG), ceruloplasmin, thyroxin binding globulin (TBG) and prealbumin using electroimmunoassay according to Laurell[4]. Vaginal cytology was judged as maturation values, giving the percentage of superficial cells the multiplication factor 1.0 and adding an intermediate-cell percentage multiplied by 0.5. Serum oestradiol and testosterone were analysed with radioimmunoassay.

RESULTS AND DISCUSSION

When a synthetic oestrogen is given, the levels of SHBG, TBG, CBG and ceruloplasmin rise and the maturation value is increased while ovarian hormone production is sometimes stimulated and sometimes depressed, depending on the dosage and type of hormone. Androgens have the opposite effect on SHBG and TBG but have very little influence on CBG and ceruloplasmin. The prealbumin level is not influenced by oestrogens but is increased when an androgenic substance is given[3-5].

In the present study serum levels of oestradiol were significantly lowered in relation to the desogestrel dose except in two women during the 0.125 mg treatment (Figure 2). Testosterone levels were also lower during treatment with desogestrel but not with lynestrenol.

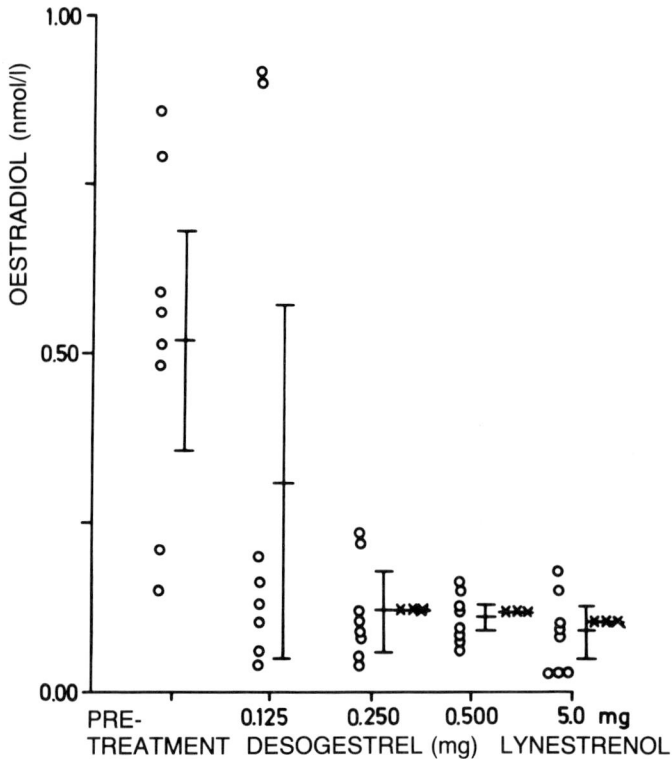

Figure 2 Individual serum levels of 17β-oestradiol in 8 fertile women before treatment on cycle day 7–9 and after 6 weeks of treatment with 5 mg lynestrenol, 0.125, 0.250 and 0.500 mg desogestrel. Treatments were given in a randomized order without intervals. Vertical bars represent means and $\pm$ 2 SEM. Statistical significances between pretreatment and treatment values are indicated with asterisks: * = $p < 1.25$, ** = $p < 0.01$ and *** = $p < 0.001$

SHBG levels were also significantly lowered during treatment (Figure 3). There was a highly significant correlation, with a correlation factor of 0.97, between SHBG and desogestrel dose except at the 0.125 mg level, while the SHBG – oestradiol correlation was weaker

($r = 0.54$). This indicates that oestradiol is not very efficient in regulating SHBG levels. This is borne out by the observation that postmenopausal and oophorectomized women have only slightly lower SHBG levels in spite of a lack of oestradiol in serum.

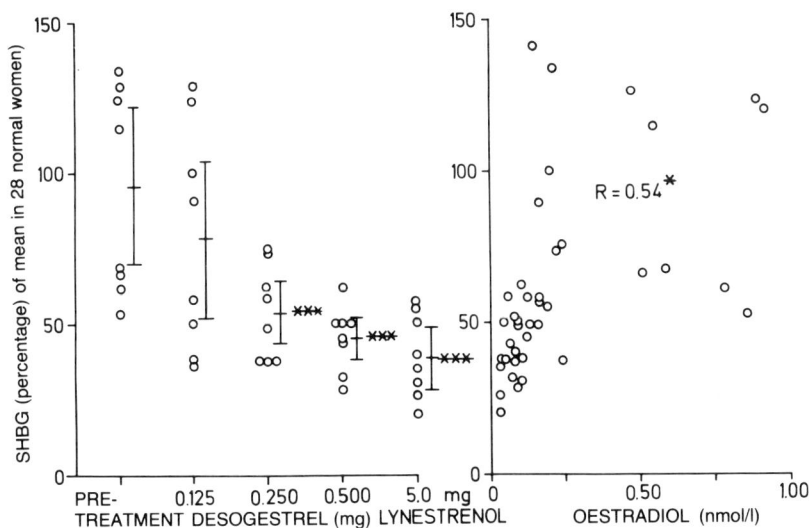

Figure 3 Left panel: Individual levels of SHBG determined by electroimmunoassay. Levels are given as percentages of a reference pool of serum from 28 untreated healthy fertile women. Volunteers, treatments and symbols as in Figure 2
Right panel: Correlation between SHBG and 17β-estradiol with pretreatment and treatment values given in Figures 2 and 4, left panel. R = correlation coefficient. * significant correlation, $p < 0.05$

It may be that the 19-nor-testosterone derivatives are blocking the SHBG-producing hepatocytes since the same has been found for levonorgestrel[6]. The 17α-hydroxyprogestogens, e.g. medroxyprogesteroneacetate, do not have this property. It is hardly an androgenic effect, since desogestrel *in vitro* has a low affinity to androgen receptors in comparison with levonorgestrel and testosterone[7]. As said in the introduction, desogestrel allows strong increases in SHBG by ethinyloestradiol in contrast to androgenic substances.

Desogestrel does not give any increase in prealbumin level (Figure

4). This is, however, seen with lynestrenol, indicating a weak androgenic rest effect in the latter.

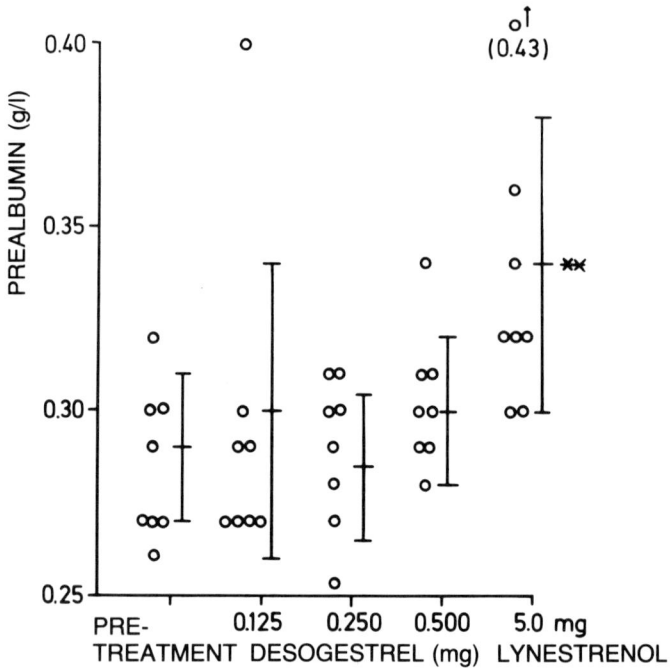

Figure 4 Individual levels of serum prealbumin in g/l. Volunteers, treatments and symbols are the same as in Figure 2

In vaginal cytology another type of reaction is seen (Figure 5). Here, despite adequate oestrogen levels in at least two cases, the maturation value is depressed strongly, hinting at an antioestrogenic effect and a lack of oestrogenic properties. The absence of an oestrogenic effect can be inferred, since no changes in oestrogen-sensitive ceruloplasmin and CBG are found.

In conclusion, we found no signs of androgenic or oestrogenic properties in desogestrel but a weak androgenic effect was detected in lynestrenol. Evidence for antioestrogenic effect was found with both substances. Desogestrel is at least 10 times as potent as lynestrenol for the variables studied.

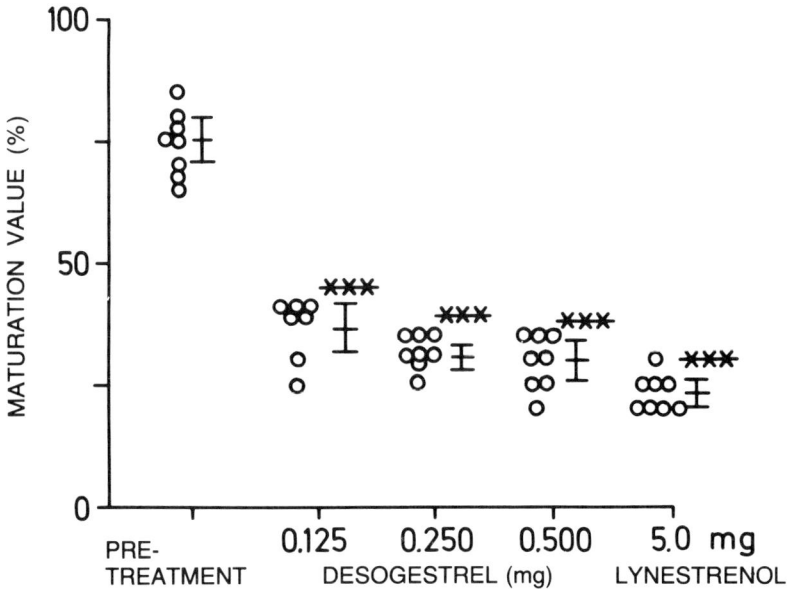

Figure 5 Individual maturation values in percent. Volunteers, treatments and symbols are the same as in Figure 2

References

1. Larsson-Cohn, U., Wallentin, L. and Zador, G. (1979). Plasma lipids and high density lipoproteins during oral contraception with different combinations of ethinylestradiol and levonorgestrel. *Horm. Metab. Res.*, **11**, 437
2. Miller, G. J. and Miller, N. E. (1975). Plasma-high-density-lipoprotein concentration and development of ischaemic heart disease. *Lancet*, **1**, 16
3. Cullberg, G., Dovre, P. A., Linstedt, G. and Steffensen, K. (1982). On the use of plasma proteins as indicators of the metabolic effects of combined oral contraceptives. *Acta Obstet. Gynecol. Scand. Suppl.*, **111**, 47
4. Laurell, C.-B. and Rannevik, G.-A. (1979). A comparison of plasma protein changes induced by danazol, pregnancy and oestrogens. *J. Clin. Endocrinol. Metab.*, **49**, 719
5. Barbosa, J., Seal, U. S. and Doe, R. P. (1971). Effects of anabolic steroids on hormone-binding proteins, serum cortisol and serum non-protein-bound cortisol. *J. Clin. Endocrinol.*, **32**, 232
6. Victor, A. and Johansson, E. D. B. (1977). Effects of d-norgestrel induced decreases in sex hormone binding globulin capacity on the d-norgestrel levels in plasma. *Contraception*, **16** (2), 115

7. Bergink, E. W., Hamburger, A. D., de Jager, E. and van der Vies, J. (1981). Binding of a contraceptive progestogen Org 2969 and its metabolites to receptor proteins and human sex hormone binding globulin. *J. Steroid Biochem.*, **14,** 175

68
Influence of a desogestrel/ ethinyloestradiol combination pill on sex hormone binding globulin and plasma androgens

E. KELLER, A. JASPER, M. ZWIRNER, H. UNTERBERG, T. SCHUMACHER and A. E. SCHINDLER

SUMMARY

It is well known that (a) the progestogen desogestrel displays low affinity for androgen receptors and (b) that ethinyloestradiol stimulates the synthesis of sex hormone binding globulin (SHBG). Thus, it was the purpose of this study to evaluate the influence of a desogestrel/ethinyloestradiol combination pill on SHBG and plasma androgens.

During three cycles, eight female volunteers took a combination pill containing 0.15 mg desogestrel and 0.03 mg ethinyloestradiol daily for 21 days followed by a hormone-free interval of 7 days. Under the pill blood sampling was done weekly; in a control cycle before and after medication blood sampling was done every other day. The following parameters were determined: SHBG, testosterone (free and total), DHT, DHEA, DHEA sulphate, prolactin, oestradiol and progesterone.

Under the desogestrel/ethinyloestradiol combination a constant increase of SHBG could be observed which decreased again during the 7 days' hormone-free intervals but without reaching pretreatment levels. Plasma free testosterone and DHT revealed inverse patterns. One month after discontinuing the pill all parameters resumed pre-treatment values.

The results presented may explain the satisfactory situation concerning undesired androgenic effects under the desogestrel/ethinyl-oestradiol combination pill.

INTRODUCTION

In the female, low levels of sexual hormone binding globulin (SHBG) and high values of free testosterone are important factors for the manifestation of signs of androgenization such as acne and/or hirsutism[1]. While oestrogens stimulate SHBG synthesis and thus indirectly cause a decrease of free testosterone, androgens and also progestogens with androgenic rest activity lower SHBG levels. Consequently, in hormonal contraception the favourable oestrogen side-effect of SHBG stimulation can be neutralized according to the type and dose of the administered progestational substance. Obviously, this circumstance is of particular importance for the increasingly used low-dose oral contraceptives (i.e. oestrogen component < 0.04 mg)[2].

Since it is well known that the progestogen desogestrel – a potent progestational 19-nortestosterone derivative[3] – displays low affinity for androgen receptors[4], it was the purpose of this study to investigate the influence of a low-dose desogestrel/ethinyloestradiol combination pill on SHBG and plasma androgens.

MATERIALS AND METHODS

During three cycles, eight female volunteers (students; on average 24.6 years, 167 cm, 57 kg, menstrual cycles of 27–35 days; two smokers; seven practising oral contraception for the first time) took a combination pill containing 0.15 mg desogestrel and 0.03 mg ethinyloestradiol (Marvelon®) daily for 21 days followed by a 7-day hormonal-free interval. During treatment, venous blood sampling from a cubital vein was done once a week (days 1, 8, 15 and 22 of the cycle). In a control cycle before (control cycle 1) and after medication (control cycle 2) blood sampling was done every other day.

The following parameters were determined in serum or plasma: SHBG, free and total testosterone, dihydrotestosterone (DHT), de-hydroepiandrosterone (DHEA), DHEA sulphate, LH, FSH, oestradiol, progesterone and prolactin.

The control cycles were centred around the day of the LH peak (indicated as day 0) as the day of presumed ovulation.

RESULTS

The control cycles before and after taking the desogestrel/ethinyloestradiol combination pill for 3 months did not reflect major differences: the duration of control cycle 1 was 32 days; the duration of control cycle 2 was 29 days (follicular phase: control cycle 1 = 20 days, control cycle 2 = 18 days; luteal phase: control cycle 1 = 12 days, control

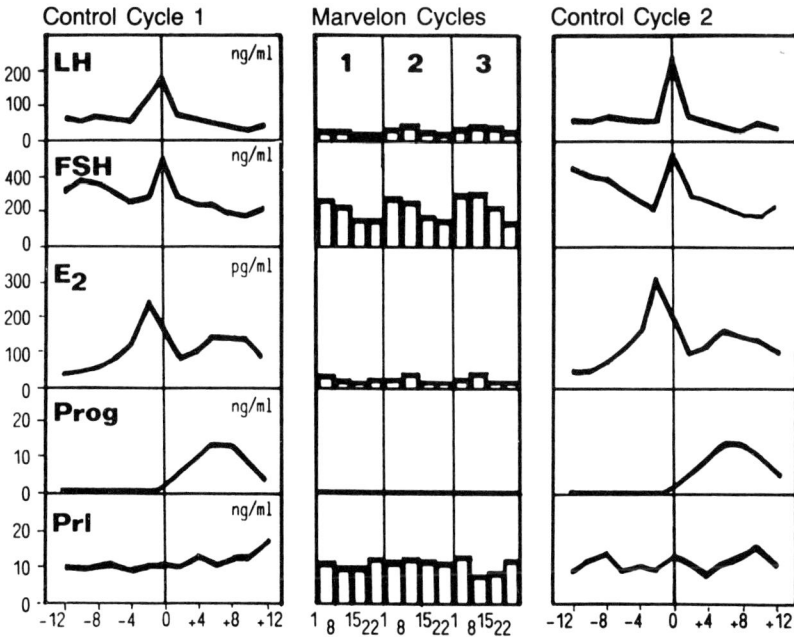

Figure 1 LH, FSH, oestradiol (E_2), progesterone (Prog), and prolactin (Prl) in a control cycle before treatment (Control Cycle 1), under three treatment cycles of a 0.15 mg desogestrel/0.03 mg ethinyloestradiol combination pill (Marvelon Cycles 1–3) and in a control cycle after treatment (Control Cycle 2); values are given as means

cycle 2 = 11 days). Both cycles revealed the classic criteria of ovulatory cycles: (1) perimenstrual FSH rise; (2) preovulatory oestradiol peak; (3) midcyclic LH and FSH peak; and (4) adequate progesterone secretion during the luteal phase (Figure 1).

633

During treatment with the pill there was a prompt suppression of LH, FSH, oestradiol and progesterone values, indicating a sufficient and reliable inhibition of ovulation already in the first treatment cycle.

In the course of all three treatment cycles a clear FSH rise after the 7-day hormonal-free interval could be observed (Figure 1).

Starting with the first treatment cycle there was a marked increase of SHBG by two-fold. During the 7-day hormonal-free interval a slight decrease of SHBG could be observed – but without reaching pretreatment values. Free testosterone and DHT revealed inverse patterns: under the pill the levels successively decreased while the levels increased during the hormonal-free interval. Total testosterone showed a similar but less marked pattern while DHEA and DHEA sulphate did not reveal characteristic changes under the pill (Figure 2).

1 month after discontinuing the pill all parameters resumed pretreatment values.

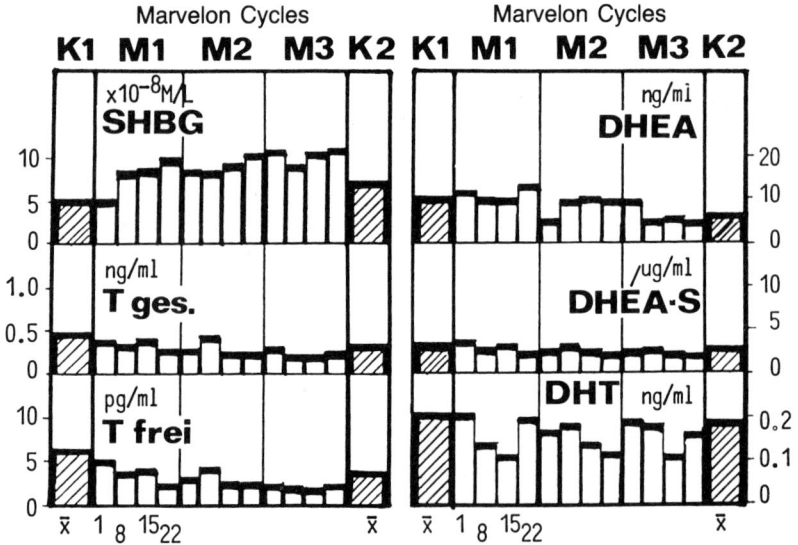

Figure 2   SHBG, total testosterone (T ges.), free testosterone (T frei), DHEA, DHEA sulphate and DHT in a control cycle before treatment (K1), under three treatment cycles of a 0.15 mg desogestrel/0.03 mg ethinyloestradiol combination pill (M1–M3), and in a control cycle after treatment (K2); values are given as means (x̄)

DISCUSSION

Already in the first treatment cycle of the desogestrel/ethinyloestradiol combination pill a reliable inhibition of ovulation was noted by a sufficient suppression of the hypothalmic–pituitary–ovarian axis. Obviously, as in amenorrhoeic patients[5] FSH was the most insensitive parameter, followed by LH and oestradiol. After discontinuing the pill no change of corpus luteum quality could be observed in comparison with the pretreatment control cycle (Figure 1).

Significantly elevated SHBG levels and thus decreased free testosterone and DHT levels – which were reported after a 3 and 6 months treatment with the desogestrel/ethinyloestradiol combination pill[6,7] – could already be detected after the first 2 weeks of treatment. Although there was a slight decrease of SHBG during the 7 days' hormone free interval after having taken the pill for 21 days, SHBG levels remained elevated in comparison with pretreatment values so that the favourable effect of preventing undesired signs of androgenization is also available during the period of withdrawal bleeding.

Furthermore, the results presented may explain the fact that 73.2% of more than 1800 women with pre-existing acne reported an amelioration or a complete disappearance of acne having taken the desogestrel/ethinyloestradiol combination pill for more than 6 months[8].

References

1. Lawrence, D. M., Kate, M., Robinson, T. W. E., Newman, M. C., McGarrigle, H. H. C., Shaw, M. and Lachelin, G. C. L. (1981). Reduced sex hormone binding globulin and derived free testosterone levels in women with severe acne. *Clin. Endocrinol.*, **15**, 87
2. Taubert, H. D. and Kuhl, H. (1981). *Kontrazeption mit Hormonen.* (Stuttgart: Georg Thieme Verlag)
3. Visser de, F., de Jager, E., de Jongh, H. P., van der Vies, J. and Feellen, F. (1975). Pharmacological profile of a new orally active progestational compound. *Acta Endocrinol. (Copenh.)*, Suppl. **199**, 405
4. Bergink, E. W., Hamburger, A. D., de Jager, E. and van der Vies, J. (1981). Binding of a contraceptive progestogen Org 2969 and its metabolites to receptor proteins and human sex hormone binding globulin. *J. Steroid Biochem.*, **14**, 175
5. Keller, E. (1981). *Hypothalamus/Hypophysen – Funktiondiagnostik bei Amenorrhoe.* (Frankfurt: Peter D. Lang Verlag)
6. Bergink, E. W., Homa, P. and Pyörälä, T. (1983). Effects of oral contraceptive combination containing Levonorgestrel and Org 2969 on serum proteins and androgen binding. *Scand. J. Clin. Lab. Invest.* (In press)
7. Mall-Haefeli, M., Werner-Fodrow, J., Huber, P. and Weijers, M. J. (1982). Klinische

und biochemische Resultate bei der Behandlung mit Marvelon – einen neuen steroidalen Ovultationshemmer. *Gebuftsh. u. Frauenheilk.*, **42,** 215

8. Geissler, K-H. (1983). Hormonelle Kontrazeption mit Marvelon. *Fortschr. Med.,* **101,** 1060

69
Comparative haematological effects of new ethinyloestradiol–progestogen combinations

M. H. BRIGGS

SUMMARY

A randomized, prospective study on metabolic effects of three oral contraceptives is presented. The products used were a low-dose triphasic formulation of levonorgestrel (LNG) and ethinyloestradiol (EE), a fixed dose combination of 0.15 mg desogestrel (DOG) + 30 µg EE, and a sequential formulation of 50 µg EE (×7), then 0.125 mg DOG + 50 µg EE (×15). Over the initial six cycles significant changes were seen in coagulation and fibrinolytic factors in users of the sequential product, but much less with the other two products. Women using the sequential formulation were therefore switched to the triphasic product. After a further three cycles the laboratory tests showed restoration towards normality.

INTRODUCTION

Large epidemiological surveys of oral contraceptive (OC) users have suggested that some of the adverse clinical associations of OCs are related to the daily oestrogen dose, though others are related to the daily progestogen dose[1]. In an attempt to produce safer and more acceptable preparations, manufacturers have introduced a range of low-dose OC formulations. Particular attention has been placed on

637

the oestrogen component and most new formulations contain a daily dose of 30 or $35\mu g$ ethinyloestradiol (EE). Recent evidence suggests that these low-oestrogen formulations have indeed reduced the incidence of some rare, but serious, side-effects of OCs[2,3]. A new progestogen (desogestrel (DOG), ORG 2969) has also been introduced and claimed to have a more favourable effect on laboratory indices of cardiovascular risk[4]. The present study was undertaken to compare the metabolic effects of three new OC formulations on young, healthy, new OC acceptors.

METHODS AND MATERIALS

The following commercial OC formulations were investigated: all contained EE combined with either levonorgestrel (LNG) or DOG.

(1) Triphasic: 0.050 mg LNG and $30\mu g$ EE ($\times 6$); 0.075 mg LNG and $40\mu g$ EE ($\times 5$); 0.125 mg LNG and $30\mu g$ EE ($\times 10$).
(2) Monophasic: 0.150 mg DOG and $30\mu g$ EE ($\times 21$).
(3) Biphasic: $50\mu g$ EE ($\times 7$); 0.125 mg DOG and $50\mu g$ EE ($\times 15$).

Criteria to enter the study included an absence of any absolute or relative contraindications to hormonal contraception, a body weight within 10% of the ideal for height, no concurrent medication, normotension, good personal motivation, age less than 30 years, and non-use of cigarettes. Written formal consent was obtained.

During the immediate pre-treatment cycle, all women used a barrier contraceptive: OCs were started on day 5 of the first treatment cycle.

Blood specimens were collected from the antecubital vein in subjects who had fasted overnight. Two specimens were taken on consecutive days during the late pre-treatment cycle (days 25–28) and during each treatment cycle on either of the last 2 days of pill taking.

Blood coagulation and fibrinolytic factors (fibrinogen, factor-VII, factor-VIII, factor-X, plasminogen, antithrombin-III) were measured every three cycles[5]. For logistic reasons, several laboratories collaborated in these measurements. All used the same quality control system.

RESULTS

At the time of preparing this report, 39 women had completed nine treatment cycles. Of these, 13 were receiving the monophasic product,

Table 1 Changes in coagulation and fibrinolytic factor activities. Results are given as percentages of pre-treatment values and are group means

Test	(150 µg DOG + 30 µg EE)			(Biphasic DOG + EE)			(Triphasic LNG + EE)		
	3	6	9	3	6	9†	3	6	9
Fibrinogen	110*	112*	113*	135***	146***	118**	108	110*	109
Coagulation factor:									
VII	108	110	111*	133***	140***	116**	104	105	103
VIII	106	107	110	121**	137***	112*	102	106	105
X	111*	113*	115*	135***	142***	115*	107	110*	108
Plasminogen	112*	116*	114*	142***	148***	116*	108	112*	110
Antithrombin-III	98	97	95	93***	88***	95	101	101	100

Cycle (treatment)

Difference between means significantly different: * $p < 0.5$; ** $p < 0.01$; *** $p < 0.001$.
†Subjects switched to triphasic treatment after cycle 6.

Table 2 Number of results outside normal reference ranges for coagulation and fibrinolytic factors

Factor	Cycle	Treatment		
		150 μg DOG + 30 μg EE ($n = 13$)	Biphasic DOG + EE[†] ($n = 14$)	Triphasic LNG + EE ($n = 12$)
Fibrinogen	0	0	0	0
	6	1	3	0
	9	2	2	0
Coagulation factor:				
VII	0	0	1	0
	6	1	4	1
	9	1	2	1
VIII	0	0	0	0
	6	2	3	0
	9	1	1	1
X	0	1	0	1
	6	1	4	0
	9	2	2	1
Plasminogen	0	0	1	1
	6	2	5	1
	9	1	2	1
AT-III	0	0	0	0
	6	1	4	1
	9	2	2	0
Total number of measurements of all factors		78	84	72
Total No. (%) of outliers	0	1 (1.3)	2 (2.4)	2 (2.8)
	6	8 (10.3)*	23 (27.4)***	3 (4.2)
	9	9 (11.5)*	11 (13.1)**	4 (5.6)

Difference between means significant: * $p < 0.05$; ** $p < 0.01$; *** $p < 0.001$.
[†]Subjects switched to triphasic treatment after cycle six.

14 the biphasic, and 12 the triphasic. As the changes in most factors in women using the biphasic were very large, it was decided for ethical reasons to transfer all of them to the triphasic product after six cycles. This should be borne in mind in interpreting the results (Table 1). In this table each woman served as her own control and results at three, six and nine cycles are expressed as a percentage of the pre-treatment cycle values.

Examination of individual values revealed a number to be outside the usual reference ranges. These are summarized in Table 2. Finally, as most women showed increases in levels of coagulation factors, but decreases in antithrombin-III, these changes can be emphasized by calculating the ratio of each factor to antithrombin-III (Table 3).

Table 3 Ratio of coagulation factors to antithrombin-III. Results are given as means and as percentages of mean values in cycle 0

	Cycle (treatment)					
	(150 μg DOG + 30 μg EE)		(Biphasic DOG + EE)		(Triphasic LNG+EE)	
	6	9	6	9†	6	9
Fibrinogen	115**	121**	166***	124**	109	109
Coagulation factor:						
VII	113*	116**	159***	122**	104	103
VIII	110	116**	156***	118**	105	105
X	116**	121**	161***	121**	109	108
Range	110–116	116–121	156–166	118–124	104–109	103–109
Mean	113*	119**	160***	121**	107	106

Difference between means significant: * $p < 0.05$; ** $p < 0.01$; *** $p < 0.001$.
†Subjects switched to triphasic treatment after cycle 6.

DISCUSSION AND CONCLUSIONS

Significant differences between the three products were apparent by cycles three and six, with large changes being seen in women using the biphasic formulation. While no cases of thrombosis were seen in any of the groups, it was considered prudent to transfer women on the biphasic to the triphasic product. As will be seen from the tables, by cycle nine there was a marked tendency for the abnormal results to become more normal, suggesting that the changes induced by the biphasic treatment are at least partially reversible by switching to a lower dose product.

While the two lower dose formulations produced much smaller changes in the various factors, fewer abnormalities were seen with the triphasic formulation containing LNG than with the monophasic product containing DOG.

On the basis of these findings, the biphasic formulation of DOG and EE does not seem suitable for routine use.

References

1. Royal College of General Practitioners (1974). *Oral Contraceptives and Health.* (London: Pitman)
2. Meade, T. W., Greenberg, G. and Thompson, S. C. (1980). Progestogens and cardiovascular reactions associated with oral contraceptives and a comparison of the safety of 50 and 30 μg oestrogen preparations. *Br. Med. J.*, **i**, 1157
3. Böttiger, L. E., Boman, G., Eklund, G. and Westerholm, B. (1980). Oral contraceptives and thromboembolic disease: effects of lowering oestrogen content. *Lancet*, **1**, 1097
4. Bergink, E. W., Hamburger, A. D., de Jager, E. and van der Vies, J. (1981). Binding of a contraceptive progestogen ORG 2969 and its metabolites to receptor proteins and human sex hormone binding globulin. *J. Steroid Biochem.*, **14**, 175
5. Triplett, D. A. and Harms, C. S. (1981). *Procedures for the Coagulation Laboratory.* (Chicago: American Society of Clinical Pathologists)

70
Oestroprogestogens and serum lipoproteins

F. R. HELLER and C. HARVENGT

SUMMARY

In the plasma, cholesterol (C) and triglycerides, are carried in five lipoprotein fractions: chylomicrons, very low density lipoproteins (VLDL), remnants, low density lipoproteins (LDL) and high density lipoproteins (HDL). Only remnants and LDL are implicated in the development of atherosclerosis; HDL, particularly HDL_2, are considered to be protective against atherosclerosis. Plasma VLDL and LDL are higher in the girls than in the boys. Women have less plasma total C and LDL-C and more plasma HDL-C than men. During the second part of the menstrual cycle, plasma levels of total C and LDL-C tend to be lower than in the first phase of the cycle. During pregnancy, plasma lipoproteins are elevated mainly during the third part of the pregnancy. In the postmenopausal period, women have a plasma lipoprotein pattern similar to that of men.

Both synthetic and natural oestrogens induced an increase in plasma VLDL and HDL (HDL_3) and a decrease in plasma LDL; these modifications could be considered as beneficial in terms of prevention of atherosclerosis. As far as the progestogens are concerned, the effects on plasma lipoproteins are opposed to those of oestrogens. The effects of the contraceptive pill on plasma lipoproteins will depend on the relative potency of its hormonal components, particularly of its progestogen component.

INTRODUCTION

After 20 years of oral contraceptive (OC) use, epidemiological data and scientific research have led to the now accepted evidence that the most important effect produced by these drugs on humans, other than the prevention of unwanted pregnancy, is an increase in the risk of cardiovascular disease. Because the incidence of cardiovascular disease is also related to disturbances of the lipoprotein metabolism, it appears to be opportune to analyse the different aspects of the interaction between female hormones and lipoprotein (LP) metabolism.

SERUM LIPOPROTEINS: METABOLISM

In the serum, lipids (cholesterol (C), triglycerides (TG), and phospholipids) are associated with peptides called apoproteins: apoproteins A-I, A-II, B, C, etc. The chylomicrons rich in TG contain Apo B48; the very low density lipoproteins (VLDL) rich in TG and the low density lipoproteins (LDL) rich in cholesterol, contain Apo B-100; and the high density lipoproteins (HDL) are rich in proteins (Apo A-I, Apo A-II) and phospholipids.

The chylomicrons and the VLDL are secreted by the intestine and the liver and transformed into intermediary lipoproteins (IDL) called remnants; the LDL and the HDL can be considered as end products of the degradation of the TG-rich LP. The interconversion of some LP is regulated by lipolytic enzymes: lipoprotein lipase (LPL) which hydrolyses TG of the TG-rich LP; hepatic lipase (HL) which hydrolyses the phospholipids of the HDL; and the lecithin:cholesterol acyltransferase (LCAT) which esterifies C contained in the HDL_3 (the heaviest fraction of HDL) which are transformed in HDL_2; in this way, LCAT probably favours the transport of C toward the liver. Some LP, when in excess in the serum, such as remnants and LDL, are associated with a high risk of coronary heart disease; a rise in VLDL and chylomicronaemia can lead to pancreatitis and osteonecrosis. In contrast, high levels of HDL (HDL_2) could lower the risk of coronary heart disease.

644

FEMALE HORMONES AND CARDIOVASCULAR DISEASE

OCs have been found to increase the risk of venous thromboembolic diseases, particularly when no predisposing conditions are present. A direct correlation exists between the risk and the oestrogen content of OCs. The pathogenesis of thromboembolic disease caused by the OC appears to be related to the proliferation of various constituents of the vessel wall and to altered blood coagulation[1]. OCs also increase the risk of myocardial infarction, thrombotic stroke and haemorrhagic stroke[2].

Compared with non-users, the relative risk for myocardial infarction is increased for current users ($\times 3$–4) and for long term (5 years or more) past users ($\times 2$) for up to 10 years after drugs have been discontinued. Moreover, the risk is increased after the age of 40 and OCs multiply the effects of other risk factors (e.g. cigarette smoking, type II hyperlipoproteinaemia, diabetes mellitus). The pathogenesis of myocardial infarction attributable to OCs comprises two components: on one hand, an increase in the platelet hyperactivity and increased production and accumulation of fibrin; on the other hand, deleterious effects on blood pressure, glucose tolerance and HDL-C.

Recently, it has been suggested that the occurrence of all arterial diseases – ischaemic heart disease, cerebrovascular diseases, peripheral vascular disease and hypertension – can be directly related to the progestogen (19-nortestosterone derivative) dosage, which is itself inversely related to the serum HDL-C concentration[3]. Thus, it appears that arterial diseases could be linked to the use of female hormones through disturbances produced by these compounds on LP metabolism.

FEMALE HORMONES AND SERUM LIPOPROTEINS: PHYSIOLOGICAL STATES

The most dramatic changes in serum LP at the different periods of life of an individual occur during the first years of life and the levels approach those of young adults by 1–2 years of age; thereafter, the serum lipids levels remain relatively stable until the onset of puberty. During sexual maturation, a decline in serum TC, LDL-C, Apo B, HDL-C and Apo A-I is observed in both sexes but mainly in boys. This is followed by an increase during the late sexual development. In girls, HDL-C increase to the prepubertal concentration while in boys the level of HDL-C remains low. In contrast, serum TG show a continued increase with age in both sexes. After sexual maturation, females have higher serum concentrations of HDL (HDL$_2$), Apo A-I and Apo A-II and lower VLDL and IDL than males. So men exhibit progressively a more atherogenic LDL/HDL ratio with age but after menopause, levels of serum LP in females are somewhat similar to those in men[4,5].

During the menstrual cycle, serum TG rise to the highest concentration at mid-cycle and fall during the luteal phase; during the late luteal phase, there is a significant fall in plasma total C, LDL-C and Apo B but no change in the HDL-C and Apo A-I[6].

During pregnancy, serum TG and total C concentrations are elevated in 95% of women; TG-LP rises progressively and the serum TG exceed 2–3 times their basal level at the end of pregnancy, with a maximal rise in VLDL-TG. Total and VLDL-Apo B are also increased; LDL-Apo B has been found to be unchanged or elevated. After delivery, serum C and TG decrease but serum C can remain high until 6–7 weeks postpartum[7]. It is important to note that, at least in the human, LDL are the lipoproteins that are used by steroidogenic tissues such as the adrenal cortex and the ovarian corpus luteum as a source of hormones.

FEMALE HORMONES AS A CAUSE OF DISORDERS IN LIPOPROTEIN METABOLISM

OCs have been shown to increase serum TG and total C concentration. Population studies from the Lipid Research Clinics Programme indicated that serum TG levels were approximately 50% higher and total-C 5–7% higher in young users of oral contraceptives, while in women aged 55 years and over, using hormone preparations (presumably oestrogens), there was a modest decline in mean cholesterol of about 5–6% and a slight but variable increase (maximum 5%) in triglycerides in comparison with non-users. Several studies have suggested that the alterations in serum levels of the different LP are related to the oestrogen/progestin potency of the contraceptive pill[8]. This was emphasized in a recent report from the Lipid Research Clinics Prevalence Study[9]. It appears that LDL-C concentrations are highest in women using low-dose oestrogen oral contraceptives (14–24%) and indistinguishable from the levels in non-users when high dose oestrogen oral contraceptives with strong progestin potency (taking into account the type and dosage) are used. With equine oestrogens, the LDL-C levels are 12% higher in younger women and 11–19% lower in postmenopausal women than in non-users.

On the other hand, the levels of HDL-C are significantly higher than in non-users and tend to be highest in users of oestrogen-dominant preparations and lowest in users of progestin-dominant preparations.

It must be remembered that the androgenic progestogens of the 19-nortestosterone (levonorgestrel) series reverse the beneficial effect of postmenopausal oestrogen treatment on HDL-C whereas among the hydroxyprogesterone derivatives, medroxyprogesterone acetate has no such effect[10]. Desogestrel, although displaying stronger progestational activity than levonorgestrel seems to produce *in vivo* effects similar to those of levonorgestrel on serum lipoproteins at the same dosage. The increase in the HDL-C observed with some contraceptive pills is accounted for primarily by an increase in HDL_3 mass in contrast with the findings in postmenopausal users of natural oestrogens, in whom increased levels of HDL are confined to the HDL_2 species[11]. On the other hand, norgestrel has been reported to lower HDL_2 concentrations.

Whole serum and LDL, HDL and VLDL triglycerides concentrations are significantly elevated in both older and younger women using sex hormones[9]. The analysis of the data clearly shows that the oestrogenic component of oral contraceptives is associated with higher TG levels[8], and that certain progestins oppose the action of the oestrogens and lower TG levels. That the changes in HDL-C and TG during oral contraceptive treatment are influenced by the total oestrogenicity of the drug is also suggested by the positive correlation found between the mean changes in HDL-C or TG levels and the mean changes in the plasma concentration of sex hormone binding globulin and with the ethinyloestradiol–levonorgestrel ratio[12].

Finally, the cholesterol content of the VLDL is elevated in women using contraceptive pills[9]; this finding may signify increased serum concentration of remnants that are associated with accelerated atherosclerosis. The low-dose triphasic contraceptive pills seem to induce little changes in the serum lipid fractions. However, recent data show that it can be misleading because the serum Apo-B levels have been found to be significantly increased by a triphasic contraceptive pill, although the changes in lipid fractions have been very small and the ratio LDL-C/HDL-C unaltered[13]. High serum Apo-B level is correlated to an increased risk of coronary heart disease. Preliminary studies have shown that the combination of desogestrel with ethinyl-oestradiol could have beneficial (increase of HDL-C and Apo A-I) or less detrimental effects (lower increase of VLDL, absence or increase of Apo B) on the serum lipoprotein pattern than other combinations[14,15], but these results have not been uniformly confirmed and more studies are needed with this compound.

In order to avoid high peaks of serum hormone concentrations and the hepatic first pass, natural oestrogens have been administered by a non-oral route. Percutaneous administration of oestradiol does not seem to alter the lipoprotein pattern[16]; with the hormone releasing vaginal rings, the LDL-C/HDL-C ratio tends to be higher when ethinyloestradiol is combined with levonorgestrel and unmodified when oestradiol is combined with the progesterone-derivatives progestins[17].

The occurrence of pregnancy and oestrogen therapy can lead to massive hypertriglyceridaemia (levels above 2000 mg dl^{-1}) with chylomicronaemia in women suffering from familial hypertriglyceridaemia but curiously not from familial combined hyperlipoproteinaemia or dysbetalipoproteinaemia.

FEMALE HORMONES AS A TREATMENT OF DISORDERS IN LIPOPROTEIN METABOLISM

In dysbetalipoproteinaemia, in fact, lower TG levels can be observed with oestrogen treatment[18]; this paradoxal effect of oestrogens could be related to an accelerated catabolism of remnants by the liver. Another beneficial effect of oestrogens may be the type II hyperlipoproteinaemia encountered in postmenopausal women[19]. Finally, two 19-nortestosterone derivatives, oxandrolone (an anabolic steroid) and norethindrone acetate (a progestogen), have been shown to reduce the plasma and VLDL-TG in various hyperlipoproteinaemias[20]. It must be remembered that oestrogens have been found to increase the risk of myocardial infarction in men (Coronary Drug Project), but to lower the same risk in post-menopausal women[21].

FEMALE HORMONES AND REGULATION OF LIPID METABOLISM

Plasma LPL activity is lower in women before puberty and becomes similar to or higher than men after puberty; plasma LH activity is lower in women after puberty although sometimes no sex-linked differences are seen in LPL and LH. During the luteal phase of the menstrual cycle, the plasma LPL activator property is increased[22]. During pregnancy, high adipose tissue LPL may facilitate increased TG uptake and fat deposition in adipose tissue; at the end of pregnancy and during lactation, the mammary tissue LPL is increased perhaps to shunt circulating TG from adipose depots to mammary tissue for milk synthesis[23]. The changes in LPL activity in these tissues seem to be related to prolactin secretion. The plasma LCAT activity is higher in males than females but the LCAT mass estimated by a radioimmunoassay (RIA) tend to be lower in males than females. Evaluated by RIA, the LCAT is similar in women with and without oestrogen replacement or oral contraceptives[24].

Rats treated with oestrogens exhibit low rates of ketogenesis and high rates of TG secretion and the hypertriglyceridaemia induced by oestrogen has been usually related to the increased TG products by the liver[25]; moreover, in roosters the Apo-B synthesis is stimulated by oestrogens. However, a decrease in plasma post-heparin lipolytic activity has been demonstrated for oestrogens and OCs, presumably due to a selective suppression in HL[26]. In men with prostatic carcinoma, the plasma LCAT activity is increased by oestrogens and cyproterone acetate, while in rats, progestogens inhibit plasma LCAT activity *in vitro* but not *in vivo*. Progestins of the 19-nortestosterone derivatives but not of the medroxyprogesterone derivatives induce an increase of HL which is significantly correlated with the decrease in plasma HDL_2[27].

The use of OCs is associated with a significant increase in biliary C saturation caused by an increase in C secretion and a decrease in bile acid secretion[28]. The saturation of bile with C is found also during the luteal phase and during the second and third trimester of pregnancy.

In rats, pharmacological doses of 17α-ethinyloestradiol cause a profound lowering of plasma C and LP by increasing the number of hepatic receptors for human LDL (Apo B), and so the rate of catabolism of LP[29]. On the other hand, in rabbits, oestrogen increases hepatic uptake of VLDL and LDL which are rich in Apo E[30].

Serum lipoproteins are modified quantitatively and qualitatively by sex and sex hormones, depending on the relative oestrogen/progestin potency. These changes could be or seem to be different whether the hormones are given as natural or synthetic compounds, whether the oral or the non-oral route is used, and sometimes are influenced by the pre-existing lipoprotein status and the menopause. In terms of atherosclerosis, evaluation of the effects of female hormones on serum lipoproteins must take into account not only the lipid content (HDL-C, LDL-C), but perhaps more importantly the peptide components of these lipoproteins (Apo A-I, Apo B). The hormonal contraception to be selected by the clinician must be proved not to impair the lipoprotein metabolism and special caution has to be taken before prescribing progestin-dominant oral contraceptives; presently, the ideal combination has still to be found.

References

1. Stadel, B. V. (1981). Oral contraceptives and cardiovascular disease (part I). *N. Engl. J. Med.*, **305**, 612
2. Stadel, B. V. (1981). Oral contraceptives and cardiovascular disease (part II). *N. Engl. J. Med.*, **305**, 672
3. Wingrave, S. J. (1982). Progestogen effects and their relationship of lipoprotein changes. *Acta Obstet. Gynecol. Scand.*, **105**, (Suppl.), 33
4. Connor, S. L., Connor, W. E., Sexton, G., Calvin, L. and Bacon, S. (1982). The effects of age, body weight and family relationships on plasma lipoprotein and lipids in men, women and children of randomly selected families. *Circulation*, **65**, 1290
5. Riesen, W. F., Mordasini, R. C. and Oetliker, O. H. (1983). Les altérations de la composition des lipoproteins sériques durant l'ontogénèse. In Van Keep, P. A. and de Gennes, J. L. (eds.). *Contraceptifs Oraux et Lipoproteines*, pp. 34–41. (Paris: Masson)
6. Kim, H. J. and Kalkhoff, R. K. (1979). Changes in lipoprotein composition during the menstrual cycle. *Metabolism*, **28**, 663
7. Hillman, L., Schonfeld, G., Miller, J. P. and Wulff, G. (1975). Apolipoproteins in human pregnancy. *Metabolism*, **24**, 943
8. Bradley, D. D., Wingerd, J., Petitti, D., Krauss, R. M. and Ramcharan, S. (1978). Serum high-density-lipoprotein cholesterol in women using oral contraceptives, estrogens and progestins. *N. Engl. J. Med.*, **299**, 17
9. Wahl, P., Walden, C., Knopp, R., Hoover, J., Wallace, R., Heiss, G. and Rifkind, B. (1983). Effect of estrogen/progestin potency on lipid/lipoprotein cholesterol. *N. Engl. J. Med.*, **308**, 862
10. Hirvonen, E., Mälkönen, M. and Manninen, V. (1981). Effects of different progestogens on lipoproteins during postmenopausal replacement therapy. *N. Engl. J. Med.*, **304**, 560
11. Krauss, R. M., Roy, S., Mishell, D. R., Jr., Casagrande, J. and Pike, M. C. (1983). Effects of two low-dose oral contraceptives on serum lipids and lipoproteins: Differential changes in high-density lipoprotein subclasses. *Am. J. Obstet. Gynecol.*, **145**, 446

12. Larsson-Cohn, U., Fahraeus, L., Wallentin, L. and Zador, G. (1981). Lipoprotein changes may be minimized by proper composition of a combined oral contraceptive. *Fertil. Steril.*, **35**, 172

13. Harvengt, C., Desager, J. P. and Lecart, C. (1983). Effects of plasma apoproteins A-I and B induced by two estrogestin preparations: monophasic versus triphasic. *Curr. Ther. Res.*, **33**, 385

14. Samsioe, G. (1982). Comparative effects of the oral contraceptive combinations 0.150 mg desogestrel + 0.030 mg ethinyloestradiol and 0.150 mg levonorgestrel + 0.030 mg ethinyloestradiol on lipid and lipoprotein metabolism in healthy female volunteers. *Contraception*, **25**, 487

15. De Jager, E. and Bergink, E. W. (1981). New progestagens for oral contraception. In Van der Molen, H. J., Klopper, A., Lunenfeld B., *et al.* (eds.). *Hormonal Factors in Fertility and Contraception. Research on Steroids*, Vol. **10**, pp. 122–31. (Amsterdam: Excerpta Medica)

16. Basdevant, A. and Guy-Grand, B. (1983). Influence de la voie d'administration sur les effets hormonaux et métaboliques de l'oestrogenotherapie. In Van Keep, P. A. and de Gennes, J. L. (eds.). *Contraceptifs Oraux et Lipoproteins*, pp. 85–9. (Paris: Masson)

17. Lithell, H., Ahren, T., Odlind, V., Weiner, E., Vessby, B., Victor, A. and Johnsson, E. D. B. (1983). Effects of progestins on lipoprotein patterns. In Bartin, C. W., Milgröm, E. and Mauvais-Jarvis, P. (eds.). *Progesterone and Progestins*, pp. 421–32. (New York: Raven Press)

18. Kushwaha, R. S., Hazzard, W. R., Gagne, C., Chait, A. and Albers, J. J. (1977). Type III hyperlipoproteinemia: paradoxical hypolipidemic response to estrogen. *Ann. Intern. Med.*, **87**, 515

19. Tikkanen, M., Nikkila, E. A. and Vartiainen, E. (1978). Natural oestrogen as an effective treatment for type-II hyperlipoproteinaemia in postmenopausal women. *Lancet*, **2**, 490

20. Tamai, T., Nakai, T., Yamada, S., *et al.* (1979). Effects of oxandrolone on plasma lipoproteins in patients with type IIa, IIb and IV hyperlipoproteinemia: occurrence of hypo-high density lipoproteinemia. *Artery*, **5**, 125

21. Bain, C., Willett, W., Hennekens, C. H., Rosner, B., Belangers, C. and Speizer, F. E. (1981). Use of postmenopausal hormones and risk of myocardial infarction. *Circulation*, **64**, 42

22. de Mendoza, S. G., Nucete, H., Salazar, E., Zerpa, A. and Kashyap, M. L. (1979). Plasma lipids and lipoprotein lipase activator property during the menstrual cycle. *Horm. Metab. Res.*, **11**, 696

23. Steingrimsdottir, L., Brasel, J. A. and Greenwood, M. R. C. (1980). Diet, pregnancy, and lactation: Effects on adipose tissue, lipoprotein lipase, and fat cell size. *Metabolism*, **29**, 837

24. Albert, J. J., Bergelin, R. O., Adolphson, J. L. and Wahl, P. W. (1982). Population-based reference values for lecithin-cholesterol acyltransferase (LCAT). *Atherosclerosis*, **43**, 369

25. Glueck, C. J., Fallat, R. W. and Scheel, D. (1975). Effects of estrogenic compounds on triglyceride kinetics. *Metabolism*, **24**, 537

26. Applebaum, D. M., Goldberg, P., Pykälistö, O. J., Brunzell, J. D. and Hazzard, W. R. (1977). Effect of estrogen on post-heparin lipolytic activity. Selective decline in hepatic triglyceride lipase. *J. Clin. Invest.*, **59**, 601

27. Nikkilä, E. A., Tikkanen, M. J. and Kuusi, T. (1983). Effects of progestins on plasma lipoproteins and heparin-releasable lipases. In Bartin, C. W., Milgröm, E. and Mauvais-Jarvis, P. (eds.). *Progesterone and Progestins*, pp. 411–20. (New York: Raven Press)

28. Kern, F., Jr., Everson, G. T., De Mark, B., McKinley, C., Showalter, R. and

Braverman, D. Z. (1982). Biliary lipids, bile acids and gallbladder function in the human female: effects of contraceptive steroids. *J. Lab. Clin. Med.*, **99**, 798

29. Kovanen, P. T., Brown, M. S. and Goldstein, J. L. (1979). Increased binding of low density lipoprotein to liver membranes from rats treated with 17α-ethinyl estradiol. *J. Biol. Chem.*, **254**, 11367

30. Floren, C. H., Kushwaha, R. S., Hazzard, W. R. and Albers, J. J. (1981). Estrogen-induced increase in uptake of cholesterol-rich very low density lipoproteins in perfused rabbit liver. *Metabolism*, **30**, 367

71
Cycle control and modern contraception: some relevant aspects

M. J. WEIJERS

SUMMARY

Literature data regarding cycle control of oral contraceptives are often unclear because of the lack of information on definitions concerning the evaluation of clinical trials. This frequently makes a valid comparison of results from different studies impossible. Information considered to be meaningful for practical purposes is discussed. Based on experience from multicentre trials with 14 000 women involving 180 000 cycles with combinations containing varying doses of a progestational and an oestrogenic substance, details are given about the role these active substances play in cycle control.

It is demonstrated that the progestational and oestrogenic components have independent influences on spotting and breakthrough bleeding. Predictions regarding cycle control, based only on the ratio progestogen to oestrogen, should not be made.

Since the introduction of oral contraceptives (OCs) in the late 1950s, the main issues with these preparations have been reliability, cycle control and safety. In comparison with other methods of contraception, OCs have an outstanding reliability[1]. Although the reliability of OCs can be assessed by various methods of calculation, the data obtained should reflect as close as possible the situation as it occurs in daily clinical practice. A relevant question raised in this context is whether pregnancies due to improper use of OCs should be included in the reporting. As appears from literature data, in daily practice up to 8% of women using OCs forget to take a tablet each day[2]. In addition it is known that the reliability of OCs may become impaired as a consequence of drug–OC interactions[3]. The implications of these aspects are growing in view of the continuing dose reductions of both the progestogen and oestrogen component of low-dose OCs[3]. This seems to be particularly valid in the case of the so-called triphasics, where dose reduction apparently has reached a critical point and, as a result, contraceptive failures begin to occur[4-7].

As far as safety is concerned, today there is a fair deal of understanding about the risks and benefits of OCs. With respect to the undesirable effects, attention has been focussed on the cardiovascular hazards, a topic that has been dealt with extensively in numerous epidemiological and biochemical studies[8,9]. Later, when the studies continued, it appeared that the risks had been overstated and were actually very small[10]. In addition it has become clear that future investigations should concentrate on the underlying mechanisms in order to identify those women who are at greater risk of developing serious adverse effects[11]. In contrast to the health risks, the health benefits of OCs have been almost ignored during the past 20 years of their use. However, fortunately times are changing and evidence is accumulating that the benefits of OC use far outweigh the risks[12].

Although there exists a vast bibliography on OCs, relatively little attention has been paid to control of bleeding, since scientifically reliable studies on cycle control are scarce. There is little meaning in presenting data on the incidence of spotting, breakthrough bleeding (BTB) and missing periods if information on the general design of the study, on the definitions of bleeding parameters and on the population concerned is inadequate or lacking. In addition, most reports have failed to provide detailed information on the various groups of women studied, for example on switchers or new starters and on the age distribution of the women. Besides, information on compliance with regular tablet intake and on the reasons for discontinuing OC treatment (drop-outs) is rare. There is also little meaning in presenting data on control of bleeding that have been 'corrected' for pre-treatment cycle irregularities[13], since this has no affinity with daily OC practice.

It needs no argument that this inadequacy of information does not present the physician with much opportunity to make a so-called 'educated selection of an oral contraceptive'[14]. To what amazing results the above-mentioned omissions and inconsistencies in reporting may lead can be illustrated best by looking at the following literature data.

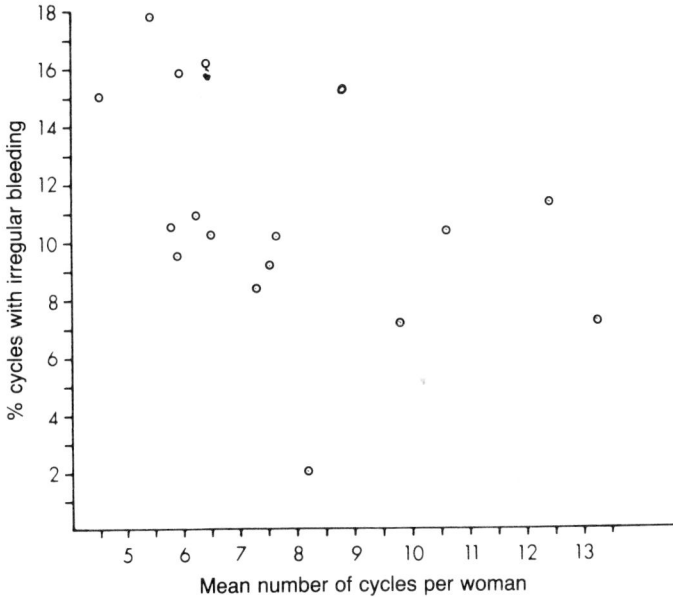

Figure 1 Mean incidence of irregular bleeding (breakthrough bleeding and spotting) as obtained with an oral contraceptive containing 0.15 mg levonorgestrel and 0.03 mg ethinyloestradiol in 16 different investigations. Reproduced by kind permission from reference 15

With a low-dose OC, containing 0.03 mg ethinyloestradiol (EE) and 0.15 mg levonorgestrel data on bleeding irregularities have been reported which were obtained in 16 different investigations[15]. Figure 1 shows the mean number of cycles with irregular bleeding (IB; calculated as a percentage over the total number of cycles per trial), in relation to the mean number of cycles per woman obtained in each trial. As can be seen the mean incidence of IB varied widely in these trials, ranging from 2 to 18%. Although cycle control may differ between different ethnic groups, it is unlikely that the wide variation in IB can be explained merely by this aspect.

In another paper, cycle control data on a so-called 'triphasic' preparation were produced referring only to the women who did not forget to take any tablet and to the women with a history of no

Table 1 The incidence of irregular bleeding with a triphasic preparation*

	Trial A (6628 cycles)[†]		Trial B (25 000 cycles)		
	All cycles, excluding women who forgot tablets	All cycles, excluding women with irregular bleeding in anamnesis	cycles[‡]		
			1	6	12
% cycles with irregular bleeding	7.8	6.5	23.8	16.0	11.5

*6 × 0.03 mg ethinyloestradiol (EE) + 0.05 mg levonorgestrel; 5 × 0.04 mg EE + 0.075 mg levonorgestrel; 10 × 0.03 mg EE + 0.125 mg levonorgestrel.
[†]From reference 13.
[‡]Without corrections. From reference 16.

bleeding irregularities[13]. Table 1 compares these 'corrected' figures with those obtained in a fairly large study by another investigator who did not apply such 'corrections'[16]. It should be noted that both studies are comparable for the mean number of treatment cycles per woman.

In view of these discrepancies, the relevance for clinical practice of presenting corrected data should be questioned seriously! In addition, it will be clear from the above that comparisons of various data on cycle control published so far will contribute neither to a better understanding nor facilitate a proper evaluation and/or selection of an OC.

It has been suggested that spotting and BTB are influenced not only by the amount of oestrogen in an OC but also by the ratio of the amount of oestrogen and progestogen[17]. Although over the years many cycle control data have been produced with a variety of high- and low-dose OCs, there is still poor understanding about the influence of the oestrogen/progestogen component of an OC on bleeding parameters.

Since March 1976 our group has collected a large number of data on cycle control, obtained in various multicentre clinical trials with 19 different experimental desogestrel/EE combinations. The studies covered 14 000 women who were treated during 180 000 cycles. Because throughout these studies the same definitions (including those for control of bleeding) were used, the data obtained can be compared and consequently the influence of the oestrogen and progestogen components on cycle control can be examined.

The following definitions for control of bleeding were applied:

(1) Spotting: a scanty bleeding, starting outside the tablet-free period, which does not require any hygienic measures or at most one sanitary towel per day.

(2) BTB: bleeding, starting outside the tablet-free period, which is not a spotting and which cannot be considered as a withdrawal bleeding.

(3) Withdrawal bleeding: a bleeding that begins in the tablet-free period.

In addition, it should be emphasized that in every study the percentage of switchers and new starters was kept fairly constant (45–55% for each group) and that at least 10 centres were involved.

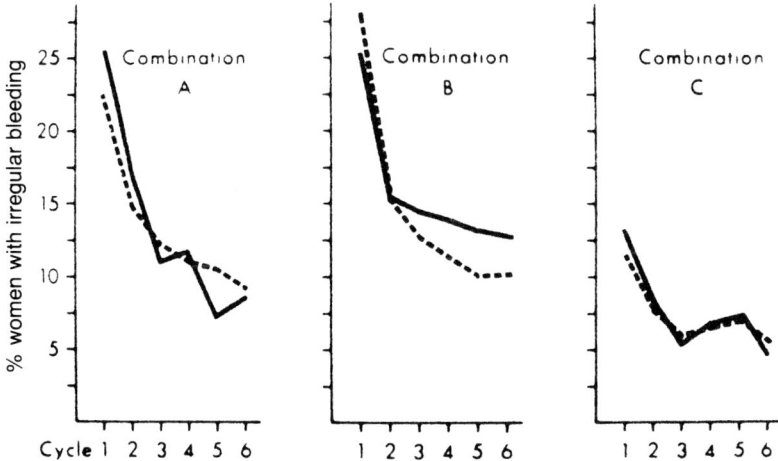

Figure 2   The influence of extension of the trial on irregular bleeding with three oral contraceptive combinations. Combination A: — = 530 women in cycle 1, 234 in cycle 6; — — — — = 1609 in cycle 1, 1244 in cycle 6. Combination B: — = 419 women in cycle 1, 298 in cycle 6; — — — — = 1044 in cycle 1, 837 in cycle 6. Combination C: — = 351 women in cycle 1, 256 in cycle 6; — — — — = 686 in cycle 1, 589 in cycle 6

657

A basic question with respect to cycle control with an OC refers to the number of data needed to obtain a fairly accurate idea about the incidence of IB. This aspect is illustrated in Figure 2 for three different OC combinations. As can be seen, extension of the trial beyond 200 women per cycle hardly influences the incidence of IB. Figure 2 also shows that with all combinations the incidence of IB is higher during the first 1–3 treatment cycles, while it stabilizes soon at much lower levels on continuation of treatment. It needs no argument in this context that for a proper judgment of an OC the prescribing physician needs a specification of the incidence of IB per cycle.

As stated above, the role of the oestrogen and progestogen components in control of bleeding is far from clear. In Figure 3 two desogestrel/EE combinations are compared that have the same progestogen:oestrogen ratio. Figure 3 shows that this ratio is not the only factor that determines the incidence of IB. Apparently, as already

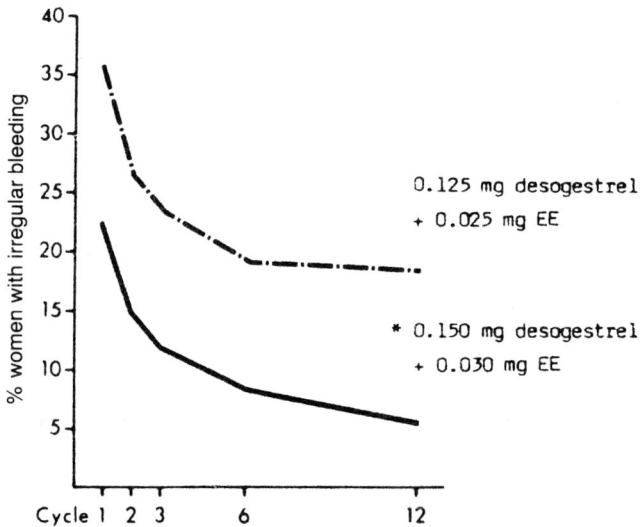

Figure 3 The influence of progestogen:oestrogen ratio on the incidence of irregular bleeding. EE = Ethinyloestradiol; *Marvelon

suggested[17], the amounts of oestrogen and/or progestogen also contribute to the ultimate effect. This is illustrated in Figures 4 and 5.

By comparing three OC combinations (Figure 4), each containing the same amount of EE (0.05 mg) but an increasing amount of desogestrel, the influence of the progestogen dose on the incidence of BTB

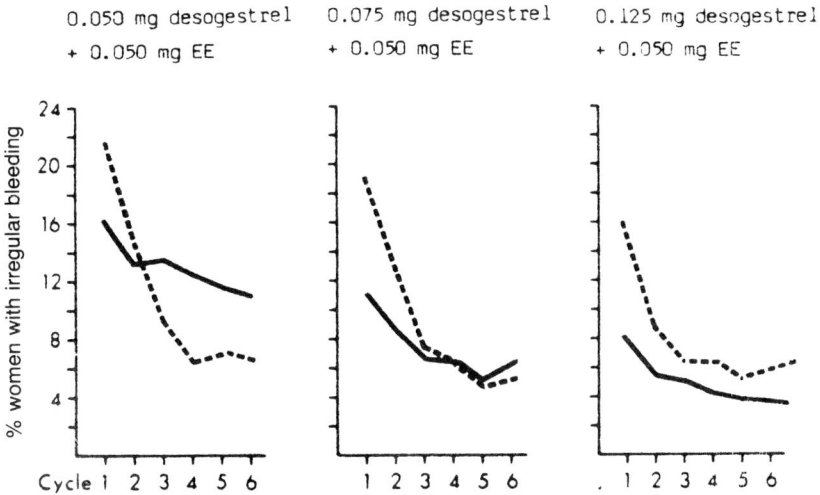

Figure 4 The influence of increasing progestogen dose on the incidence of irregular bleeding with oral contraceptive combinations containing 0.05 mg ethinyloestradiol (EE). — = Breakthrough bleeding; — — — — = spotting

and spotting could be examined. As can be seen from Figure 4, the incidence of BTB decreases when the progestogen dose increases. The consistency of this phenomenon has been demonstrated also in the case of combinations that contain a dose of 0.03 mg EE and an increasing amount of desogestrel. This strongly suggests that it is primarily the amount of progestogen in an OC that influences the occurrence of BTB.

On the other hand, it appears that the oestrogen dose is the major determining factor for spotting. This is very well illustrated by Figure 5, which shows that in the presence of the same dose of desogestrel, spotting substantially decreases when the oestrogen dose is increased from 0.03 mg EE to 0.05 mg EE.

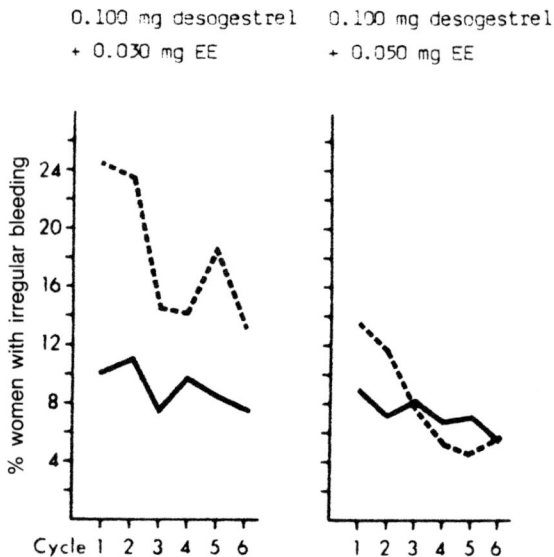

Figure 5 The influence of an increasing oestrogen dose (ethinyloestradiol, EE) on the incidence of irregular bleeding with oral contraceptive combinations containing 0.1 mg desogestrel. — = Breakthrough bleeding; — — — = spotting

Summarizing with respect to control of bleeding the following conclusions can be made:

(1) Reports should contain all definitions applied to the study.
(2) No corrections should be made for events that are known to

exist during the daily use of OCs, such as forgetting tablets and a history of irregular bleeding.

(3) For adequate assessment of cycle control with an OC, the data should refer to at least 200 women, treated during six cycles, and should be obtained in at least 10 centres. Extension of a trial from 200 to 600 or more women per cycle changes the mean incidence of IB only by 2–3%.

(4) The oestrogen and progestogen components of OCs each play a separate role in the occurrence of BTB and spotting. No indication was found for a so-called 'optimal oestrogen/progestogen-dose relationship'.

References

1. Vessey, M. (1982). Efficacy of different contraceptive methods. *Lancet*, **1**, 841
2. N.I.S.S.O. (Nederlands Instituut voor Sociaal Sexuologisch Onderzoek) (1975). *Anticonceptiegedrag. Verslag van een onderzoek bij 1200 nederlandse vrouwen en mannen naar de wijze waarop men een zwangerschap probeert te voorkomen.* (Report on an investigation in 1200 Dutch women and men with respect to their ways of preventing pregnancy). (Zeist: N.I.S.S.O.)
3. Orme, M. L. E. (1982). The clinical pharmacology of oral contraceptive steroids. *Br. J. Clin. Pharmacol.*, **14**, 31
4. Fay, R. A. (1982). Failure with the new triphasic oral contraceptive Logynon. *Br. Med. J.*, **284**, 17
5. Graham, H. (1982). Failure with the new triphasic oral contraceptive Logynon. *Br. Med. J.*, **284**, 422
6. Cullberg, G., *et al.* (1982). Two oral contraceptives, efficacy, serum proteins, and lipid metabolism. *Contraception*, **26**, 229
7. Cullberg, G. (1983). Säkerheten hos lagdoserade p-piller-metodfel en biverkning? (Reliability of low-dose contraceptive pill-method error a side effect?) *Läkartidningen*, **80**, 2484
8. Johns Hopkins University (1982). *Population Reports. Oral Contraceptives in the 1980s*, Series A, No. **6**, A189–A221. (Baltimore: Johns Hopkins University)
9. Briggs, M. H. and Briggs, M. (1981). Metabolic effects of oral contraceptives. In Fen, C. C., *et al.* (eds.). *Recent Advances in Fertility Regulation.* Proceedings of a symposium on recent advances in fertility regulation. Beijing 2–5 September 1980, pp. 83–111. (Geneva: S. A. Atar)
10. Wiseman, R. A. and MacRae, K. D. (1981). Oral contraceptives and the decline in mortality from circulatory disease. *Fertil. Steril.*, **35**, 277
11. Kay, C. R. (1980). The happiness pill? *J. R. Coll. Gen. Pract.*, **30**, 8
12. Mishell, D. R. (1982). Noncontraceptive health benefits of oral steroidal contraceptives. *Am. J. Obstet. Gynecol.*, **142**, 809
13. Lachnit-Fixson, U. (1979). Erstes Dreistufenpraeparat zur hormonalen Konzeptionsverhuetung, Klinische Ergebnisse. *Muench. Med. Wochenschr.*, **121**, 1421
14. Woutersz, T. B. (1981). A low-dose combination oral contraceptive. *J. Reprod. Med.*, **26**, 615
15. Bergstein, N. A. M. (1976). Clinical efficacy, acceptability and metabolic effects of new low dose combined oral contraceptives. *Acta Obstet. Gynecol. Scand. Suppl.*, **54**, 51

16. Upton, G. V. (1982). Clinical experience with triphasics. Presented at the *San Francisco Congress, October 17–22*

17. Lawson, J. S. (1979). Optimum dosage of an oral contraceptive. *Am. J. Obstet. Gynecol.,* **134,** 315

72
Studies with desogestrel for fertility regulation

J. R. NEWTON

INTRODUCTION

Over the past 20 years Organon have been involved in developing a new series of progestogens characterized by the absence of an oxygen at position 3 of the steroid skeleton. Following lynestrenol, the most promising compound in early trials was desogestrel, a 13-ethyl-11-methylene-3-desoxy compound, which is a more specific progestogen than both norethisterone and levonorgestrel[1]. Receptor binding studies have demonstrated a lower affinity of the main metabolite of desogestrel for androgen receptors than levonorgestrel[1].

A large multicentre trial indicated that a combination of $150\,\mu g$ desogestrel and $30\,\mu g$ ethinyloestradiol (Marvelon) was an effective oral contraceptive (pregnancy rate $0.1\,(\text{woman-year})^{-1}$) and caused a low level of irregular bleeding and side-effects[2]. Further work has suggested that this combination elevates HDL-cholesterol levels compared with a combination of $150\,\mu g$ levonorgestrel and $30\,\mu g$ oestradiol (Microgynon)[3,4].

In January 1982, prior to its introduction in the UK, a limited acceptability trial of Marvelon was initiated. The aim was to investigate the efficacy and tolerance of this new pill in the British family planning clinic population.

Recently considerable interest has been directed towards the effect of different hormonal contraceptive formulations on HDL cholesterol.

Epidemiological studies have demonstrated an inverse relationship between this parameter and ischaemic heart disease[5]. For this reason a randomized comparative study of Marvelon and Microgynon was conducted on a sub-group of patients participating in the acceptability trial.

PATIENTS AND METHODS

Twelve family planning clinics participated in the acceptability trial and recruited 238 suitable patients within a 3-month period.

In four centres 70 of these patients were randomly allocated to either Marvelon or Microgynon only for comparison of the effects on serum lipoproteins and SHBG.

Patients selected were healthy, of fertile age, having a regular cycle and with risk of pregnancy. No patient who had employed any hormonal preparation within 3 months was included. Other exclusion criteria were those standard contraindications to oral contraceptives, including breast-feeding women and those receiving any drug with a known interaction with oral contraceptives. Informed consent was obtained before treatment.

Marvelon tablets containing $150 \mu g$ desogestrel and $30 \mu g$ ethinyl-oestradiol were taken daily for 21 days, commencing on the first day of menstrual bleeding. There was a 7-day treatment-free interval before the next treatment cycle and each patient was assessed over six treatment cycles. Microgynon was administered in an identical manner.

After selection for the trial a brief gynaecological history was taken and a physical examination, which included measurement of blood pressure and weight, was performed.

Follow-up visits were after one, three and six cycles, at which blood pressure, weight and side-effects were recorded. Patients were required to complete diary cards for recording bleeding patterns and tablet compliance and these were collected at each clinic visit.

The following definitions were used:

(1) Withdrawal bleeding: bleeding beginning during the tablet-free period (days 22–28).
(2) Spotting: scanty bleeding occurring during tablet intake, requiring a minimum of sanitary protection.

(3) Breakthrough bleeding: bleeding occurring during tablet intake, requiring two or more sanitary pads per day.

The patients who agreed to participate in the serum lipoprotein study
also provided a fasting (12 hour) blood sample before treatment and
after three and six cycles. Wherever possible, during treatment blood
samples were collected in the third week of each cycle.

After centrifugation serum was collected and stored at $-20°C$
until analysis for total cholesterol, HDL cholesterol, triglycerides and
SHBG. All serum protein and lipid analysis was performed in one
laboratory and the samples from all centres were assayed at the same
time.

SHBG concentrations were measured as described by Bergink et
al.[6]. HDL fractions were prepared using the phosphotungstate/magne-
sium chloride sedimentation method of Burnstein et al.[7]. Total cholesterol and triglycerides were determined using the Boehringer test
method.

The measured values of all laboratory parameters were replaced
by their logarithms to obtain normally distributed data, and were
subjected to an analysis of co-variance using baseline measurements
as co-variates, employing Winer's repeated measures design[8]. Owing
to this choice of design, only those patients for whom complete data
were available at every time point could be included in the analysis.

RESULTS

208 women treated with Marvelon completed 931 cycles within the
trial period. The age structure is shown in Table 1. Nearly 50% of

Table 1 Age distribution

Age (years)	Number (%)
< 20	101 (48.6)
20–24	46 (22.1)
25–29	34 (16.3)
30–34	19 (9.1)
35–39	8 (3.8)
> 39	0 (0.0)

the patients were less than 20 years old, a high proportion of whom
were new pill users.

Contraceptive efficacy appeared to be good. There was only one pregnancy, despite a high incidence (8.3% of all cycles) of forgotten tablets. This pregnancy started in cycle 3 – the patient did not admit to any forgotten tablets but reported suffering mid-cycle diarrhoea and vomiting for several days whilst on holiday abroad.

Table 2 Incidence of withdrawal bleeding on Marvelon

Cycle	No. of women completing cycle	Women experiencing withdrawal bleeding (%)
3	145	91.2
6	117	97.5

Incidences of withdrawal and unscheduled bleeding are shown in Figure 1 and Table 2. In the majority of patients the amount of

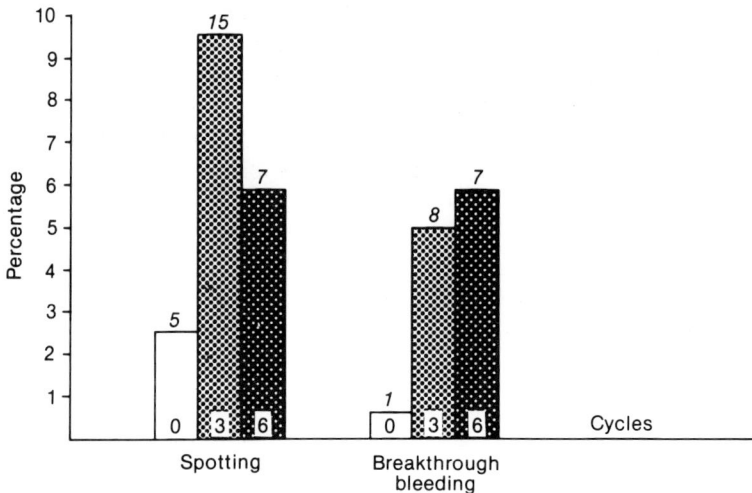

Figure 1 Incidence of unscheduled bleeding on Marvelon

withdrawal bleeding was the same or less than before treatment and the duration in days was also generally reduced. By cycle 6, 95% of withdrawal bleeds were starting between days 23 and 26.

40% of the unscheduled bleeding reported was experienced during the last 5 days of tablet taking. Only four patients found their irregular bleeding sufficiently inconvenient to discontinue Marvelon treatment, and two of these dropped out during the first cycle. In more than 17% of all cycles in which unscheduled bleeding occurred, the patient reported forgetting between one and five tablets. However, during 60% of cycles in which one or two tablets were omitted, no unscheduled spotting or bleeding was reported.

No serious side-effects occurred. Various minor complaints were reported, both before and during treatment. The incidence of pre-treatment complaints together with those newly emergent complaints

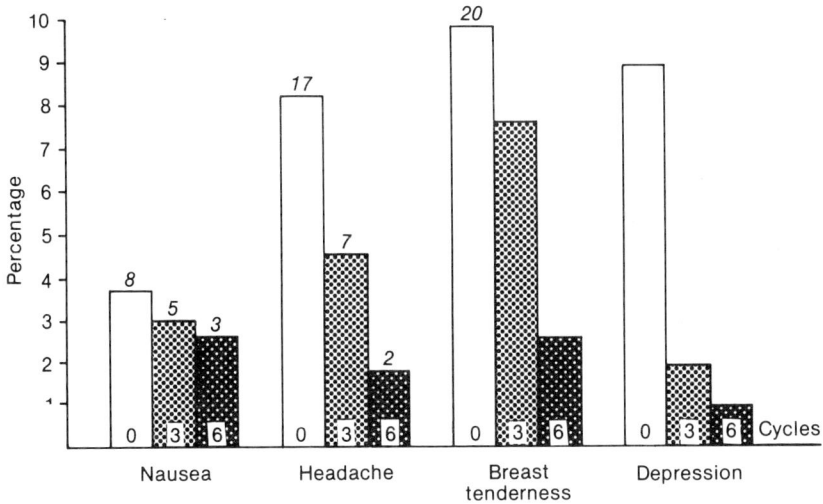

Figure 2 Incidence of newly emergent minor complaints on Marvelon

not recorded before treatment is shown in Figure 2. Fifteen patients withdrew from the trial as a result of side-effects, half of these during the first cycle. The only other complaint of interest was change in libido – a small number of women (< 5%) reporting either an increase or a decrease.

Table 3 Changes in blood pressure during Marvelon treatment

Cycle		Average deviation from pre-treatment cycle values (mm Hg)	
	No. of women	Systolic	Diastolic
3	127	−3.0	−1.2
6	118	−4.0	−1.9

667

Blood pressure and body weight changes are shown in Tables 3 and 4. Although the data is limited, effects on blood pressure were apparently minimal. A small weight increase is evident, but half of the trial patients were less than 20 years old and therefore still have growth potential.

Table 4 Changes in body weight during Marvelon treatment

Cycle	No. of women	No change, No. (%)	Average change from pre-treatment cycle (kg)
3	127	99 (78)	+0.5*
6	118	78 (66.1)	+0.8*

*Includes patients aged under 20 years.

The results of the randomized comparison of Marvelon and Microgynon and their effects on SHBG and serum lipoproteins are shown in Table 5. Examination of the baseline measurements showed no observable differences between the treatment groups on entry to the study. Mean values for all patients were not different from mean values of patients included in the analysis.

Table 5 Geometric mean values for serum proteins and lipid variables

Variable	Marvelon group			Microgynon group		
Cycle	0	3	6	0	3	6
No. of women	40	34	27	30	24	20
Total cholesterol (mmol l^{-1})	5.43	6.27	5.55	5.34	5.47	5.03
HDL cholesterol (mmol l^{-1})	1.38	1.63	1.46	1.39	1.33	1.12
Triglycerides (mmol l^{-1})	0.73	1.02	1.08	0.80	0.80	0.80
SHBG (nmol l^{-1})	69	187	184	63	71	64

HDL = High-density lipoprotein; SHBG = Serum hormone binding globulin.

There was no difference between treatments on effect on total cholesterol – both groups experienced a transient rise which had returned to pre-treatment values by 6 months. However, there were significant differences in HDL cholesterol values ($p \leq 0.0001$) between treatment groups. In the Marvelon-treated group the changes paralleled those seen in total cholesterol, with a transient rise at 3 months. In the Microgynon-treated group there was no change at 3 months but HDL-cholesterol levels had fallen considerably by 6 months.

Triglyceride levels were higher ($p \leqslant 0.005$) in the Marvelon treatment group.

SHBG levels were significantly increased ($p \leqslant 0.0001$) in the Marvelon-treated group as compared with the Microgynon group.

The effect of smoking was examined in relation to each parameter, but no significant differences between smokers and non-smokers could be found.

DISCUSSION

Extensive trials in Europe with the combination of 150 μg desogestrel and 30 μg ethinyloestradiol have yielded a Pearl Index for tablet failure of 0.0 and for patient failure[2] of 0.1. It was therefore unexpected to find a pregnancy in a small trial, although this patient's prolonged diarrhoea and vomiting may have resulted in malabsorption of the hormones.

The incidence of unscheduled bleeding during oral contraceptive use is known to decrease considerably during the first six cycles. By following up the patients for only six cycles it must be realized that a higher level of bleeding disturbances will be seen and should not therefore be compared with results of longer trials expressed as a percentage of total cycles. However, spotting and breakthrough bleeding were more common in this trial than in larger trials with Marvelon[2] where less than 5% spotting and 4.3% breakthrough bleeding were reported at six cycles. The data of this study were compatible with similar studies in Scandinavia[9,10].

The irregular bleeding reported in this trial was often during the last few days of pill taking and was closely related to a high incidence of forgotten pills. Despite this, it was encouraging to notice that on more than half the occasions when a patient forgot one or two tablets in a cycle there was no spotting or breakthrough bleeding.

Marvelon appeared to be well tolerated with respect to the common pill-induced side-effects and only a small proportion of patients discontinued the trial for reasons related to the treatment.

It is well known that a multiplicity of factors affect serum proteins and lipid levels[11]. Most studies have therefore been performed on volunteers, but this trial was conducted on routine clinic patients. Every reasonable effort was made to control for time of cycle and smoking habits were recorded. Allocation to treatment was according to a random list and assays were performed 'blind' in one laboratory.

Considerable interest has been generated in recent years as to the possibility of finding an oral contraceptive that might confer beneficial long-term effects by elevating HDL-cholesterol fractions[12]. Oestrogens are known to cause elevation of HDL-cholesterol values whilst progestogens commonly oppose this effect. In this trial a transient rise in HDL-cholesterol level was reported similar to that found in Scandinavian trials[3,4], compared with a fall in the Microgynon-treated group. The clinical relevance of these changes in the long term must remain unclear until epidemiological studies have been undertaken.

It has been suggested that an oral contraceptive that raised SHBG would confer advantages to women who suffer androgen-related side-effects such as hirsutism and acne[13]. This trial confirmed that Marvelon increases SHBG significantly, compared both with pre-treatment levels and Microgynon treatment. Although specific trials in acne and hirsutism would be desirable, it may well be that Marvelon would be a reasonable alternative to a levonorgestrel-containing pill in susceptible patients.

CONCLUSION

Preliminary experience of 12 British family planning clinics confirmed the choice of Marvelon as a useful new combined pill with minimal side-effects and potentially beneficial metabolic effects.

Acknowledgements

The author thanks his medical, nursing and administrative colleagues, without whom the study would not have been feasible; Dr W. Bergink for laboratory estimations; and Ir. J. Voerman and Mr D. Nelson for statistical analysis. The study was supported by Organon Laboratories Ltd.

References

1. Bergink, E. W., Hamburger, A. D., De Jager, E. and van der Vies, J. (1981). Binding of a contraceptive progestogen Org 2969 and its metabolites to receptor proteins and human sex hormone binding globulin. *J. Steroid Biochem.*, **14**, 175
2. Weijers, M. J. (1982). Clinical trial of an oral contraceptive containing $150\,\mu g$ desogestrel and $30\,\mu g$ ethinyloestradiol. *Clin. Ther.*, **4**, 359
3. Samsioe, G. (1982). Comparative effects of the oral contraceptive combinations

0.0150 mg desogestrel + 0.030 mg ethinyloestradiol and 0.150 mg levonorgestrel + 0.030 mg ethinyloestradiol on lipid and lipoprotein metabolism in healthy female volunteers. *Contraception*, **25**, 487

4. Bergink, E. W., Borglin, N. E., Klottrup, P. and Liukko, P. (1982). Effects of desogestrel and levonorgestrel in low-dose oestrogen oral contraceptives on serum lipoproteins. *Contraception*, **25**, 477

5. Gordon, T., Castelli, W. P. and Njortland, M. (1977). HDL as a protective factor against CHD – The Framingham study. *Am. J. Med.*, **62**, 707

6. Bergink, E. W., Holma, P. and Pyorala, T. (1981). Effects of oral contraceptive combinations containing levonorgestrel or desogestrel on serum proteins and androgen binding. *Scand. J. Clin. Lab. Invest.*, **41**, 663

7. Burstein, M., Scholnik, H. R. and Morfin, R. (1978). Rapid method for the isolation of lipoproteins from human serum by precipitation with polyanions. *J. Lipid. Res.*, **11**, 583

8. Winer, B. J. (1971). *Statistical Principles in Experimental Design*. (New York: McGraw Hill)

9. Borglin, N. E., Christensen, O. J. E., Culberg, G. *et al.* (1982). Scandinavian trial of an oral contraceptive containing 0.150 mg desogestrel and 0.03 mg ethinyloestradiol. *Acta Obstet. Gynecol. Scand. Suppl.*, **111**, 39

10. Culberg, G., Samsioe, G., Andersen, R. F., *et al.* (1982). Two oral contraceptives, efficacy, serum proteins and lipid metabolism. *Contraception*, **26**, 229

11. Bradley, D. D., Wingerd, J., Petitti, D. B., *et al.* (1978). Serum high density lipoproteins cholesterol in women using oral contraceptives, estrogens and progestins. *N. Engl. J. Med.*, **299**, 17

12. Kay, C. R. (1980). The happiness pill? *J. R. Coll. Gen. Pract.*, **30**, 8

13. el Makzangy, M. N., Wynn, V. and Lawrence, D. M. (1979). Sex hormone binding globulin capacity as an index of oestrogenicity or androgenicity in women on oral contraceptive steroids. *Clin. Endocrinol.*, **10**, 39

671

Part III

Section 4

Reproductive Health in Adolescence*

* Held under the auspices of WHO, Maternal and Child Health Department

73
Introductory remarks

B. LUNENFELD

I am honoured and glad to welcome you and chair this symposium of Reproductive Health in Adolescence

Adolescents of today will be the active citizens of tomorrow. From the pool of adolescents today will come tomorrow's world leaders. The adolescent of today will be the parent of tomorrow. A healthy adolescent will provide a healthier world of tomorrow and this will be in line with the World Health Organization's declared aim of 'Health for All' by the year 2000.

The approach to adolescent health has to be holistic, taking into account mental and physical aspects of health including the diverse psycho-social aspects in the diverse ethnic groups and regions.

Adolescents, who constitute more than 20% of the World Population, have survived the diseases of childhood and are not yet affected by the degenerative changes and diseases of adulthood and the aged.

Mortality and morbidity of the adolescent population are mainly due to accidents, suicide, drugs and sexually transmitted diseases and, in the female population, to teenage pregnancies with all their sequences.

WHO realized the importance of adolescent health many years ago and has given the mandate concerning adolescent health to its Division of Family Health, and in particular, to one of its major units, the Unit of Maternal and Child Health.

The main objectives of the programme are preventive in nature and include:

(1) Creation of effective health services for this underprivileged population;
(2) Prevention of sexually transmitted diseases;
(3) Prevention of teenage pregnancies.

This, of course, necessitates: (1) in depth studies of adolescent sexual behaviour; (2) identification and needs of contraceptive methods; (3) development of cost-effective and appropriate methods of contraception with minimal health risks.

All this necessitates an in-depth understanding of the mental, physical and endocrinological events leading to and following puberty.

Today's symposium is the natural fore-runner of the International Youth Year declared by the United Nations for 1985, and will cover some aspects of the stated priorities of this programme.

The symposium will cover:

(1) The Endocrine Maturation of the Girl at Puberty* – by Dr P. Sizonenko
(2) Adolescent Sexual Behaviour – by Dr Hathaway
(3) Adolescent Health Services – by Dr Teper
(4) Teenage Contraception – by Dr Barwin
(5) Adolescent Pregnancies – by Dr Cates.

These comments and proposals were submitted to Dr A. Petros-Barvazian, Director, Division of Family Health, who was invited to the meeting for this purpose. Dr Petros-Barvazian told the Working Group that she understands the problems and since the programme is highly interested in the success and continuation of this programme, will help to solve the difficulties which have arisen.

*This paper was not available for inclusion in the published Proceedings.

74
Adolescent sexual behaviour

H. S. HATHAWAY

Increasing numbers of paediatric patients aged 13–18 years will be seeking the services of obstetricians and gynaecologists rather than those of the paediatrician. Parents and clinicians frequently feel a sense of uneasiness when dealing with the sexual behaviour of youth. This is due in part to a lack of reliable knowledge in this area.

Adolescence, defined herein as the period between 10 and 19 years of age, is a period of rapid change from childhood to adulthood; physical, intellectual and emotional. The maturation process proceeds with changes in attitudes and values, changing relationships with parents and peers and the development of new freedoms and responsibilities. Unfortunately, society does not offer clear guidelines for this process. This places a heavy burden on every adolescent or young adult to decide what is acceptable behaviour during this period of becoming a man or woman.

To reach maturity, the adolescent must progress through four theoretical developmental tasks[1]. The first task begins with movement away from the family, toward becoming independent, the beginning stages of teenage rebellion. The second task is the formation of future plans, college, a job, marriage, and acquisition of skills for future economic independence from parents. The development of a sexual identity with responsible relationships – a stage not completed until intimacy and caring are present, several steps away from experimentation and curiosity – is the third task. And finally is the establishment of a realistic, stable, and positive self-identity with a sense of social responsibility, a task which is basic to all aspects of adolescent health and functioning.

Most young people experience this period without mental illness or disabling physical trauma. Yet many problems arise because of the stresses related to the developmental tasks of adolescence and the normal degree of risk taking and experimenting that occurs.

The third task of adolescence, the development of a sexual identity, is not a new task of the 70s or 80s; however, the visibility of this task, the controversial attitudes concerning abortion, teenage pregnancy and the use of contraception, plus the spending of governmental dollars dictates that the sexual behaviour of the adolescent is a primary social concern.

Table 1 Percentage of never-married women aged 15–19, who ever had intercourse, by age and race, United States, 1971 and 1979

Age	1971			1979		
	White (%)	Black (%)	Total (%)	White (%)	Black (%)	Total (%)
15	11.3	31.2	14.4	18.3	41.4	22.5
19	40.9	78.3	46.4	64.9	88.5	69.0

Source: Zelnik, M. and Kantner, J. F. (1980). Sexual activity, contraceptive use and pregnancy among metropolitan area teenagers: 1971-1979. *Family Planning Perspectives*, **12**, 229

Adolescent sexual behaviour in the United States was the focus of national sampling surveys in 1971, 1976 and 1979[2,3]. Table 1 shows that sexual activity among unmarried metropolitan females rose from 46.4% who reported sexual intercourse by age 19 in 1971 to 69% in 1979[2,3]. Sixty-nine per cent of unmarried males aged 17–21 years also reported sexual activity. Perhaps one might say that equality of the sexes exists in this area, if nowhere else.

The age at first intercourse among unmarried metropolitan area females dropped by 4 months, from a mean of 16·6 years in 1971 to 16.2 years in 1979[2]. Along with the increased prevalence of sexual experience, there has been a fairly substantial increase in the number of partners teenage women have had. Table 2 shows that 6.2% of women had six or more partners by age 19 in 1971, 14.3% in 1976[3]. This may be related to a longer premarital period secondary to younger age at first intercourse as well as a greater postponement of marriage.

Several reasons for this increase in sexual activity have been cited. The growing economic independence of women and the diminishing influence of religion affect the sexual behaviour of all ages. The availability of effective and safe contraception can remove the fear of pregnancy. The legalization of abortion, government funding for family planning clinics, and aid to dependent children have been implicated as cause of increased adolescent sexual activity and promiscuity, teenage pregnancy and out-of-wedlock births. Studies have refuted this assumption[4]. Women on welfare have been shown to regulate their fertility as well as other women when given access to birth control. Birth rates are lower in states which support Family Planning clinics and have higher payments to low income mothers. It is true that the availability of contraception and legal abortion have prevented unwanted pregnancies and botched abortions for many young women.

Table 2 Percentage of sexually experienced never-married women aged 15–19, according to number of partners ever, 1971 and 1976

No. of partners	1971		1976	
	15–17 y (%)	18–19 y (%)	15–17 y (%)	18–19 y (%)
1	66.5	56.1	54.0	45.3
2–3	22.7	27.7	31.5	31.3
4–5	5.9	9.9	8.4	9.1
6 or more	4.9	6.3	6.1	14.3

Source: Furstenberg, F. F., Jr., Lincoln, R. and Menken, J. (1981). *Teenage Sexuality, Pregnancy, and Childbearing.* p. 17. (Philadelphia: University of Pennsylvania Press)

The social environment in the United States contributes to early sexual activity. The media provides constant bombardment with the attractiveness of sexuality on television, radio, records, and magazines. Sex is being used to sell everything from underwear to sailboats. Feminine spray, tampons, deodorant, toothpaste, everything one could possibly use is presented, except any item that concerns birth control and responsible sexual behaviour. There are few role models in the entertainment media who attempt to promote responsible sexual behaviour. The right to say 'no' is seldom presented.

The transition to non-virginity is seldom premeditated, unless it occurs after marriage. It is usually accompanied by a desire for spontaneity, doing what comes naturally. Some of the reasons[5] adolescent females may give for engaging in sexual activity are: (1) Most will cite 'affection', see sex as necessary for the social rewards of dating; sometimes as payment to a male if a female is to be popular. (2) Having a boyfriend is proof to self and others of prowess as a female; having sex may be considered as a rite of passage. (3) Engaging in sexual activity may be necessary to solidify a relationship. (4) Sex may be a means of satisfying natural drives and curiosity. (5) Sex may simply be an expression of physical pleasure; if it feels good, do it.

The national survey of 1979 showed that the first sexual encounter usually occurs in the teenager's home[3]. The older the girl, the more likely the encounter will occur in the partner's home. Parents can hardly be unaware of this activity, though not necessarily condoning it.

Early adolescent childbearing, ages 12–16 years, has been identified as initiating a syndrome of failure[6]. This syndrome includes failure to complete the developmental tasks of adolescence, failure to remain in school, failure to limit family size, failure to establish a stable family, and failure to establish a vocation. The young parent may bypass important stages of psychosocial maturation as she is expected to fulfil the role of parenthood, a difficult role for the mature woman. The young female adolescent may perceive no more attractive options. The baby may represent something of her own or a means to combat loneliness. The pregnancy may be a method of acting out, wanting to get away from home, or simply following the role model of mother or sibling.

Several programmes have been established in an attempt to address the social concerns and problems associated with adolescent sexual behaviour.

To enable all persons who desire to obtain family planning care access to such services, the United States Congress enacted the Family Planning Act of 1970. Abortion was first legalized in 1967. Federal support for abortions for low income women was granted in the early 60s. Recently that support was discontinued. Colorado is one of the five states which provides abortion funds for low income women. Thirty per cent of Colorado abortions were for adolescents in 1981[7]. The increasing availability of contraception and abortions has undoubtedly played a significant role in the birth rates for women of all ages. Table 3 shows that births per 1000 white women aged 15–19 years decreased from 79.1 in 1955 to 44.6 in 1977[8]. Out-of-wedlock births increased during this period from 6.0 per 1000 unmarried white females to 13.6

The Tri-County Health Department with which I am affiliated offers four Family Planning Clinics on an ability-to-pay fee scale. Forty-five per cent of users are teens and 80% of users have incomes below the poverty level. The clinics offer evening hours to accommodate working parents and students. Medical services offered include (1) annual gynecological examinations, (2) Papanicolau's test, (3) breast examination, (4) vaginitis treatment, (5) venereal disease test and treatment, (6) pregnancy testing, and (7) birth control methods and supplies. Counselling for birth control, vasectomy, gynecological problems, tubal ligation, problem pregnancy, sexually transmitted disease, prenatal care, infertility and nutrition are also offered. Community education is of high priority. One of the pamphlets distributed contains this message on the cover: How to do it Right: Birth Control[9]. Doing it right means being honest with yourself; either not having sex at all, or, if you do not want a child, having sex with good

Table 3 Birthrates and out-of-wedlock birthrates for women under age 20, by race, United States, 1950–1977

Age and race	1950	1955	1960	Year 1965	1970	1975	1977
A. Birthrates (per 1000 women)							
15–19							
White	70.0	79.1	79.4	60.7	57.4	46.8	44.6
Black	163.5*	167.2*	156.1	140.6	147.7	113.8	107.3
18–19							
White	—	—	—	—	101.5	74.4	71.1
Black	—	—	—	—	204.9	156.0	147.6
15–17							
White	—	—	—	—	29.2	28.3	26.5
Black	—	—	—	—	101·4	86·6	81·2
10–14							
White	0.2	0.3	0.4	0.3	0.5	0.6	0.6
Black	5.1*	4.8*	4.3	4.3	5.2	5.1	4.7
B. Rates of out-of-wedlock births (per 1000 unmarried women)							
15–19							
White	5.1	6.0	6·6	7.9	10.9	12.1	13.6
Black	68.5*	77.6*	76.5*	75.8*	96.9	95.1	93.2

*Rates for non-whites.
Sources: DHEW, National Center for Health Statistics, Vital Statistics, Vol. 1, 1955, 1960, 1965, 1970 and 1975; —————, "Teenage Childbearing: United States, 1966–1975." Monthly Vital Statistics Report 26(5)Suppl(9/8/77); —————, "Advance Report, Final Natality Statistics, 1977." Monthly Vital Statistics Report 27(11)Suppl(2/5/79).

birth control. Doing it right means planning for birth control ahead of time, thinking ahead about what having a baby or another baby means, can you afford it financially, emotionally, or physically? Will it affect other plans you have for the future?

There are two 'Teen Clinics' in Denver, Colorado, which offer comprehensive health care to adolescents only. The clinics are headed by an adolescent specialist physician. Additional personnel are mid-level practitioners, counsellors, and social workers especially selected for their skill and interest in teenagers. In addition to services provided by the Family Planning Clinics, the Teen Clinics offer physical examination for school and sports, adolescent peer education, mental health counselling, nutritional counselling and adolescent peer education. Confidentiality, if desired, may be obtained for pregnancy testing, birth control and sexually transmitted diseases without parental consent as provided by Colorado law. Twenty-seven per cent of the visits in 1982 were for medical illness or routine physical examination, 37% were for family planning, pregnancy test, gynaecological service or venereal disease check, and 36% were obstetric visits. Each of the 2000 users averaged five visits per year.

There remains a significant number of teenagers who have unprotected intercourse. In 1976, half of sexually active teenagers less than 14 years of age delayed using contraception until months after becoming sexually active[3]. Half of teenage pregnancies occur in the first 6 months after beginning sexual activity[3]. Very few teenagers intend to get pregnant and most think romantically, 'It can't happen to me.'

Reasons that teenagers give for not using contraception are as follows. (1) Didn't expect to have intercourse. (2) Didn't think I could get pregnant. (3) Contraceptives were not available. (4) Believed it wrong or dangerous to use contraceptives. (5) Believed it would spoil mood or pleasure. (6) Other reasons are romanticism, denial of intent or risk, guilt reaction, and a desire to fulfil a pregnancy wish. These reasons demonstrate that accurate sex education before sexual intercourse occurs could impact significantly on responsible sexual behaviour resulting in the appropriate and timely use of contraception.

Comparison of contraceptive users in 1971 and 1976 showed that the greatest increase in users occurred at age 15, from 30% in 1971 to 50% in 1976. At age 19, 52% were users in 1971 and 70% in 1976[3].

Type of contraceptive used most frequently in 1971 and 1976 is compared in Table 4[3]. A rise in the more effective methods of contraception occurred and use of the pill doubled. Use of withdrawal decreased by more than 50%.

The use of contraception seems to be a function of commitment to sex, to the incorporation of sex into the self-image[12].

In an attempt to incorporate sex education, family planning and comprehensive health care for adolescents into the educational system, the Maternity Infant Project in Saint Paul, Minnesota, opened an in-school health care programme in 1977[11]. After 3 years the clinic was being used by two-thirds of the 12th grade students and nine out of ten pregnant students. Birth rates fell from 60 per thousand to 45 per thousand in the first year. The school dropout rate among females was reduced from 45% to 10%. No repeat pregnancies occurred among those students who delivered with the project and returned to school. More students who received their care through the high school clinic remained on contraception than those using the

Table 4 Percentage of ever-contracepting never-married women aged 15–19, according to methods ever used, by age, 1971 and 1976

	1971		1976	
	15–17 y (%)	18–19 y (%)	15–17 y (%)	18–19 y (%)
Pill	17.4	36.3	45.1	72.9
Condom	61.6	59.7	41.2	37.4
Douche	32.0	32.0	6.8	11.4
Withdrawal	62.9	65.6	39.1	20.7
Foam, jelly, cream	7.7	12.7	4.4	14.8
IUD	1.7	3.8	2.5	7.8
Diaphragm	2.6	3.8	1.3	2.4
Rhythm	5.6	5.5	14.3	14.5
Other	0.2	0.0	0.1	0.5

Source: Zelnik, M. and Kanter, J. F. (1981). Sexual and contraceptive experience of young unmarried women in the United States, 1976 and 1971. In Furstenberg, F. F., Jr., Lincoln, R. and Menken, J. (eds.) *Teenage Sexuality, Pregnancy, and Childbearing.* pp. 68-92. (Philadelphia: University of Pennsylvania Press)

Family Planning Clinic. Review of the pregnancy complications experienced by the young women revealed that 15% had mild or severe pre-eclampsia, more than two times the proportion (7%) found among the older clinic users whose average age was 21.6 years. The incidence of premature and low birth-weight infants was not significantly different between the two age groups. Gonorrhoea was diagnosed in 12% but was present in only 5% of the older group.

Anaemia (Hb less than 11 g/dl) was present in 20% of younger women and in 11% of older women.

There is no similar programme in a Colorado high school; however, there is a programme named 'Teen Parents' operational in one of the high schools in the Tri-County area. The students remain in school during pregnancy and return post-partum as soon as possible. The infants and toddlers accompany their mothers to school. Part of the day is spent in the Child Care Classroom where students learn parenting skills, career guidance, management and the economics of rearing a child. The remainder of the day is spent in a regular or special classroom enabling the teen parent to complete the educational requirements for graduation. One of the educational goals is to provide courses and learning experiences which help to reinforce the student's self-worth. Of the 78 graduates since 1977, only three are on Welfare, 65% are working full-time, and five are attending college. This programme is an exception. Only 10–40% of our Colorado schools offer any form of sex education, and very little is offered when the student is less than 16 years old. Most is too late and not enough.

A conservative estimate is that 5000 adolescents aged 10–18 run away each year in the Denver area[7]. More girls than boys are runaways. In many of these cases there is suspicion of sexual abuse as a child. A significant number of runaways become adolescent prostitutes. There is a programme in Denver, Colorado, which offers residential and outreach care to these adolescents. Workers in the 'Outreach Program' frequent the bars and streets contacting the youth and offering a safe place to stay. Psychological counselling, peer and parent group rap sessions and continued education are offered.

A complication of sexual activity at any age is sexually transmitted disease. This is primarily a problem among the young. Education of the public, particularly adolescents, to understand early signs of disease and the kinds of sexual behaviour which increases risk, encouraging males with multiple partners to use condoms, screening high-risk groups, and appropriate treatment of primary care and contacts is essential.

In conclusion, there have been significant social changes in the United States during the past two decades. One of these changes has been an increase in adolescent sexual activity. Consequences of such behaviour may be an unwanted child born to young people who have not developed their self-esteem and personal identity. We as professionals must recognize that this change has occurred. We must strive to ensure that adolescents have the knowledge, skills and opportunities that enable informed choice of responsible sexual behaviours. We must emphasize primary prevention by helping families, communities, and professionals develop and strengthen the coping skills adolescents must have to address needs being met through sexual behaviour[13].

References

1. Fine, L. L. (1973). What's a normal adolescent? A guide for the assessment of adolescent behavior. *Clin. Pediatr.*, **12**, 1
2. Zelnik, N. and Kantner, J. F. (1980). Sexual activity, contraceptive use and pregnancy among metropolitan area teenagers: 1971–1979. *Fam. Plann. Perspect.*, **12**, 230
3. Zelnik, M. and Kantner, J. F. (1981). Sexual and contraceptive experience of young unmarried women in the United States, 1976 and 1971. In Furstenberg, F. F., Jr., Lincoln, R. and Menken, J. (eds.) *Teenage Sexuality, Pregnancy, and Childbearing.* pp. 68-92. (Philadelphia: University of Pennsylvania Press)
4. Moore, K. A. and Caldwell, S. B. (1981). The effect of government policies on out-of-wedlock sex and pregnancy. In Furstenberg, F. F., Jr., Lincoln, R. and Menken, J. (eds.) *Teenage Sexuality, Pregnancy, and Childbearing.* pp. 126-35. (Philadelphia: University of Pennsylvania Press)
5. Klein, L. (1978). Antecedents of teenage pregnancy. *Clin. Obstet. Gynecol.*, **21**, 1151
6. Waters, J. L. (1969). Pregnancy in adolescents: a syndrome of failure. *South. Med. J.*, **62**, 655
7. Montgomery, A. and Scales, P. (1981). *Adolescent Health in Colorado: Status, Implications, Directions.* (Colorado Department of Health Press)
8. Furstenberg, F. F., Jr., Lincoln, R. and Menken, J. (1976). *Teenage Sexuality, Pregnancy, and Childbearing.* p. 4. (Philadelphia: University of Pennsylvania Press)
9. *How to do it Right: Birth Control.* (Community Health Education, Family Planning, and OB/GYN Services of the Denver Department of Health and Hospitals)
10. Zelnik, N. and Kantner, J. F. (1979). Reasons for non-use of contraception. *Fam. Plann. Perspect.*, **2**, 289
11. Lindeman, C. (1975). *Birth Control and Unmarried Young Women.* (New York: Springer)
12. Edwards, L. E., Steinman, M. E., Arnold, K. A. and Hakanson, E. Y. (1980). Adolescent pregnancy prevention services in high school clinics. *Fam. Plann. Perspect.*, **12**, 6
13. Beach, R. K. (1982). The sexually active teenager: clinical concerns. Presented at the *25th Annual General Pediatric Summer Course*, August 1-5, Aspen, Colorado

75
Adolescent health services

S. TEPER

Population estimates suggest that by 1985 a little over 20% of the world's population will be aged between 10 and 19 – 10–19 being a useful working definition for adolescence. Children aged under 10 will account for almost a further 24% of the world population. In some countries – Bangladesh, Afghanistan and the Democratic Republic of Yemen, for example – the two age groups will comprise a higher proportion, 50% or more, of the total population. In rare cases, in countries which have experienced high fertility in the recent past together with low or moderate mortality, the population aged under 20 will account for a remarkable 60% of population by 1985; Kenya is one such country. In the light of recent experiences in developing societies, it seems unlikely that significant reductions in the fertility of all women (including adolescents) will occur in the next few years. In any case, the size of the cohorts of women who will be at risk of childbearing between now and the end of the century means that large *numbers* of births will occur *irrespective of fertility levels*. Third World countries must, therefore, prepare to face the various consequences – economic, social, political and health – of continuing rapid population growth. In the industrialized countries, the problem to be faced is a different one. In these countries, young people form a smaller percentage of the population (the 1985 estimate for the under 20s is around 30%), and the group which will dominate changes in population size and structure in the next two decades are the elderly, those aged 65 and over.

Adolescents are an important group because they obviously constitute a numerically significant proportion of the population. Equally obviously, they are important because they are the parents of the future. In addition, as we move from putting emphasis on curative medicine to stressing preventive aspects and lifestyle, we are beginning to recognize the adolescent age group as a positive health resource. It is known that 'the determinants of later health are laid down at these ages'. It is crucial, therefore, that contacts between adolescents and health personnel provide information and care which promote positive attitudes and behaviour in relation to health.

Adolescence is traditionally seen as a period of life which is relatively free from health problems. However, in terms of development, it is a time during which malnutrition and disease can have a devastating impact on the individual, in both the short- and long-term. In relation to reproductive health, pregnancy and delivery complications and sexually transmitted diseases can affect future reproductive capacity as well as family health. Adolescent-orientated services have tended to focus on specific health problems: biological, psychosocial, emotional and mental, or arising through disability or from sexual activity. In relation to this last area, early pregnancy has been seen almost universally as a life-event with severe and undesirable consequences.

Pregnancy during adolescence involves medical and psychosocial problems, and these are greater the younger the age of the girl. Medically, the use of contraception may be problematic. In part, this reflects biological factors – for example, the small size of the uterus in the first 1–2 years after menarch makes the use of the IUD difficult and irregular cycles make the use of the rhythm method particularly unreliable. The risks to an adolescent from a termination of pregnancy are no higher than those for an older woman if gestation at termination is controlled. However, young girls are more likely than older women to present for a late abortion, so that their *total* complication rates tend to be higher. During pregnancy, the young girl has a greater risk than her older counterpart of anaemia and toxaemia; she is at greater risk of complications at delivery and of a premature birth; and she is more likely to have a stillborn infant or to have a liveborn baby die in the early neonatal period. Socially, childbirth can mean that the girl loses the opportunity for more schooling and as a result is disadvantaged in the employment market. The adolescent's baby will be affected, and so too may the father to be – especially if he is also a teenager. The girl may be ostracized or a precipitous marriage arranged. Seeking an abortion may be particularly dangerous if only clandestine, illegal operations are available.

Sadly, there are a number of reasons to expect the situation to become worse in the future. First, there is the prospect of continuing population growth and its implications in many parts of the world. Secondly, some of the social changes which have already occurred in developed countries are now beginning to occur – or to occur to a greater extent – in the developing world. These changes include increasing urbanization, the growth of slum cities, alterations in sexual mores, the weakening of family ties, uncertainties in the parenting role and the increasing use of drugs. A decline in the mean age at menarche and a later age at marriage delay the formation of a family unit and prolong the time from puberty to functional adulthood. Finally, when young people have nothing to face except unemployment, girls may deliberately seek to bear a child in order to establish adult status and acquire an identity.

To date, one of the main objectives of adolescent reproductive health services has been to prevent pregnancy by offering contraception. Despite massive efforts in this direction, the number of pregnancies to teenagers continues to give cause for grave concern. Even in Sweden – where we would expect progress to be made and where, in fact, much has been achieved – there were still 4156 live births and nearly 6000 (5933) abortions to girls under the age of 20 in 1981, accounting for some 8% of all pregnancies. There is some evidence that girls who now become pregnant in Sweden form a special risk group, and this suggests that efforts at education and service provision can – *in the interim stage of reducing a health problem* – actually *increase* inequalities in health.

It is relatively simple to describe the clinical services needed for/available to adolescents (Table 1).

Table 1 Adolescent status and services offered

Adolescent status	Services offered
Sexually active	Contraception, cervical cytology, clinics for sexually transmitted diseases
Pregnant	Induced abortion (where legalized), antenatal care, delivery services, postpartum care, paediatric care for the infant
All adolescents	Gynaecological services

Sex education, education on babycraft and for parenthood, and counselling are usually regarded as quite separate from clinical services. This fits the model for 'adult' services, in which curative and preventive medicine are two distinct entities. Because adolescence is a period of rapid biological, psychological and social development, this second group of 'educational' services may be of as much importance, if not more important, to adolescents as the clinical services, and certainly the two should be integrated. Both types of care are in short supply – or are non-existent – for most of the world's young people, the majority of whom experience this phase of their life in economically and socially deprived conditions. Both types of service are also often in short supply – or, again, are non-existent – in parts of the industrialized world. Where services do exist, they are underutilized, and sometimes *un*utilized. In part, this non-use is a function of the structure of the services, which is in turn a function of the fact that, more often than not, the structure is determined by the perceptions of adults. Most medical services are, nor surprisingly, planned by adults, are adult orientated and are used by adults. When services and programmes aimed at adolescents exist, they usually deal with specific problems and there is little or no opportunity for feedback. Policy makers and service providers do not acquire an insight into the users' reactions to services.

The most cogent argument for abandoning the adult model of services for adolescents is that the approach has not been successful in reducing the incidence of adolescent pregnancy to any large degree. A further very real problem in this field is that we persist in seeing the reproductive (and other) health problems of adolescents as adult problems which are occurring early – that is, they are occurring in adolescence rather than in adulthood. In fact, these problems need to be seen in the context of the psychology that is peculiar to adolescence. Our failure to operate on this premise is one fundamental reason for the lack of success in reducing adolescent fertility.

Many other reasons have contributed, and still contribute, to this failure. For example:

(1) Adults may fear that offering information on sexual and reproductive matters and/or providing clinics leads to sexual experiments and 'promiscuity'. These attitudes obviously conflict with the adolescents' needs to gain knowledge.

(2) Legal constraints may exist which make it difficult or impos-

sible for health personnel to treat minors or unmarried adolescents – or to treat them in confidence.

(3) Parents with inadequate knowledge may expect to be the source of information for their children, despite the taboos and barriers to communication which often exist between parent and child.

(4) School programmes are likely to contribute relatively little when compulsory education ends at an early age (say, at around 11 years of age), when enrolment is far from universal and when there is a bias towards educating male children. Materials are also likely to be in short supply in these circumstances, and to have an inappropriate (Western) orientation.

(5) Teachers are not always suitably trained, or suitable for training, to transmit this information. They must be able to deal with factual information, and with the emotional aspects of human relationships and sexual, contraceptive and reproductive behaviour. Teachers (or others) need to be available and able to counsel young people, and they must be knowledgeable about available services. Many children learn from their peers, their siblings or from the mass media rather than from specialist educators.

(6) Many adolescents are outside the school system, and are particularly hard to reach with education or services. These young people are probably in greatest need.

These are some of the structural factors which affect adolescent knowledge and behaviour which in turn affect the success of clinics and programmes. The list above does not pretend to be comprehensive; problems will vary from country to country, within a country and over time. The development of health services usually involves a 'response' mechanism – services are needed to cope with specific diseases. On the whole, the 'response' to adolescent fertility has been to provide obstetric services and family planning clinics. The needs of adolescents are more complicated than this. Adolescents must make complex decisions about fragile personal and sexual relationships during a time in which they are highly vulnerable. At the same time, they are trying to develop their roles in the family, at school or work and in the wider community. Sometimes they need reassurance

691

from health personnel rather than medical care. Young people sometimes feel abnormal because they are *not* sexually active!

Most of us would like health care to be delivered by staff who are
non-judgemental in their attitudes. Most of us want our confidentiality and privacy to be respected in the consultation and in
relation to medical records. Most of us want to use clinics which are
geographically accessible and are open at convenient times. We
can be certain that adolescents want these condtions too. Indeed,
confidentiality, privacy and accessibility may be of even greater
importance to them than they are to us. However, beyond these
obvious conditions little is known of the *real* needs of adolescents –
'real' in the sense that they are seen as needs by the adolescents
themselves. This is an area in which research is needed. Such research
involves a dialogue between adolescents and those who plan and
deliver health services, possibly with research workers as intermed-
iaries. The process means establishing a rapport so that adolescents
feel able to express their needs. This dialogue is itself a mechanism
by which young people can be integrated into the actual planning
and provision of services.

Research along these lines is already underway in a number of
countries under the auspices of the World Health Organization.
Steered by its Task Force on Reproductive Health in Adolescence,
WHO has been active in many aspects of this field over the past
decade. Studies have been undertaken on menstrual patterns, ovulatory patterns, on the onset of sperm ejaculation, on factors affecting
the choice and use of contraception, on risk factors in maternal
and child health in adolescence, on outcome of pregnancy, on sex
education as well as on health services.

A useful framework has been developed covering the time from
sexual maturation to pregnancy, motherhood and voluntary or involuntary infertility (Figure 1). By identifying the points at which services (used as a broad term) can be introduced to cope with or modify
behaviour, it is a useful tool for those involved in policy and planning
and also for the evaluation of health services.

It would be naïve to suggest that it is easy – or even that it is
feasible – to reduce adolescent sexual activity and its outcomes
substantially. What is certainly necessary is that, through the provision of services, we minimize the adverse effects associated with
early sexual activity and pregnancy. To do this it is essential to
acknowledge and accept the strength of adolescent sexuality, and to

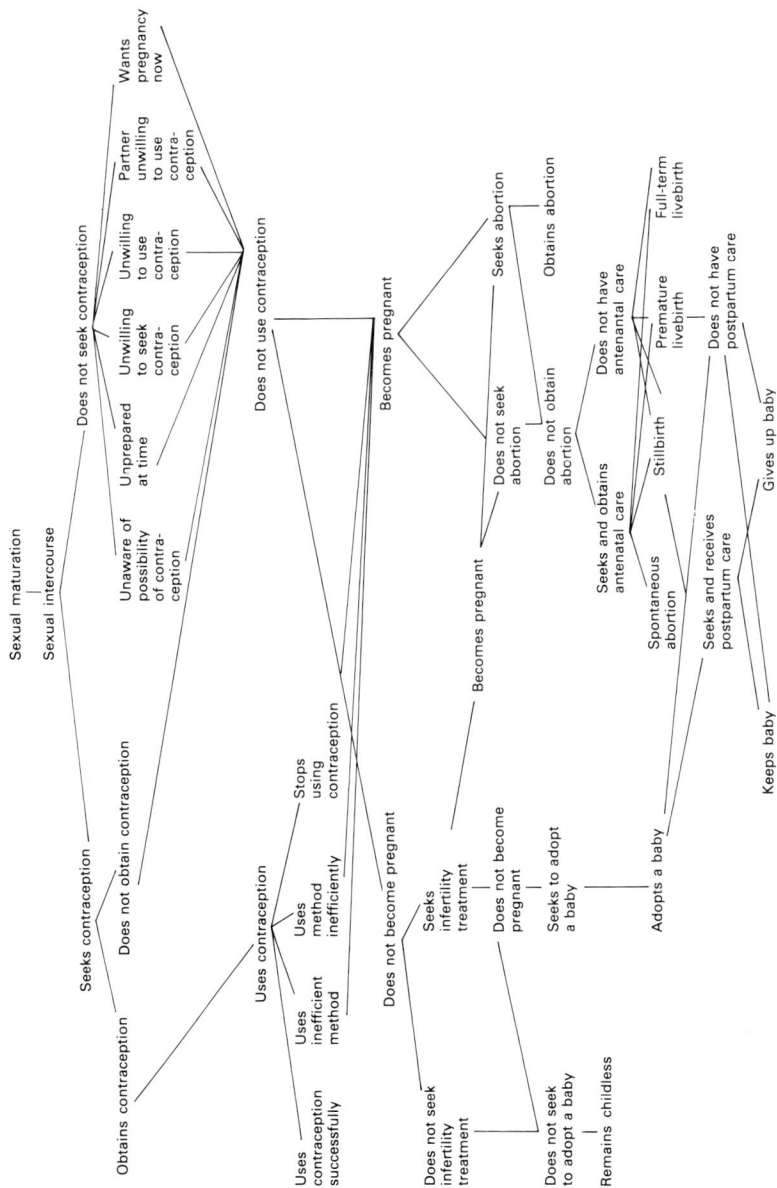

Figure 1 Potential points of intervention in sequential pathways to motherhood. Reproduced with permission from *Research Needs and Approaches in Adolescent Reproductive Health in Developing Countries of the WHO European Region.* Document ICP/MCH 023 4676B. (WHO: Geneva)

recognize that a substantial proportion of adolescents will be sexually active during adolescence.

Similarly, one of the objectives of service provision must be the creation of environments in which adolescents feel able to discuss problems that they have, and in which balanced attitudes towards sexuality, contraceptive use, childbearing and other aspects of health behaviour can be developed. Encouraging positive attitudes and behaviour, plus further efforts at service provision, should lead to *some* reduction in the incidence of pregnancy in the current adolescent population. However, the broader approach may have a dramatic impact on the incidence of adolescent pregnancy in the *children* of this same population. The ultimate impact of the holistic approach to adolescent reproductive health may be very much greater than can be achieved by the provision of family planning clinics when such clinics seek to treat contraceptive behaviour as an isolate, and in doing so deny the power of adolescent sexuality and ignore the complexity of the unique process through which each one of us goes in the transition from childhood to adulthood.

The General Assembly of the United Nations has designated 1985 as International Youth Year, with the themes 'participation, development and peace', and has called for specific actions for and with young people. This provides us with a natural focus for initiating the involvement of young people in their own health care. Nevertheless, we should be aware that the demographic factors outlined at the start of this paper have very real practical implications. Specifically, rapid population growth in developing countries and drastic ageing in the industrialized world mean that the resources allocated for health services are likely to be given to adults rather than to adolescents during the remaining years of this century.

Bibliography

Eisen, P. (1983). *Adolescent and Youth Health: Perspectives, Problems, Priorities.* Paper prepared for WHO: Geneva
Friedman, H. L. and Edstrom, K. (1982). *Adolescent Reproductive Health: An Approach to Health Service Research.* Paper prepared for WHO: Geneva
Hofman, A. D. (1982). *Biological and Psychological Correlates of Contraception in Adolescence: A Review.* Paper prepared for WHO: Geneva
World Health Organization (1977). *Health Needs of Adolescents.* Technical Report Series, No. **609.** (WHO: Geneva)
World Health Organization (1978). *Service Oriented Research in Adolescent Fertility.* EURO Reports and Studies, No. **1.** (WHO: Copenhagen)

76
Teenage contraception – a Canadian perspective

B. N. BARWIN

Sexually active teenagers, like adults, need protection against unwanted pregnancy; and the same array of jellies are effective for both. Providing birth-control services to teenagers so as to maintain their interest in contraception in the face of their changing needs confronts professionals in the field with a new set of challenges. Promoting contraception does not necessarily imply condonation of intercourse; rather it prevents untimely and unwanted pregnancies. Adolescents need medically safe and socially relevant contraception.

30% of 15-year-old boys and 41.6% of the 16- and 17-year-old boys reported having experienced sexual intercourse. Only 8.3% of the Canadian 15-year-old girls were sexually active while 18.6% of the 16-year-old and 17-year-old girls had been sexually active. 95% of Canadian teenagers going to birth-control clinics reportedly have experienced sexual intercourse before seeking contraception. The younger the girl, the more likely she will delay seeking contraceptive advice. Risk taking is probably most prevalent amongst adolescents.

Adolescent medical care should include health maintenance, venereal disease prevention and treatment and sexual and contraceptive counselling. Adolescent females are in need of relevant, effective, contraceptive services. Effective care begins by respecting an adolescent as a person with constantly changing physical and emotional states. We must learn to respect and work with the adolescent's peer group. Use of a contraceptive method increases the risk that a young

Table 1 Mechanical and barrier methods of contraception

Method	Advantages	Disadvantages
Coitus interruptus	Useful in unprotected intercourse, no medical risk, secrecy possible	High risk of failure, poor gratification, premature ejaculation
Rhythm/Billings method	No prescription, no medical risk	Cycles too irregular, requires motivation, requires intelligence, high risk of failure
Condom	Non-prescription, male responsibility, protection against VD, inexpensive, no medical complication, secrecy possible, low risk of failure	Strong motivation, Occasional breakage, some loss of sensation, pre-coital interference
Vaginal creams, foams and suppositories	Non-prescription, minimal medical risk, secrecy possible, protects against VD, low failure rate	Strong motivation, occasional allergy, messy, pre-coital interference
Diaphragm	Highly effective with cream, protects against VD, relatively low failure rate	Motivation required, messy, pre-coital interference, requires intelligence, instruction necessary, privacy for insertion

Table 2 Methods most suited to teenage contraception

Method	Advantages	Disadvantages
IUD	Secrecy possible, initial motivation only, low failure rate	Menorrhagia, dysmenorrhoea, minimal increase in pelvic infection
Morning-after pill	Unprotected intercourse, emergency only, low failure rate	Side-effects, possible teratogenic effects
Depot-Provera	Minimal motivation, amenorrhoea, effective	Spotting, weight gain, possible breast lesions, post-therapy amenorrhoea
Birth control pill	Minimal risk of major side-effects, effective, alleviates dysmenorrhoea, regulates cycle	Strong motivation (daily), minimal side-effects, breakthrough bleeding, amenorrhoea, secrecy difficult

woman's sexual activity may be discovered but non-use entails the substantial risk that a pregnancy may ensue. Table 1 shows the mechanical and barrier methods of contraception. Table 2 shows those methods most suited to adolescents.

Bibliography

Barwin, B. N. (1982). Teenage Contraception. In Barwin, B. N. and Belisle, S. (eds.). *Adolescent Gynecology and Sexuality*, p. 81. (New York: Mason)

77
Teenage pregnancy and abortion

W. CATES, Jr.

INTRODUCTION

During the last decade, the 'epidemic' of teenage pregnancy was widely heralded both in the USA and other areas of the world[1-5]. As increasing numbers of young women born during the baby boom of the 1950s began to enter adolescence in the late 1960s, the number of births to teenagers increased annually until 1970[4]; the proportion of births represented by teenagers increased through 1973[6]. In 1973, the fertility rate for 14-year-old women reached its highest level since 1920, and the rate for 15 year olds had again increased to its peak level of the late 1950s[7]. The USA was reported to have one of the highest teenage fertility rates in the world[8].

Surveys of teenage reproductive behaviour in the United States from 1971 to 1979 documented increasing proportions of premaritally sexually experienced teenagers at every year of age from 15 to 19[9]. At the same time, use of contraception increased among premaritally sexually active 15–19-year-old women[9], and legal abortion became increasingly available – first on a limited regional basis in the early 1970s and then on a national level in 1973[10]. As legal abortion statistics became more complete and accurate, the total number of reported pregnancies to teenagers (legal abortions plus live births) continued to increase. Thus, because the number of births and the fertility rates to teenagers were declining, legal abortion played an important role in teenage fertility control.

In 1978, approximately 1.2 million reported pregnancies (including 460 000 abortions) occurred among the 5 million sexually active women aged 13–19 years in the USA[5]; an additional 200 000 pregnancies in these women were estimated to have ended in spontaneous miscarriages and stillbirths. Most (77%) of the pregnancies were unintended[5] and almost half (44%) of the births were delivered out of wedlock[8]. At 1976 rates, almost 40% of today's 14 year olds in the USA will experience one pregnancy before they are 20, and 15% will have a legal abortion.

In this Chapter I will focus on secondary prevention of unplanned teenage births – namely, the use of legal abortion rather than contraception. The other authors in the symposium on adolescent reproductive health have described the physiology and practice of teenage contraception. Thus, I will complement their approach by discussing the changing patterns of abortion use by teenagers in the USA, the medical risks of abortion for teenagers, and the public health impact in the USA of the increasing availability of legal abortion for teenagers.

PATTERNS OF TEENAGE ABORTION

Between 1972 and 1978, the reported pregnancy rate for teenagers in the USA increased relatively slowly (+13%), but the abortion rate more than doubled. The proportion of reported teenage pregnancies ending in legal abortion also doubled, from 20% to 38%[11]. Similar trends occurred in England and Wales after the passage of the Abortion Act in 1967[12]. In general, the developed countries of North America and Western Europe have shown increasing rates of legal abortion to teenagers during the 1970s[13].

A disproportionate number of abortions is obtained by teenagers. Since 1972, 15–19-year-old women have formed about 20% of the population of childbearing women aged 15–44 years, but have accounted for approximately one-third of legal abortions.

Abortion ratios (abortions/1000 live births) are one indicator of the proportion of pregnancies which are unplanned. In this Chapter, I used abortion ratios by age at conception because artificially high ratios result for teenagers when calculated by age at occurrence[13]; age at time of abortion was reduced by 3 months and age at time of birth by 9 months. Even after this age correction, from 1972 to 1976 the abortion ratios for teenagers in the USA were higher than those for every age except 35–39 and 40 and older. In 1977 and 1978, the most recent years for which statistics are available, the abortion ratios for teenagers had become higher than those for every age except 40 and over[13].

In 1972, among women less than 20 years of age, the youngest white teenagers had the highest legal abortion ratio. The abortion ratio for white teenagers decreased with increasing age[11]. Legal abortion ratios for black and other teenagers in each age category were lower than those for white teenagers of corresponding ages. By 1978, all abortion ratios had increased, and age- and race-specific differences in abortion ratios had narrowed; the ratios ranged from 37% to 40% of reported pregnancies ending in abortion. In 1978, the least race-specific difference in abortion ratios occurred for the youngest teenagers, where abortion ratios were essentially equal[11].

Older teenagers in both race categories had slightly higher abortion ratios in 1978 than did the youngest teenagers. This difference in abortion ratio patterns occurred because we used the abortion ratios by age at conception, rather than by age at occurrence. Since essentially all of the pregnancies to teenagers less than 15 years of age in 1978 were unplanned[5] and 87% of their births were out of wedlock, factors other than planning status must contribute to their lower frequency of abortion. In this regard, young teenagers have been found to be more negative about abortion than are older teenagers, have a greater tendency to delay abortion[15] and are more dependent on parents for source of payment.

The higher a teenager's socioeconomic status, the more likely she is to terminate a pregnancy by abortion. In 1978 in Rhode Island, 56% of all pregnancies to teenagers living in the highest socioeconomic-status areas were terminated by abortion as compared with 22% of those among teenagers living in poverty areas.

MEDICAL RISKS OF ABORTION FOR TEENAGERS

Like any other surgical procedure, abortion entails some risk. However, teenagers are at no greater risk of complications than are older women; moreover, teenagers have a lower risk of death.

Short-term morbidity

Teenagers have major complication rates similar to those for older women for surgical evacuation methods (suction curettage and dilatation and evacuation), but have significantly lower rates for saline

701

Table 1 Major complication rates* for legal abortion, by woman's age and abortion method, 1971–75†

Abortion method	Age (years)				
	≤17	18–19	20–24	25–29	≥30
Suction curettage (≤12 weeks' gestation)	0.3	0.3	0.3	0.4	0.3
Dilatation and evacuation (13–24 weeks' gestation)	0.4	0.7	0.5	0.7	0.9
Saline instillation (13–24 weeks' gestation)	1.1	1.4	1.8	1.8	3.5

* Major complications per 100 procedures.
† Reproduced from reference 16, with permission.

instillation (Table 1). For suction curettage procedures performed at 12 weeks' gestation or earlier, the major complication rate varies between 0.3 and 0.4 per 100 procedures regardless of the woman's age.

However, the specific type of complication after suction curettage varies by age of the woman (Table 2). Teenagers have significantly lower rates of uterine perforation, transfusions for haemorrhage and

Table 2 Specific complication rates* associated with legal abortion, by woman's age and abortion method, 1971–75†

Abortion method and type of complication	Age (years)				
	≤17	18–19	20–24	25–29	≥30
Suction curettage:					
Fever ≥3 days	0.14	0.17	0.09	0.16	0.03
Transfusion	0.02	0.0	0.06	0.11	0.09
Major surgery	0.0	0.01	0.06	0.07	0.15
Cervical injury	1.68	0.94	1.09	0.80	0.84
Uterine perforation	0.09	0.11	0.20	0.27	0.23
Dilatation and evacuation:					
Fever ≥3 days	0.0	0.22	0.16	0.43	0.45
Transfusion	0.0	0.15	0.11	0.14	0.45
Major surgery	0.17	0.22	0.0	0.43	0.45
Saline instillation:					
Fever ≥3 days	0.23	0.65	0.47	0.64	0.69
Transfusion	0.55	0.54	0.79	1.1	2.54
Major surgery	0.05	0.0	0.11	0.28	0.35

* Major complications or treatments per 100 procedures.
† Reproduced from reference 16, with permission.

unintended major surgery, but have higher rates for cervical injury. Even after controlling for other factors associated with cervical injury, women 17 years and younger still have a significantly greater risk[16].

Preservation of cervical competence is felt to be important for a woman's future childbearing ability. Possible means to reduce the incidence of cervical injury would include the use of Pratt rather than Hegar dilators and the routine use of laminaria in young and/or nulliparous patients. Use of local rather than general anaesthesia during suction curettage has also been associated with significantly lower rates of cervical injury, haemorrhage and uterine perforation[17]; however, total major complication rates for local and general anaesthesia were similar because local anaesthesia was associated with higher rates for convulsions and postabortal pyrexia.

After 12 weeks' gestation, the type of method used also affects the rates of short-term major complications for teenagers. Abortions performed by dilatation and evacuation (D&E) have significantly lower short-term major complications for teenagers (0.5/100 D&E procedures) than do those performed by either saline instillation (1.2/100 saline procedures) or prostaglandin instillation (2.0/100 $PGF_{2\alpha}$ procedures). Although rates for cervical injury are higher after D&E than instillation, routine use of laminaria apparently reduces the rate of cervical trauma after D&E[16].

Delay

Two types of delay are associated with increased medical risk of abortion for teenagers: (1) delay in seeking the abortion procedure; and (2) delay in seeking treatment for post-abortion complications. Distance from the abortion facility and legal requirements for parental notification or approval are among the factors contributing to delay in obtaining abortions[19]. Almost one-third of the abortion facilities in the USA in 1980 required parental consent or notification for women 17 years of age or younger[5]. However, a large proportion of delay was related to individually oriented factors[20]; a history of irregular periods was the strongest single determinant for seeking a late abortion. Thus, continued efforts are needed to make late abortion procedures safer, cheaper and more readily available.

After the abortion procedure, teenagers have a particular need to be counselled about the signs and symptoms of infection and should be urged to obtain treatment promptly; treatment facilities that can respond to complications in a confidential manner without involving teenagers' parents might reduce any delay in seeking treatment.

Emotional complications

Even though deciding to have an abortion may be difficult for them, most teenagers feel comfortable after the event, with a sense of relief at having terminated an unplanned pregnancy[21]. In comparison with older women, teenagers are apparently at higher risk of the short-term psychological sequelae: anxiety, depression, sadness, guilt and regret[22]. However, in Denmark, psychiatric admissions after abortion were lower for teenagers than for older women[23]. A stable partner relationship was the most important variable protecting against post-abortion psychosis. Other factors influencing a teenager's reaction to abortion are the level of parental support, her pre-abortion psychological states, attitudes and support of the attending medical staff, the degree of her ambivalence about abortion, and the opportunity for her to make her own decision regarding the abortion[21].

The type of abortion procedure also affects the psychological sequelae; uterine curettage procedures are associated with more favourable post-abortion reactions than are instillation procedures[24]. Since teenagers are more likely to delay abortion until the later gestational ages when instillation procedures may be used, clinicians should be aware of the emotional impact of the particular method they use.

Long-term effects

An issue of great concern to teenagers is whether induced abortion will threaten subsequent desired pregnancies. Studies of such adverse outcomes as low birth-weight, short gestation, and spontaneous abortion in subsequent planned pregnancies after previous induced abortions, have arrived at conflicting conclusions[25]. Those investigations which have found significantly increased risks of adverse outcomes after just one prior abortion have primarily involved surgical (sharp) curettage as the abortion procedure[25]. Suction curettage is apparently not associated with the same level of increased risks of adverse outcomes in subsequent pregnancies.

However, whether multiple abortion procedures threaten future pregnancies may be another matter. Two recent studies have shown increased rates of spontaneous abortion in young women who had more than one pregnancy terminated by induced abortion. In other studies, the higher risks associated with multiple abortions disappear when the data are re-analysed to take confounding factors into account[25]. These factors include behavioural characteristics (i.e., smoking), the sequence of previous pregnancy outcomes, the interval between a previous pregnancy ending in the repeat abortion and a subsequent pregnancy continued to term, and whether any complications had occurred in the previous abortion (i.e. requiring re-curettage) or the current pregnancy[25].

Although the issue of the late effects of induced abortion is unresolved, several recommendations can be made to aid clinicians[15]. First, teenagers considering abortion should be encouraged to make their decision as early as possible; this will reduce both the short- and possible long-term risks of the abortion or will allow proper prenatal care early in pregnancy. Second, if a nulliparous teenager with an immature cervix requests an abortion that would require dilatation of 11 mm or more, serious consideration should be given to the use of laminaria tents. Third, teenagers who have had one induced abortion should be counselled regarding the safety and effectiveness of the various contraceptive approaches and cautioned about relying on abortion as their primary method of birth control.

PUBLIC HEALTH IMPACT OF LEGAL ABORTION ON TEENAGERS

The availability of legal abortion for teenagers has had an important impact on four public health parameters: deaths, births, contraception, and marriage.

Deaths

Since 1973, the reported number of teenage deaths after illegal abortion declined in the USA (Table 3). Most teenagers are apparently now choosing to terminate unplanned pregnancies through safer legal channels rather than resorting to the less safe self-induced or non-physician-induced procedures. In addition, the risk of death following legal abortion has also declined as physicians become more experienced with abortion procedures and management of complications. Thus, the number of deaths to teenagers from both illegal and legal abortions combined is approximately one-half that of the era when legal abortion was unavailable.

Despite the widespread use of legal abortion by teenagers, deaths from illegal abortion continue to occur. Between 1975 and 1978, four teenagers died from illegal abortions (Table 3). Close examination of the factors leading these young women to attempt illegal rather than legal abortions demonstrated ignorance and desire for secrecy as precipitating reasons[26]. Because many women seek illegal abortion for personal and sociocultural factors apparently unrelated to cost or availability, a small number of illegal abortion deaths will probably continue to occur even when access to legal abortion is generally unrestricted.

Table 3 Number of teenage abortion-related deaths, by category and year, United States, 1972-1978*

Year	Legally induced	Illegally induced
1972	6	7
1973	2	3
1974	5	0
1975	9	1
1976	0	0
1977	4	1
1978	3	2
Total	29	14

* Excludes deaths from ectopic pregnancy.

Births

In the first half of the 1970s, legalization of abortion was temporally associated with declines in total birth rates for young teenagers[7] and with declines in out-of-wedlock birth rates both locally and nationally[27]. Although out-of-wedlock birth rates for teenagers have recently increased, the proportion of intended births among teenage out-of-wedlock first births has also increased, from one in five in 1971 to one in three in 1976[28]. The most likely explanation is the increase in the proportion of unintended pregnancies that are terminated by abortion.

Use of abortion has also been associated with the level of a State's teenage fertility rate. In 1974, State-to-State variation in fertility rates for 15–19 year olds was significantly associated with abortion-to-live birth ratios for the same age group; States with the highest abortion ratios had the lowest teenage fertility rates[29].

Contraception

Teenagers have apparently not directly substituted use of abortion for contraception, but have used a combination of both to lower their birth rates, especially considering the increasing teenage sexual activity[9]. The proportion of premaritally sexually experienced 15–19-year-old women who always use contraception increased during the 1970s, and the proportion of never-users declined[9]. A study of the interstate variation in fertility of teenage women showed that the availability of both contraception and abortion played a role in reducing levels of teenage fertility rates between 1970 and 1974[29]. In 1976, young unmarried women who became pregnant and had an abortion were no less likely to be using contraception at the time of conception than young women who became unintentionally pregnant and did not have an abortion[30]. Similar findings about teenagers using contraception have been reported from England[31].

Case series reports have shown that teenagers whose first pregnancies end in abortion have increased use of effective contraception 6 months after the procedure and do not come to rely on abortion as their primary method of birth control[32]. Contraceptive use after abortion apparently increased during the 1970s since young unmarried women whose first pregnancy ended in abortion in 1976 showed a substantial reduction in the risk of repeat pregnancy over the 24-month period following the abortion in comparison with this risk in 1976[33].

Although more teenagers are using contraception, the average delay between a teenager's initiation of sexual activity and her first visit to a family planning clinic was found to be 16 months[34]. More than one-third of the teenagers suspect pregnancy on their initial visit. The two major reasons given for this delay are procrastination and fear their parents will find out. Since half of all initial premarital pregnancies occur in the first 6 months of sexual activity, and more than one-fifth in the first month, current programmes providing contraceptive services for teenagers will not eliminate the need for abortion.

In addition, the risk of a premarital first pregnancy for teenage contraceptive users increased between 1976 and 1979[9]. Part of the increase has been due to a decline in oral contraceptive use by teenagers since 1976 and a corresponding increase in use of the less effective non-prescription methods[9]. Without the option of legal abortion, these women would have to choose between illegal abortion or an unplanned birth.

Marriage

The availability of legal abortion has also affected teenage marriage rates. In the USA, before 1969, trends in crude marriage rates among States with different levels of legal abortion services were similar[35]. Beginning in 1970, States with high abortion ratios had significantly greater declines in teenage marriage rates than did States with low ratios[35]. Since 1973, the proportion of 14–19-year-old women who are married in the USA has slowly declined[5]. In 1979, the proportion of premaritally pregnant teenagers who married during their first pregnancy was half that of the proportion who married in 1971[9]. This suggests that liberalized abortion policies might be providing teenagers with a new alternative to marriage forced by premarital pregnancy.

Because marriage and childbearing during the teenage years have greater health and social repercussions than later marriage and child-bearing[36], these lower marriage rates may have an important public health impact. Teenage parents acquire less education than their contemporaries, their marriages are less stable, and they eventually have more children than they consider ideal[36]. The effect of truncated education on later job satisfaction and income is more serious for the adolescent mother than father. As long as education and childbearing continue to be mutually exclusive activities, it will be difficult for young women with children to catch up either with their female peers or with their male counterparts. The adverse consequences of early childbearing can be partially mitigated by parental assistance. More unwed teenager mothers who live with parents or other relative complete high school and obtain employment than do those who live alone[5].

CONCLUSION

Teenagers are apparently more likely to use legal abortion than older women to prevent unplanned births. The most important variable affecting teenagers who have abortions is that the procedures are performed later in pregnancy, thus increasing the crude risks and costs of pregnancy termination. After adjusting for this factor, teenagers have generally lower morbidity and mortality rates than do older women from legally induced abortion. The scientific literature is inconclusive about whether abortion methods used for today's teenagers will be associated with any harmful effects on later desired pregnancies. Rather than discouraging the use of contraception, the availability of legal abortion since 1970 has been associated with increased use of contraceptives by teenagers.

Acknowledgements

I thank Dee Woodard for her help in completing this manuscript.

References

1. The Alan Guttmacher Institute (1976). *11 Million Teenagers – What can be Done about the Epidemic of Adolescent Pregnancies in the United States?* (New York: Alan Guttmacher Institute)
2. Baldwin, W. H. (1976). *Adolescent Pregnancy and Childbearing – Growing Concerns for Americans.* Population Bulletin 31. (Washington, DC: Population Reference Bureau)
3. Fielding, J. E. (1978). Adolescent pregnancy revisited. *N. Engl. J. Med.,* **299,** 893
4. National Center for Health Statistics (1977). *Teenage Childbearing: United States 1966–75. Monthly Vital Statistics Report: Natality Statistics 26.* DHEW publication No. (HRA) 77-1120. (Washington, DC: US Government Printing Office)
5. The Alan Guttmacher Institute (1981). *Teenage Pregnancy: The Problem that hasn't Gone Away.* (New York: Alan Guttmacher Institute)
6. Klerman, L. V. (1980). Adolescent pregnancy: A new look at a continuing problem. *Am. J. Publ. Hlth.,* **70,** 776
7. Baldwin, W. (1981). Adolescent pregnancy and childbearing – An overview. *Semin. Perinatol.,* **5,** 1
8. Westoff, C. F., Calot, G. and Foster, A. D. (1983). Teenage fertility in developed nations: 1971–1980. *Fam. Plann. Perspect.,* **15,** 105
9. Zelnik, M. and Kanter, J. F. (1980). Sexual activity, contraceptive use and pregnancy among metropolitan-area teenagers: 1971–1979. *Fam. Plann. Perspect.,* **12,** 230
10. Cates, W., Jr. (1982). Legal abortion: the public health record. *Science,* **215,** 1586
11. Ezzard, N. V., Cates, W., Jr., Kramer, D. G. and Tietze, C. (1982). Race-specific patterns of abortion use by American teenagers. *Am. J. Publ. Hlth.,* **72,** 809
12. Teper, S. (1974). Recent trends in teenage pregnancy in England and Wales. *J. Biosoc. Sci.,* **7,** 141
13. Tietze, C. (1981). *Induced Abortion: A World Review.* (New York: The Population Council)
14. Zelnik, M. and Kantner, J. F. (1975). Attitudes of American teenagers toward abortion. *Fam. Plann. Perspect.,* **7,** 89
15. Cates, W., Jr. (1980). Adolescent abortions in the United States. *J. Adolesc. Hlth. Care,* **1,** 18.

709

16. Cates, W., Jr., Schulz, K. F. and Grimes, D. A. (1983). The risk associated with teenage abortion. *N. Engl. J. Med.,* **309,** 621
17. Grimes, D. A., Schulz, K. F., Cates, W., Jr. and Tyler, C. W., Jr. (1979). Local versus general anesthesia: Which is safer for performing suction curettage abortions? *Am. J. Obstet. Gynecol.,* **135,** 1030
18. Cates, W., Jr. and Grimes, D. A. (1981). Deaths from second-trimester abortion by dilatation and evacuation: causes, prevention, facilities. *Obstet. Gynecol.,* **58,** 631
19. Bracken, M. B. and Kasl, S. V. (1975). Delay in seeking induced abortion: A review and theoretical analysis. *Am. J. Obstet. Gynecol.,* **121,** 1008
20. Burr, W. A. and Schulz, K. F. (1980). Delayed abortion in an area of easy accessibility. *J. Am. Med. Assoc.,* **244,** 44
21. Cates, W., Jr., Schulz, K. F., Grimes, D. A. and Tyler, C. W., Jr. (1979). Short-term complications of uterine evacuation techniques for abortion at 12 weeks' gestation or earlier. In Zatuchni, Sciarra, and Speidel (eds.) *Pregnancy Termination: Procedures, Safety and New Developments,* pp. 127–35. (Hagerstown, Md.: Harper and Row)
22. Bracken, M. B., Hachamovitch, M. and Grossman, G. (1974). The decision to abort and psychological sequelae. *J. Nerv. Ment. Dis.,* **158,** 154
23. David, H. P., Rasmussen, N. K. and Holst, E. (1981). Postpartum and postabortion psychotic reactions. *Fam. Plann. Perspect.,* **13,** 88
24. Kaltreider, N. B., Goldsmith, S. and Margolis, A. J. (1979). The impact of midtrimester abortion techniques on patients and staff. *Am. J. Obstet. Gynecol.,* **133,** 235
25. Hogue, C. J. R., Cates, W., Jr., and Tietze, C. (1982). Reproductive outcomes after induced abortion. *Epidemiol. Rev.,* **4,** 66
26. Binkin, N. J., Gold, J. and Cates, W., Jr. (1982). Illegal abortion deaths in the United States: Why are they still occurring? *Fam. Plann. Perspect.,* **14,** 163
27. Sklar, J. and Berkov, B. (1974). Abortion, illegitimacy and the American birth rate. *Science,* **185,** 909
28. Zelnik, M. and Kantner, J. F. (1978). First pregnancies to women aged 15–19: 1976 and 1971. *Fam. Plann. Perspect.,* **10,** 11
29. Brann, E. A. (1979). A multivariate analysis of interstate variation in fertility of teenage girls. *Am. J. Publ. Hlth.,* **69,** 661
30. Zelnik, M. and Kantner, J. F. (1978). Contraceptive patterns and premarital pregnancy among women aged 15–19 in 1976. *Fam. Plann. Perspect.,* **10,** 135
31. Francome, C. (1983). Unwanted pregnancies among teenagers. *J. Biosoc. Sci.,* **15,** 139
32. Margolis, A., Rindfuss, R., Coghlan, R. and Rochat, R. W. (1974). Contraception after abortion. *Fam. Plann. Perspect.,* **6,** 56
33. Zelnik, M. (1980). Second pregnancies to premaritally pregnant teenagers, 1976 and 1971. *Fam. Plann. Perspect.,* **12,** 69
34. Zabin, L. S. and Clark, S. D., Jr. (1981). Why the delay – A study of teenage family planning clinic patients. *Fam. Plann. Perspect.,* **13,** 205
35. Bauman, K. E., Anderson, A. E., Freeman, J. L. and Koch, G. G. (1977). Legal abortions and trends in age-specific marriage rates. *Am. J. Publ. Hlth.,* **67,** 52
36. Menken, J. (1972). The health and social consequences of teenage childbearing. *Fam. Plann. Perspect.,* **4,** 45

Index

711

712

719